Electromyography in Clinical Practice

A Case Study Approach

Electromyography in Clinical Practice
A Case Study Approach

Second Edition

Bashar Katirji, M.D., F.A.C.P.
Professor of Neurology
Case Western Reserve University School of Medicine
Director, Neuromuscular Center and Electromyography Laboratory
Neurological Institute
University Hospitals Case Medical Center
Cleveland, Ohio

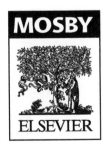

MOSBY

ELSEVIER

1600 John F. Kennedy Blvd.
Suite 1800
Philadelphia, PA 19103-2899

ELECTROMYOGRAPHY IN CLINICAL PRACTICE ISBN: 978-0-323-02899-8
Copyright © 2007 by Mosby, Inc., an affiliate of Elsevier Inc.

Previous editions copyrighted 1997

Library of Congress Cataloging-in-Publication Data

Katirji, Bashar.
    Electromyography in clinical practice: a case study approach/Bashar Katirji—2nd ed.
       p.; cm
    Includes bibliographical references and index.
    ISBN 978-0-323-02899-8
    1.Electromyography. 2.Neuromuscular diseases—Diagnosis—Case studies. I. Title.
    [DNLM: 1. Neuromuscular Diseases—diagnosis—Case Reports. 2. Electromyography—Case Reports.
    WE 550 K19e 2007]
RC77.5.K38 2007
616.7'407547—dc22   2007018876

Acquisitions Editor: Susan F. Pioli
Editorial Assistant: Joan Ryan
Senior Project Manager: David Saltzberg
Design Direction: Steve Stave

Printed in the United States of America

Last digit is the print number: 10 9 8 7 6 5 4 3 2 1

Dedication
To my wife Patricia, my children Linda and Michael, and my parents Malak and Zakaria
Without their love, encouragement and blessing, this work could not be achieved.

Preface to the Second Edition

I have been delighted with the enthusiastic reception given by physicians to the first edition of this book since its publication 10 years ago (1997). The aim of the book was to provide case-based learning of the most commonly encountered neuromuscular disorders in the EMG laboratory. The second edition maintains the main mission of reducing the gap between theory and practice in the field of electrodiagnostic medicine. In this edition, a new section (Part I) was added pertaining to the fundamentals of EMG. This section serves as an orientation and a quick guide to the readers who are not familiar with the techniques, terminology and basic concepts. It is divided into four chapters: Chapter 1 introduces the field of electrodiagnostic medicine and its scope; Chapter 2 covers the basic concepts of nerve conduction studies and needle EMG;

Chapter 3 discusses latent responses and repetitive nerve stimulations; and Chapter 4 describes the findings in various neuromuscular diseases. Part II contains all the cases. Though most cases were unchanged from the first edition, a few new ones were added and many were enriched with new and improved waveforms, tables and updated references. The discussions are longer in this edition and include new advances in the field, such as the increased use of comparison internal nerve conduction studies in the diagnosis of carpal tunnel syndrome, inching techniques in the diagnosis of ulnar nerve lesions, and quantitative motor unit analysis in the diagnosis of myopathy and neurogenic disorders.

Bashar Katirji

Preface to the First Edition

A disease known is half cured.
    Proverb (regarding diagnosis)

The electromyographic examination is a powerful diagnostic tool for assessing diseases of the peripheral nervous system. Electromyography (EMG) is an extension of the neurologic examination and is essential for the diagnosis and prognosis of most neuromuscular disorders.

Electromyography in Clinical Practice is the result of almost 15 years of teaching EMG. I came to the conclusion, a few years ago, that fellows, residents, and medical students enjoy the exercise of EMG problem solving. This usually is accomplished by discussing cases and analyzing the various data obtained first on nerve conduction studies and then on needle EMG to reach a final diagnosis. *The objective of this book is to provide practical discussions of the most commonly encountered disorders in the EMG laboratory, using typical and real case studies.* The book is not intended to teach techniques, and it presumes certain basic knowledge of clinical neurophysiology.

The book is composed of 27 cases, selected from a teaching file I kept for the purpose of training in EMG. To create a sense of unknown, these cases are organized randomly but placed into three large categories: (1) focal disorders of the lower extremity, (2) focal disorders of the upper extremity, and (3) generalized disorders. Because I expect that many readers will read this book at their leisure (such as when they are confronted with a similar patient), I intentionally have repeated some of the important tables and figures to prevent a painful search into other chapters.

The organization of the chapters is kept uniform, with minimal variability. Each case starts with a history and physical examination, in which the pertinent findings are presented. After each case presentation, there are a few questions, with corresponding answers placed at the end of the discussion. The questions are not meant to be extensive (or preparatory for examination) but are included mostly to stimulate the reader before he/she proceeds into the discussion. A summary and analysis of the EMG and clinical findings with final EMG diagnosis follows the case presentation. At the beginning of the discussion, anatomy, pathophysiology, or pathology relevant to the case presented are always incorporated. Clinical features are always discussed, but less extensively than the EMG findings. The electrodiagnostic discussions are emphasized and kept practical to reflect the objective of the book. A follow-up and final diagnosis complete the case. I have supplemented the discussions with many tables and figures, which I find extremely useful for both the novice and experienced clinician. Main articles are referenced as suggested readings and kept to the most useful publications and reviews.

Bashar Katirji, M.D., F.A.C.P.
Cleveland, Ohio

Preface to the First Edition

Acknowledgments

I am indebted to my mentor and friend, the late Dr. Asa J. Wilbourn, who inspired me into the field, often complemented me about the first edition and encouraged me to write the second. I also thank all the staff, colleagues and current and former fellows at University Hospitals Case Medical Center. I am also grateful to all the staff at the EMG laboratory, especially Peggy Neal, Karen Spencer, and Bobbie Phelps. I would also like to thank Susan Pioli, Elsevier editor, for her continuous support and encouragement into the publication of this second edition. Her assistants, Joan Ryan and Laurie Anello, played a pivotal role in helping me keep track of the various chapters, figures and tables.

Contents

Contents

Part I
Introduction to Clinical Electromyography

1

The Scope of the EMG Examination

Electromyography (EMG) is a term that was first coined by Weddell et al in 1943 to describe the clinical application of needle electrode examination of skeletal muscles. Since then, and at least in North America, the nomenclature "*EMG*" or "*clinical EMG*" has been used by physicians to refer to the electrophysiologic examination of peripheral nerve and muscle that include the *nerve conduction studies (NCS)* as well as the needle evaluation of muscles. These terms continue to cause confusion that hinders communication among physicians and healthcare workers. Some physicians refer to the study as EMG/NCS, reserving the name EMG solely to the needle EMG evaluation and adding the term NCS to reflect the nerve conduction studies separately. Others have used the title *needle EMG* or *needle electrode examination* to reflect the needle evaluation of muscles, while keeping the term EMG to describe the entire evaluation of nerve and muscle. More recently, a nonspecific term, the "*electrodiagnostic (EDX) examination*," has gained popularity to serve as an umbrella covering both the needle EMG and NCS. Other nomenclature used worldwide includes the electrophysiologic examination, which may be confused with the cardiac electrophysiological studies, and the *electroneuromyographic (ENMG) examination* which is the most accurate description of the study, yet unfortunately not widely used. Finally, physicians performing and interpreting these studies are called electromyographers (EMGers), electrodiagnosticians, or EDX consultants.

Regardless, the designations, EDX, EMG, clinical EMG, or ENMG examinations are best used interchangeably to reflect the entire electrophysiological study of nerve and muscle (NCS and needle EMG), while the terms "needle EMG" or needle electrode examination should be reserved for the specific testing which involves needle electrode evaluation of muscle. This author uses the terms EMG examination and EDX examination interchangeably, and refers to the needle examination of muscle as needle EMG.

The EDX examination comprises a group of tests that are usually complementary to each other and often necessary to diagnose or exclude a neuromuscular problem (Table 1–1). These include principally the *nerve conduction studies (NCS)*, that are sensory, motor, or mixed, and the *needle EMG*, sometimes referred as "conventional" or "routine" needle EMG to distinguish this test from other needle EMG studies including single fiber EMG and quantitative EMG. Also, "concentric" or "monopolar" needle EMG is sometimes utilized to reflect the type of needle electrode used. In addition to the two main components of the EMG examination, three late responses are often incorporated with the NCSs and have become an integral part of the NCSs. These include the *F waves* also referred to as F responses, the *H reflexes* also known as H responses, and the *blink reflexes*. Two specialized tests are often added to the routine EDX study mainly in patients with suspected neuromuscular junction disorders. These include the *repetitive nerve stimulations* and the *single fiber EMG*. Finally, a group of specialized studies that require special expertise as well as sophisticated equipment and software, used as a clinical and research tool in the assessment of the microenvironment of the motor unit, include *motor unit action potential (MUAP) morphology analysis, MUAP turns and amplitudes analysis, macro EMG, motor unit number estimate (MUNE)*, and *near-nerve recording studies*.

THE REFERRAL PROCESS TO THE EMG LABORATORY

Patients are referred to the EMG laboratory for EDX studies following a clinical assessment by a physician who suspects a disorder of the peripheral nervous system. For example, a patient with intermittent hand paresthesias and positive Phalen's signs may be referred to the EMG

Table 1–1. The Spectrum of Clinical Electromyography (Electrodiagnosis)

1. Nerve conduction studies
   - Sensory
   - Motor
   - Mixed
2. Needle electromyography (routine, conventional)
   - Concentric
   - Monopolar
3. Late responses
   - F waves
   - H reflexes
   - Blink reflexes
4. Specialized electrodiagnostic tests
   - Repetitive nerve stimulation
   - Single fiber electromyography
   - Quantitative electromyography
     - Quantitative motor unit action potential morphology analysis
     - Turns and amplitude analysis
     - Macro electromyography
     - Motor unit number estimate (MUNE)
   - Near-nerve recording studies

laboratory to evaluate a possible carpal tunnel syndrome. The background and specialty of the referring physician plays a significant role in the planning and execution of the EDX study. In the experience of this author, this usually follows one of these three scenarios:

1. The referring physician is also the EDX consultant (electromyographer). In other words, the patient is examined first by the EDX consultant (usually a neurologist or physiatrist) who performs and interprets the EDX study. The advantage of this situation is that the neurological examination is often thorough and the differential diagnosis is limited. Hence, the selection of NCSs and the choice of sampled muscles on needle EMG are well guided by the neurological findings. Though this situation is ideal, it is not common or practical in a busy EMG laboratory. Also with this approach, the electromyographer may encounter one or two pitfalls. The first is that he/she may perform a very limited and suboptimal study and become excessively biased by the clinical information, resulting in a significant number of diagnostic errors. The second hazard is that the EDX consultants may change the interpretation of similar findings among different studies to suit and support the clinical diagnosis. For example, a diabetic patient with denervation of quadriceps, iliacus, thigh adductors, and lumbar paraspinal muscles may be diagnosed in the EMG laboratory as consistent with lumbar radiculopathy or diabetic amyotrophy depending on the temporal course of the symptoms, pain characteristics, status of diabetic control, or findings on imaging of the spine.

2. The referring physician is well versed with the anatomy and disorders of the peripheral nervous system and the EDX examination. The physician is often a neurologist or physiatrist, but occasionally a neurosurgeon or an orthopedist. In this situation, the referral information includes brief, yet focused, clinical information, and a limited differential diagnosis. In these situations, the EDX consultant performs an EDX study on the symptomatic limb(s) to confirm or exclude the suspected diagnosis or, sometimes, makes an alternative diagnosis which may have not been considered by the referring physician.

3. The referring physician is not well versed with disorders of the peripheral nervous system. Often, the referral working diagnoses in these patients are vague, nonspecific, or extensive. Since the EDX study has limitations related to patient discomfort, expense, and time constraints, a directed neurological history and a brief neurological examination is often mandatory before planning and executing the EDX study. Unfortunately, contacting the referring physician to extract more specific information is often not fruitful.

THE EMG LABORATORY PROCEDURES

Testing an Adult

Patients referred to the EMG laboratory should have a *referral form* completed by the referring physician with relevant clinical information and preferably a pertinent neurological differential diagnosis (Figure 1–1). Referring physicians should also describe the EDX study to their adult patients, particularly in regard to the discomfort associated with it, without creating unnecessary heightened anxiety. If unclear about the technical details of the procedure, they should encourage their patients to contact the EMG laboratory prior to the test date, to get a verbal or written description of the procedure. Such written *descriptions* should be widely available in all referring physicians' offices (Table 1–2).

Upon arrival at the EMG laboratory for testing, the patient should be informed in detail of the procedures planned based on the referral information and clinical manifestations. Reading a written description is useful, but a verbal description of the procedure by the EDX technologist, the electromyographer, or both is usually more comforting and reassuring to the patient.

The practice of electrodiagnosis is widely regarded as a practice of medicine. The electromyographer must have a good fund of knowledge of the anatomy, physiology, and disorders of the peripheral nervous system, and be familiar

EMG Laboratory Referral Form

Patient Name:_____Hospital ID Number _____

Patient Telephone (Home):_____Work_____

Appt. Date:_____ Time:_____ a.m./p.m.

Reason for EMG (indicate symptoms, findings, working diagnosis and/or check appropriate box below):

_____

_____

_____

_____

Referring Physician Name:_____

FOCAL PROBLEMS (SELECT LIMB - RIGHT OR LEFT - IF BOTH, INDICATE WORSE SYMPTOMATIC SIDE)					
UPPER EXTREMITY	*Right*	*Left*	*LOWER EXTREMITY*	*Right*	*Left*
Cervical Radiculopathy			Lumbosacral Radiculopathy		
Carpal Tunnel Syndrome (CTS)			Lumbar Canal Stenosis		
Median Neuropathy (except CTS)			Femoral Neuropathy		
Ulnar Neuropathy			Peroneal Neuropathy		
Radial Neuropathy			Sciatic Neuropathy		
Brachial Plexopathy			Tarsal Tunnel Syndrome (TTS)		
Thoracic Outlet Syndrome (TOS)			Lumbosacral Plexopathy		
Axillary Neuropathy			*OTHER*		
Musculocutaneous Neuropathy			Facial Neuropathy (Bell's Palsy)		
Suprascapular Neuropathy			Vagal Neuropathy (Laryngeal Palsy)		
			Phrenic Neuropathy		
			Thoracic Radiculopathy		
GENERALIZED PROBLEMS (SELECT RIGHT OR LEFT - BOTH UPPER & LOWER EXTREMITIES WILL BE EXAMINED)					
Peripheral Polyneuropathy			Myasthenia Gravis		
Motor Neuron Disease (ALS, ...)			Myopathy		

Special Instructions: At the time of the EMG appointment, the patient's skin should be clean without lotions, oils or creams. No other special preparation is required. The patient can take all their medications as prescribed. Please indicate if the patient is taking a blood thinner, or is on medication for myasthenia gravis, or has a pacemaker or stimulator. There are no aftereffects and the patient can return to their usual activities immediately upon leaving the laboratory. The results of the EMG examination are faxed and mailed to the referring physician, who in turn, will explain the results to the patient. If you have further questions, please call the EMG laboratory at .....

Figure 1–1. *A sample of the referring request for an EMG examination. (Adapted from Katirji B. The clinical electromyography examination. An overview. Neurol Clin N Am 2002;20:291–303.)*

Table 1–2. A Sample of a Descriptive Explanation of the EMG Examination to be Given to Patients before Undergoing Testing

WHAT YOU SHOULD KNOW ABOUT YOUR EMG TESTING

The EMG (ElectroMyoGraphy) Examination

The EMG examination is a diagnostic examination of nerve and muscle function. Your doctor has arranged this test to assist in establishing a diagnosis and plan treatment. The EMG examination includes (1) nerve conduction studies and (2) muscle testing.

Nerve conduction studies are performed by placing discs on the skin over nerves and muscles and recording the responses to electrical stimulation of the nerves. The nerves are stimulated with mild electrical impulses that give an unusual and surprising sensation (much like the sensation in the fingers experienced when you hit you elbow on a desk).

The muscle testing involves direct recording of muscle activity at rest and during contraction by inserting small needles into various muscles. A pinprick sensation is experienced when the needle is inserted and sometimes a mild, dull ache is noted while the needle is in place. No electrical shocks are given. The needle picks up the electrical activity generated by normally by the muscle. This electrical activity is displayed on a screen and over a loudspeaker so that the physician can see and hear it.

The EMG examination is safe, well tolerated, and involves only minor discomfort. It takes about one and a half hours to complete the study. However, it is not unusual for more time to be required.

Special Instructions

At the time of your EMG appointment, your skin should be clean and without lotions, oils, or creams. No special preparation is required. You can take all your medications as prescribed by your doctor. Please notify the technologist if you are taking a blood thinner (warfarin or Coumadin), are on medication for myasthenia gravis (Mestinon), or have a pacemaker or stimulator. There are no after effects and you may return to your usual activities upon leaving the EMG laboratory.

Test Results

The results of the EMG examination are sent to your doctor, who, in turn, will explain them to you and plan the appropriate treatment.

Reprinted with permission from Katirji B. The clinical electromyography examination. An overview. Neurol Clin N Am 2002;20:291–303.

with the techniques that are necessary for performing the EDX study. Although a formal training in clinical EMG is necessary, the skills of the electromyograper are usually based on the number and type of patients studied. In practice, the electromyographer functions similar to a radiologist, by providing diagnostic studies directed by the patient clinical symptoms and working diagnosis. Hence, the EMG study should be as independent as possible, by providing an objective physiological assessment of the neuromuscular system.

NCSs and repetitive nerve stimulations (RNSs) may be performed by the electromyographer, EDX technologist, or both. Well-trained, preferably certified, EDX technologists should work under close supervision of the electromyographer. All NCSs and RNSs should be viewed by the physician before proceeding with the needle EMG. Additional NCS may be added pending the needle EMG findings. For example, the superficial peroneal sensory NCS should be added to the routine NCS of the lower extremity, if the needle EMG examination reveals denervation in L5 innervated muscles, to confirm the location of the lesion to the intraspinal canal as seen with an L5 radiculopathy.

Needle EMG is performed by the electromyographer. The data are obtained live and are not easily stored or reviewed. A concentric or monopolar needle electrode with the smallest diameter possible should be utilized, to reduce the pain and discomfort associated with needle insertion. The patient should be comforted throughout the procedure; if requested, a pause should be granted in the midst of the study.

Testing a Child

The EMG examination often creates extreme anxiety in young children and their parents. If possible, children should be accompanied by at least one nonanxious parent throughout the study for comfort purposes. The parent may hold the child's hand or sit next to the child. Occasionally, both parents may not withstand observing the test performed on their child, and in these situations, they are better kept away during the active component testing.

Most teenagers tolerate the test well. High current nerve stimulations that are excessively supramaximal should be avoided to reduce the pain and discomfort. In an extremely anxious child (and occasionally adult), the needle EMG should focus on muscles with the highest likelihood of abnormality, since only few muscles may be ultimately sampled. For example, sampling the vastus lateralis and deltoid may be the only possible muscles examined in an anxious child with possible proximal myopathy.

Sedation of young children, particularly those between the ages of 2 and 10 years, is advocated but still debated. Sedation has the advantage of allowing the performance of

NCSs and repetitive nerve stimulation without any concern about movement artifacts. However, sedation has the disadvantage of rendering the needle EMG more difficult, if the child does not activate enough MUAPs needed for accurate analysis. In these situations, the evaluation of both MUAP morphology and recruitment may be suboptimal. Sedation of young children is not without risks and should be done under physician and nurse supervision and constant monitoring of vital signs and oxygenation. The use of chloral hydrate in the past was not always successful and occasionally resulted in deep and prolonged sedation. This drug has been replaced by agents that induce rapid hypnosis without excitation such as midazolam hydrochloride (Versed®) or propofol (Diprivan®).

Propofol (Diprivan®) is the most popular intravenous sedative-hypnotic anesthetic widely used in the United States since 1989 because of its rapid onset of action and recovery. Plasma levels decline quickly as a result of high metabolic clearance and prompt distribution to the tissues. These properties account for propofol's rapid onset and short duration of action. Clinically, maintenance of adequate sedation requires a constant infusion of propofol. Discontinuation of propofol anesthesia usually results in a rapid decrease in plasma concentrations and prompt awakening. Although the terminal elimination half-life of the drug is 1 to 3 days, the sedative effects typically dissipate within 5 to 10 minutes after the infusion is discontinued. Longer anesthesia cases or sedation in the intensive care unit may produce higher plasma concentrations and thus prolong awakening time. With the advent of propofol, the use of sedation of young children undergoing EMG testing has become more feasible since the time to awakening after a one- to two-hour infusion is extremely short. Also, it is possible to titrate the dose to allow partial awakening that is good enough to assess MUAP morphology and recruitment.

In infants, using a pediatric stimulator is recommended since the distance between the cathode and anode is smaller. Shock artifacts that occasionally obliterate the response partially or completely or prevent accurate measurement of amplitude or latency are common with distal stimulations at the wrists and ankles. This is due to the very short distance between the cathodes and recording electrodes with distal stimulations.

Testing in the Intensive Care Unit

EDX testing of critically ill patients with suspected neuromuscular disorders in the intensive care unit (ICU) is often difficult and may be frustrating because of several limitations (Table 1–3). Particular attention should be given to the patient's skin temperature since peripheral vasoconstriction is common and may lower skin temperature. A core temperature of greater than 36°C or skin temperature greater than 32°C should be aimed for, since lower temperatures result in slowing of distal latencies and conduction velocities. Excessive tissue edema may be associated with low amplitude sensory or motor responses or interferes with supramaximal stimulations and giving a false impression of axonal loss. The edema may be generalized (as with hypoalbunimemia) or limited to the legs (such as with congestive heart failure), hands (such as with extravasation of fluids from intravenous lines), or neck (such as following tracheostomy or central line placement). Many ICU patients have a bleeding diasthesis or are on anticoagulation that prevents extensive needle EMG testing. Excessive sweating, skin breakdown, central lines, pacemakers, monitoring devices, or communicable diseases also influence the type of procedure, the particular site, and extremity tested.

Table 1–3. Limitations of Electrodiagnostic Testing in the Intensive Care Unit

Limitation	Result
Nerve conduction studies	
Cool extremities	Delayed distal latencies and conduction velocities
Edema	Low amplitude or unevoked sensory and motor responses
Excessive sweating	Artifacts and inadequate or unevoked responses
Skin breakdown	Inability to stimulate or record
Central line	Inability to stimulate near the line in fear of cardiac stimulation
Pacemaker	Inability to stimulate near the wires or pacer in fear of cardiac stimulation
Anterior neck swelling	Inability to percutaneously achieve supramaximal simulation of the phrenic nerves
Needle EMG	
Bleeding diasthesis	Inability to complete a thorough needle EMG
Coma or deep sedation	Inability to accurately assess MUAP morphology or recruitment
Agitation	Inability to accurately assess the insertional and spontaneous activities
Intubation/ventilation	Inability to turn the patient to needle test the paraspinal muscles

In spite of these limitations, EDX testing, including needle EMG, NCS, and repetitive nerve stimulation, may be performed safely in the ICU, and often provide significant assistance in neuromuscular diagnosis and prognosis. Reviewing the history, physical examination, and medication history as well as discussing the queries and testing plan with the ICU team may prove beneficial to avoid possible pitfalls. Except in rare situations, the EDX tests done in the ICU are often less extensive than the studies done in the EMG laboratory, often with less NCS and needle EMG sampling. However, enough details are usually obtained to diagnose or exclude certain neuromuscular disorders that may be encountered in the ICU. In acute situations, serial studies are often necessary for final diagnosis and prognosis.

Testing of the respiratory system in the ICU is another important part of the application of EDX testing that has not been used frequently. Its major role is to investigate the cause of respiratory insufficiency or failure to wean off mechanical ventilation by testing components of the peripheral nervous system involved in ventilation, including the diaphragm and phrenic nerve. Phrenic motor NCS by surface stimulation, recording from the skin over the diaphragm, may be performed in the ICU setting, but are not uncommonly limited by neck swelling, central lines, and pacemaker wires. Diaphragmatic needle EMG examination of the diaphragm may be performed, but is cumbersome in the ICU and patients may not be alert enough to cooperate with testing.

EMG LABORATORY REPORT

When completed, the EDX consultant should explain the findings in brief to the patient, bearing in mind that the electromyographer is often not the referring or treating physician. Discussion of a serious illness, such as amyotrophic lateral sclerosis, may be best left to the referring physician. Suggestions for clinical management should not be discussed with the patient (except in general terms if necessary) unless the referring physician has requested a formal neuromuscular consultation.

The results of the EDX study should be conveyed promptly to the referring physician(s). An EMG laboratory report is the best way to transmit the results of the EDX assessment to the referring physician. Occasionally, the EDX consultant should contact the referring physician if the EMG findings reflect a grave disease or if a planned surgery needs to proceed or be cancelled due to these findings.

Generating a concise and understandable EMG laboratory report is an important function of the electromyographer. The EDX report should be typed (not hand written) since it constitutes an integral part of the patient's medical records. The report should contain all the pertinent data acquired during the study, despite that some referring physicians are only interested in the final conclusion (Figure 1–2). In addition to the demographic data (patient name, age, birth date, sex, hospital number, date of study, and referring physician), the EMG laboratory report should include the following:

1. *Reason for referral to the EMG laboratory.* This should include a brief and pertinent clinical summary, the temporal course of the illness (with date of onset if applicable), and the complicating factors which may influence the EDX findings. These factors include diabetes mellitus, local swelling, limb deformity, history of poliomyelitis, or previous lumbar or cervical spinal surgery. An example of a statement outlining a brief history and the reason for referral is the following: "Acute right wrist drop noted after recent abdominal surgery on 6/4/2004. The patient has had diabetes mellitus for 3 years and a remote history of anterior cervical diskectomy. Evaluate for right radial neuropathy and brachial plexopathy."

2. *Nerve conduction studies.* This segment of the report should always be part of the EMG laboratory report, and is particularly directed to physicians who are well versed with the EDX examination. Recording and revealing limb(s) temperature is extremely useful, since many of the NCS parameters are greatly affected by cool limbs. Since F wave and H reflex latencies are length-dependent, the patient's height should be also shown on the report. The tabulated NCS form should be detailed but not overcrowded with unnecessary data. Nerves stimulated, stimulation sites, and recording points are extremely important. Amplitudes (distal and proximal), latencies, conduction velocities, and F wave latencies should be noted. Normal laboratory values should also be shown if possible (Figure 1–2A).

3. *Needle EMG.* This should list all the muscles examined with their detailed findings. The insertional activity (increased, decreased, myotonic discharges, etc.), spontaneous activity (fibrillation potentials, fasciculation potentials, complex repetitive discharges, etc.), MUAP activation (normal, fair, poor) and recruitment (normal, decreased, early), and MUAP morphology (amplitude, duration, percentage polyphasia) should be all reported (Figure 1–2B). If an advanced EMG study is done (quantitative MUAP analysis, MUNE, single fiber EMG, etc.), the data should be outlined in detail.

4. *Summary.* It is a good practice to recap the pertinent aspects of the EDX study in one or two paragraphs. All the abnormalities and relevant negatives should be highlighted. This summary sets the stage for formulating a meaningful impression.

Electromyography Laboratory Report

University Hospitals Health System
University Hospitals of Cleveland

University Hospitals of Cleveland
EMG Laboratory
11100 Euclid Avenue
Cleveland, Ohio 44106-5098
(216) 844-1923
(216) 844-7624 (fax)

Name:
Hospital No: 1420589
Sex: Male
Height: 67 (in)
Referring Physician: Dr.

Date: 3/4/04
Birth date: 9/14/57
Age: 46
Temp: 33.1 (C) Hand
Temp: 31.5 (C) Foot

CASE WESTERN RESERVE UNIVERSITY
School of Medicine

Reason for Referral :

Nerve Conduction Studies

Nerve Stimulated	Stimulation Site	Recording Site	Amplitude Motor=mV; Sensory=µV			Distal/Peak Latency msec			Conduction Velocity m/sec			F-wave Latency msec	
			Rt	Lt	NL	Rt	Lt	NL	Rt	Lt	NL	Rt	Lt
Median (S)	Wrist	Index	46		>20	2.8		<3.4					
Median (S)	Wrist	Middle	40		>20	2.8		<3.4					
Ulnar (S)	Wrist	Little	32		>12	2.3		<3.1					
Radial (S)	Forearm	Snfbox	22		>18	2.5		<2.7					
Sural (S)	Calf	Ankle	19		>5	3.4		<4.5					
Superficial Peroneal (S)	Leg	Ankle	11		>5	3.2		<4.5					
Median (M)	Wrist	APB	11.9		>6	3.3		<3.9				27.5	
Median (M)	Elbow	APB	11.4			7.2			59		>50		
Ulnar (M)	Wrist	ADM	13.8		>7	2.8		<3.1				27.3	
Ulnar (M)	Ab Elb	ADM	11.3			7.8			66		>50		
Peroneal (M)	Ankle	EDB	7.5		>3	4.7		<5.5				49.5	
Peroneal (M)	Ab Knee	EDB	6.4			12.8			48		>40		
Tibial (M)	Ankle	AH	13.2		>8	4.8		<6.0				51.5	
Tibial (M)	Knee	AH	10.9			13.8			43		>40		
Tibial (H - Reflex (M))	Knee	Soleus	13.7			6.4							
Tibial (H - Reflex)	Knee	Soleus	2.5			32.5							

(NR = No Response; Rt = right; Lt = Left; APB = Abductor Pollicis Brevis; ADM = Abductor Digiti Minimi; EDB = Extensor Digitorum Brevis; AH = Abductor Hallucis).

A

Figure 1–2. *Sample of an EMG report.* **A:** *Nerve conduction studies.*

Continued

Needle Examination

Muscle	Insertional Activity	Spontaneous Activity		Voluntary Motor Unit Potentials					Comment
				Recruitment pattern		Configuration			
		Fibs	Fascs	Recruitment	Activation	Duration	Amplitude	Polyphasia	
Right									
FDI-1st Dorsal Int	Normal	0	0	Normal	Normal	Normal	Normal	Normal	
FPL-Flex poll long	Normal	0	0	Normal	Normal	Normal	Normal	Normal	
PT-Pronator teres	Normal	0	0	Normal	Normal	Normal	Normal	Normal	
Biceps	Normal	0	0	Normal	Normal	Normal	Normal	Normal	
Triceps	Normal	0	0	Normal	Normal	Normal	Normal	Normal	
Deltoid (middle)	Normal	0	0	Normal	Normal	Normal	Normal	Normal	
AHB-Abd hall brev	Normal	0	0	Normal	Normal	Normal	Normal	Normal	
EDB-Ext dig brevis	Normal	0	0	Normal	Normal	Normal	Normal	Normal	
TA-Tib Anterior	Normal	0	0	Normal	Normal	Normal	Normal	Normal	
EHL-Ext hall longus	Normal	0	0	Normal	Normal	Normal	Normal	Normal	
MG-Medial Gastroc	Normal	0	0	Normal	Normal	Normal	Normal	Normal	
TP-Tib posterior	Normal	0	0	Normal	Normal	Normal	Normal	Normal	
VL-Vastus lateralis	Normal	0	0	Normal	Normal	Normal	Normal	Normal	
TFL-Tensor fasc lata	Normal	0	0	Normal	Normal	Normal	Normal	Normal	

(CRD = Complex repetitive discharge; N-Myoton = Neuromyotonia; SL Decr = Slightly Decreased; MO Decr = Moderately Decreased; MkDecr = Markedly Decreased; +1, +2, +3 = slightly, moderately, markedly increased; -1, -2, -3 = slightly, moderately, markedly reduced; N/+1 = borderline increased; N/-1 = borderline reduced).

Summary :

Impression :

Figure 1–2, cont'd. B: *Needle EMG.*

B

5. *Impression (or conclusion)*. This is the most important component of the EMG report since it represents the final link between the electromyographer and referring physician. The impression should be brief, yet clear and disclose as much information as possible. The EDX examination often makes an anatomic or physiologic diagnosis but not a final clinical diagnosis. For example, the EDX study often diagnoses a median mononeuropathy at the wrist but not a carpal tunnel syndrome, or a necrotizing myopathy but not polymyositis. In these situations, the electromyographer may report that the finding are "consistent with or compatible with" the appropriate suspected clinical syndrome. When a peripheral nerve lesion is detected, the site of pathology with its severity, chronicity, and pathophysiology, should be delineated. The EMGer may also provide a brief list of differential diagnoses that are based on the EDX findings. For example, if myotonia is detected on needle EMG, a list of the common inherited myotonic disorders and the drug-induced myotonias may be useful to the referring physician. Rarely, such as with the Lambert-Eaton myasthenic syndrome, the EDX examination may be diagnostic of a specific disorder.

If the EDX study is normal, the impression should also state that the study did not find evidence of the specific disorder(s) for which the patient was referred. If the EDX examination was limited or incomplete, such as due to poor patient tolerance, this should be explicitly explained in the impression. In situations where multiple EDX findings are detected, they should preferably be listed relevant to their individual relation to the suspected diagnosis, followed by the likely incidental or asymptomatic findings. If a repeat EMG study is needed, the report's impression should state the proposed time frame for such a study.

The electromyographer should be as objective as possible and not rely fully on the clinical information in making a diagnosis that is not substantiated by the EDX findings. For example, the EDX of a patient with a remote elbow fracture and suspected tardy ulnar palsy may show an axon-loss ulnar mononeuropathy without focal slowing or conduction block but with denervation of the ulnar innervated muscles in the forearm. The electromyographer should report that the ulnar mononeuropathy is localized at or above the elbow and refrain from localizing the lesion to the elbow. Apart from prognostication in patients with nerve injuries, the EDX report should not include treatment or management recommendations. In situations where the electromyographer is the treating physician or is asked to provide a neuromuscular consultation, a detailed neurological history, examination, diagnosis, management, and prognosis should be included in a distinct neurological consultation report.

SUGGESTED READINGS

Aminoff MJ. Electromyography in clinical practice, 3rd ed. New York: Churchill-Livingstone, 1998.

Dumitru D. Electrodiagnostic medicine, 2nd ed. Philadelphia: Hanley and Belfus, 2001.

Katirji B. Clinical electromyography. In: Bradley WG, Daroff RB, Fenichel GM, Jankovic J, eds. Neurology in clinical practice, 4th ed. Boston: Butterworth-Heinemann, 2004, pp. 491–520.

Katirji B. (ed.). Clinical electromyography. Neurology clinics. Philadelphia: WB Saunders, 2002.

Katirji B. The clinical electromyography examination. An overview. Neurol Clin N Am 2002;20:291–303.

Kimura J. Electrodiagnosis in diseases of nerve and muscle: principles and practice, 3rd ed. New York: Oxford University Press, 2001.

Preston DC, Shapiro BE. Electromyography and neuromuscular disorders. Philadelphia: Elsevier/Butterworth-Heinemann, 2005.

Shapiro BE, Katirji B, Preston DC. Clinical electromyography. In: Katirji B, Kaminski HJ, Preston DC, Ruff RL, Shapiro EB, eds. Neuromuscular disorders in clinical practice. Boston: Butterworth-Heinemann, 2002, pp. 80–140.

Smith SJM. Electrodiagnosis. In: Birch R, Bonney G, Wynn Parry CB, eds. Surgical disorders of the peripheral nerves. Edinburgh: Churchill-Livingstone, 1998, pp. 467–490.

Wilbourn AJ, Ferrante MA. Clinical electromyography. In: Joynt RJ, Griggs RC, eds. Baker's clinical neurology on CD-ROM. Philadelphia: WB Saunders, 2000.

2

Routine Clinical Electromyography

NERVE CONDUCTION STUDIES

There are three types of NCS that are used in clinical practice: motor, sensory, and mixed NCS. The motor fibers are assessed indirectly by stimulating a nerve while recording from a muscle and analyzing the evoked compound muscle action potential (CMAP), also referred to as the motor response or the M wave (M for motor). The sensory fibers are evaluated by stimulating and recording from a nerve and studying the evoked sensory nerve action potential (SNAP), also referred to as the sensory response. Mixed NCSs are less commonly used and assess directly the sensory and motor fibers in combination by stimulating and recording from a mixed nerve and analyzing the evoked mixed nerve action potential (MNAP).

Stimulation Principles and Techniques

Percutaneous (surface) stimulation of a peripheral nerve is the most widely used nerve conduction technique in clinical practice. The output impulse is a rectangular wave with a duration of 0.1 or 0.2 ms, although this may be increased up to 1 ms in order to record a maximal response. Two different types of percutaneous (surface) electric stimulators are used: both are bipolar having a cathode (negative pole) and anode (positive pole). The first type is a *constant voltage stimulator* that regulates voltage output so that current varies inversely with the impedance of the skin and subcutaneous tissues. The second type is a *constant current stimulator* that changes voltage according to impedance, so that the amount of current that reaches the nerve is specified within the limits of skin resistance. In bipolar stimulation, both electrodes are placed over the nerve trunk. As the current flows between the cathode and anode, negative charges accumulate under the cathode depolarizing the nerve, and positive charges gather under the anode hyperpolarizing the nerve.

With bipolar stimulation, the cathode should be, in most situations, closer to the recording site. If the cathode and anode of the stimulator are inadvertently reversed, anodal conduction block of the propagated impulse may occur. This is due to hyperpolarization at the anode that may prevent the depolarization that occurs under the cathode from proceeding past the anode. In situations where it is intended for the volley to travel proximally (such as with F wave or H reflex recordings), the bipolar stimulator is switched and the cathode is placed more proximally.

Supramaximal stimulation of nerves that results in depolarization of all the available axons is a paramount prerequisite to all NCS measurements. To achieve supramaximal stimulation, current (or voltage) intensity is slowly increased until it reaches a level where the recorded potential is at its maximum. Then, the current should be increased an additional 20–30% to ensure that the potential does not increase in size further (Figure 2–1). Stimulation via a needle electrode deeply inserted near a nerve is used less often in clinical practice. This is usually reserved for circumstances where surface stimulation is not possible, such as in deep-seated nerves (e.g., sciatic nerve or cervical root stimulation).

Recording Electrodes and Techniques

Surface electrodes are most often used for nerve conduction recordings. Surface recording electrodes are often made as small discs that are placed over the belly of the muscle or the nerve (Figure 2–2). The advantages of surface recording are that the evoked response is reproducible and changes only slightly with the position of the recording electrode. Also, the size (amplitude and area) of the response is a semiquantitative measure of the number of axons conducting between the stimulating and recording electrodes.

5 mV/D   3 ms/D

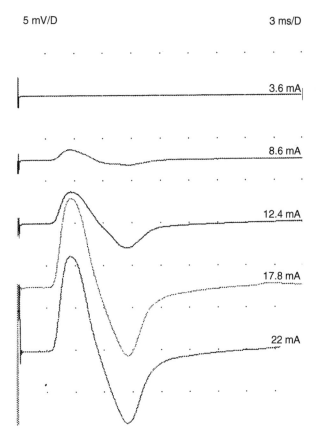

Figure 2–1. *Supramaximal stimulation of a peripheral nerve during a motor nerve conduction study (median nerve stimulating at the wrist while recording abductor pollicis brevis). With a subthreshold stimulus of 3.6 mA (top response), none of the fibers were stimulated and no response was evoked. With a higher stimulus of 8.6 mA (second response), few fibers are stimulated and a low-amplitude compound muscle action potential (CMAP) is recorded. A further increase in the current to 12.4 mA (third response) reveals a larger CMAP that is still submaximal. A 17.4 mA stimulus results in a maximal CMAP (fourth response). This can only be confirmed after increasing the stimulus intensity by 20–25% (supramaximal stimulus of 22 mA, fifth response) and evoking a CMAP that is identical to the maximal CMAP. With maximal and supramaximal stimulations, all nerve fibers are stimulated.*

With motor conduction studies, the active recording electrode is placed over the belly of the muscle that correlates with the endplate zone. This ensures that muscle activity at the moment of depolarization is recorded as soon as the nerve action potential has arrived at the endplate. Ring electrodes are convenient to record the antidromic sensory potentials from hand digital nerves over the proximal and distal interphalangeal joints (Figure 2–3). These ring electrodes could act as stimulation points with orthodromic recording from hand digits.

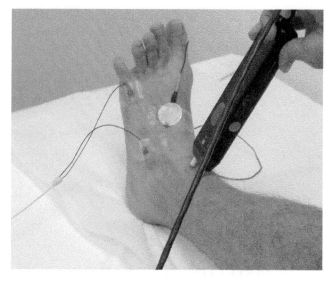

Figure 2–2. *Belly-tendon recording of compound muscle action potential. The settings are for peroneal motor conduction study recording the extensor digitorum brevis and stimulating distally at the ankle. Note that the active electrode (G1) is over the belly of the muscle while the reference electrode (G2) is over the tendon. The ground electrode is placed nearby.*

Needle recording is also possible but is less popular and reserved for situations where the recording sites are deep-seated muscles or nerves. Needle recordings are also useful to improve the recording from small atrophic muscles or a proximal muscle not excitable in isolation. In contrast to surface recording, needle electrode recording registers only a small portion of the muscle or nerve action potentials and

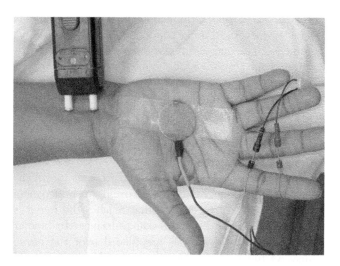

Figure 2–3. *Ring electrodes used in recording sensory nerve action potential (SNAP). The settings are for antidromic median SNAP recording index finger.*

the amplitude of the evoked response is extremely variable and highly dependent on the exact location of the needle. Hence, amplitude and area measurement are not reproducible which renders this technique not clinically valuable such as in assessing conduction block or estimating the extent of axonal loss (see below).

Recording Settings and Filters

Filters are set in the recording equipment to reject low- and high-frequency electrical noise. Low-frequency (high-pass) filters exclude signals below a set frequency, while high-frequency (low-pass) filters exclude signals above a certain frequency. Filtering results in some loss or alteration of the signal of interest. For instance, as the low-frequency filter is reduced, more low-frequency signals pass through, and the duration of the recorded potential increases slightly. Likewise, as the high-frequency filter is lowered, more high-frequency signals are excluded, and the amplitude of the recorded potential usually decreases. Hence, all potentials should be obtained with standardized filter settings, and only compared to normal values collected using the same filter settings. The recommended low and high filter settings for motor conduction studies are 10 Hz and 10 kHz, respectively. The high-frequency filter is set lower for sensory nerve conduction studies than for motor nerve conduction since high-frequency noise (>10 kHz) commonly obscures high-frequency sensory potentials. For sensory conduction studies, the low- and high-frequency filters settings are typically 20 Hz and 2 kHz.

The amplifier sensitivity determines the amplitude of the potential. Overamplification of the response truncates the response, which results in false measurements of evoked response amplitude and area, while underamplification prevents accurate measurements of the takeoff point from baseline. Typically, sensory studies are recorded with a sensitivity of 10–20 μV/division and motor studies with a sensitivity of 2–5 mV/division.

Recording Procedure

A prepulse preceding the stimulus triggers the sweep on a storage oscilloscope. A stimulus artifact occurs at the beginning of the sweep, and serves as an indicator of the time when the shock occurred from which point latencies are measured. Digital averaging is a major improvement in recording low-amplitude responses by eliminating artifacts and noise. Signals time-locked to the stimulus summate at a constant latency and appear as an evoked potential, distinct from the background noise. The signal-to-noise ratio increases in proportion to the square root of the trial number. For example, four trials give twice as big a response as a single stimulus, whereas nine trials give three times

the amplitude. Modern instruments digitally indicate the latency and amplitude when the desired spot on the waveform is marked.

Sensory Nerve Conduction Studies

Sensory NCSs are performed by stimulating a nerve while recording the transmitted potential from the same nerve at a different site. Hence, SNAPs are true nerve action potentials. *Antidromic* sensory NCSs are performed by recording potentials directed toward the sensory receptors while *orthodromic* studies are obtained by recording potentials directed away from these receptors. Sensory latencies and conduction velocities are identical with either method, but SNAP amplitudes are higher in antidromic studies and, hence, more easily obtained without the need for averaging techniques. Since the thresholds of some motor axons are similar to those of large myelinated sensory axons, superimposition of muscle action potentials may obscure the recorded antidromic SNAPs. These volume-conducted muscle potentials often occur with mixed nerve stimulation or may result from direct muscle co-stimulations. Fortunately, SNAPs can still be measured accurately in most cases because the large-diameter sensory fibers conduct 5–10% faster than motor fibers. This relationship may change in disease states that selectively affect different fibers. In contrast to the antidromic studies, the orthodromic responses are small in amplitude, more difficult to obtain, and might require averaging techniques (Figure 2–4).

SNAPs may be obtained by (1) stimulating and recording a pure sensory nerve (such as the sural and radial sensory responses), (2) stimulating a mixed nerve while recording distally over a cutaneous branch (such as the antidromic median and ulnar sensory responses), or (3) stimulating a distal cutaneous branch while recording over a proximal mixed nerve (such as the orthodromic median and ulnar sensory studies). The active recording electrode (G1) is placed over the nerve and the reference electrode (G2) is positioned slightly more distal with antidromic recordings or slightly more proximal with orthodromic techniques. The distance between G1 and G2 electrodes should be fixed (usually at about 3–4 cm), since it has a significant effect on SNAP amplitude. The SNAP is usually triphasic with an initial small positive phase, followed by a large negative phase and a positive phase. Several measurements may be recorded with sensory NCSs (Figure 2–5):

1. *SNAP amplitude.* This is a semiquantitative measure of the number of sensory axons that conduct between the stimulation and recording sites. It is usually calculated from the baseline (or the initial positive peak,

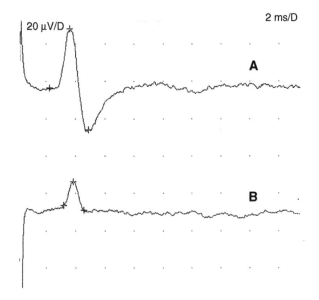

Figure 2–4. *Antidromic and orthodromic median sensory nerve action potentials. The response in (**A**) is antidromic, i.e., stimulating the wrist and recording the index finger. The response in (**B**) is orthodromic, i.e., stimulating the index and recording at the wrist. Note that the peak latencies are comparable while the antidromic response is much larger in amplitude than its orthodromic counterpart.*

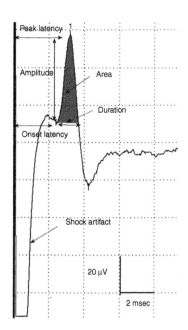

Figure 2–5. *Antidromic median sensory nerve action potential stimulating wrist while recording middle finger revealing commonly measured parameters including a shock (stimulation) artifact.*

if present) to the negative peak (baseline-to-peak amplitude). It may also be measured from negative peak to positive peak (peak-to-peak amplitude). SNAP amplitudes are expressed in microvolts (μV). SNAP duration and area may be measured but are not useful because of significant temporal dispersion and phase cancellation that accompany sensory NCSs (see temporal dispersion and phase cancellation).

2. *SNAP latencies.* Sensory distal latencies may be measured (in ms) from the stimulus artifact to the onset of the SNAP (*onset latency*) or from the stimulus artifact to the peak of the negative phase (*peak latency*). Onset latency may be obscured by a large shock artifact, a noisy background, and wavy baseline. Though peak latency does not reflect the fastest conducting sensory fibers, it is easily defined and more precise than onset latency.

3. *Sensory conduction velocity.* This requires stimulation at a single site only because the latency consists of only the nerve conduction time from the stimulus point under the cathode to the recording electrode. Sensory conduction velocities are calculated using onset latencies (not peak latencies), in order to calculate the speed of the fastest conducting fibers, and the distance between the stimulating cathode and the active recording electrode (G1).

$$\text{Sensory conduction velocity} = \frac{\text{Distance}}{\text{Onset latency}}$$

Sensory conduction velocity may also be calculated after a distal and a proximal stimulation and measurement. For example, the median sensory SNAPs are obtained at the wrist and elbows and the conduction velocity is measured as follows:

$$\text{Sensory conduction velocity} = \frac{\text{Distance}}{\substack{\text{Proximal onset latency} - \\ \text{distal onset latency}}}$$

Motor Nerve Conduction Studies

Motor NCS is performed by stimulating a motor or mixed peripheral nerve while recording the CMAP from a muscle innervated by that nerve. The CMAP is the summated recording of synchronously activated muscle action potentials. The advantage of this technique is a magnification effect based on motor unit principles: Stimulation of each motor axon results in up to several hundred muscle action potentials with this number depending on the innervation ratio (number of muscle fibers per axon) of the examined muscle.

A belly-tendon recording is a typical electrode placement to obtain a CMAP: a pair of recording electrodes are used with an active lead (G1) placed on the belly of the muscle and a reference lead (G2) on the tendon (see Figure 2–2). Both active and reference electrodes locations are an essential determinant of the CMAP size, shape, and latency. The propagating muscle action potential, originating near the motor point and under G1, gives rise to a simple biphasic waveform with an initial large negative phase followed by a smaller positive phase. With incorrect positioning of the active electrode away from the endplate, the CMAP will show an initial positive phase that corresponds to the approaching electrical field of the impulses from muscle fibers toward the electrode. Similar initial positivity is also recorded with a volume-conducted potential from distant muscles activated by anomalous innervation or by accidental spread of stimulation to other nerves.

Whenever possible, the nerve is stimulated at two or more points along its course. Typically, it is stimulated distally near the recording electrode and more proximally to evaluate its proximal segment. Several measurements are evaluated with motor NCSs (Figure 2–6):

1. *CMAP amplitude.* This is usually measured from baseline to negative peak and expressed in millivolts (mV). CMAP amplitude, recorded with surface electrodes, is a semiquantitative measure of the number of axons conducting between the stimulating and the recording points. CMAP amplitude is also dependent on the relative conduction speed of the axons, the integrity of the neuromuscular junctions, and number of muscle fibers that are able to generate action potentials.
2. *CMAP duration.* This is usually measured as the duration of the negative phase of the evoked potential and is expressed in milliseconds (ms). It is a function of the conduction rates of the various motor axons within the

tested nerve and the distance between the stimulation and recording electrodes. The CMAP generated from proximal stimulation has a longer duration and a lower amplitude than that obtained from distal stimulation (see temporal dispersion and phase cancellation).
3. *CMAP area.* This is usually restricted to the negative phase area under the waveform and shows linear correlation with the product of the amplitude and duration. It is measured in mV ms and requires electronic integration using computerized equipment. The ability to quantify CMAP area has almost replaced the need to measure its duration since the duration is incorporated in the area calculation.
4. *CMAP latencies.* This is the time interval between nerve stimulation (shock artifact) and the onset of the CMAP. It is expressed in ms and reflects the conduction rate of the fastest conducting axon. Since the nerve is typically stimulated at two points, *distal latency* is measured following a stimulation at a distal point near the recording site, and a *proximal latency* is obtained with a more proximal stimulation point. Both latencies are dependent mostly on the length of the nerve segment but also include the slower conduction along the terminal nerve segments and neuromuscular transmission time, and possibly some conduction time along muscle fibers.
5. *Conduction velocity.* This is a computed measurement of the speed of conduction and is expressed in meters per second (m/s). Measurement of conduction velocity allows the comparison of the speed of conduction between different nerves and subjects, irrespective of the length of the nerve and the exact sites of stimulations. Also, motor conduction velocity reflects the pure speed of the largest motor axon and, in contrast to distal and proximal latencies, does not include any neuromuscular transmission time nor propagation time along the muscle membrane. Motor conduction velocity is calculated after incorporating the length of the nerve segment between distal and proximal stimulation sites. The nerve length is estimated by measuring the surface distance along the course of the nerve and should be more than 10 cm to improve the accuracy of surface measurement. Motor conduction velocity is calculated as follows:

$$\text{Motor conduction velocity} = \frac{\text{Distance}}{\text{Proximal latency} - \text{distal latency}}$$

Mixed Nerve Conduction Studies

Mixed NCSs are done by stimulating and recording from nerve trunks with sensory and motor axons. Often, these tests are done by stimulating a nerve trunk distally and

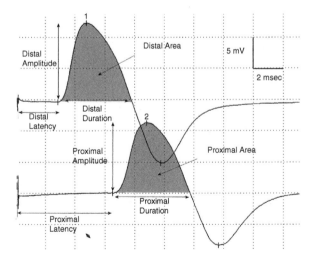

Figure 2–6. *Median motor nerve conduction study revealing commonly measured parameters following distal (top) and proximal (bottom) stimulations.*

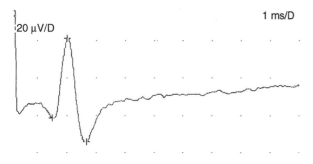

20 µV/D   1 ms/D

Figure 2–7. *Mixed nerve action potential. This is a median palmar response stimulating the mixed median nerve in the palm and recording orthodromically the median nerve at the wrist.*

recording more proximally, since the reverse is often contaminated by large CMAP that obscures the relatively low-amplitude MNAPs. In situations where the nerve is deep (such as the elbow or knee), the MNAP may be very low in amplitude or unelicitable, due to considerable tissue interposing between the nerve and recording electrode. Hence, these studies are not popular in clinical practice and are restricted to evaluating mixed nerves in distal nerve segments, such as in the hand or foot during the evaluation of carpal tunnel syndrome and tarsal tunnel syndrome, respectively (Figure 2–7).

Segmental Stimulation in Short Increments

Routine NCSs are often sufficient to localize the site of lesion in entrapment neuropathies. However, during the evaluation of a focal nerve lesion, inclusion of the unaffected segments in conduction velocity calculation dilutes the effect of slowing at the injured site and decreases the sensitivity of the test. Therefore, incremental stimulation across the shorter segment helps localize an abnormality that might otherwise escape detection. More precise localization requires moving the stimulus in short increments along the course of the nerve while keeping the recoding site constant. This procedure is often labeled inching (or actually centimetering) since 1 cm increment is a common distance measurement. The large per-step increase in latency more than compensates for the inherent measurement error associated with stimulating multiple times in short increments. The analysis of the waveform usually focuses on sudden changes in latency values or abrupt drop in amplitude.

The inching technique is particularly useful in assessing patients with carpal tunnel syndrome, ulnar neuropathies at the elbow or wrist, or peroneal neuropathy at the fibular neck. For example, with stimulation of a normal median nerve in 1 cm increments across the wrist, the latency changes approximately 0.16–0.21 ms per cm from

midpalm to distal forearm. A sharply localized latency increase across a 1 cm segment indicates a focal abnormality of the median nerve.

Physiologic Variabilities

Temperature. Nerve impulses propagate slower by 2.4 m/s or approximately 5% per degree Celsius as the limb cools from 38 to 29°C. Also, cooling results in a higher CMAP and SNAP amplitude and longer duration probably because of accelerated and slowed Na^+ channel inactivation. Hence, a CMAP or SNAP with high amplitude and slow distal latency or conduction velocity should be highly suspicious of a cool limb (Figure 2–8).

To reduce this type of variability, skin temperature is measured with a plate thermistor that correlates linearly with the subcutaneous and intramuscular temperatures. If the skin temperature falls below 33 to 34°C, it is necessary to warm the limbs by immersion in warm water. Warming packs or a hydroculator can also be used, particularly in bedridden or intensive care unit patients. Adding 5% of the calculated conduction velocity for each degree below 33°C theoretically normalizes the result. However, such conversion factors are based on experience with healthy individuals and do not apply to patients with abnormal nerves.

Age. Nerve conduction velocities are slow at birth since myelination is incomplete. They are roughly one-half the adult value in full-term newborns and one-third that of

20 µV/D   2 ms/D

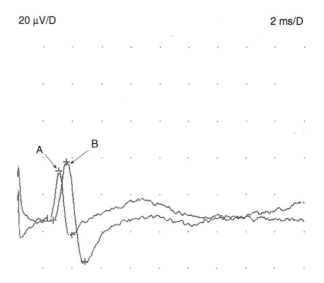

Figure 2–8. *The effect of temperature on antidromic median sensory nerve action potential stimulating at the wrist and recording the index finger. Response obtained with a skin palm temperature of (**A**) 33.5°C and (**B**) 29.5°C. Note that cool limb results in a SNAP with slower onset and peak latencies and higher amplitude.*

term newborns in 23- to 24-week premature newborns. They reach adult values at 3–5 years. Then, motor and sensory nerve conduction velocities tend to slightly increase in the arms and decrease in the legs during childhood up to 19 years. With aging, conduction velocities slowly decline after 30–40 years of age, that the mean conduction velocity is reduced about 10% at 60 years of age.

Aging also causes a diminution in SNAP and CMAP amplitudes, which decline slowly after the age of 60 years. This affects SNAP amplitudes more prominently, that normal upper limb SNAP amplitude drops up to 50% by age 70, and lower limb SNAPs in healthy subjects above the age of 60 years are low in amplitude or unevokable. Hence, absent lower extremity SNAPs in the elderly must always be interpreted with caution, and are not necessarily considered abnormal without other confirmatory data.

Height and nerve segments. An inverse relationship between height and nerve conduction velocity suggests that longer nerves generally conduct slower than shorter nerves. For example, the nerve conduction velocities of the peroneal and tibial nerves are 7–10 m/s slower than the median and ulnar nerves. This cannot be explained entirely by the small reduction in temperature of the legs as compared with the arms. Possible factors to account for the length-related slowing include abrupt distal axonal tapering, progressive reduction in axonal diameter, or shorter internodal distances. For similar reasons, nerve impulses propagate faster in proximal than in distal nerve segments. Hence, adjustments of normal values must be made for individuals of extreme height, which is usually no more than 2–4 m/s below the lower limit of normal.

Anomalies. Anomalous peripheral innervations may mislead the electrodiagnostic physician and occasionally lead to erroneous diagnosis and treatment. There are several anomalous peripheral innervations that are important to recognize since they have a significant effect on NCS.

1. *Martin-Gruber anastomosis.* This is an anomalous connection between the median and the ulnar nerves in the forearm that usually consists of motor axons. Two or three communicating branches in the forearm leave the median nerve and join the ulnar nerve to innervate the ulnar-innervated intrinsic hand muscles, in particular the first dorsal interosseous muscle (the most common target), the hypothenar muscles (abductor digiti minimi), the thenar muscles (adductor pollicis, deep head of flexor pollicis brevis), or a combination of these muscles. Martin-Gruber anastomosis, also referred to as median-to-ulnar anastomosis in the forearm, is present in approximately 15–20% of the population, and is sometimes bilateral. This anomaly manifests during ulnar or median NCSs depending on where the anomalous fibers terminate.

- In situations where the communicating fibers terminate in the first dorsal interosseous muscle or the hypothenar muscles, the ulnar NCS, recording first dorsal interosseous or abductor digiti minimi (ADM), manifests with a drop in the ulnar CMAP amplitude between distal and proximal stimulation sites (conduction block). With distal stimulation at the wrist, the CMAP reflects all ulnar motor fibers, while proximal stimulations (usually below and above elbow) activate only the uncrossed fibers which are fewer in number and resulting in lower CMAP amplitudes. This anomaly can be confirmed by median nerve stimulation at the elbow that evokes a small CMAP from the abductor digiti minimi, which is not present on median nerve stimulation at the wrist (Figure 2–9). With median stimulation at the wrist recording the first dorsal interosseous, there is often a small

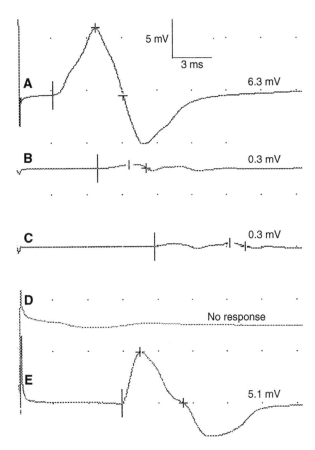

Figure 2–9. *Martin-Gruber anastomosis with evidence of prominent median to ulnar anastomosis recording hypothenar muscle (ADM). The figure shows an ulnar motor conduction study recording hypothenar muscle (ADM), stimulating the ulnar nerve at the wrist (**A**), below elbow (**B**) and above elbow (**C**). It also reveals the response following stimulating the median nerve at the wrist (**D**) and the elbow (**E**).*

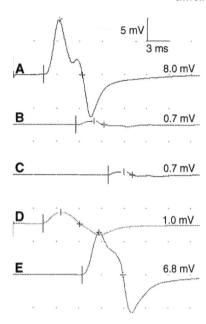

Figure 2–10. *Martin-Gruber anastomosis with evidence of prominent median to ulnar anastomosis recording first dorsal interosseous muscle. The figure shows an ulnar motor conduction study recording first dorsal interosseous muscle, stimulating the ulnar nerve at the wrist (**A**), below elbow (**B**) and above elbow (**C**). It also reveals the response following stimulating the median nerve at the wrist (**D**) and the elbow (**E**).*

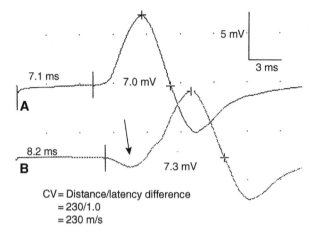

CV = Distance/latency difference
= 230/1.0
= 230 m/s

Figure 2–11. *Martin-Gruber anastomosis with evidence of median to ulnar anastomosis recording thenar muscle in a patient with moderate carpal tunnel syndrome. The figure shows a median motor conduction study recording abductor pollicis brevis (**A**, distal; **B**, proximal). Note the slowing of the distal latency (7.1 ms, N < 4.0 ms) which is compatible with carpal tunnel syndrome. There is a spuriously rapid conduction velocity with a larger proximal thenar CMAP exhibiting a positive dip (arrow).*

evoked CMAP that reflects volume conduction from the neighboring median thenar muscles (Figure 2–10).

- When anomalous fibers innervate the thenar muscles, stimulation of the median nerve at the elbow activates the nerve and the crossing ulnar fibers resulting in a large CMAP, often with a initial positivity caused by volume conduction of action potential from ulnar thenar muscles to the median thenar muscles. In contrast, distal median nerve stimulation evokes a smaller thenar CMAP without the positive dip since the crossed fibers are not present at the wrist. Also, the median nerve conduction velocity in the forearm is spuriously fast, particularly in the presence of a carpal tunnel syndrome, since the CMAP onset represents different population of fibers at the wrist compared to the elbow (Figure 2–11). An accurate conduction velocity may be obtained by using collision studies that abolish action potentials of the crossed fibers.

2. *Accessory deep peroneal nerve.* This anomaly is present in about 20% of the population. The anomalous nerve is a branch of the superficial peroneal nerve that usually arises as a continuation of the muscular branch to the peroneus longus and brevis muscles. It passes behind the lateral malleolus and terminates in the extensor digitorum brevis on the dorsum of the foot. During peroneal motor NCS recording the extensor digitorum brevis, the peroneal CMAP amplitude is larger stimulating proximally than distally since the anomalous fibers are not present at the ankle. This anomaly can be confirmed by stimulating behind the lateral malleolus. This yields a CMAP (not present in normal situations) that, when added to the distal CMAP, is approximately equal or higher than the CMAP obtained with proximal peroneal nerve stimulations (Figures 2–12 and 2–13).

3. *Riche-Cannieu anastomosis.* This is a communication between the recurrent motor branch of the median nerve and the deep branch of the ulnar nerve. This results in dual innervation of some of the intrinsic hand muscles such as the first dorsal interosseous, adductor pollicis, and abductor pollicis brevis. Riche-Cannieu anastomosis is rather common but often not clinically or electrophysiologically apparent. When this anomaly is prominent, denervation in ulnar muscles may be present following a median nerve lesion and vice versa. Also, a complete median or ulnar nerve lesion may be associated with relative sparing of some median innervated muscles or ulnar innervated muscles in the hand respectively.

4. *Pre- and postfixed brachial plexus.* In most individuals, the brachial plexus arises from the C5 to T1 cervical roots. In some, the plexus origin shifts up one level, arising from C4 to C8, and in others it shifts one level down, originating from C6 to T2. The former situation

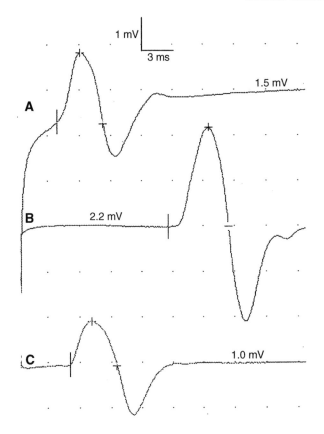

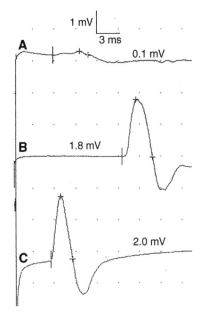

Figure 2–13. *Prominent accessory deep peroneal nerve anomaly. Note here that the distal CMAP was extremely low in amplitude (**A**) while the proximal CMAP is higher (**B**). Similar to Figure 2–12, stimulation behind the lateral malleolus yielded a relatively large CMAP (**C**). However, in this example, most fibers were directed to the extensor digitorum brevis through the accessory deep peroneal nerve, leaving only a few to travel through the main trunk of the deep peroneal nerve.*

Figure 2–12. *Accessory deep peroneal nerve anomaly shown while performing a peroneal motor conduction study recording extensor digitorum brevis. The distal stimulation at the ankle (**A**) results in a CMAP that was lower in amplitude that the proximal response following knee stimulation (**B**). Stimulation behind the lateral malleolus yielded a CMAP (**C**). Note that the summation of the CMAPs at (**A**) and (**C**) were higher than the CMAP at (**B**).*

is referred to as a prefixed brachial plexus, while the latter is a postfixed brachial plexus. These anomalies have implication on the precise localization of cervical root lesions based on myotomal representation. In a prefixed plexus, the location of the cervical lesion is one level higher than concluded based on the clinical examination and electrodiagnostic studies. In contrast, with a postfixed plexus, the cervical root lesion is one level lower.

Temporal dispersion and phase cancellation. The CMAP, evoked by supramaximal stimulation, represents the summation of all individual muscle action potentials directed to the muscle through the stimulated nerve. Typically, as the stimulus site moves proximally, the CMAPs slightly drop in amplitude and area and increase in duration. This is caused by temporal dispersion where the

velocity of impulses in slow-conducting fibers lags increasingly behind those of fast-conducting fibers as conduction distance increases. With dispersion, there is also a slight positive/negative phase overlap and cancellation of MUAP waveforms. The final result of temporal dispersion and phase cancellation is a reduction of CMAP amplitude and area and prolongation of its duration.

Physiological temporal dispersion affects the SNAP more than the CMAP. This is related to two factors. First is the disparity between sensory fiber and motor fiber conduction velocities. The range of conduction velocities between the fastest and slowest individual human myelinated sensory axons is almost double that of the motor axons (25 m/s versus 12 m/s). This results in more dispersion of individual action potentials and leads to more prominent phase cancellation. The second factor is the difference in duration of individual unit discharges between nerve and muscle. With short-duration biphasic sensory spikes, a slight latency difference could line up the positive peaks of the fast fibers with the negative peaks of the slow fibers and cancel both. In longer duration motor unit potentials, the same latency shift would only partially superimpose peaks of opposite polarity, and cancellation would be less of a factor (Figures 2–14 and 2–15).

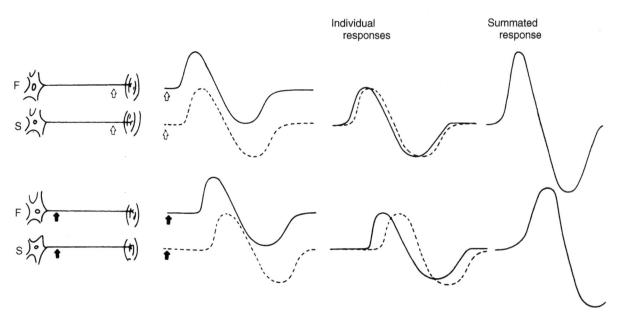

Figure 2–14. *Temporal dispersion and phase cancellation of two surface-recorded motor unit potentials at distal and proximal sites. This can be translated into many similar biphasic potentials, which contribute to the compound muscle action potential (CMAP). (Reproduced from Kimura J et al. Relation between size of compound sensory or muscle action potentials, and length of nerve segment. Neurology 1986;36:647–652, with permission.)*

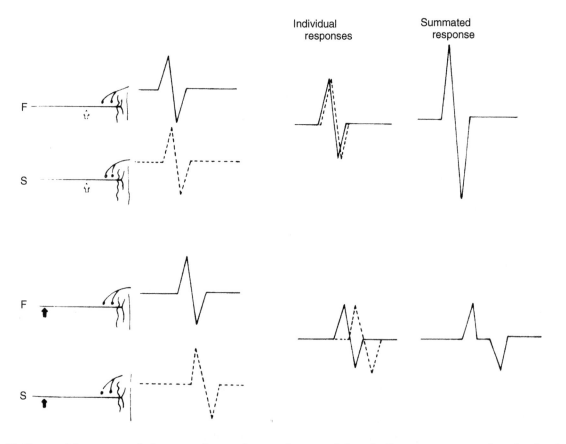

Figure 2–15. *Temporal dispersion and phase cancellation of two surface-recorded single-fiber sensory potentials at distal and proximal sites. This can be translated into many similar biphasic potentials, which contribute to the sensory nerve action potential (SNAP). (Reproduced from Kimura J et al. Relation between size of compound sensory or muscle action potentials, and length of nerve segment. Neurology 1986;36:647–652, with permission.)*

Intertrial variability. Principal factors contributing to an intertrial variability include errors in determining surface distance and in measuring latencies and amplitudes of the recorded response. A slight shift in recording site results in significant amplitude variability. NCSs are more reproducible when done by the same examiner, because of the significant degree of inter-examiner variability.

Common Sources of Error

Several major pitfalls in NCS may result in erroneous measurements, calculations, and conclusions. These are usually due to technical errors related to a large obscuring stimulus artifact, increased background electrical noise, submaximal stimulations at distal or proximal sites or both, spread of the stimulating current to a nerve not under study, eliciting an unwanted potential from distant muscles, misplacement of recording or reference electrodes, or errors in the measurement of nerve length and conduction time.

Large Stimulus Artifact

The stimulus artifact may obscure the onset of the recorded potential if its trailing edge overlaps with that potential leading to inaccurate measurements of both amplitude and latency. This occurs most commonly with sensory nerve conduction studies and is exacerbated when the recording electrode and the stimulating probe are too close or when the stimulus intensity is high. The shock artifact will have a decreasing negative effect on the recorded potential by increasing the distance between stimulator and recording electrodes, or by decreasing the stimulation intensity. This artifact may also be reduced by slight rotation of the stimulator's anode while maintaining the cathode in place, placing the ground electrode between the stimulator and recording electrodes, and ensuring that the stimulator and recording electrode cables do not overlap.

Increased Electrode Noise

Electrode noise usually interferes with recording small potentials, such as SNAPs or fibrillation potentials. The most common cause of electrical noise in the EMG laboratory is 60 or 50 Hz interference generated from other electrical devices. Impedance is an electrical term combining the effects of resistance to flow for a DC current and capacitance for an AC current. As per Ohm's law, the voltage (E) from electrical noise equals the current (I) induced from the electrical noise multiplied by the resistance (R) or impedance ($E = IR$). Signals recorded during the NCSs (and needle EMG) are the result of differential amplification, in which the difference between the signals at the active (G1) and reference (G2) electrodes is amplified and displayed. Therefore, if the same electrical noise is present at both the active and reference electrodes (such as with closely placed G1 and G2 electrodes), it is subtracted out, and only the signal of interest is amplified (i.e., common mode rejection). However, if the resistance or impedance is different at each electrode, then the same electrical noise will induce a different voltage at each electrode input. This difference is then amplified and displayed, often obscuring the signal of interest. Hence, preventing electrode impedance mismatch is the best way to achieve identical electrical noise at each electrode.

To prevent electrode noise, intact electrodes without frayed or broken connections should be used, and the skin cleaned with either alcohol or acetone. Conducting electrode jelly is then applied to the electrode before it is attached to the skin. The recording electrodes should be held firmly against the skin with tape or a Velcro band.

Submaximal Stimulation

An erroneous diagnosis of conduction block may occur if submaximal stimulation was not achieved at a proximal stimulation site only while the distal stimulation site was supramaximal. Conversely, a submaximal stimulation at a distal site with a supramaximal stimulation at a proximal site may erroneously suggest an anomalous innervation. A misdiagnosis of axonal loss may be made if a nerve is not supramaximally stimulated at both its distal and proximal sites.

In addition to their effect on CMAP and SNAP amplitudes, submaximal stimulations at all stimulation sites result in prolonged latencies and conduction velocities, since the largest fibers have the highest threshold for stimulation and are evoked last.

Co-stimulation of Adjacent Nerves

The stimulating current may spread to excite nearby nerves, which may result in a spuriously large amplitude potential. Inadvertent co-stimulation of adjacent nerves distally but not proximally may be mistaken for conduction block, while proximal without distal co-stimulation, may erroneously suggest an anomalous innervation. To avoid co-stimulation of adjacent nerves, the examiner should watch the morphology of the waveform carefully, and for the muscle twitch with each stimulation. If there is an abrupt change in waveform configuration or in muscle twitch pattern, especially at higher currents, co-stimulation of adjacent nerves may have occurred. Common sites of nerve co-stimulation are the median and ulnar nerve stimulations at the wrist, elbow or axilla, and the common peroneal and tibial nerves stimulations at the knee. Co-stimulation of multiple nerve elements is unavoidable with percutaneous stimulation of the supraclavicular elements of the brachial plexus at Erb's point.

Recording or Reference Electrode Misplacement

With the belly-tendon method of recording, the CMAP shows an initial positive deflection if the active (G1) recording electrode is not placed over the endplate. This occurs since the volume-conducted depolarization potential first occurs at a distance from the recording electrode. This electrode misplacement results in error in measuring the latency and the CMAP amplitude may be reduced.

The SNAP or MNAP may be low in amplitude when the recording electrode is inadvertently placed lateral or medial to the nerve trunk, since the amplitude of the potential decays dramatically with increasing distance from the generator. This occurs most frequently with sensory conduction studies of anatomically variable sensory nerve trunks, such as the sural, superficial peroneal, medial, and lateral antebrachial cutaneous nerves.

The location of the reference electrode (G2), when accurately placed over the muscle tendon, has little influence on the CMAP since it is almost inactive at that site. However, the distance between these electrodes influences the SNAPs and MNAPs, since the active and reference electrodes are both typically placed over the nerve trunk. Accordingly, the nerve segment under the active electrode depolarizes first, followed by depolarization of the segment underneath the reference electrode. If the active and reference electrodes are too close, they may briefly become electrically active at the same time, resulting in a lower amplitude. Taking into account the normal range of nerve conduction velocities, the preferred inter-electrode distance between the active and reference recording electrodes for sensory and mixed nerve recordings is 3–4 cm, which ensures that depolarization will not occur under both electrodes simultaneously.

Distance Measurement Error

The surface distance is a fair estimate of the true length of the studied nerve. However, nerves may run an oblique course or turn around a bony structure. This may result in a large discrepancy between the measured and actual length of the nerve and lead in erroneous conduction velocity. Estimating the true length of the ulnar nerve across the elbow is the most notable representative of measurement error that continues to be debated. The ulnar nerve in most subjects is redundant when the arm is in the extended elbow position and stretched to its full distance during the extended position. If measurements of the ulnar nerve are made in the extended position, the true length of the underlying nerve is underestimated resulting in erroneous focal slowing across the elbow. With the elbow in a flexed position, the measured surface distance across the elbow better reflects the true underlying length of the nerve resulting in a more valid calculation of

conduction velocity. Other examples of nerve segments that are subject to surface measurement errors include the radial nerve around the spiral groove, the peroneal nerve around the fibular neck, and the median and ulnar nerves between the axilla and Erb's point (supraclavicular fossa).

NEEDLE ELECTROMYOGRAPHIC EXAMINATION

Motor Units and Muscle Fibers

The motor unit consists of a single motor neuron and all the muscle fibers it innervates. The number of muscle fibers innervated by a single motor axon is the *innervation ratio*, which is variable ranging from 3 to 1 for extrinsic eye muscles to several hundreds to 1 for limb muscles. A low ratio occurs in muscles with greater ability for fine gradations of movement, and is typically found in the extraocular, facial, and hand muscles.

Muscle fibers are classified based on their mechanical properties and resistance to fatigue. Based on the speed of the actin–myosin reaction and the Ca^{2+}-dependent activation and relaxation regulatory systems, muscle fibers are either slow or fast. They are also either fatigue-resistant with higher mitochondrial content, or fatigable. Hence, muscle fibers are usually labeled as type I (slow and fatigue-resistant), type II A (fast and fatigue-resistant), or type II B (fast and fatigable) fibers (Table 2–1). All muscle fibers of each individual motor unit are of one specific type. The distribution of muscle fibers of a single motor unit within a muscle is wide with considerable overlap among the territories of motor units.

All muscle fibers in one motor unit discharge simultaneously when stimulated by synaptic input to the lower motor neuron or by electrical stimulation of the axon. Based on the "size principle," the smallest motor neurons are activated first with larger motor neurons recruited later with progressive increase in force. This order of recruitment correlates with the functional properties of the motor units, i.e., the small motor units are slow and fatigue-resistant and are activated first and for longer periods of time than the large motor units that are fast and fatigable and recruited later and for shorter periods of time.

Principles

The skeletal muscle fiber has a resting potential of 90 mV, with negativity inside the cell. These fibers, as well as neurons and other excitable cells, generate action potentials when the potential difference across the plasma membrane is depolarized past a specific threshold. This follows an "all-or-none" rule, which means that increasing the

Table 2–1. Skeletal Muscle Fiber Types

	Slow Type I	Fast, Fatigue-Resistant Type IIA	Fast, Fatigable Type IIB
Diameter	+	++	+++
Capillary supply	+++	+++	+
Mitochondrial content	+++	+++	+
SR volume	+	+++	+++
Myofibrillar ATPase	+	+++	++++
Myofibrillar Ca^{2+} sensitivity	+++	+	+
SR Ca^{2+} uptake	Slow	Fast	Fast
Myoglobin content	+++	+++	+
NADH dehydrogenase	+++	+++	+
Succinate dehydrogenase	+++	+++	+
Glycerophosphate dehydrogenase	+	+++	+++
Lactate dehydrogenase	+	+++	+++
Twitch kinetics	Slow	Fast	Fast
Speed of shortening	Slow	Fast	Fast
Fatigue resistant	Yes	Yes	No

stimulus does not change the shape of the action potential. The generation of an action potential reverses the transmembrane potential, which then becomes positive inside the cell. An extracellular electrode, as used in needle EMG, records the activity resulting from this switch of polarity as a predominantly negative potential (usually triphasic, positive–negative–positive waveforms). However, when recording near a damaged region, action potentials consist of a large positivity followed by a small negativity.

The needle EMG study is an essential component of the EDX evaluation. It provides an efficient and rapid mean of testing the electrical activity of motor units in a widespread number of muscles. The selection of muscle to be sampled is based on the working and differential diagnoses as determined by the clinical manifestations and NCS findings. The accessibility of the muscle, the ability to activate it, and the degree of pain associated with needle insertion particularly in children and anxious adults also play a role in that choice.

Concentric and Teflon-coated monopolar needle electrodes are equally satisfactory in recording muscle potentials, with few appreciable differences (Table 2–2). Though monopolar needles are less painful, they require an additional reference electrode nearby which often results in greater electrical noise due to electrode impedance mismatch between the intramuscular active electrode and the surface reference disk.

Techniques

Knowledge of the anatomy of muscles is a prerequisite for needle EMG. This includes their exact location, segmental and peripheral innervations, and activation maneuvers. The electromyographer first identifies the needle insertion point by recognizing the proper anatomical landmark of the sampled muscle. The initial insertion of the needle electrode should occur when the muscle is relaxed and not contracted since this is less painful. Needle EMG evaluation is performed in three steps:

1. Inserting or slightly moving the needle within the relaxed muscle causes insertional activity that results from needle injury of muscle fibers. This also assesses spontaneous activity by moving the needle a small distance and pausing a few seconds. At least 4–6 brief needle movements should be made in four quadrants of the muscle to assess insertional and spontaneous activity.

2. A minimal contraction is obtained to assess the morphology of several MUAPs that are measured on the

Table 2–2. Difference Between Monopolar and Concentric Needle Electrodes

Concentric	Monopolar
Does not requires an independent reference electrode	Requires an independent reference electrode
More painful	Less painful
More expensive	Less expensive
Low baseline noise	High baseline noise
Lower MUAP amplitude	Higher MUAP amplitude
Sharper MUAP rise time	MUAP rise time not as sharp
Shorter MUAP duration	Longer MUAP duration

oscilloscope or hard copy. If sharp MUAPs are not seen with minimal contraction, the needle should be moved slightly (pulled back or moved slightly deeper).

3. The intensity of muscle contraction is increased to assess the recruitment pattern of MUAPs. Maximal contraction normally fills the screen, producing the interference pattern.

Oscilloscope sweep speeds of 10 ms per division bests define spontaneous and voluntary activities. A 50 μV/division sensitivity is the usual amplification for the evaluation of insertional and spontaneous activities, while 200 μV/ division is used for analysis of voluntary motor activity.

Insertional and Spontaneous Activity

Normal Insertional and Spontaneous Activity

Brief bursts of electrical discharges accompany insertion and repositioning of a needle electrode into the muscle, slightly outlasting the movement of the needle, and usually not lasting more than 300 ms. Insertional activity appears as a cluster of positive or negative repetitive high-frequency spikes, which make a crisp static sound over the loudspeaker.

At rest, muscle is silent. It is, however, noisy in the motor endplate region (the site of neuromuscular junctions), which is usually located near the center of the muscle belly. Two types of normal endplate spontaneous activity occur together or independently: endplate spikes and endplate noise.

Endplate spikes. These are intermittent spikes and represent discharges of individual muscle fibers generated by activation of intramuscular nerve terminals irritated by the needle. Their characteristic irregular firing pattern distinguishes them from the regular-firing fibrillation potentials (Figure 2–16). The waveform of endplate spike is also distinguished by its initial negative deflection since the generator of the potential is usually underneath the needle's tip. Endplate spikes fire irregularly at 5–50 impulses per second, and measures 100–200 μV in amplitude, and 3–4 ms in duration. They have a cracking sound on the loudspeaker, imitating "sputtering fat in a frying pan."

Endplate noise. The tip of the needle approaching the endplate region frequently registers recurring irregular negative potentials, 10–50 μV in amplitude and 1–2 ms in duration (Figure 2–17). These potentials are the extracellularly recorded miniature endplate potentials that, in turn, are nonpropagating depolarizations caused by spontaneous release of acetylcholine quanta. Endplate potentials produce a characteristic sound on loudspeaker much like a "seashell held to the ear."

Abnormal Insertional Activity

Increased insertional activity. An abnormally prolonged (increased) insertional activity, that lasts longer than 300 ms and does not represent endplate potentials, indicates instability of the muscle membrane. It is often seen in conjunction with denervation, myotonic disorders, or necrotizing myopathies.

Myotonic-like or pseudomyotonic discharges. These are insertional positive waves, initiated by needle movements only and lasting few seconds. This isolated activity is distinguished from true myotonic discharges by the stability of the positive waves that do not wax or wane in amplitude or frequency. These discharges are usually seen during early denervation of muscle fibers such as one to two weeks after acute nerve injury.

50 μV/D   20 ms/D

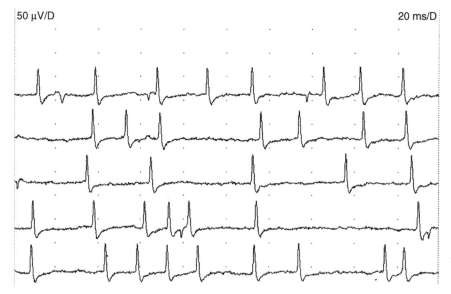

Figure 2–16. *Endplate spikes. Note the irregular firing pattern and the biphasic morphology with an initial negative deflection that separates this from the brief spike form of fibrillation potentials. (Compare the waveforms in this figure with those in Figure 2–18.)*

50 µV/D   20 ms/D

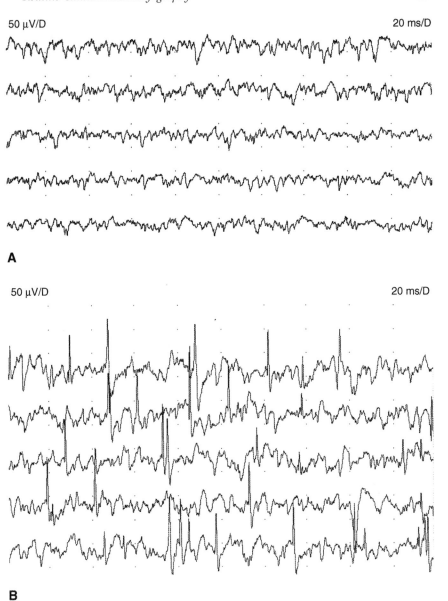

A

50 µV/D   20 ms/D

B

Figure 2–17. *Endplate noise. Note the low-amplitude, high-frequency and predominantly negative potentials (**A**). These may be seen in conjunction with the endplate spikes (**B**).*

Decreased insertional activity. A reduction or absence of insertional muscle activity suggests either fibrotic or severely atrophied muscles. Rarely, this represents functionally inexcitable muscles such as during the acute attacks of periodic paralysis.

Abnormal Spontaneous Activity

Fibrillation potentials. Fibrillation potentials are spontaneous action potentials generated by recently denervated muscle fibers. They often are triggered by needle insertion and persist more than 3 seconds after the needle movement stops. Fibrillation potentials typically fire in a regular pattern at a rate of 1–30 impulses per second. They produce a sound reminiscent of the sound caused by "rain on

the roof" or "the tick/tock of a clock." They consist of one of two types of waveforms with distinctive morphologies (positive waves and brief spikes), which likely reflect the relation between the position of the needle electrode and the muscle fiber.

1. *Positive waves* have an initial positivity and subsequent slow negativity with a characteristic sawtooth appearance (Figure 2–18). It is likely that the needle mechanically deforms the muscle fiber, and the action potential that move toward the damaged part of the muscle fiber is incapable of propagate further. This accounts for the positive wave morphology and absence of negative spike.

50 µV/D   20 ms/D

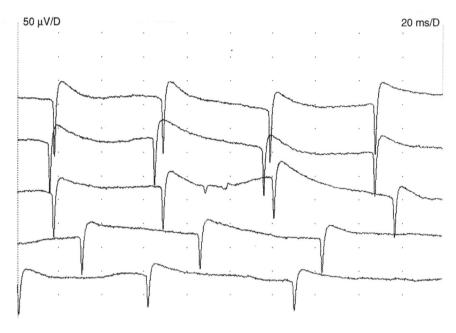

Figure 2–18. *A positive waveform of fibrillation potentials shown in raster form. Note that the discharge frequency is quite regular but decreases slightly and steadily starting the third trace.*

2. *Brief spikes* are usually triphasic with initial positivity (Figure 2–19). They range from 1 to 5 ms in duration and are 20–200 µV in amplitude when recorded with a concentric needle electrode. If the needle electrode is placed near the endplate zone, brief spikes fibrillation potentials may resemble physiologic endplate spikes with an initial negativity. Although often seen together, positive sharp waves tend to precede brief spikes after nerve injury, possibly because they can be triggered by the insertion of a needle in already irritable muscle membrane.

Fibrillation potentials are seen following muscle denervation that occurs with motor axon loss lesions to the anterior horn cells of the spinal cord, root, plexus, or peripheral nerve. Fibrillation potentials appear after 1–2 weeks of

50 µV/D   20 ms/D

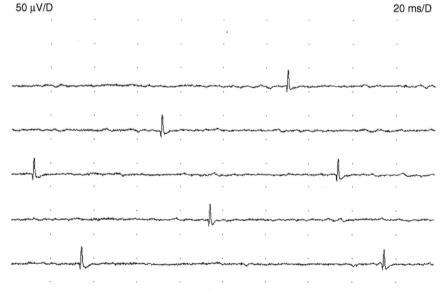

Figure 2–19. *A brief spike form of fibrillation potential shown in raster form. Note that the discharge is brief in duration, triphasic with an initial positivity and a regular rate.*

acute denervation but do not become full till after 3 weeks after nerve injury. They disappear late in the course of denervation when muscle fibers become reinnervated or fibrotic and severely atrophied. Hence, fibrillation potentials may be absent in very acute or chronic denervation.

Fibrillation potentials are also commonly encountered in necrotizing myopathies, such as the inflammatory myopathies, critical illness myopathies and muscular dystrophies. This is likely due to segmental necrosis of muscle fibers, leading to effective denervation of the distant segments as they become physically separated from the neuromuscular junction. Also, damage to the terminal intramuscular motor axons, presumably by the inflammatory process, may also result in muscle fiber denervation. In disorders of the neuromuscular junction such as myasthenia gravis or botulism, fibrillation potentials are rare. They are best explained by a chronic neuromuscular transmission blockade, resulting in "effective" denervation of muscle fibers.

Fibrillation potentials are graded from 0 to +4 as follows: 0, no fibrillation potentials; +1 persistent single trains of potentials (>2–3 seconds) in at least two areas; +2, moderate number of potentials in three or more areas; +3, many potentials in all areas; +4, abundant spontaneous potentials nearly filling the oscilloscope. This conventional grading is semiquantitative since the density of fibrillation potentials represents only a rough estimate of the extent of denervated muscle fibers.

Fasciculation potentials. Fasciculation potentials are spontaneous (involuntary) discharges of a motor unit. They originate from the anterior horn cell or motor axon anywhere along its length. Fasciculation potentials fire randomly and irregularly, with variable waveform morphology, and much slower firing rate than voluntary MUAPs. They may be associated with a visible muscle twitch and, rarely, in slight movement of a small joint in the fingers of toes. When abundant, fasciculation potentials give a "popping corn" sound on the loudspeaker.

Fasciculation potentials are encountered most commonly in motor neuron diseases, but are seen also in radiculopathies, entrapment neuropathies, peripheral polyneuropathies, and the cramp-fasciculation syndrome. They are seen also in tetany, thyrotoxicosis, and overdose of anticholinesterase medication. In addition, they may occur in healthy individuals, and there is no reliable method of distinguishing "benign" from "malignant" fasciculation potentials except that the fasciculation potentials in motor neuron disease tend to fire slower, are more complex, and less stable. Most importantly, benign fasciculation potentials are not associated clinically with weakness and wasting, or with other electrophysiologic signs of denervation including fibrillation potentials and neurogenic MUAP changes (Figure 2–20).

Complex repetitive discharges. A complex repetitive discharge is often referred to as CRD and was formerly known as bizarre repetitive discharge. It is a composite

0.1 mV/D   20 ms/D

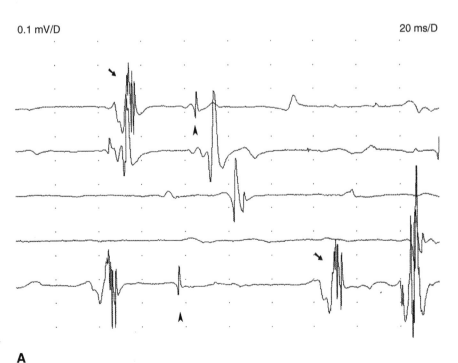

Figure 2–20. *Fasciculation potentials recorded, in raster mode, from the vastus lateralis in a patient with motor neuron disease. In (**A**) the sweep speed is set at 20 ms/division while in*

A

Continued

50 µV/D   200 ms/D

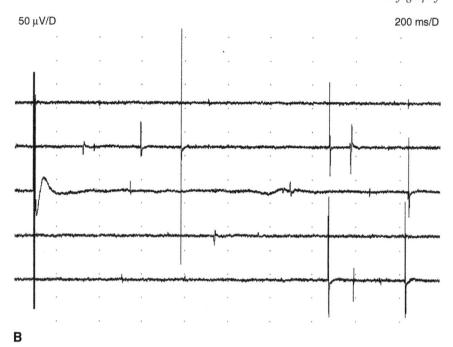

B

Figure 2–20, cont'd. *(B) it is set at a long sweep speed of 200 ms/division. Note that the morphology of the potentials is of motor units but with extreme variability in configuration among the individual discharges and their irregular firing pattern. Individual fasciculation potential may recur irregularly (arrows and arrowheads in (A)).*

waveform that contains several distinct spikes and often fires at a constant and fast rate of 30 to 50 Hz. Occasionally, the discharge frequency is slow or extremely fast, ranging from 5 to 100 Hz. The individual CRD ranges from 50 µV to 1 mV in amplitude and up to 50–100 ms in duration. It remains uniform from one discharge to another, a feature that helps distinguishing it from myokymic discharge (Figure 2–21). CRDs typically begin

and cease abruptly. On loudspeaker, CRD produces a noise that mimics the sound of a "machine." Pathophysiologically, CRD results from the near synchronous firing of a group of muscle fibers that communicates ephaptically. One fiber in the complex serves as a pacemaker, driving one or several other fibers so that the individual spikes within the complex fire in the same order as the discharge recurs. One of the late-activated fibers re-excites the principal

50 µV/D   50 ms/D

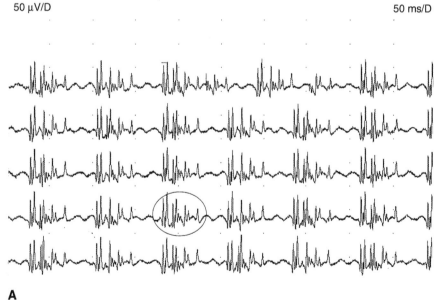

A

Figure 2–21. *Complex repetitive discharge recorded from the deltoid muscle in a patient with chronic C6 radiculopathy. Note that the complex (circled) is stable and remains exactly the same between discharges with a constant firing rate. In (A) the discharge is shown as a triggered rastered form and in*

50 μV/D   50 ms/D

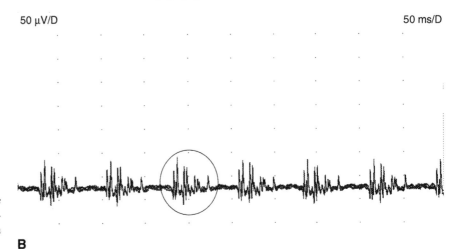

Figure 2–21, cont'd. (**B**) *the five rasters are superimposed. Note that the complex superimposes perfectly reflecting its uniform configuration.*

B

pacemaker to repeat the cycle. The chain reaction eventually blocks resulting in abrupt cessation. CRDs are abnormal discharges but rather nonspecific since they accompany a variety of chronic neurogenic as well myopathic disorders. They may also be found in the iliopsoas or cervical parapsinal muscles of apparently healthy individuals, probably implying a clinically silent neuropathic process.

Myokymic discharges. Myokymic discharge is defined as groups of motor unit potentials that fire repetitively in a quasi-rhythmical fashion with intervening period of silence. The burst composed of about 2–15 spikes with frequent variability in the number of spikes per discharge (Figure 2–22). The intraburst frequency is about 30–40 Hz, while the interburst frequency is much slower and ranges from 1 to 5 Hz, which gives myokymia the sound of "marching soldiers" on the loudspeaker. Clinically, myokymic discharges often give rise to sustained muscle contractions, which have an undulating appearance beneath the skin (bag of worms). Myokymic discharges probably originate ectopically in motor fibers and decrease in intensity with progressively distal nerve blocks. They may be amplified by increased axonal excitability, such as after hyperventilation-induced hypocapnia.

0.2 mV/D   200 ms/D

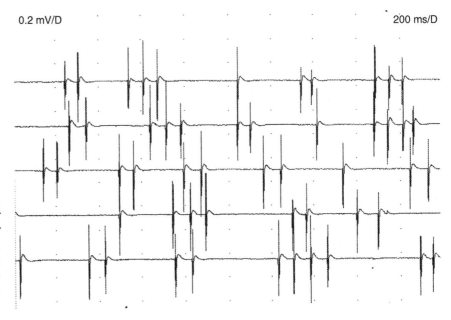

Figure 2–22. *Myokymic discharge shown in a raster mode with a long sweep speed of 200 ms/division. Note that the number of potentials often changes from one burst to another, varying in this example from one to four potentials. Note also the relatively slow interburst frequency of about 2 Hz while the intraburst frequency is about 18–20 Hz.*

Table 2–3. Causes of Myokymic Discharges

Focal		Generalized
Facial	**Limb**	**Generalized**
Multiple sclerosis	Radiation plexopathy (brachial or lumbosacral)	Thyrotoxicosis
Brainstem tumors	Carpal tunnel syndrome	Thymoma
Syringobulbia	Ulnar neuropathy	Guillain-Barré syndrome
Bell's palsy	Chronic radiculopathy	Gold intoxication
Guillain-Barré syndrome	Spinal stenosis	Penicillamine
Basilar invagination	Guillain-Barré syndrome	Timber rattlesnake poisoning
Cerebellopontine angle tumor	CIDP*	Isaac's syndrome
Cardiac arrest	HNPP†	
Hydrocephalus		
Lymphocytic meningitis		

*CIDP = chronic inflammatory demyelinating polyneuropathy.
†HNPP = hereditary neuropathy with liability to pressure palsy (tomaculous neuropathy).

Myokymic discharges may be restricted to focal areas such as the in face with brainstem glioma or multiple sclerosis, a single extremity with radiation plexopathy, or the thenar eminence with carpal tunnel syndrome. They also may be generalized as encountered in association with gold toxicity or the syndrome of continuous motor unit activity (Isaac syndrome) (Table 2-3).

Neuromyotonic discharges. Neuromyotonic discharges are extremely rare discharges in which motor units fire repetitively at high frequency (150–250 Hz), either continuously or in recurring decrementing bursts, producing a "pinging sound" on loudspeaker (Figure 2–23). The discharge continues during sleep, and diminishes in intensity with progressively distal nerve blocks, implicating the entire axon as the site of generation. The syndrome of continuous motor unit activity (Isaac syndrome) which may have an autoimmune etiology, with the target antigen likely being peripheral nerve potassium channels, is often associated with neuromyotonia and myokymia. Other conditions associated with neuromyotonia include anticholinesterase poisoning, tetany, and chronic spinal muscular atrophies.

Myotonic discharges. Like fibrillation potentials, myotonic discharges appear either as a sustained run of sharp positive waves or brief spikes (Figure 2–24). Positive sharp waves are initiated by needle insertion injuring muscle membrane, whereas the brief spikes tend to occur at the beginning of slight volitional contraction. Both types of discharges typically wax and wane in amplitude (range = 10 μV–1 mV), and frequency (range = 20–150 Hz), which

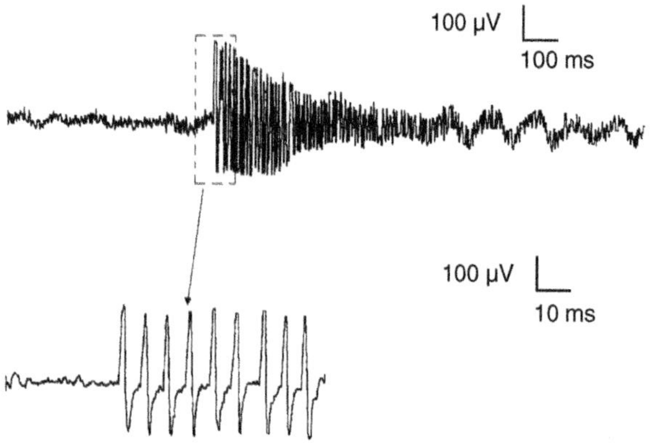

Figure 2–23. *Neuromyotonic discharge. Note the decrementing response. The top is recorded with a long sweep speed of 100 ms/division while the insert is at a regular sweep speed of 10 ms/division. Note the very high frequency (150–250 Hz) repetitive discharge of a single motor unit. (Reproduced from Preston DC, Shapiro BE. Electromyography and neuromuscular disorders. Boston, MA: Butterworth-Heinemann, 1998, with permission.)*

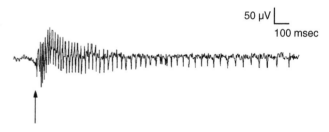

Figure 2–24. *Myotonic discharge recorded with a sweep speed of 100 ms/division. The arrow depicts the time of needle insertion that triggers the discharge from a muscle fiber. Note the waxing and waning of both amplitude and frequency. (Reproduced from Preston DC, Shapiro BE. Electromyography and neuromuscular disorders. Boston, MA: Butterworth-Heinemann, 1998, with permission.)*

Table 2–4. Common Causes of Electrical Myotonia

Myotonic Dystrophies
Type I, II and PROMM (proximal myotonic myopathy)

Myotonia Congenita
Thomsen disease
Becker disease

Other Myotonic Disorders
Atypical painful myotonia
Myotonia fluctuans

Muscle Channelopathies
Paramyotonia congenita
Hyperkalemic periodic paralysis (between attacks)

Other Myopathies
Acid maltase deficiency (Pompe's disease)
Myotubular myopathy
Colchicine
Inflammatory myopathies (rarely)

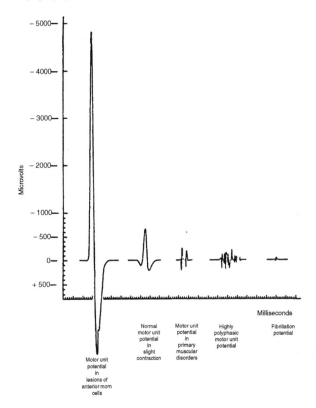

Figure 2–25. *Relative average durations and amplitudes of some MUAPs seen in myopathic and neurogenic disorders. (Reproduced from Daube J. Needle electromyography in clinical electromyography. Muscle Nerve 1991;14:685–700, with permission.)*

gives rise to a characteristic noise over the loudspeaker, simulating a "dive-bomber" or an "accelerating–decelerating motorcycle or chain saw."

Myotonic discharges may occur with or without clinical myotonia in the myotonic dystrophies, myotonia congenital, and paramyotonia congenita. They may also accompany acid maltase deficiency, colchicine myopathy, myotubular myopathy, and hyperkalemic periodic paralysis (Table 2–4).

Cramp discharges. On needle EMG, a cramp discharge consists of MUAPs involuntarily and regularly firing extremely fast at a rate of 40–60 Hz, with abrupt onset and cessation. Cramps most often occur in healthy individuals, but are exaggerated by hyponatremia, hypocalcemia, thyroid disorders, pregnancy, postdialysis state, and the early stages of motor neuron disease. Clinically, cramps are sustained muscle contractions and resemble muscle contractures that accompany several of the metabolic muscle diseases, but the latter are characterized by complete electrical silence on needle EMG.

Voluntary Motor Unit Action Potentials

Motor Unit Action Potential Morphology

The motor unit action potential (MUAP) is the sum of the extracellular potentials of muscle fiber action potentials of a motor unit. The waveform is dictated by the inherent properties of the motor unit and the spatial relationships between the needle and individual muscle fibers. The extracellularly recorded MUAP, recorded along the length of the muscle fibers and away from the endplate region, has a triphasic waveform (Figure 2–25). The initial positive

deflection represents the action potential propagating towards the electrode. As the potential passes in front of the electrode the main positive–negative deflection is recorded. When the action potential propagates away from the electrode the potential returns to the baseline. Slight repositioning of the electrode causes major changes in the electrical profile of the same motor unit. Therefore, one motor unit can give rise to MUAPs of different morphology at different recording sites. If the electrode is placed immediately over the endplate area, the initial positive defection will not be recorded and the potential will have a biphasic waveform with an initial negative deflection.

Amplitude. MUAP amplitude is the maximum peak-to-peak amplitude and ranges from several hundred microvolts to a few millivolts with a concentric needle, and is substantially greater with a monopolar needle. At a short distance between the recording electrode and the potential generators (muscle fibers), the MUAP has a short rise time and high amplitude with a "crisp" or "sharp" sound on the loudspeaker. In contrast, the MUAP recorded from distant muscle fibers has a long rise time and a low amplitude that sounds "dull" or "muffled" on the loudspeaker.

For example, the MUAP amplitude decreases to less than 50% at a distance of 200–300 μm from the source and to less than 1% a few millimeters away. Therefore, only a small number of individual muscle fibers located near the tip of the recording electrode determine the amplitude of an MUAP (probably less than 20 muscle fibers lying within a 1 mm radius of the electrode tip). In general, amplitude indicates muscle fiber density and not the motor unit territory. High MUAP amplitude, when isolated, is considered a nonspecific abnormality except when it is significantly increased (more than twice the upper normal limit); then, it indicates a neurogenic process.

Duration. MUAP duration reflects the electrical activity generated from most muscle fibers belonging to a motor unit. Muscle potentials generated more than 1 mm away from the electrode contribute to the initial and terminal low-amplitude portions of the potential. The duration also indicates the degree of synchrony among many individual muscle fibers with variable length, conduction velocity, and membrane excitability. MUAP duration is a good index of the motor unit territory and is the parameter that best reflects the number of muscle fibers within a motor unit. A shift in needle position has much less effect on MUAP duration than amplitude. The duration is measured from the initial deflection away from baseline to the final return to baseline, and normally varies from 5 to 15 ms, depending on the sampled muscle and the age of the subject. In normal subjects, large muscles tend to have long-duration MUAPs and MUAP duration increases with age after the sixth decade.

Long-duration MUAPs are the best indicators of reinnervation. They occur with increased number or density of muscle fibers, or a loss of synchrony of fiber firing within a motor unit as seen with lower motor neuron disorders. These MUAPs may also show high amplitude (see Figure 2–25). In contrast, short-duration MUAPs often have low amplitude and are indicators of muscle fiber loss as seen with necrotizing myopathies.

Phases. An MUAP phase constitutes the portion of a waveform that departs from and returns to the baseline. The number of phases equals the number of negative and positive peaks extending to and from the baseline, or the number of baseline crossings plus one. Normal MUAPs have four phases or less, though about 5–15% of MUAPs in distal muscles have five phases or more, and this may be up to 25% in proximal muscles, such as the deltoid, iliacus, and gluteus maximus. Increased polyphasia is an abnormal yet nonspecific MUAP abnormality since it is encountered in myopathies as well as in neuropathies. An increased number of polyphasic MUAPs suggests a desynchronized discharge, loss of individual fibers within a motor unit, or temporal dispersion of muscle fiber potentials within a motor unit. Excessive temporal dispersion, in turn, results

from differences in conduction time along the terminal branch of the nerve or over the muscle fiber membrane. After severe denervation when the newly sprouting axons only reinnervate few muscle fibers, the MUAP may also be polyphasic with short duration and low amplitude ("nascent" MUAP).

Some MUAPs have a serrated pattern with several *turns* or directional changes without crossing the baseline; this also indicates desynchronization among discharging muscle fibers. *Satellite potential* (linked potential or parasite potential) is a late spike of MUAP, which is distinct, but time locked with the main potential. It implicates early reinnervation of muscle fibers by collateral sprouts from adjacent motor units.

Motor Unit Action Potential stability
Motor units normally discharge semirhythmically, with successive potentials showing nearly identical configuration due to firing of all muscle fibers of the motor unit during every discharge. The morphology of a repetitively firing unit may fluctuate if individual muscle fibers intermittently block within the unit. This instability may be evident in neuromuscular junction disorder, such as myasthenia gravis, the myasthenic syndrome, or botulism. Also during reinnervation such as motor neuron disease, subacute radiculopathy, or polyneuropathy, the newly formed endplates are immature and demonstrate poor efficacy of neuromuscular transmission. This results in unstable MUAP waveforms with moment-to-moment MUAP variability (Figure 2–26). The MUAP instability disappears when reinnervation is complete and well established and helps to distinguish between a subacute and chronic neurogenic process.

Motor Unit Action Potential Firing Patterns
During constant contraction, a healthy individual initially excites only 1–2 motor units semirhythmically. The motor units activated early are primarily those with small, type I muscle fibers. Large, type II units participate later during strong voluntary contraction. Greater muscle force brings about not only recruitment of previously inactive units, but also more rapid firing of already active units, both mechanisms operating simultaneously.

The *firing rate* of the motor unit equal to the number of MU discharges in a one second time interval, and is measured in hertz (Hz). When several MUAPs are discharging they superimpose, which makes MUAP identification and firing rate analysis difficult requiring automated methods. When one or two MUAPs are firing, such as during minimal voluntary effort or when there is marked decrease in the number of MUAPs firing, this analysis become quite easy. The firing rate may be estimated manually by freezing a 100 ms epoch and multiplying the number of discharges

0.2 mV/D   20 ms/D

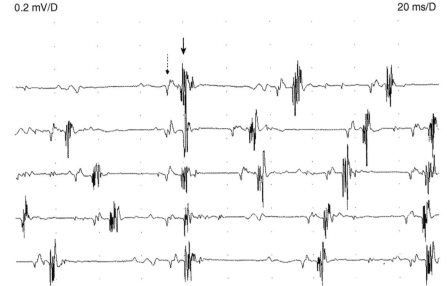

Figure 2–26. *Unstable polyphasic motor unit action potential with a satellite potential. Both the main component of the potential (solid arrow) and the satellite potential (dashed arrow) are unstable. This complex potential is triggered upon using a trigger, delay line and a raster mode. Note the extreme variation in the morphology of the unit and its satellite potential between subsequent discharges.*

of an MUAP by 10 to obtain a one second epoch. For example, a motor unit appearing twice in a 100 ms sweep has a firing rate of $2 \times 10 = 20$ Hz. The multiplication factor can be adjusted depending on the analyzed epoch, being 5 for a 200 ms epoch and 2 for a 500 ms epoch (Figure 2–27). Another way of calculating the firing rate of a motor unit is by dividing 1000 by the time interval between successive MUAP discharges in ms. For example, a firing rate of a unit with an interval of 50 ms is 20 Hz.

Motor unit firing is a dynamic process that involves a balance between the number of motor units recruited and their firing rate. With minimal contraction, one MUAP is first recruited and its firing rate when it begins to discharge is called its onset frequency. When the subject gradually increases the force of contraction, the motor unit firing rates increases slightly and eventually a second motor unit is recruited. *Recruitment frequency* is defined

as the firing frequency just before the time an additional unit is recruited. In normal muscles, the onset frequency varies between 6 and 10 Hz while the recruitment frequency ranges between 8 and 15 Hz, and the reported ranges for healthy individuals and those with neuromuscular disorders overlap considerably. *Recruitment ratio* is the average firing rate divided by the number of active units. This ratio should normally not exceed 5, for example, three units each firing less than 15 impulses per second. A ratio of 10, with two units firing at 20 impulses per second each, indicates a pathologic lower motor neuron process.

Activation is the central control of motor units that allows an increase in the firing rate and force. Failure of descending impulses also limits recruitment, although here the excited motor units discharge more slowly than expected for normal maximal contraction. Thus, a decreased number of voluntary MUAPs with a slow firing rate (*poor activation*) is a feature of an upper motor neuron disorder

0.2 mV/D   20 ms/D

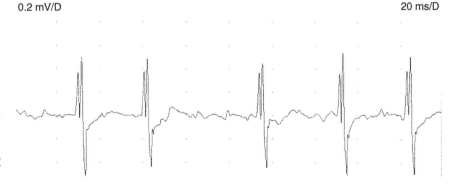

Figure 2–27. *A slightly increased duration motor unit action potential firing rapidly. The sweep speed is set at 20 ms/division, resulting in an epoch of 200 ms. The firing rate is $5 \times 5 = 25$ Hz.*

(such as stroke or myelopathy) but may be seen with volitional lack of effort (such as due to pain, conversion reaction, or malingering). This stands in sharp contrast to a fast firing rate associated with a disorder of the lower motor neuron (*decreased recruitment*).

With greater contraction, many motor units begin to fire rapidly, making recognition of individual MUAPs difficult, hence the name *interference pattern*. This is assessed by its sound on the loudspeaker and the number of spikes and their amplitude. The interference pattern depends on the descending input from the cortex, number of motor neurons capable of discharging, firing frequency of each motor unit, waveform of individual potentials, and phase cancellation. An incomplete interference pattern may be due to either poor activation or reduced recruitment. Recruitment may be assessed during maximum contraction by examining the interference pattern, or during moderate levels of contraction by estimating the number of MUAPs firing for the level of activation. Evaluating MUAPs during maximal effort is most valuable in excluding mild degrees of decreased recruitment.

In myopathy, the motor unit pool produces a smaller force per unit than a normal pool. These usually low-amplitude, short-duration MUAPs must be recruited instantaneously to support a slight voluntary effort in patients with moderate to severe weakness. *Early recruitment* refers to the greater than expected number of discharging MUAPs for the force of contraction. With early recruitment, a full interference pattern is attained at less than maximal contraction, but its amplitude is low because fiber density is decreased in individual motor units. In advanced myopathies with severe muscle weakness and atrophy (such as in advanced muscular dystrophy), loss of muscle fibers may be so extensive that whole motor units effectively disappear, resulting in a decreased recruitment and an incomplete interference pattern, mimicking a neuropathic recruitment.

SUGGESTED READINGS

Chaudhry V, Cornblath DR, Mellits ED, et al. Inter- and intra-examiner reliability of nerve conduction measurements in normal subjects. Ann Neurol 1991;30:841–843.

Daube J. Needle electromyography in clinical electromyography. Muscle Nerve 1991;14:685–700.

Erim Z, de Luca CJ, Mineo K, et al. Rank-ordered regulation of motor units. Muscle Nerve 1996;19:563–573.

Gutmann L. Important anomalous innervations of the extremities. Muscle Nerve 1993;36:899–990.

Hammer K. Nerve conduction studies. Springfield, IL: C Thomas Publishers, 1982.

Harik SI, Baraka AS, Tomeh GF, et al. Autonomous peripheral nerve activity causing generalized muscle stiffness and fasciculations: report of a case with physiological, pharmacological, and morphological observations. Johns Hopkins Med J 1976; 139(S):49–60.

Hart IK, Waters C, Vincent A, et al. Autoantibodies detected to expressed K+ channels are implicated in neuromyotonia. Ann Neurol 1997;41:238–246.

Iyer V, Fenichel GM. Normal median nerve proximal latency in carpal tunnel syndrome: a clue to coexisting Martin-Gruber anastomosis. J Neurol Neurosurg Psychiatry 1976;39:449–452.

Katirji B. Clinical electromyography. Neurology clinics. Philadelphia, PA: WB Saunders, 2002.

Katirji B. Clinical electromyography. In: Bradley WG, Daroff RB, Fenichel GM, Jankovic J, eds. Neurology in clinical practice, 4th ed. Boston, MA: Butterworth-Heinemann, 2004, pp. 491–520.

Kimura J. Collision technique. Physiologic block of nerve impulses in studies of motor nerve conduction velocity. Neurology 1976;26:680–682.

Kimura J. The carpal tunnel syndrome: localization of conduction abnormalities within the distal segment of the median nerve. Brain 1979;102:619–635.

Kimura J. Facts, fallacies, and facies of nerve conduction studies: twenty-first annual Edward H. Lambert lecture. Muscle Nerve 1997;20:777–787.

Lambert EH. The accessory deep peroneal nerve: a common variation in innervation of extensor digitorum brevis. Neurology 1969;19:1169–1176.

McDonald WI. The physiological consequences of demyelination. In: Sumner AJ, ed. The physiology of peripheral nerve disease. Philadelphia, PA: WB Saunders, 1980, pp. 265–286.

McIntosh KA, Preston DC, Logigian EL. Short segment incremental studies to localize ulnar entrapments at the wrist. Neurology 1998;50:303–306.

Petajan JH. Motor unit recruitment. Muscle Nerve 1991;14: 489–502.

Preston DC, Shapiro BE. Needle electromyography. Fundamentals, normal and abnormal patterns. Neurol Clin N Am 2002;20:361–396.

Rutkove SB, Kothari MJ, Shefner JM. Nerve, muscle, and neuromuscular junction electrophysiology at high temperature. Muscle Nerve 1997;20:431–436.

Sander HW, Quinto C, Chokroverty S. Median-ulnar anastomosis to thenar, hypothenar, and first dorsal interosseous muscles: collision technique confirmation. Muscle Nerve 1997;20: 1460–1462.

Shapiro BE, Katirji B, Preston DC. Clinical electromyography. In: Katirji B, Kaminski HJ, Preston DC, Ruff RL, Shapiro EB, eds. Neuromuscular disorders in clinical practice. Boston, MA: Butterworth-Heinemann, 2002.

St lberg E, Antoni L. Electrophysiological cross section of the motor unit. J Neurol Neurosurg Psychiatry 1980;43:469–474.

Wilbourn AJ. Nerve conduction studies. Types, components, abnormalities and value in localization. Neurol Clin 2002;20: 305–338.

3

Specialized Electrodiagnostic Studies

LATE RESPONSES

Late responses are obtained using special techniques that are not possible with conventional nerve conduction studies. The settings are usually changed to allow the examiner to capture these responses. This include using longer sweep speed of 5–10 ms/division and lower amplifier gain of 200–500 µV/division which could be adjusted depending on the limb studied, site of stimulation and magnitude of response. Since it is intended for the action potentials to travel proximally with the late response recording, the bipolar stimulator is switched to place the cathode more proximally and the anode distally.

F Wave

F waves were named in reference to "foot" since they were originally recorded in small foot muscles, though they may be generated by the stimulation of any motor or mixed nerve. A supramaximal stimulus applied at any point along the course of a motor nerve elicits an F wave in a distal muscle that follows the CMAP (M response). The impulse travels antidromically to the spinal cord and the F wave is produced by backfiring of motor neurons. An average of 5–10% of the motor neurons available in the motor neuron pool backfire after each stimulus. The afferent and efferent loops of the F wave are motor with no intervening synapse. Hence, the F waves test the integrity of the entire motor axons, including the ventral roots.

The F waves are low-amplitude and ubiquitous responses that are typically variable in latency, amplitude, and morphology (Figure 3–1A and B). Their variability is explained by differing groups of motor neurons generating the recurring discharge with each individual group of neurons having different number of motor neurons and conducting properties. Several parameters may be analyzed, but the *minimal F wave latency* is the most reliable and useful

measurement since it represents conduction of the largest and fastest motor fibers. Since F wave latencies vary from one stimulus to the next, an adequate study requires that about 10 F waves be clearly identified. The minimal F wave latency is also dependent on the length of motor axons which correlates with the patient's height and limb length. The most sensitive criterion of abnormality in a unilateral disorder is a latency difference between the two sides, or between two similar nerves in the same limb. Absolute latencies are most useful only for sequential reassessment of the same nerve. *F wave persistence* is a measure of the number of F waves obtained for the number of stimulations. This varies between individuals and is inhibited by muscle activity while it is enhanced by relaxation or the use of Jendrasik maneuver. It is usually above 50% except when stimulating the peroneal nerve while recording the extensor digitorum brevis. *F wave chronodispersion* is the degree of scatter among consecutive F waves and is determined by the difference between the minimal and maximal F wave latencies. It indicates the range of motor conduction velocities between the smallest and largest myelinated motor axon in the nerve. The *F wave conduction velocity* may be calculated after distal and proximal supramaximal stimulations and provides a better comparison between proximal and distal (forearm or leg) segments.

F wave latencies are prolonged in most polyneuropathies, particularly the demyelinating type, including Guillain-Barré syndrome and chronic inflammatory demyelinating polyneuropathy (CIDP) (Figure 3–1C and D). F wave latencies in radiculopathies have a limited use. They may be normal despite partial motor axonal loss because the surviving axons conduct normally, and in single radiculopathies since most muscles have multiple root innervation. Finally, focal slowing at the root level may get diluted by the relatively long motor axon.

A Wave

The A wave (axonal wave) is a potential that is seen occasionally during recording of F waves at supramaximal stimulation. The A wave follows the CMAP and often precedes, but occasionally follows, the F wave. The A wave may be mistakenly considered for an F response but its constant latency and morphology in at least 10 out of 20 stimulations differentiates it from the highly variable morphology and latency of the F wave (Table 3–1).

The A wave may be seen in up to 5% of asymptomatic individuals, particularly while studying the tibial nerve (Figure 3–2A and B). In contrast, recording multiple or complex A waves from several nerves is often associated with acquired or inherited demyelinating polyneuropathies (Figure 3–3). A waves are sometimes seen in axon-loss polyneuropathies, motor neuron disease, and radiculopathies. The exact pathway of the A wave is unknown but it may be generated as a result of ephaptic transmission between two axons with the action potential conducting back down the nerve fiber to the muscle. The A wave may also appear following sprouting and reinnervation along the examined nerve. The constant morphology and latency of the A wave is best explained by the fixed point of a collateral sprout or ephapse. When the A wave follows rather than precedes the F response, it suggests that the regenerating collateral fibers are conducting very slowly.

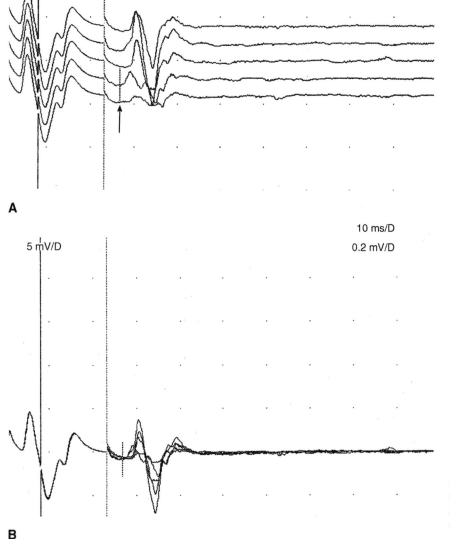

A

B

Figure 3–1. *Median F waves, stimulating the median nerve at the wrist while recording abductor pollicis brevis. (**A**) Normal 22-year-old subject shown in a raster mode. (**B**) Normal 22-year-old subject shown superimposed.*

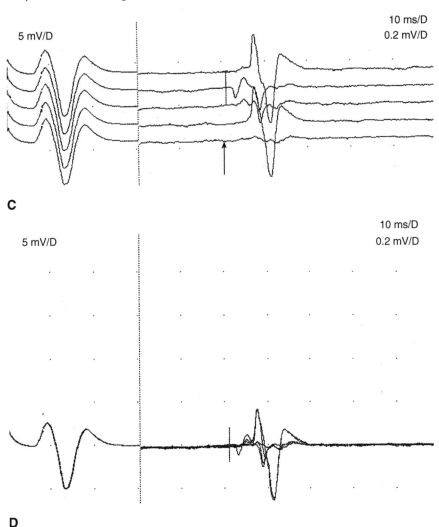

Figure 3–1. cont'd (**C**) *A 20-year-old with Guillian-Barré syndrome shown in a raster mode.* (**D**) *A 20-year-old with Guillian-Barré syndrome shown superimposed. Arrows in* (**A**) *and* (**C**) *denotes the minimal f wave latency. Note that the variability in F wave morphology and latency and the significant delay in F wave latencies in Guillian-Barré syndrome compared to normal.*

H Reflex

The H reflex, named after Hoffmann for his original description, is an electrical counterpart of the stretch reflex which is elicited by a mechanical tap. Group 1A sensory fibers constitute the afferent arc which monosynaptically or oligosynaptically activate the alpha motor neurons that in turn generate the efferent arc of the reflex through their motor axons. The H reflex amplitude may be occasionally as high as the M amplitude but it is often lower with the H/M amplitude ratio usually not exceeding 0.75.

The H reflex and F wave can be distinguished by increasing stimulus intensity (see Table 3–1). The H reflex is best elicited by a long-duration stimulus which is *submaximal* to produce an M response, whereas the F wave requires *supramaximal* stimulus Also, the F wave can be elicited from any limb muscle while the H reflex is most reproducible with stimulating the tibial nerve while recording the soleus muscle which assess the integrity of the S1 arc reflex and is equivalent to the Achilles reflex (Figure 3–4). Finally, the H reflex latency (and often amplitude) is constant when elicited by the same stimulus intensity, since it reflects activation of the same motor neuron pool.

The H reflex is most useful as an adjunct study in the diagnosis of peripheral polyneuropathy or S1 radiculopathy. The H reflex latency and amplitude is the most sensitive, yet nonspecific, among the nerve conduction studies in the early phases of Guillain-Barré syndrome. The H reflex may be absent in healthy elderly subjects and isolated abnormalities of the H reflex are nondiagnostic since they may reflect pathology anywhere along the reflex arc.

Blink Reflex

The blink reflex generally assesses the facial and trigeminal nerves and their connections within the pons and medulla.

Table 3–1. Comparisons Between the Common Late Responses Recorded in Limb Muscles

	F Wave	A Wave	H Reflex
Physiologic basis	Not a reflex. Antidromic discharge of anterior horn cells	Not a reflex. An ephaptic transmission or reinnervation sprout	A true reflex
Afferent pathway	Antidromic motor fibers	Antidromic motor fibers	Orthodromic sensory fibers
Efferent pathway	Orthodromic motor fibers	Orthodromic motor fibers	Orthodromic motor fibers
Optimal stimulus	Supramaximal	Supramaximal	Submaximal (subthreshold)
Recording sites in normal subjects	Following stimulation of almost any motor nerve. May be absent stimulating peroneal nerve recording extensor digitorum brevis	Following stimulation of tibial nerve recoding abductor hallucis mostly	Following stimulation of tibial nerve at the knee recording soleus/gastrocnemius. Following stimulation of distal nerves recoding hand and foot muscles in newborns. May be absent in elderly patients
Latency	Variable	Constant	Constant
Morphology	Variable	Constant	Constant (except for amplitude change)
Amplitude	Much lower than M response (less than 5% of the M response)	Variable but usually similar to the F wave	≤M response (H/M ratio usually 0.75)
Clinical significance	Delayed or absent in peripheral polyneuropathies particularly the demyelinative types	Appears in several nerves in peripheral polyneuropathies and may be complex in the demyelinative types	Absent or delayed in peripheral polyneuropathies and S1 radiculopathy

It has an afferent limb, mediated by sensory fibers of the supraorbital branch of the ophthalmic division of the trigeminal nerve, and an efferent limb mediated by motor fibers of the facial nerve and its superior motor branches.

The supraorbital nerve is stimulated over the supraorbital notch and the blink responses are recorded from the orbicularis oculi bilaterally using a two channel recording setting. The blink reflex has two components, an early R1 and a late R2 response. The R1 response is present only ipsilateral to the stimulation and is usually a simple triphasic waveform with a di-synaptic pathway between the main trigeminal sensory nucleus in the midpons and the ipsilateral facial nucleus in the lower pontine tegmentum. The R2 response is a complex waveform and is the electrical counterpart of the corneal reflex. It is typically present bilaterally with an oligosynaptic pathway between the nucleus of the trigeminal spinal tract in the ipsilateral pons and medulla, and interneurons forming connections to the ipsilateral and contralateral facial nuclei.

The blink reflex is most useful in unilateral lesions such as facial palsy, trigeminal neuropathy, or lower brainstem lesion. With *facial nerve lesions*, the R1 and R2 potentials are absent or delayed with supraorbital stimulation ipsilateral to the lesion, while the R2 response on the contralateral side is normal. With *trigeminal nerve lesions*, the

ipsilateral R1 and R2, contralateral R2 are absent or delayed with ipsilateral stimulation while all responses are normal with contralateral stimulation. With a *midpontine lesion* involving the main sensory trigeminal nucleus or the pontine interneurons to the ipsilateral facial nerve nucleus or both, supraorbital stimulation on the side of the lesion results in an absent or delayed R1, but an intact ipsilateral and contralateral R2. Finally, with a *medullary lesion* involving the spinal tract and trigeminal nucleus or the medullary interneurons to the ipsilateral facial nerve nucleus or both, supraorbital stimulation on the affected side results in a normal R1 and contralateral R2, but an absent or delayed ipsilateral R2. In demyelinating polyneuropathies such as the Guillain-Barré syndrome or Charcot-Marie-Tooth disease type 1, the R1 and R2 responses may be markedly delayed, reflecting slowing of motor fibers, sensory fibers, or both.

REPETITIVE NERVE STIMULATION

Repetitive nerve stimulation (RNS) of motor or mixed nerves is performed for the evaluation of patients with suspected neuromuscular junction disorders, including myasthenia gravis, Lambert-Eaton myasthenic syndrome, botulism, and congenital myasthenic syndromes. The design and plans for RNS depends on physiologic facts inherent to the

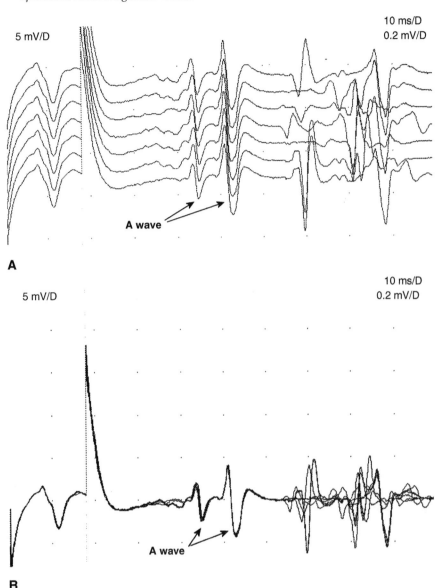

5 mV/D

10 ms/D
0.2 mV/D

A wave

A

5 mV/D

10 ms/D
0.2 mV/D

A wave

B

Figure 3–2. *Tibial A wave, stimulating the tibial nerve at the ankle while recording the abductor hallucis muscle. (**A**) Waveforms shown in a raster mode. (**B**) Waveforms superimposed. Note that the response has a constant morphology and latency, which results in perfect superimposition.*

neuromuscular junction that dictate the type and frequency of stimulations utilized in the accurate diagnosis of neuromuscular junction disorders.

Physiology and Principles

A *quantum* is the amount on acetylcholine packaged in a single vesicle, which contains approximately 5000 to 10 000 acetylcholine molecules. Each quantum (vesicle) released results in a 1 mV change of postsynaptic membrane potential. During rest, spontaneous release of individual quanta forms the basis of miniature endplate potential.

The number of quanta released after a nerve action potential depends on the number of quanta in the *immediately available (primary) store* and the probability of release, i.e., $m = p \times n$, where m = the number of quanta released during each stimulation, p = the probability of release (effectively proportional to the concentration of calcium and typically about 0.2, or 20%), and n = the number of quanta in the immediately available store. In normal conditions, a single nerve action potential triggers the release of 50–300 vesicles (quanta) with an average equivalent to about 60 quanta (60 vesicles). In addition to the immediately available store of acetylcholine located beneath the presynaptic nerve terminal membrane, *a secondary (or mobilization) store* starts to replenish the immediately available store after 1–2 seconds of repetitive nerve action potentials. A large *tertiary (or reserve) store* is also available in the axon and cell body.

10 ms/D

1 mV/D

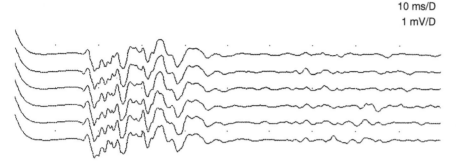

Figure 3–3. *Complex A wave stimulating the median nerve at the wrist while recording abductor pollicis brevis in a patient with Guillian-Barré syndrome shown in a raster form. Note that the complex response has a constant morphology and latency.*

The *end plate potential* is the potential generated at the postsynaptic membrane following a nerve action potential. Since each vesicle released causes a 1 mV change in the postsynaptic membrane potential, this results in about 60 mV change in the amplitude of the membrane potential.

In normal conditions, the number of quanta (vesicles) released at the neuromuscular junction by the presynaptic terminal far exceeds the postsynaptic membrane potential change required to reach the *threshold* needed to generate a postsynaptic muscle action potential. This *safety factor* ensures an endplate potential that is always above threshold and results in muscle fiber action potential. In addition to quantal release, several other factors contribute to the safety factor and endplate potential including acetylcholine receptor conduction properties, acetylcholine receptor density, and acetylcholinesterase activity.

Following depolarization of the presynaptic terminal, voltage-gated calcium channels open leading to calcium influx. Through a calcium-dependent intracellular cascade, vesicles are docked into active release zones and acetylcholine molecules are released. Calcium then diffuses slowly out of the presynaptic terminal in 100–200 ms.

The rate at which motor nerves are repetitively stimulated dictates whether calcium accumulation plays a role in enhancing the release of acetylcholine. At slow rate of RNS (i.e., a stimulus than every 200 ms or more, or a stimulation rate of <5 Hz), the role of calcium in acetylcholine release is not enhanced and subsequent nerve action potentials reach the nerve terminal long after calcium has dispersed. In contrast, with rapid RNS (i.e., a stimulus every 100 ms or less, or stimulation rate >10 Hz), calcium influx is greatly enhanced and the probability of release of acetylcholine quanta increases.

The surface-recorded CMAP obtained during routine motor NCS represents the summation of all muscle fiber action potential generated in a muscle following supramaximal stimulation of all motor axons.

Slow Repetitive Nerve Stimulation

Slow RNS is usually performed by applying 3–5 supramaximal stimuli to a mixed or motor nerve at a rate of 2–3 Hz.

This rate is low enough to prevent calcium accumulation, but high enough to deplete the quanta in the immediately available store before the mobilization store starts to replenish it. A total of 3–5 stimuli are adequate since the maximal decrease in acetylcholine release occurs during the first 3–5 stimuli.

Calculation of the decrement with slow RNS requires comparing the baseline CMAP amplitude to the lowest CMAP amplitude (usually the third or fourth). The CMAP decrement is expressed as a percentage and calculated as follows:

$$\% \text{ decrement} = \frac{\text{Amplitude (1st response)} - \text{amplitude (3rd/4th response)}}{\text{Amplitude (1st response)}} \times 100$$

In normal conditions, slow RNS does not cause a CMAP decrement. Although the second to fifth endplate potentials fall in amplitude, they remain above threshold (due to the normal safety factor) and ensure generation of muscle fiber action potential with each stimulation. In addition, the secondary store begins to replace the depleted quanta after the first few seconds with a subsequent rise in the endplate potential. Hence, all muscle fibers generate muscle fiber action potentials and the CMAP does not change (Figures 3–5 and 3–6A). In postsynaptic neuromuscular junction disorders (such as myasthenia gravis), the safety factor is reduced since there are fewer available acetylcholine receptors. Hence, the baseline endplate potential is reduced but usually still above threshold. Slow RNS results in a decrease in endplate potential amplitudes at many neuromuscular junctions. As endplate potentials become subthreshold, there is a decline in the number of muscle fiber action potentials, leading to a CMAP decrement (see Figures 3–5 and 3–6B). In presynaptic disorders (such as Lambert-Eaton myasthenic syndrome), the baseline end plate potential is low, with many endplates not reaching threshold. Hence, many muscle fibers do not fire, resulting in a low baseline CMAP amplitude. With slow RNS, there is further CMAP decrement, due to the further decline of acetylcholine release with the subsequent

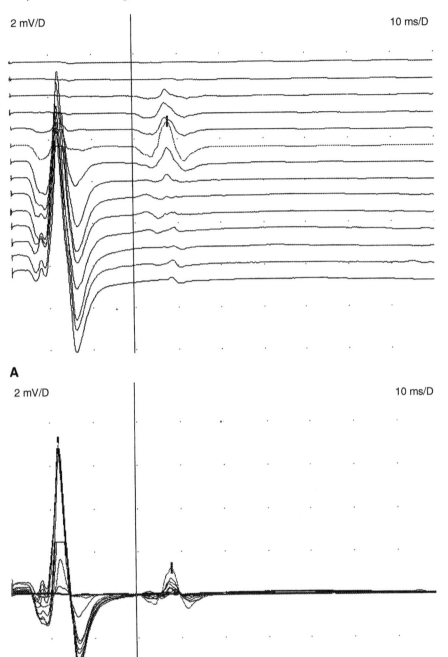

2 mV/D   10 ms/D

A

2 mV/D   10 ms/D

B

Figure 3–4. *H reflex stimulating the tibial nerve at the popliteal fossa while recording the soleus/gastrocnemius muscles. (**A**) Waveforms in a raster form. (**B**) Waveforms superimposed. Note that the response appears with submaximal stimulations and disappears with supramaximal stimulations.*

stimuli, resulting in further loss of many endplate potentials and muscle fiber action potentials (see Figures 3–5 and 3–6C).

Rapid Repetitive Nerve Stimulation

Rapid RNS is most useful in patients with suspected presynaptic neuromuscular junction disorders such as Lambert-Eaton myasthenic syndrome or botulism. The optimal frequency is 20–50 Hz for 2–10 seconds. A typical rapid RNS applies 200 stimuli at a rate of 50 Hz (i.e., 50 Hz for 4 seconds). Calculation of CMAP increment after rapid RNS is as follows:

$$\% \text{ increment} = \frac{\text{Amplitude (highest response)} - \text{amplitude (1st response)}}{\text{Amplitude (1st response)}} \times 100$$

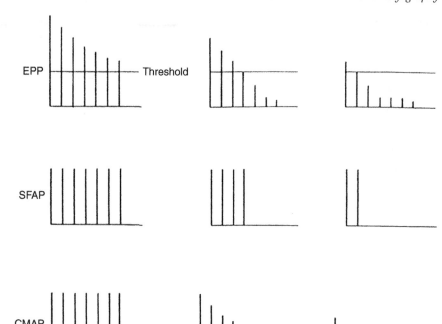

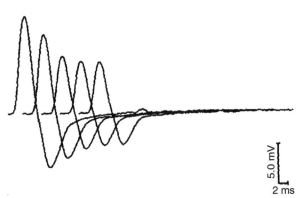

Figure 3–5. *Slow repetitive stimulation effect on end plate potential (EPP), single fiber action potential (SFAP), also referred as muscle action potential (MAP), and compound muscle action potential (CMAP) in normal, myasthenia gravis (MG) and Lambert-Eaton syndrome (ELS). (Adapted from Oh S. Clinical electromyography, neuromuscular transmission studies. Baltimore, MD: Williams and Wilkins, 1988, with permission.)*

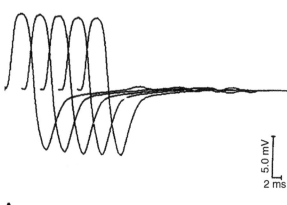

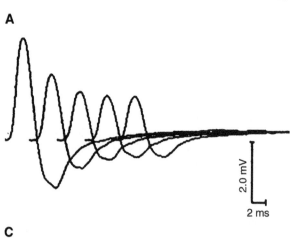

Figure 3–6. *Slow repetitive nerve stimulation at 3 Hz of the median nerve at the wrist while recoding the abductor pollicis brevis. (A) Normal. (B) Patient with severe generalized myasthenia gravis showing a significant CMAP decrement. (C) Patient with Lambert-Eaton myasthenic syndrome showing also a significant CMAP decrement. Note that the baseline (first) CMAP in myasthenia gravis is normal (12 mV) while it is low in amplitude in the Lambert-Eaton myasthenic syndrome (3.5 mV).*

With rapid RNS or postexercise CMAP evaluation, there are two competing forces that are acting on the nerve terminal. First, stimulation tends to deplete the pool of readily available synaptic vesicles. This depletion reduces transmitter release by reduction of the number of vesicles that are released in response to a nerve terminal action potential. Second, calcium accumulates within the nerve terminal, thereby increasing the probability of synaptic vesicle release. In a normal nerve terminal, the effect of depletion of readily available synaptic vesicles usually predominates, so that with rapid RNS, the number of vesicles released decreases. However, the endplate potential does not fall below threshold due to the safety factor. Hence, the supramaximal stimulus generate muscle fiber action potentials at all endplates and no CMAP decrement occurs (Figures 3–7 and 3–8A).

A brief (10 second) period of maximal voluntary isometric exercise is much less painful and has the same effect as rapid RNS at 20–50 Hz. A single supramaximal stimulus is applied to generate a baseline CMAP. Then, the patient performs a 10 second maximal isometric voluntary contraction which is followed by another stimulus and a postexercise CMAP.

In a presynaptic disorder (such as Lambert-Eaton myasthenic syndrome), very few vesicles are released and many muscle fibers do not reach threshold, resulting in

low baseline CMAP amplitude. With rapid RNS, the calcium concentrations in the nerve terminal can rise high enough to stimulate synaptic vesicle fusion for a sufficient number of synaptic vesicles to result in an endplate potential capable of action potential generation. This leads to many muscle fibers reaching threshold and firing and results in a CMAP increment (see Figures 3–7, 3–8B and 3–9). The increment is typically higher than 200% in Lambert-Eaton myasthenic syndrome, and is usually 30–100% in patients with botulism (Table 3–2).

In a postsynaptic disorder (such as myasthenia gravis), rapid RNS causes no change of CMAP since the depleted stores are compensated by the calcium influx. In severe postsynaptic blockade (such as during myasthenic crisis), the increased quantal release cannot compensate for the marked neuromuscular block resulting in a drop in endplate potential amplitude. Hence, fewer muscle fiber action potentials are generated with an associated CMAP decrement (see Table 3–2).

SINGLE FIBER ELECTROMYOGRAPHY

Single fiber EMG is a tool in which individual muscle fiber action potentials are isolated and analyzed *in vivo*.

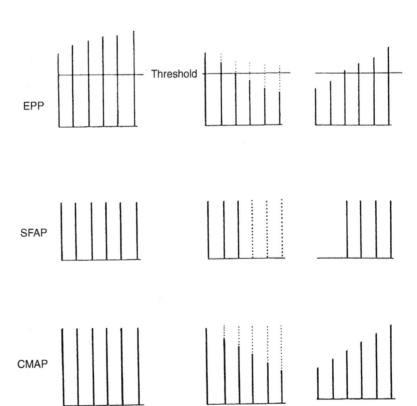

Figure 3–7. *Rapid repetitive stimulation effect on end plate potential (EPP), single fiber action potential (SFAP), also referred as muscle action potential (MAP), and compound muscle action potential (CMAP) in normal, myasthenia gravis (MG) and Lambert-Eaton syndrome (ELS). (Adapted from Oh S. Clinical electromyography, neuromuscular transmission studies. Baltimore, MD: Williams and Wilkins, 1988, with permission.)*

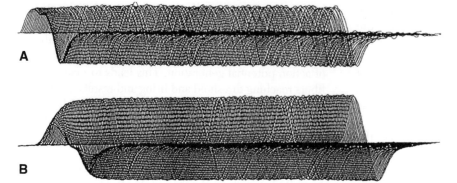

Figure 3–8. *Rapid repetitive stimulation at 50 Hz of the median nerve at the wrist while recoding the abductor pollicis brevis. (**A**) Normal. (**B**) Patient with Lambert-Eaton myasthenic syndrome showing significant increment of the CMAP.*

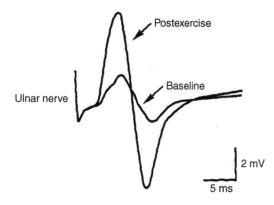

Figure 3–9. *Pre- and postexercise CMAPs of the ulnar nerve following stimulation at the wrist while recoding the abductor digiti minimi in a patient with Lambert-Eaton myasthenic syndrome. The responses are superimposed. Note that the CMAP at rest (baseline) is low in amplitude but there is a prominent (about 200%) increment after 10 seconds of exercise.*

There are several technical requirements for performing single fiber EMG:

1. A concentric single fiber needle electrode allows the recording of single muscle fiber action potentials. The small side port on the cannula of the needle serves as the pickup area. Single fiber needle electrode records from a circle of 300 μm radius, as compared with the 1 mm radius of a conventional EMG needle.
2. The amplifier must have an impedance of 100 megohms or greater to counter the high electrical impedance of the small lead-off surface, and the filter should have a 500 Hz low frequency to attenuate signals from distant fibers. Also, the gain is set higher and the sweep speed is faster for single fiber EMG recordings than for conventional needle EMG.
3. An amplitude threshold trigger allows recording from single muscle fiber, and a delay line permits the entire waveform to be viewed even though the single fiber potential triggers the sweep.
4. Single fiber potentials suitable for study must have a peak-to-peak amplitude greater than 200 μV, rise time less than 300 μs, and a constant waveform.
5. Computerized equipment assists in data acquisition, analysis, and calculation.

Single muscle fiber action potentials may be obtained with voluntary activation or following peripheral nerve stimulation. *Voluntary (recruitment) single fiber EMG* is a common method for activating muscle fibers. A mild voluntary contraction produces a biphasic potential with a duration of approximately 1 ms and an amplitude that varies with the recording site. The needle is rotated, advanced, and retracted until a potential meets these criteria. *Stimulation single fiber EMG* is a relatively newer technique performed by inserting another monopolar needle electrode near the intramuscular nerve twigs and stimulating at a low current and constant rate. This method does not require patient participation and, thus, may be completed on children and uncooperative or comatose patients. Single fiber EMG is useful in assessing fiber density or in jitter analysis.

Table 3–2. Baseline Compound Muscle Action Potential (CMAP) and Repetitive Nerve Stimulation (RNS) Findings of Common Neuromuscular Junction Disorders

NMJ Defect	Typical Disorder	CMAP	Slow RNS	Fast RNS or Postexercise CMAP
Postsynaptic	Myasthenia gravis	Normal	Decrement	Normal or decrement
Presynaptic	Lambert-Eaton myasthenic syndrome	Low	Decrement	Increment

Fiber Density

Fiber density is determined by the number of single fiber potentials firing almost synchronously with the initially identified single fiber potential. Increased muscle fiber clustering indicates collateral sprouting. Simultaneously firing single fiber potentials within 5 ms after the triggering single fiber unit are counted at 20–30 sites. For example, in the normal extensor digitorum communis muscle, single fibers fire without nearby discharges in 65–70% of random insertions; with only two fibers discharging in 30–35%; and with three fibers discharging in 5% or fewer. An average number of single muscle fiber potentials per recording site can be calculated. In conditions with loss of mosaic distribution of muscle fibers from a motor unit, such as reinnervation, fiber density increases.

Jitter

Jitter analysis is most useful in the assessment of neuromuscular junction disorders. The jitter represents the variability of the time interval between two muscle fiber action potentials (muscle pair) that are innervated by the same motor unit. In other words, it is the variability of the interpotential intervals between repetitively firing paired single fiber potentials (Figure 3–10). Jitter can be determined by using a commercially available computer software program. It is calculated as the mean value of consecutive interval difference, over a number of 50–100 discharges as follows:

$$\text{MCD} = \frac{[\text{IPI } 1 - \text{IPI } 2] + [\text{IPI } 2 - \text{IPI } 3] + \cdots [\text{IPI } (N-1) - \text{IPI } N]}{N-1}$$

where MCD is the mean consecutive difference, IPI 1 is the interpotential interval of the first discharge, IPI 2 of the second discharge, etc., and N is the number of discharges recorded.

Neuromuscular blocking is the intermittent failure of transmission of one of the two muscle fiber potentials. This reflects the failure of one of the muscle fibers to transmit an action potential due to the failure of the endplate potential to reach threshold. Blocking represent the most extreme abnormality of the jitter and is measured as the percentage of discharges of a motor unit in which a single fiber potential does not fire. For example, in 100 discharges of the pair, if a single potential is missing 30 times, the blocking is 30%. In general, blocking occurs when the jitter values are significantly abnormal.

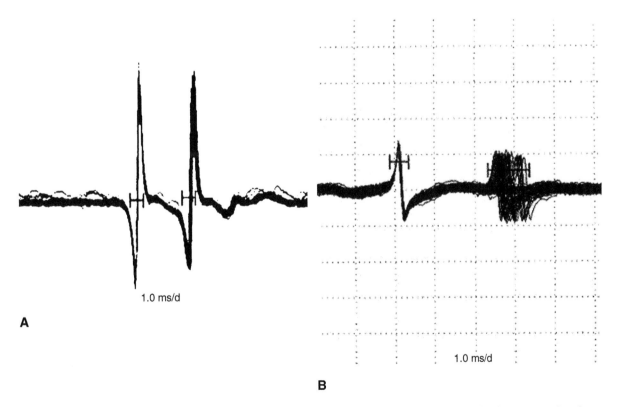

1.0 ms/d

A

1.0 ms/d

B

Figure 3–10. *Jitter single fiber EMG study of the frontalis muscle shown in a superimposed mode. The first potential is the triggered potential while the second is the slave potential. (**A**) Normal. (**B**) Patient with myasthenia gravis. Note the significant jitter of the slave potential (**B**) compared to (**A**).*

The results of single fiber EMG jitter study are expressed by: (1) the mean jitter of all potential pairs, (2) the percentage of pairs with blocking, and (3) the percentage of pairs with normal jitter. Since jitter may be abnormal in 1 of 20 recorded potentials in healthy subjects, the study is considered to indicate defective neuromuscular transmission if (1) the mean jitter value exceeds the upper limit of the normal jitter value for that muscle, (2) more than 10% (more than two pairs) exhibits jitter values above the upper limit of the normal jitter, or (3) there is any neuromuscular blocking.

Jitter analysis is highly sensitive but not specific. Although it is frequently abnormal in myasthenia gravis and other neuromuscular junction disorders (see Figure 3–10), it may also be abnormal in a variety of neuromuscular disorders including motor neuron disease, neuropathies, and myopathies. Thus, the diagnostic value of jitter has to be considered in the contest of the patient's clinical manifestations, and routine electrodiagnostic findings.

SUGGESTED READINGS

Boonyapisit K, Kaminski HJ, Ruff RL. The molecular basis of neuromuscular transmission disorders. Am J Med 1999;106:97–113.

Fisher MA. H reflex and F waves. Fundamentals, normal and abnormal patterns. Neurol Clin N Am 2002:20;339–360.

Katirji B, Weissman JD. The ankle jerk and the tibial H-reflex: a clinical and electrophysiological correlation. Electromyogr Clin Neurophysiol 1994;34:331–334.

Katirji B, Kaminski HJ. Electrodiagnostic approach to the patient with suspected neuromuscular junction disorder. Neurol Clin N Am 2002:20;557–586.

Katirji B. Electrodiagnosis of neuromuscular transmission disorders. In: Kaminski HJ, ed. Myasthenia gravis and related disorders. New York: Humana Press, 2003, pp. 149–175.

Kimura J. Clinical uses of the electrically elicited blink reflex. Adv Neurol 1983;39:773–786.

Nishida T, Kompoliti A, Janssen I, et al. H reflex in S-1 radiculopathy: latency versus amplitude controversy revisited. Muscle Nerve 1996;19:915–917.

Oh SJ. Electromyography: neuromuscular transmission studies. Baltimore, MD: Williams and Wilkins, 1988.

Rowen J, Meriggioli MN. Electrodiagnostic significance of supramaximally stimulated A-waves. Muscle Nerve 2000; 23:1117–1120.

Shields RW Jr. Single-fiber electromyography is a sensitive indicator of axonal degeneration in diabetes. Neurology 1987;37:1394–1397.

Stålberg E, Trontelj JV. The study of normal and abnormal neuromuscular transmission with single fibre electromyography. J Neurosci Meth 1997;74:145–154.

Tim RW, Sanders DB. Repetitive nerve stimulation studies in the Lambert-Eaton myasthenic syndrome. Muscle Nerve 1994;17: 995–1001.

4

Electrodiagnostic Findings in Neuromuscular Disorders

Details of the electrodiagnostic findings in various neuromuscular disorders are outlined within the case studies in this book. The following is a brief summary of these findings in the most common neuromuscular disorders.

FOCAL MONONEUROPATHIES

Compression, traction, laceration, thermal, or chemical injury may damage one or more components of the peripheral nerves, including the myelin, axons, or supporting nerve structures (endoneurium, epineurium, and perineurium). The pathophysiologic responses to peripheral nerve injuries have a limited repertoire; that is demyelination, axon loss, or a combination of both.

Demyelinative Mononeuropathy

With focal injury to myelin, conduction along the affected nerve fiber is altered. This may result in slowing of conduction or conduction block along the nerve fibers or a combination of both.

1. *Focal slowing.* This is usually the result of widening of the nodes of Ranvier (paranodal demyelination). Focal slowing may be *synchronized* when demyelination affects all the large myelinated fibers equally. When the focal lesion is distal, there is prolongation of distal and proximal latencies while the proximal conduction velocity remains normal. If the focal lesion is between the distal and proximal stimulation sites, there is prolongation of proximal latency only resulting in slowing in proximal conduction velocity while the distal latency remains normal (Figure 4–1). With lesions manifesting as focal synchronized slowing, the CMAP amplitudes, durations, and areas remain normal and do not change significantly following proximal and distal stimulation.

Desynchronized (differential) slowing occurs when conduction time is reduced at the lesion site along a variable number of the medium or small nerve fibers (average or slower conducting axons). Here, the CMAP is dispersed with prolonged duration on stimulations proximal to the lesion (Figure 4–2). The latency and conduction velocity along the injury site remain normal, since at least some of the fastest conducting axons are spared. When the largest axons are also affected, the dispersed CMAP with prolonged duration is also

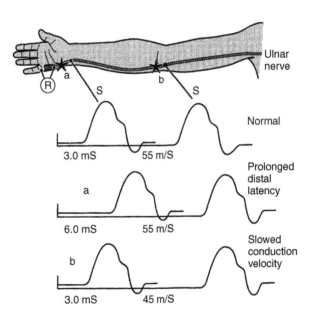

Figure 4–1. *Nerve conduction studies showing focal slowing in distal segment (a) resulting in slowing of distal latency only, and in proximal segment (b) resulting in slowing of conduction velocity only. (Reprinted from Wilbourn AJ. Nerve conduction studies. Types, components, abnormalities and value in localization. Neurol Clin 2002;20:305–338, with permission.)*

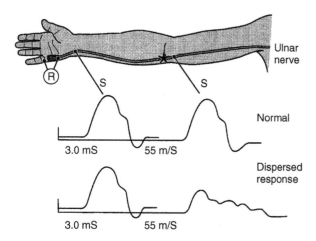

Figure 4–2. *Nerve conduction studies showing desynchronized slowing. The response with proximal stimulation is dispersed consistent with differential slowing of nerve fibers in the proximal nerve segment. (Reprinted from Wilbourn AJ. Nerve conduction studies. Types, components, abnormalities and value in localization. Neurol Clin 2002;20:305–338, with permission.)*

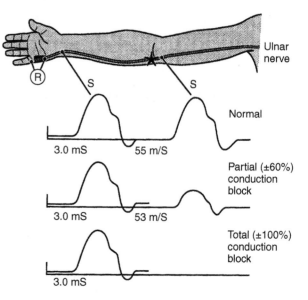

Figure 4–3. *Nerve conduction studies showing partial or complete conduction blocks in the proximal segment of the nerve. (Reprinted from Wilbourn AJ. Nerve conduction studies. Types, components, abnormalities and value in localization. Neurol Clin 2002;20:305–338, with permission.)*

accompanied by slowing of distal latency (in distal lesions) or conduction velocity (in proximal lesions).

2. *Conduction block.* This is usually the result of focal loss of one or more myelin segment (segmental or internodal demyelination) which leads to interruption of action potential transmission. A nerve lesion manifesting with conduction block is best localized when it can be bracketed by two stimulation points, one distal to the site of injury and one proximal. In conduction block, stimulation distal to the lesion elicits a normal CMAP, whereas proximal stimulation elicits a response with reduced amplitude (partial conduction block) or absent response (complete conduction block) (Figure 4–3). The percentage drop in amplitude and area (amplitude or area decay) are calculated as follows:

Amplitude decay (conduction block) =
$$100 \times \frac{\text{Distal amplitude} - \text{proximal amplitude}}{\text{Distal amplitude}}$$

Area decay (conduction block) =
$$100 \times \frac{\text{Distal area} - \text{proximal area}}{\text{Distal area}}$$

There are several limitations to the definitive diagnosis of demyelinative conduction block:

(A) A reduced CMAP size may result from phase cancellation between action potentials peaks of opposite polarity because of abnormally increased temporal dispersion. Such excessive desynchronization often develops in acquired demyelinative neuropathies. If the distal and proximal responses have dissimilar waveforms, the discrepancy in amplitude between the two may represent in part a phase cancellation rather than true conduction block. Hence, in true partial conduction block, the significant drop of CMAP amplitude, with stimulation proximal to the lesion site compared with the CMAP distal to it, should not be accompanied by significant (>15%) prolongation of CMAP duration and should be supported by significant drop in CMAP area. In general, more than 50% decrease of the CMAP amplitude across the lesion along with more than 50% drop in CMAP area, are definitive signs of conduction block. A 20–50% drop CMAP amplitude and area may be consistent with conduction block in situations when the two stimulation sites are close (usually 10 cm or less) such as across the fibular neck or elbow (Table 4–1).

(B) A distal demyelinating lesion, causing conduction block of the nerve segment between the most distal possible stimulating point and the recording site, manifest as unelicitable or low CMAP amplitude at both distal and proximal stimulation sites. This finding mimics the findings encountered with axonal degeneration (see axon-loss mononeuropathy). Such a demyelinative lesion could only be distinguished from axon loss lesion by repeating the NCS

Table 4–1. Electrodiagnosis of Conduction Block

Definite in Any Nerve*

1. ≥50% drop in CMAP amplitude with a 15% prolongation of CMAP duration and with ≥50% drop in CMAP area
2. ≥30% drop in amplitude and area over a short nerve segment (e.g., radial across the spiral groove, ulnar across the elbow, peroneal across the fibular head)

Possible in Median, Ulnar, and Peroneal Nerves Only

1. 20–50% drop in CMAP amplitude with ≤15% prolongation of CMAP duration and with 20–50% drop in CMAP area

---

*Caution should be taken in evaluating the tibial nerve, where stimulation at the knee can be submaximal, resulting in 50% or at times greater than 50% drop in amplitude and area, especially in overweight and very tall patients.

after several weeks. Often in demyelinative lesions, the distal CMAP improves rapidly, a finding that is not consistent with axon loss.

(C) With proximal demyelinative conduction block lesions, it may not be technically possible to bracket the lesion with two stimulation sites since the lesion is extremely proximal. Examples include demyelinating lesions at the root level, femoral nerve, facial nerve, sciatic nerve, or lumbosacral plexus. In these situations, stimulation distal to the lesion can only be achieved. The diagnosis of conduction block is made only by inference, when a normal or nearly normal CMAP is coupled with significant reduction of recruitment on needle EMG of the recorded muscle.

(D) The prominent temporal dispersion due to phase cancellation seen in evaluating normal SNAPs precludes the use of these potentials in the diagnosis of conduction block (see Chapter 2, Figure 2–15).

(E) Conduction block pattern is often seen with acute axonal loss nerve lesions before the completion of wallerian degeneration (see axon-loss mononeuropathy).

3. *Focal slowing with conduction block.* Demyelinating lesions presenting with both focal slowing and partial conduction block are not common. They are usually seen at chronic entrapment sites such ulnar nerve lesions across the elbow. In such situations, a significant number of fibers have internodal demyelination resulting in conduction block (drop in amplitude and area across the abnormal segment) while other fibers have paranodal demyelination manifesting as focal slowing of the same nerve segment.

Axon-Loss Mononeuropathy

Following acute focal axonal damage, the distal nerve segment undergoes wallerian degeneration. However, early after axonal transection, the distal axon remains excitable.

Hence, stimulation distal to the lesion elicits a normal CMAP, whereas proximal stimulation elicits an absent response (complete conduction block) when the lesion is total and reduced CMAP amplitude (partial conduction block) when the lesion is incomplete (Figure 4–4). In an attempt to distinguish this pattern from a demyelinative conduction block, some refer to this pattern as an axonal noncontinuity, early axon loss, or axon discontinuity conduction block.

Wallerian degeneration of the axons distal to the nerve lesions is completed in 7–11 days. In the first 1–2 days, the distal CMAP and SNAP are normal. The distal CMAP amplitude then decreases and reaches its nadir in 5–6 days, while the distal SNAP amplitude lags slightly behind. It starts declining in amplitude after 4–5 days and reaches its nadir in 10–11 days (Figure 4–5). The earlier decline of the CMAP amplitude comparing to the SNAP amplitude following axon-loss nerve lesion is likely related to the early neuromuscular transmission failure that affects the recording of the CMAP amplitudes only. This is supported by the fact that MNAPs, recorded directly from nerve trunks, follow the time course of SNAPs.

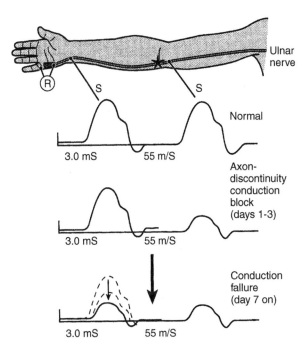

Figure 4–4. *Nerve conduction studies in partial axon loss lesion. Initially, there is an axon discontinuity conduction block. Following wallerian degeneration, the distal response drop in amplitude and the subsequent study showed uniformly low amplitude CMAP irrespective of the site of stimulation. (Reprinted from Wilbourn AJ. Nerve conduction studies. Types, components, abnormalities and value in localization. Neurol Clin 2002;20:305–338, with permission.)*

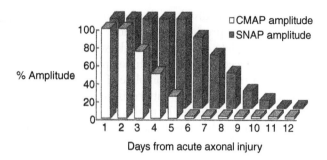

% Amplitude

□ CMAP amplitude
■ SNAP amplitude

Days from acute axonal injury

Figure 4–5. *Effect of wallerian degeneration on distal CMAP and SNAP amplitudes following acute nerve lesion.*

On motor NCS, a conduction block is present soon after axonal injury. However, as the distal axons undergo wallerian degeneration, this is replaced by unelicitable or low CMAP amplitudes with both distal and proximal stimulations corresponding to complete or partial motor axonal loss lesions respectively (see Figure 4–4). At this time, the distal CMAP amplitude is a reliable semiquantitative estimate of the amount of axonal loss in peripheral nerve lesions. In the chronic phases of partial axonal nerve lesions with reinnervation via collateral sprouting, the CMAP may improve to reach normal or near normal values giving a false indication of a milder degree of original axonal loss.

When the electrodiagnostic study is done early after an acute peripheral nerve lesion, it should be repeated at 10–11 days or later (or 5 days or later in purely motor nerves) in order to distinguish between conduction block caused by demyelination versus axonal loss, and to assess the extent of axon loss if present. Following this period of wallerian degeneration, stimulating the nerve below the lesion results in absent or reduced CMAP amplitude since degenerating axons would have lost their excitability. An absent or reduced CMAP amplitude from stimulation above or below the lesion indicates complete or partial axonal loss respectively. In demyelinating lesions, the distal CMAP remains unchanged with persistent conduction block across the lesion. In mixed lesions, the distal CMAP drops but remains significantly higher than the proximal implying both axon loss and segmental demyelination.

In partial axon-loss peripheral nerve lesions, the distal latencies and conduction velocities remain normal or are borderline. Selective loss of fast-conducting fibers associated with more than a 50% reduction in mean CMAP amplitude can slow conduction velocity to 80% of normal value because the velocity represents the remaining slow-conducting fibers. Motor conduction velocity may be occasionally slowed to 70% of normal value, when there is severe axonal loss with marked reduction of CMAP amplitude to less than 10% of normal.

Needle EMG is useful in assessing the progress of *reinnervation* of axon loss peripheral nerve lesions that may occur spontaneously or after nerve repair. Although collateral sprouting in partial axon loss lesions starts as early as 1–2 days after a nerve lesion, the early signs of reinnervation may first become evident on needle EMG one month later, but are usually definite by 2–3 months postinjury. MUAP morphology helps assessing the process of muscle fiber reinnervation that occurs following collateral sprouting and proximodistal regeneration of nerve fibers from the site of the injury. Collateral sprouting causes first an increased number of MUAP turns and phases followed by an increased duration and amplitude of MUAPs, while early proximodistal regeneration of nerve fibers in severe axon loss lesions often manifests by recording brief, small, and highly polyphasic (nascent) MUAPs. MUAPs tend to become longer in duration and higher in amplitude with the passage of time due to improved synchrony of muscle fiber action potentials.

In contrast to demyelinating or mixed mononeuropathies, pure axon-loss peripheral nerve lesions cannot be localized by NCSs when studied after the completion of wallerian degeneration, since they are not associated with focal conduction slowing or block. The identification of conduction block in the early days of axonal loss is extremely helpful in localizing a peripheral nerve injury. Waiting for the completion of wallerian degeneration results in diffusely low or unevoked CMAPs (regardless of stimulation site), which does not allow for accurate localization of the injury site. Localizing a purely axon-loss mononeuropathy after the completion of wallerian degeneration depends on needle EMG, with principles that are similar to manual muscle strength testing used during the neurological examination. Typically, the needle EMG reveals neurogenic changes (fibrillation potentials, reduced MUAP recruitment, chronic neurogenic MUAP morphology changes) that are limited to muscles innervated by the injured nerve distal to the site of the lesion (Figure 4–6). In contrast, muscles innervated proximal to the lesion remain normal. Unfortunately, attempting to localize axon loss lesions solely by needle EMG has several shortcomings that may result in poor localization or, sometimes, mislocalization of the site of the nerve lesion. These include the following scenarios:

1. *Nerve lesions along segments with no motor branches.* The inherent anatomy of the injured nerve plays an important role in the precise localization of nerve lesions. Many nerves travel substantial distances without giving out any motor branches (Figure 4–7). For example the median and ulnar nerves have long segments in the arm from which no motor branches arise. Hence, it is often that the electromyographer

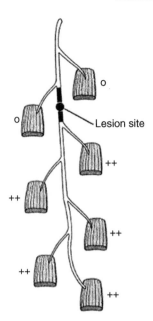

Figure 4–6. *Localization of peripheral nerve lesion using needle EMG. Muscles distal to the lesion reveals abnormal neurogenic findings (++) while proximal muscles are normal (O). (Adapted from Wilbourn AJ. Nerve conduction studies. Types, components, abnormalities and value in localization. Neurol Clin 2002;20: 305–338, with permission.)*

localize such a lesion to a long segment that may offer little assistance to the referring physician or surgeon, simply because the focal lesion may be at any point along this long nerve segment. In contrast to the median and ulnar nerves, the radial nerve is more ideal for localization by needle EMG since it gives off multiple motor branches at fairly regular and short intervals.

2. *Fascicular nerve lesions.* Nerve fascicles remain distinct for most of their course within the nerve trunk and may be selectively injured. Also, peripheral nerve lesions may spare nerve fascicles resulting in muscles that escape denervation despite being located distal to the lesion site (Figure 4–8). The spared fascicle may occupy a protected location of the nerve at the lesion site or may be exiting the nerve trunk at or near the lesion site. This fascicular nerve lesion may falsely suggest that the lesion is localized more distal to its actual site. Examples of this fascicular involvement include sparing of ulnar muscles in the forearm (flexor carpi ulnaris and ulnar part of flexor digitorum profundus) following an axon loss ulnar nerve lesions at the elbow, and sparing the superficial peroneal-innervated muscles (peroneus longus and brevis) following an axon loss common peroneal nerve lesion at the knee or fibular neck.

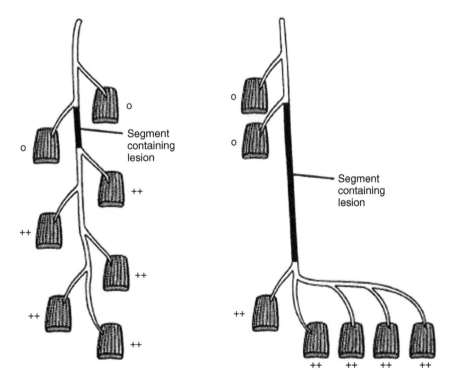

Figure 4–7. *Localization of peripheral nerve lesion using needle EMG. The diagram on the left shows an "ideal" nerve with branches separated by short nerve segments (e.g., the radial nerve) allowing precise localization. In contrast, the diagram on the right depicts a nerve with a long segment that gives no motor branches (e.g., the median nerve in the arm) resulting in a suboptimal localization of lesion to a long nerve segment (++ are denervated muscles while O are normal muscles). (Adapted from Wilbourn AJ. Nerve conduction studies. Types, components, abnormalities and value in localization. Neurol Clin 2002;20: 305–338, with permission.)*

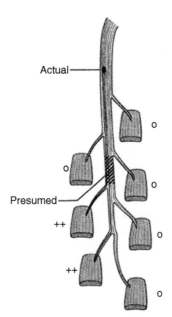

Figure 4–8. *Fascicular peripheral nerve lesion leading to mislocalization of lesion more distally (+ + are denervated muscles while O are normal muscles). (Adapted from Wilbourn AJ. Nerve conduction studies. Types, components, abnormalities and value in localization. Neurol Clin 2002;20:305–338, with permission.)*

3. *Chronic nerve lesions.* The process of reinnervation includes proximodistal regeneration of nerve fibers from the site of the injury, collateral sprouting, or both. With partial axon loss lesions that are mild or modest, reinnervation via proximodistal regeneration may be efficient in proximally located muscles resulting in remodeling of the motor units. Hence, a needle EMG done several years after such a lesion may only detect the neurogenic changes in the more distal muscles and result in mislocalizing the lesion more distally (Figure 4–9).

RADICULOPATHIES AND PLEXOPATHIES

Radiculopathies are, by definition, lesions of the ventral or dorsal roots or both occurring within the spinal canal space. In contrast, plexopathies are lesions that involve the peripheral nerve extraspinally. Since the dorsal root ganglia are usually located outside of the spinal canal and within the intervertebral foramina, radiculopathies are considered preganglionic lesions while plexopathies are postganglionic.

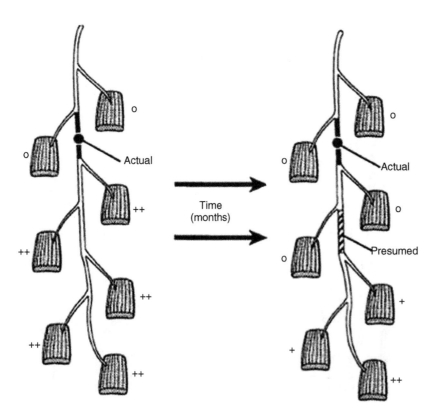

Figure 4–9. *Chronic nerve lesion. The diagram on the left shows that muscles located distal to the lesion and tested in the acute and subacute phase of nerve injury showed signs of denervation. In contrast, the diagram on the right reveals with the passage of time (months to years) effective reinnervation and remodeling of several muscles close to the lesion site leading to mislocalization of the lesion more distally (+ and ++ are denervated muscles while O are normal muscles). (Adapted from Wilbourn AJ. Nerve conduction studies. Types, components, abnormalities and value in localization. Neurol Clin 2002;20:305–338, with permission.)*

The dorsal root ganglia contain unipolar sensory neurons with a peripheral and a central axon. In radiculopathies associated with axonal loss due to lesions of the proximal sensory axons, the distal sensory axons do not degenerate since the dorsal root neurons usually escape injury. Hence, the SNAP remains normal despite sensory loss and degeneration of proximal sensory axons. When the motor axons within the ventral roots are also injured, radiculopathies exhibits signs of motor axon degeneration including abnormal needle EMG and, when severe, low-amplitude CMAPs.

Needle EMG is the most sensitive and specific electrodiagnostic test for the identification of cervical and lumbosacral radiculopathies, particularly those associated with axon loss. Needle EMG is also useful in the accurate localization of the level of the root lesion. Finding signs of denervation and reinnervation (fibrillation potentials, decrease recruitment, and long-duration, high-amplitude polyphasic MUAPs) in a segmental myotomal distribution (i.e., in muscles innervated by the same roots via more than one peripheral nerve), with or without denervation of the paraspinal muscles localize the lower motor neuron lesion to the root level. A normal SNAP of the corresponding dermatome ensures that the lesion is within the spinal canal (i.e., proximal to the dorsal root ganglia). For example, in a C7 radiculopathy, the triceps (radial nerve) and pronator teres (median nerve) are often abnormal on needle EMG, with or without the cervical paraspinal muscles, and the median SNAP recording middle finger is normal.

In contrast to intraspinal canal root lesions, axon-loss extraspinal plexopathies affect the CMAP as well as the SNAP amplitudes when mixed nerves undergo wallerian degeneration. Abnormal SNAPs are not compatible with root lesions (preganglionic), but consistent with lesions affecting the brachial plexus (postganglionic). These findings are particularly important in brachial plexus traction injuries that may mimic root avulsions. In avulsions, the dorsal root ganglia remain intact despite severe sensory loss and the peripheral sensory axons do not undergo wallerian degeneration. Hence, the SNAPs in root avulsions are spared while they are low in amplitude or absent in brachial plexopathies.

GENERALIZED POLYNEUROPATHIES

Nerve conduction studies are essential in the diagnosis of peripheral polyneuropathies, and in establishing the type of fiber(s) affected (large fiber sensory, motor, or both). Most importantly, NCSs often can identify the primary pathological process of peripheral polyneuropathy (axonal loss or segmental demyelination), an important step in establishing the etiological diagnosis of the various peripheral polyneuropathies.

Demyelinating Polyneuropathies

The electrophysiologic hallmark of these polyneuropathies is a widespread increase in conduction time due to impaired saltatory conduction. Hence, the NCSs are characterized by significant slowing of conduction velocities (<75% of lower limit of normal) and distal latencies (>130% of upper limit of normal).

With distal stimulation, the CMAP amplitude is mildly or moderately reduced because of abnormal temporal dispersion and phase cancellation, and the distal latency is delayed because of demyelination. With more proximal stimulation, the CMAP amplitude is lower due to temporal dispersion and conduction block along some fibers. The proximal conduction velocity is markedly slowed because of increased probability for the nerve action potentials to pass through demyelinated segments (Figure 4–10C).

Chronic demyelinating polyneuropathies may be further distinguished by NCS into *inherited* and *acquired* polyneuropathies. Inherited demyelinating polyneuropathies such as Charcot-Marie-Tooth disease type I, are characterized by uniform slowing along various segments of individual nerves and adjoining nerves. The abnormalities are usually symmetrical without accompanying conduction blocks (except possibly at compressive sites). In contrast, acquired demyelinating polyneuropathies, such as chronic inflammatory demyelinating polyneuropathy, often have asymmetric nerve conductions, even when there is no apparent clinical asymmetry. In addition, multifocal conduction blocks and excessive temporal dispersions at nonentrapment sites are characteristics for acquired demyelinating polyneuropathies.

In demyelinating polyneuropathies, the needle EMG may show signs of mild axonal loss manifested by fibrillation potentials and reinnervated MUAPs.

Axonal Polyneuropathies

Axonal polyneuropathies produce length-dependent dying-back degeneration of axons. The major change on NCS is a decrease of the CMAP and SNAP amplitudes, more marked in the lower extremities (see Figure 4–10B). In contrast, conduction velocities and distal latencies are normal. As with axon loss mononeuropathies, selective loss of many fast-conducting fibers associated with more than a 50% reduction in mean CMAP amplitude can slow conduction velocity to 70–80% of normal value.

In axon-loss polyneuropathy, the needle EMG is most useful in depicting the temporal profile of the illness. Fibrillation potentials typically develop within 2–3 weeks

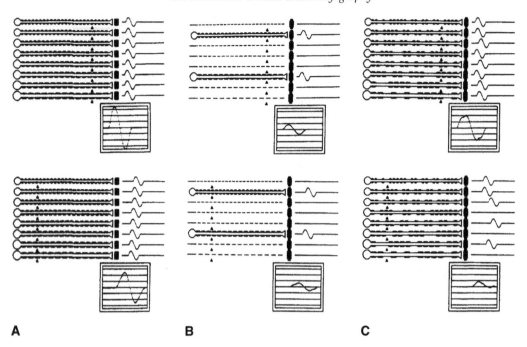

Figure 4–10. *Computerized model of peripheral motor nerve in normal (**A**), axonal degeneration (**B**), and segmental demyelination (**C**). (Reprinted from Brown WF, Bolton CF, eds. Clinical electromyography. Boston, MA: Butterworth-Heinemann, 1989, with permission.)*

of an acute neuropathy, and reinnervated MUAPs become apparent within 1–2 months. In acute polyneuropathies, needle EMG during the first few weeks of illness may show only reduced recruitment of MUAPs in weak muscles with normal MUAP morphology and no spontaneous activity. In relatively active or progressive axon-loss polyneuropathies, a combination of fibrillation potentials with reduced recruitment of reinnervated MUAPs is most prominent distally. In chronic and very slowly progressive polyneuropathies, reinnervation may completely keep pace with active denervation yielding little or no fibrillation potentials but reduced recruitment of reinnervated MUAPs.

ANTERIOR HORN CELL DISORDERS

There are three reasons for performing electrodiagnostic studies in patients with suspected amyotrophic lateral sclerosis: (1) to confirm lower motor neuron dysfunction in clinically affected regions; (2) to detect electrophysiologic evidence of lower motor neuron dysfunction in clinically uninvolved regions; and (3) to exclude other pathophysiologic processes. A disadvantage of the clinical EMG study is that it can only evaluate lower motor neuron degeneration while upper motor neuron degeneration can only be assessed clinically. Hence, the diagnosis of amyotrophic lateral sclerosis with evidence of upper and lower

motor neuron degeneration is often based on the clinical evaluation with the electrodiagnostic study playing only a supporting role.

In patients with suspected motor neuron disease, sensory NCSs are usually normal. Motor NCSs are either normal or yield low CMAP amplitudes consistent with motor neuronal loss. There are no motor conduction blocks and the motor conduction velocities are normal or slightly slowed not below 70% of the lower limits of normal. In patients with suspected motor neuron disease, NCSs are most useful in excluding other neuromuscular diagnosis such as polyneuropathies, multifocal motor neuropathy, or neuromuscular junction disorders.

Needle EMG is the most important electrodiagnostic study for providing evidence of generalized lower motor neuron degeneration. Early in the course of the illness, denervation in clinically normal muscles and limbs is most useful in establishing early dissemination of denervation. Needle EMG in amyotrophic lateral sclerosis often shows signs of active denervation (fibrillation and fasciculation potentials), chronic denervation (reinnervated and unstable MUAPs), and reduced MUAP recruitment. Lambert's original criteria for diagnosis include detecting fibrillation and fasciculation potentials in muscles of the lower as well as the upper extremities or in the extremities as well as the head. These criteria evolved over the years into denervation at least three extremities or two extremities and cranial muscles (the head and neck considered an extremity). Although lower motor neuron degeneration ultimately affects almost the entire neuraxis (brainstem and cervical, thoracic, or lumbosacral segments of spinal cord), the early phases of the illness are often characterized by limited and more focal weakness. The revised El Escorial criteria recommend that needle EMG signs of lower motor neuron degeneration should be present in at least two of the four central nervous system regions, i.e., the brainstem, cervical, thoracic, or lumbosacral regions.

MYOPATHIES

Insertional activity is usually normal or increased except in the late stage of the disease when it is reduced by atrophy and fibrosis. Spontaneous activity is absent except in necrotizing myopathies (such as inflammatory myopathies and muscular dystrophies). MUAP amplitude and duration are reduced because of random loss of fibers from the motor unit. Split muscle fibers and regeneration of muscle fibers sometimes accounts for satellite potentials and polyphasia. Early recruitment is common because more motor units are needed to maintain a given force in compensation for the small size of individual units.

A disadvantage of the electrodiagnosis of myopathies is that the EMG findings in myopathy are not always specific to make a final diagnosis. Exceptions include conditions that are associated with (1) myotonia such as myotonic dystrophies, myotonia congenita, paramyotonia congenita, hyperkalemic periodic paralysis, acid maltase deficiency, and some toxic myopathies (such as colchicine), or (2) fibrillation potentials which occur in inflammatory myopathies, critical illness myopathy, and progressive muscular dystrophies. Another disadvantage of the needle EMG is that it is either normal or has only subtle abnormalities in many myopathies particularly those not usually associated with myonecrosis, such as the metabolic and endocrine myopathies. Hence, a normal needle EMG does not exclude a myopathy.

In polymyositis and dermatomyositis, it is essential to recognize the changing pattern on needle EMG at diagnosis, following treatment, and during relapse. Fibrillation potentials appear first at diagnosis or relapse and disappear early during remission. Abnormal MUAP morphology becomes evident later and lasts longer to resolve. The presence of fibrillation potentials is also helpful in differentiating exacerbation of myositis from a corticosteroid-induced myopathy.

NEUROMUSCULAR JUNCTION DISORDERS

In myasthenia gravis as well as other postsynaptic neuromuscular junction disorders, the baseline (resting) CMAP is normal. Slow repetitive nerve stimulation (RNS) results

a CMAP decrement that often improves or corrects after brief exercise. The diagnostic sensitivity of RNS is much higher recording proximal than distal muscles. The decrement often improves or is repaired after exercise ("*posttetanic facilitation*"), and worsens several minutes after exercise ("*postexercise exhaustion*"). If done, rapid RNS (or postexrecise CMAP) causes no change of CMAP or, in severe situations, a CMAP decrement.

In Lambert-Eaton myasthenic syndrome, botulism, and other presynaptic disorders, the baseline (resting) CMAP amplitude is low. With slow RNS, there is further CMAP decrement. However, with rapid RNS or postexercise CMAP, there is a CMAP increment, which is typically higher than 200% in Lambert-Eaton myasthenic syndrome, and is usually 30–100% in patients with botulism.

UPPER MOTOR NEURON LESIONS

Patients with upper motor neuron lesions have normal NCSs and needle EMG including normal insertional activity, no spontaneous activity at rest, and normal MUAP morphology. The only abnormality is a reduced interference pattern with poor activation of MUAPs (slow rate of motor unit discharge). Recruitment, measured by either recruitment frequency or ratio, is normal. Hysterical weakness or poor effort produces a similar pattern, except that motor unit firing may be irregular.

SUGGESTED READINGS

Brooks BR, Miller RG, Swash M, Munsat TL, for the World Federation of Neurology Group on Motor Neuron Diseases. El Escorial revisited: revised criteria for the diagnosis of amyotrophic lateral sclerosis. Amyotroph Lateral Scler Other Motor Neuron Disord 2000;1:293–299.

Campbell WW, Pridgeon RM, Sahni KS. Short segment incremental studies in the evaluation of ulnar neuropathy at the elbow. Muscle Nerve 1992;15:1050–1054.

Gordon PH, Wilbourn AJ. Early electrodiagnostic findings in Guillain-Barré syndrome. Arch Neurol 2001;58: 913–917.

Katirji MB, Agrawal R, Kantra TA. The human cervical myotomes. An anatomical correlation between electromyography and CT/myelography. Muscle Nerve 1988;11:1070–1073.

Kimura J. The carpal tunnel syndrome: localization of conduction abnormalities within the distal segment of the median nerve. Brain 1979;102:619–635.

Lacomis D. Electrodiagnostic approach to the patient with suspected myopathy. Neurol Clin N Am 2002:20;587–603.

Lambert EH, Mulder DW. Electromyographic studies in amyotrophic lateral sclerosis. Mayo Clin Proc 1957; 32:441–446.

McIntosh KA, Preston DC, Logigian EL. Short segment incremental studies to localize ulnar entrapments at the wrist. Neurology 1998;50:303–306.

Lambert EH. Electromyography in amyotrophic lateral sclerosis. In: Norris FH, Jr, Kurland LT, eds. Motor neuron diseases. New York: Grune and Stratton, 1969, pp. 135–153.

Chad DA. Electrodiagnostic approach to the patient with suspected motor neuron disease. Neurol Clin N Am 2002: 20;527–555.

Rhee RK, England JD, Sumner AJ. Computer simulation of conduction block: effects produced by actual block versus interphase cancellation. Ann Neurol 1990;28: 146–159.

Wilbourn AJ. The electrodiagnostic examination in myopathies. J Clin Neurophysiol 1993;10:132–148.

Wilbourn AJ and Aminoff MJ. The electrodiagnostic examination in patients with radiculopathies. Muscle Nerve 1998;21: 1612–1631.

Part II
Focal Disorders

Lower Extremity

Case 1

HISTORY AND PHYSICAL EXAMINATION

A 29-year-old white man noted an acute right footdrop. He was otherwise in excellent health, with no history of diabetes or trauma. He was referred to the electromyography (EMG) laboratory.

Neurologic examination revealed severe weakness (Medical Research Council [MRC] 2/5) of right ankle and toe dorsiflexion and moderate weakness of right ankle eversion (MRC 4/5). Ankle inversion and plantar flexion were normal. Deep tendon reflexes, including Achilles reflexes, were normal. The patient had slight impairment of pain sensation over the dorsum of the right foot. Tinel's sign could not be induced by percussion of the peroneal nerve around the fibular neck.

EMG examination was performed 4 weeks after the onset of acute footdrop.

Please now review the Nerve Conduction Studies and Needle EMG tables.

QUESTIONS

1. Based on clinical grounds only:
   A. The prognosis is poor and recovery will be delayed.
   B. The prognosis is excellent and recovery will be rapid.
   C. The prognosis cannot be predicted.
2. The predominant pathophysiologic process involved here is:
   A. Demyelination, with anticipated protracted recovery.
   B. Axon loss, with anticipated rapid recovery.
   C. Demyelination, with anticipated rapid recovery.
   D. Axon loss, with anticipated protracted recovery.
3. A conduction block pattern on nerve conduction study accompanies the following condition(s):
   A. Segmental demyelination.

B. Axonal loss preceding wallerian degeneration.
C. Axonal loss following wallerian degeneration.
D. A and B.
E. A and C.

4. The prognosis for recovery of footdrop in this patient is:
   A. Poor because of prominent fibrillation potentials.
   B. Poor because of the near absence of voluntary motor unit potentials.
   C. Excellent because of normal distal peroneal compound muscle action potential (CMAP) amplitudes.
   D. Poor because of very low proximal peroneal CMAP amplitudes.
5. Which of the following is not usually encountered in a purely demyelinating focal nerve lesion?
   A. A decrease in amplitude with proximal stimulation, compared with distal stimulation.
   B. Significant dispersion of motor response with proximal stimulation, compared with distal stimulation.
   C. Focal slowing of conduction.
   D. Fibrillation potentials in weak muscles.

EDX FINDINGS AND INTERPRETATION OF DATA

The pertinent electrodiagnostic EDX features in this case include the following:

1. Prominent right peroneal conduction block across the fibular neck, recording both the extensor digitorum brevis (EDB) and the tibialis anterior. As is shown in the Nerve Conduction Table, the right peroneal CMAP amplitude, recording the EDB, decreased from 5.3 mV to 1.4 mV (73.5%) with stimulation below the fibular neck and at the knee, respectively (Figure C1–1). This was supported by a similar drop in CMAP area across the fibular neck from 19.5 mV/ms to 4.5 mV/ms (77%). There is no definite focal slowing across the fibular

Case 1: Nerve Conduction Studies

Nerve Stimulated	Stimulation Site	Recording Site	Amplitude (m = mV, s = μV)			Distal/Peak Latency (ms)			Conduction Velocity (m/s)			F Latency (ms)	
			Right	Left	Normal	Right	Left	Normal	Right	Left	Normal	Right	Left
Sup. peron. (s)	Leg	Ankle	6	6	≥6	3.4	3.0	≤4.4					
Sural (s)	Calf	Leg	16		≥6	4.2		≤4.4	41		≥40		
Peroneal (m)*	Ankle	EDB	5.6	6	≥3	4.9	4.2	≤5.5				NR	43
Peroneal (m)	Bel. fib. head	EDB	5.3	5					46	49	≥40		
Peroneal (m)	Knee	EDB	**1.4**						41		≥40		
Peroneal (m)	Bel. fib. head	Tibialis anterior	5.0	6	≥4	3.6	3.3	≤4.0					
Peroneal (m)	Knee	Tibialis anterior	**0.5**	6					**23**	41	≥40		
Tibial (m)	Ankle	AH	15		≥8	5.4		≤5.8				44	
Tibial (m)	Knee	AH	18						51		≥40		
H reflex	Knee	Soleus	4.5	6		30.0	28.8						
M response	Knee	Soleus	14	18		5.2	4.8						

AH = abductor hallucis; Bel. fib. head = below fibular head; EDB = extensor digitorum brevis; m = motor; NR = no response; s = sensory; Sup. peron. = superficial peroneal.
Data in bold type are abnormal.
*See Case Figure C1–1.

Case 1: Needle EMG

Muscle	Insertional Activity	Spontaneous Activity		Voluntary Motor Unit Action Potentials (MUAPs)							
		Fibs	Fasces	Recruitment				Configuration			
				Normal	Activation	Reduced	Early	Duration	Amplitude	% Polyphasia	Others
R. tibialis anterior	↑	1+	0			↓↓↓		Normal	Normal	Normal	
Extensor hallucis	↑	1+	0			↓↓↓		Normal	Normal	Normal	
Extensor digitorum brevis	↑	1+	0			↓↓↓		Normal	Normal	Normal	
Peroneus longus	↑	Few	0			↓↓		↑	Normal	↑	
Flexor digitorum longus	Normal	0	0	X				Normal	Normal	Normal	
Medial gastrocnemius	Normal	0	0	X				Normal	Normal	Normal	
Vastus lateralis	Normal	0	0	X				Normal	Normal	Normal	
Biceps femoris (short head)	Normal	0	0	X				Normal	Normal	Normal	
Gluteus medius	Normal	0	0	X				Normal	Normal	Normal	
Mid-lumbar paraspinal	Normal	0	0	–							
Lower lumbar paraspinal	Normal	0	0	–							

Fasces = fasciculations; Fibs = fibrillations; R. = right; ↑ = increased; ↓↓ = moderately reduced; ↓↓↓ = severely reduced.

neck (conduction velocities of 41 m/s versus 46 m/s). Also, the peroneal CMAP amplitude, recording the tibialis anterior, decreased from 5.0 mV to 0.5 mV (90%) with stimulation below the fibular neck and at the knee, respectively. The conduction velocity here is slowed, especially when compared with the asymptomatic left side (23 m/s on the right versus 41 m/s on the left).

2. Preservation of the distal peroneal CMAP amplitudes (recording both the EDB and the tibialis anterior) and of the superficial peroneal sensory nerve action potential (SNAP), both in absolute values and when compared with the asymptomatic side.

3. Fibrillation potentials and neurogenic recruitment of all deep and superficial peroneal innervated muscles below the knee (worse in the deep peroneal distribution), with a normal biceps femoris, short head.

These findings imply that the predominant pathologic process is segmental demyelination (conduction block with normal distal peroneal CMAPs and SNAP), with minimal axonal loss (fibrillation potentials). The prognosis for

recovery is excellent because it is dependent primarily on remyelination.

DISCUSSION

The anatomy and clinical and electrodiagnostic (EDX) presentations of peroneal mononeuropathy are discussed in detail, along with an accompanying case of peroneal nerve lesion (Case 8). The discussions here are limited to peripheral nerve injury and the electrodiagnostic findings of such injury.

Structure of Peripheral Nerve

The peripheral nerve consists of both unmyelinated and myelinated fibers and their supporting elements. The unmyelinated axons are surrounded only by the plasma membrane of a Schwann cell. The myelinated axons are engulfed by a Schwann cell that wraps around the axons

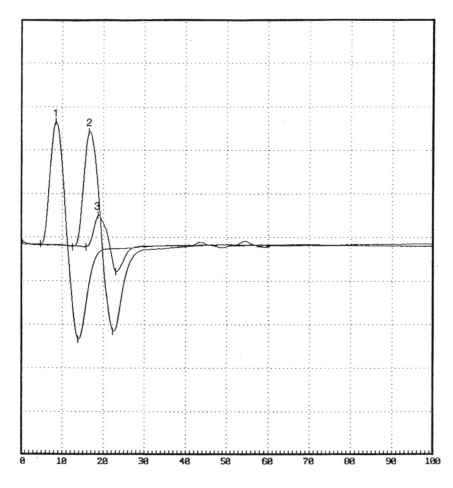

Figure C1–1. *Peroneal motor nerve conduction studies recording the extensor digitorum brevis and stimulating the ankle (1), below the fibular neck (2), and the knee (3). Note the significant decrease in compound muscle action potential (CMAP) amplitude and area between the second and third tracings, without prolongation of negative peak duration. (Amplitudes are 5.6, 5.3, and 1.4 mV, respectively, and areas are 20.5, 19.5, and 4.5 mV/ms, respectively. Sensitivity, using a vertical scale, is 2 mV.)*

multiple times, thereby insulating the axon with multiple layers of cell membrane, which is rich in lipid sphingomyelin. The myelinated axon is surrounded completely by myelin and Schwann cells, except at certain gaps. In adults, the gaps between myelin segments, called the *nodes of Ranvier*, measure approximately 1 μm, while myelinated segments between nodes, called the *internodal segments*, measure approximately 1 mm each.

The relatively thick myelin sheath has a low capacitance and a large resistance to the electrical current that attempts to escape from the axon to the extracellular space. Also, the axons contain a high concentration of voltage-gated sodium channels at the nodes of Ranvier, which are essential for the propagation of action potentials. These characteristics of myelinated fibers (myelin and Na channels at the nodes of Ranvier) result in a rapid saltatory conduction between consecutive nodes of Ranvier.

Pathology of Peripheral Nerve Injury

Transient neurologic symptoms related to minor peripheral nerve compression are extremely common and are rapidly reversible. They probably result from action potential propagation failure caused by ischemia. They are not associated with structural alteration of the axon, myelin, or supporting structure. In contrast, prolonged or severe compression, traction, laceration, thermal, or chemical injury may damage the myelin, axon, or the supporting components of the peripheral nerves and results in significant disability from which the patient may not recover completely.

Nerve injuries that are associated with focal interruption of the continuity of the axons cause significant changes in the structure of the peripheral nerve distal to the lesion (Table C1–1). The distal axons undergo a degenerative process, known as *wallerian degeneration*. This occurs since all the necessary building blocks needed for maintaining the axon are made in the cell body (peikaryon) and cannot reach the distal stump. The rate at which wallerian degeneration proceeds varies depending on the nerve injured, axon diameter, and the length of distal stump (the larger and the longer the distal stump the more time is

Table C1–1. Consequences of Focal Axonal Injury Distal to the Lesion

Wallerian (axonal) degeneration
Myelin breakdown
Neuromuscular transmission failure
Endoneurial tube shrinkage
Fascicular atrophy
Denervation atrophy of muscles

needed for wallerian degeneration to be completed). Within hours of most nerve injuries, myelin begins to retract from the axons at the nodes of Ranvier. This is followed by swelling of the distal nerve segment, leakage of axoplasm, and subsequently the disappearance of neurofibrils. Within days, the axon and myelin fragment, and digestion of nerve components starts. By the end of the first week, the axon and myelin become fully digested and Schwann cells start to bridge the gap between the two nerve segments. In chronic nerve lesions, the endoneurial tubes in the distal stump shrink, the nerve fascicles atrophy distal to the lesion, and, in complete nerve transection, the severed ends retract away from each other.

In contrast to the severe changes that occur distal to the lesion, only minor changes occur proximally. Though most of the proximal stump survives and maintains its ability to regenerate, there is often a slight retrograde degeneration of axons, up to several centimeters from the site of injury depending on the severity of the lesion. Also, the neuron cell body reacts to the axonal injury, by revealing an eccentric nucleus and marginally placed rough endoplasmic reticulum (Nissl's substance). These changes are worse with proximal than with distal nerve lesions.

Classification of Peripheral Nerve Injury

Many classifications of peripheral nerve injury have been suggested, but Seddon's and Sunderland's classifications are the most widely used in clinical practice. These are based on the functional status of the nerve and on histologic findings. They are shown in Table C1–2 and in Figure C1–2, with their corresponding electrophysiologic findings.

1. *Neurapraxia (first degree nerve injury).* Focal pressure on the peripheral nerve, when brief and modest, may distort the myelin near the nodes of Ranvier, producing segmental block of conduction without wallerian degeneration. The nerve conducts normally distally but not across the lesion, resulting in conduction block which is the electrophysiologic correlate of neurapraxia (see below). There are no or little changes in the muscles and recovery is usually complete following remyelination that occur within 1–3 months if the offending cause is removed.

2. *Axonotmesis.* With increasing compression or other physical injuries, the axons are focally damaged resulting in secondary wallerian degeneration distal to the site of injury. However, with this type of injury, there is variable disruption of the supporting structures (endoneurium, perineurium, and epineurium) that carries variable prognosis. Hence, Sunderland advocated that axonotmesis lesions be divided into three further

Table C1–2. Classification of Peripheral Nerve Injury

Seddon classification	Neurapraxia	Axonotmesis			Neurotmesis
Sunderland classification	First degree	Second degree	Third degree	Fourth degree	Fifth degree
Electrodiagnostic findings	Conduction block	Axonal loss			
Pathologic findings	Segmental demyelination with intact axons and supporting structures	Loss of axons and myelin with intact supporting structures	Loss of axons and myelin with disrupted endoneurium only	Loss of axons and myelin with disrupted endoneurium and perineurium	Loss of axons and myelin with disruption of all supporting structures (transection)
Prognosis	Excellent. Recovery is usually complete in 2–3 months	Slow but good recovery. Dependent on sprouting and reinnervation	Protracted improvement that may fail due to misdirected axonal sprouts	Unlikely improvement without surgical repair	Impossible improvement without surgical repair

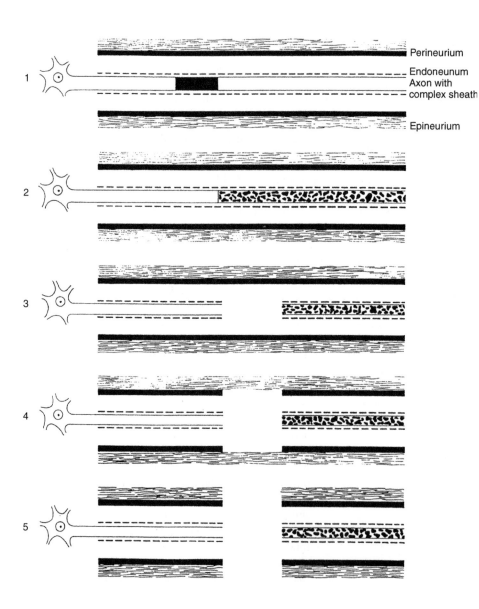

Figure C1–2. *Sunderland classification of peripheral nerve injury. 1, First degree: conduction block. 2, Second degree: wallerian degeneration secondary to a lesion confined to the axon, with preservation of the endoneurial sheath. 3, Third degree: disruption of the axon and endoneurial tube with an intact perineurium. 4, Fourth degree: disruption of all neural elements except the epineurium. 5, Fifth degree: transection with complete discontinuity of the entire nerve trunk. (Reprinted with permission from Sunderland S. Nerve injuries and their repair: a critical appraisal, Edinburgh: Churchill Livingstone, 1991.)*

subtypes, depending on what component of the surrounding nerve stroma is affected:

a. *Second degree nerve injury*, in which axon loss is associated with intact endoneurial tubes, perineurium, and epineurium. These lesions have better prognosis than other axon loss lesions since axonal regneration is well guided by the intact endoneurial tubes.

b. *Third degree nerve injury*, in which the axons, Schwann cell tubes, and endoneurium are damaged leaving the perineurium and epineurium intact. These lesions have poor prognosis and may require surgical intervention since axonal regeneration is often misdirected and may lead to neuroma formation.

c. *Fourth degree nerve injury*, where the perineurium is also disrupted, but the epineurium is intact. These lesions have very poor prognosis and surgery is often required.

3. *Neurotmesis (fifth degree nerve injury)*. This is the most severe type of nerve injury manifesting as complete disruption of the nerve with all the supporting structures. The nerve is transected with loss of continuity between its proximal and distal stumps. These lesions have no chance for improvement without surgical repair.

Diagnosis of Peripheral Nerve Injury

Injuries to peripheral nerves are highest in prevalence in young adults between the ages of 18 and 35 years and result in substantial degree of disability. They are often accompanied by other bodily injuries including fractures, dislocations, or soft tissue damage. When associated with head or spine injury, peripheral nerve lesions may be overlooked until late during the rehabilitative phase of treatment. Traumatic nerve injuries may be direct (such as with a stab wound to the sciatic nerve) or indirect (such as with radial neuropathy following humeral fracture). These lesions are much more common during wartime, but they also accompany civilian trauma that results from vehicular accidents, industrial accidents, gunshots, or knife wounds. Also, a significant percentage of peripheral nerve injuries encountered in clinical practice are iatrogenic, occurring in the setting of surgical or radiological procedures, or following needle insertion or medical therapy such as with the use of anticoagulation.

The diagnosis of peripheral nerve injury often requires a detailed history and neurologic examination, with the EDX studies and surgical findings playing important roles in diagnosis and management. The history and physical examination are extremely important in predicting the location, type, and severity of the nerve lesion. For example, a stab wound injury to a nerve is often associated with axonal interruptions and grade three to five nerve injuries,

while intraoperative nerve compression distant from the site of surgical field is usually a grade one (neurapraxic and demyelinating) or two (axonal) nerve injury.

Electrodiagnosis of Peripheral Nerve Injury

The EDX studies are the cornerstone in the diagnosis and management of nerve injuries by providing valuable information as to the location of the lesion, and its severity, pathophysiology, and prognosis (Table C1–3). Intraoperatively, the EDX studies guide the surgeon during the procedure and help assess the status of the regenerating axons within the injured nerve segment. During the recovery stage of peripheral nerve injury that may occur spontaneously or after surgical repair, the EDX studies are also essential in the evaluation of remyelination, regeneration, and reinnervation.

In contrast to the anatomical classification of nerve injuries, the pathophysiologic responses to peripheral nerve injuries have a limited repertoire: that is, axon loss, demyelination, or a combination of both. The EDX studies evaluate the integrity of the myelin sheath and the axon exclusively, and can only distinguish a neurapraxic injury (myelin injury) from all other degrees of injury that are associated with axonal damage and wallerian degeneration.

Localization of Nerve Lesions Using Nerve Conduction Studies

There are essentially three electrophysiologic consequences to peripheral nerve injury that can be assessed by nerve conduction studies. Two of them, namely focal slowing of conduction and conduction block, are caused by myelin disruption; the third is a manifestation of axonal loss (conduction failure).

Focal Slowing

Focal slowing in peripheral nerve injuries represents a convenient method of localizing lesions. When focal slowing is an isolated finding such as of the ulnar nerve across the elbow, the patient is not symptomatic and has no weakness or sensory loss. In symptomatic peripheral nerve injuries, focal slowing is associated with conduction block due to internodal demyelination, axon loss, or both.

Table C1–3. Role of Electrodiagnostic Studies in Peripheral Nerve Injury

Localize the site of nerve injury
Determine the pathophysiology of the lesion
Estimate the severity of the injury
Determine the prognosis
Assess the progress of remyelination and reinnervation

Focal slowing of conduction usually is caused by widening of the nodes of Ranvier (paranodal demyelination) and, sometimes, focal axonal narrowing. It is evident on NCSs by slowing of conduction of a specific nerve segment, while other segments of the same nerve as well as neighboring nerves remain normal. When the large myelinated fibers are slowed to essentially the same extent, focal slowing across the involved nerve segment is *synchronized*. This is manifested by either a prolongation of distal latencies (in distal lesions) or slowing in conduction velocities (in proximal lesions), while the CMAP amplitude, duration, and area are not affected and do not change when the nerve is stimulated proximal to the lesion. When variable number of the medium or small nerve fibers (average or slower conducting axons) are affected only, *desynchronized* (differential) slowing of conduction across the nerve segment is evident. In this situation, the CMAP is dispersed on stimulation proximal to the lesion and has prolonged duration, with normal (nondispersed) response on distal stimulation. If this finding is isolated, the distal latency or conduction velocity, which represent the speed of the largest (fastest) axons, are normal. However, in most clinical situations, the large fibers are often involved also, desynchronized slowing is usually accompanied by slowing at the involved segment, resulting in concomitant slowing of distal latency or conduction velocity.

Conduction Block

Normally, the action potential is generated by sufficient temporal and spatial summation of excitatory inputs to motor or sensory axons. The nerve potential travels a myelinated axon in a saltatory fashion, passing hundreds of nodes of Ranvier without failure. The axonal regions at the site of the nodes of Ranvier are rich in Na channels. An abrupt change in Na conductance forms the basis for the generation of nerve action potential and the maintenance of saltatory conduction. Loss of myelin can involve one or more segments of these axons (*segmental demyelination*). Segmental demyelination can result from in widening of the nodes (*paranodal demyelination*) or the loss of one or more internodal segments (*internodal demyelination*). Both forms of demyelination can result in slowing or block of conduction. However, at least in compressive/entrapment neuropathy, focal slowing of conduction is characteristic of paranodal demyelination, whereas conduction block is a manifestation of internodal demyelination.

Before one can understand the electrophysiologic diagnosis of conduction block, the normal conduction studies of nerves, especially in reference to *temporal dispersion and phase cancellation*, and, ultimately, conduction block, must be discussed.

Three physiologic facts play a pivotal role in the generation of the CMAP which is obtained with surface recording.

1. The CMAP is produced by supramaximal stimulation of peripheral nerve and represents the summation of all individual muscle fiber action potentials directed to the muscle through the stimulated nerve.
2. The surface-recorded motor units are biphasic, with an initial negative phase followed by a positive phase, and a total duration of 5 to 15 ms in most human muscles.
3. The motor axons are not uniform but differ in size, thickness of myelin, and conduction velocities. The range of conduction velocities of individual human motor axons is 12 to 13 m/s.

Because of this physiologic variability, the CMAP configuration changes according to the site of stimulation. Typically, as the stimulus site moves proximally, the CMAP increases in duration and decreases in amplitude and, to a lesser extent, area. With more proximal stimulation, action potentials generated by motor units of slowly conducting fibers are increasingly dispersed in time with respect to those from fast-conducting fibers. This results in positive/negative phase overlap and cancellation of some components of the motor unit waveforms, thus prolonging its duration and reducing the amplitude and area of the summated response (CMAP).

Temporal dispersion and phase cancellation are more prominent in sensory nerve conduction studies due to (1) the disparity of sensory fiber conduction velocities which are almost double that of the motor axons (25 m/s) and (2) the surface recorded nerve action potentials are triphasic. The SNAP may normally decrease in amplitude and area by 50% or more and its duration can increase by 100% or more with proximal stimulation in antidromic studies (or with proximal recording with orthodromic studies). Hence, it is a common practice not to rely on sensory studies in the diagnosis of conduction block. Figures C1–3 and C1–4 depict the concept of temporal dispersion and phase cancellation using computer modeling.

Impeding transmission of action potentials is the basis of conduction block. This usually results from internodal demyelination, but can occur in axonal loss before wallerian degeneration ("axonal" conduction block). Blockage of the transmission of electrical impulses anywhere throughout the course of motor axons results in motor weakness that is often indistinguishable from weakness that results from loss of motor neurons or motor axons. Experimental evidence on tourniquet paralysis on baboon hind limb showed that conduction block is reversible and the distal nerve remains normal and excitable (Figure C1–5).

In practice, conduction block is defined as a relative decrease in the CMAP amplitude and area with proximal stimulation, when compared with the CMAP on distal stimulation, without significant prolongation of

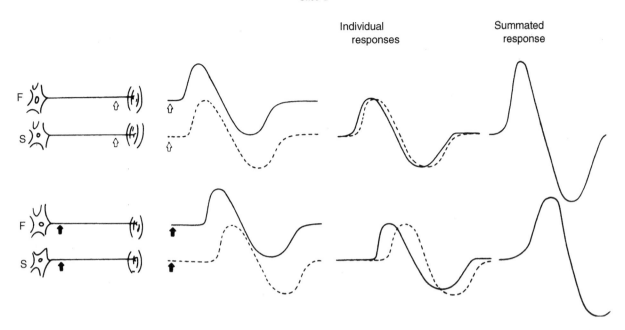

Figure C1–3. *Temporal dispersion and phase cancellation of two surface-recorded motor unit potentials at distal and proximal sites. This can be translated into many similar biphasic potentials, which contribute to the compound muscle action potential (CMAP). (Reprinted with permission from Kimura J et al. Relation between size of compound sensory or muscle action potentials, and length of nerve segment. Neurology 1986;36:647–652.)*

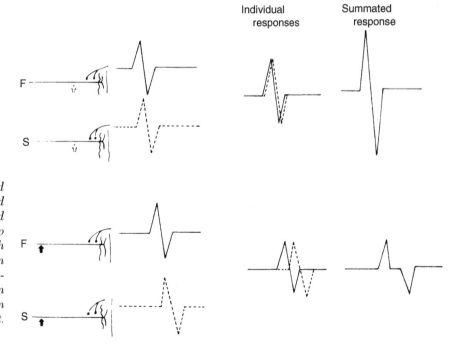

Figure C1–4. *Temporal dispersion and phase cancellation of two surface-recorded single-fiber sensory potentials at distal and proximal sites. This can be translated into many similar biphasic potentials, which contribute to the sensory nerve action potential (SNAP). (Reprinted with permission from Kimura J et al. Relation between size of compound sensory or muscle action potentials, and length of nerve segment. Neurology 1986;36:647–652.)*

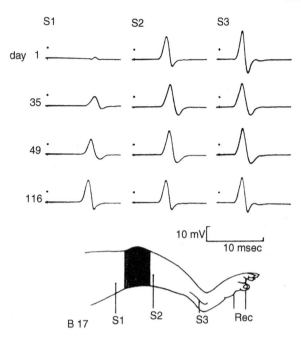

Figure C1–5. *Evoked compound muscle action potential (CMAP) from the abductor hallucis muscle of a baboon at different intervals after a tourniquet was inflated for 95 minutes to 1000 mmHg around the knee. S1, S2, and S3 are the sites of stimulation, as is shown in the schematic (bottom). (Reprinted with permission from Fowler CJ, Danta G, Gilliatt RW. Recovery of nerve conduction after a pneumatic tourniquet: observation on the hind-limb of the baboon. J Neurol Neurosurg Psychiatry 1972;35: 638–647. © BMJ Publishing Group.)*

CMAP duration. Conduction block should be distinguished from physiologic or abnormal temporal dispersion. Based on experimental studies, differential slowing along medium and thinly myelinated fibers may result in temporal dispersion and phase cancellation manifesting as significant drop of amplitude that may occasionally reach up to 80%. This is often associated with obvious and marked prolongation of CMAP duration. In contrast to amplitude decay, differential slowing does not drop the area beyond 50%. Hence, in true conduction block a significant drop in amplitude should always be corroborated by a similar drop in CMAP area.

There are no uniformly accepted criteria for the identification of conduction block. Table C1–4 reveals some of the common errors made in the EMG laboratory in the diagnosis of true conduction block. Table C1–5 lists practical criteria for the diagnosis of conduction block. In general, an amplitude change should be always supported by area change, since a significant drop in amplitude up to 50% or more may occasionally be due solely to abnormal temporal dispersion while an area drop of more than 50% is always due to conduction block. In clinical practice, the

Table C1–4. Common Errors in the Diagnosis of Conduction Block

Technical

Submaximal percutaneous stimulations (proximal sites, obesity, edema)

Examination of long peripheral nerves (tibial nerve, tall subjects)

Anomalous innervation (e.g., Martin-Gruber anastomosis)

Pathological

Abnormal temporal dispersion with phase cancellation

identification of demyelinative conduction block is an excellent tool for precisely localizing peripheral nerve lesions. Conduction block is often caused by acute nerve compression such as peroneal mononeuropathy at the fibular neck or radial mononeuropathy across the spiral groove. It is also a common finding in immune-mediated peripheral neuropathies such as acute inflammatory demyelinating polyneuropathy, chronic inflammatory demyelinating polyneuropathy, or multifocal motor neuropathy. Finally, conduction block usually is reversible and amenable to treatment, by removing the offending compression factor from the injured nerve or immunotherapy.

Axonal Loss

In cases where there has been *axonal damage following the completion of wallerian degeneration*, the NCSs characteristically result in unelicitable or uniformly low CMAP amplitude, which is not dispersed, at all stimulation points. This pattern unfortunately cannot localize the site of injury to a specific segment of the nerve, and other measures need to be considered in localization such as the history, clinical examination, and needle EMG.

Table C1–5. Electrodiagnosis of Conduction Block*

Definite in Any Nerve[†]

≥50% decrease in CMAP amplitude, with <15% prolongation of compound muscle action potential (CMAP) duration, and

≥50% decrease in CMAP area, or

≥30% decrease in area or amplitude over a short nerve segment (e.g., radial across the spiral groove, ulnar across the elbow, peroneal across the fibular neck)

Likely in Median, Ulnar, and Peroneal Nerves Only

20–50% decrease in CMAP amplitude, with <15% prolongation of CMAP duration, and

20–50% decrease in CMAP area

CMAP = compound muscle action potential.
*All amplitudes, areas, and durations reflect negative-peak areas, amplitudes, and durations.
[†]Caution should be used in evaluating the tibial nerve since stimulation at the knee may result in more than 50% decrease in amplitude, especially in obese patients.

NCSs, done on patients who harbor *axonal damage before the completion of wallerian degeneration*, require special attention since they can be a source of error in localizing, characterizing, or prognosticating nerve lesions. However, these early studies are useful since they often help localizing lesions better than if NCSs are done after the completion of wallerian degeneration.

Early after axonal damage, the distal stump remains excitable for a variable period with some differences between the motor and sensory responses. The distal CMAP remains normal for 1 to 2 days after injury, giving rise to a pattern of conduction block on NCS that mimics the one seen with segmental demyelination. This pattern is sometimes referred to as "axonal noncontinuity, early axon loss, and axon discontinuity" conduction block. It is important to recognize this pattern since it carries poor prognosis, in contrast to the conduction block that is caused by segmental demyelination which usually recovers rapidly and completely. As wallerian degeneration progresses following axon injury, the distal CMAP then falls precipitously to reach its nadir by 5–6 days postinjury. After this time, the conduction block pattern is replaced by unelicitable CMAPs in complete lesions or low-amplitude CMAPs in partial lesions that are independent of the stimulation sites. In contrast to the motor studies, the distal sensory nerve remains excitable for a slightly longer period. The distal SNAP remains normal for 5–6 days and then decreases rapidly to reach its nadir in 10–11 days (Figure C1–6). Thus, repeat studies performed after the completion of wallerian degeneration prove that the lesion is due to axonal loss, by revealing a decrease in distal CMAP to values very similar to proximal CMAP values, along with low or absent SNAP.

Identification of motor conduction block in the early days of axonal loss is extremely helpful for localization, particularly in closed nerve injury, in which the exact site of trauma is not clear on clinical grounds. Thus, nerve conduction studies must be obtained if possible as soon as the patient seeks medical attention. Waiting for the completion of wallerian degeneration results in low CMAPs, regardless of stimulation sites, thus not allowing for any localization of the injury site.

Mixed (Axonal and Demyelinating) Lesions

Mixed lesions exhibit a mixture of pathophysiology including axon loss and segmental demyelination. In acute nerve lesion, this often manifests as axon loss and conduction block, while focal slowing tends to be a feature of more chronic lesions (e.g., entrapment neuropathies). By analyzing distal and proximal CMAPs as well as the distal SNAP, the EDX study can semiquantitatively estimate the number of axons that have undergone wallerian degeneration and those that have segmental demyelination.

Localization of Nerve Lesions Using Needle Electromyography

The earliest finding on needle EMG following a nerve injury is a complete loss of voluntary activity (with a complete lesion) or a decrease in MUAP recruitment (with a partial lesion) in weak muscles. This is the result of failure of nerve action potentials to reach the target muscle that follows nerve lesions associated with axon loss or segmental demyelination. Hence, a decrease MUAP recruitment per se cannot distinguish between axon loss and demyelinating lesions. Also, the degree of impaired MUAP recruitment correlates with the extent of clinical weakness, and is proportional to the number of lost or demyelinated axons.

Axon loss lesions studied by NCSs prior to wallerian degeneration, as well as demyelinating (neurapraxic) lesions, are often precisely localized to a short segment of the nerve due to the presence of conduction block across that segment. Hence, localization of lesions by needle EMG is most important in axon loss lesions that are first studied following the completion of wallerian degeneration

Figure C1–6. *Distal compound muscle action potential (CMAP) and sensory nerve action potential (SNAP) after acute axonal nerve injury.*

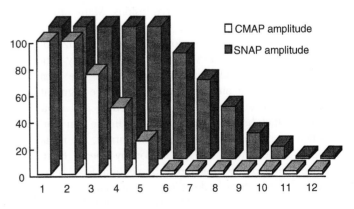

% Amplitude

Days from acute axonal injury

☐ CMAP amplitude
■ SNAP amplitude

of motor axons (more than 5–6 days postinjury). These lesions are associated with nonlocalizable NCSs that are characterized by low-amplitude or unelicitable CMAPs from all nerve simulation sites.

The concept of localization by needle EMG is similar to clinical localization using manual muscle strength testing which is part of the motor system evaluation during the neurologic examination. Muscles innervated by branches arising from the nerve distal to the lesion are often weak, while those innervated by branches proximal to the lesion are normal. Clinical localization of the site of the lesion is usually accurate in sharp penetrating injuries that are well defined such as nerve laceration. However, clinical localization may not be possible or inaccurate in patients with extensive bodily injury that may limit the neurological examination or involve several nerves or elements of a plexus.

Localization by needle EMG relies on electrophysiological changes that occur in denervated muscles, namely fibrillation potentials, reduced MUAP recruitment, and MUAP changes characteristic of reinnervation. It should be noted that fibrillation potentials appear after 1–2 weeks of acute denervation but do not become full until after 3 weeks after nerve injury. They disappear late in the course of denervation when muscle fibers become reinnervated or fibrotic and severely atrophied. Hence, fibrillation potentials may be absent in very acute or chronic denervation. Also, reinnervation MUAPs are first apparent after one month of injury in partial axonal lesions and become widespread with increasing time.

The concept of localization by needle EMG follows the same rules as the manual muscle examination, namely muscles innervated by branches arising from the nerve distal to the lesion are denervated, while those innervated by branches proximal to the lesion are normal. Unfortunately, several types of axon loss lesions may pose problems when attempting to localize the site of the injury solely by needle EMG.

1. *Nerve lesions along segments with no motor branches.* The anatomy of the injured nerve plays a pivotal role in the precise localization of nerve lesions. Many nerves travel substantial distances without giving out any motor branches. Hence, long segment localization along one of these nerves may be of relatively little assistance to the clinician, simply because the focal lesion may be at any point along the nerve segment. Examples of such nerves are the median and ulnar nerves which have very long segments in the arm from which no motor branches arise. In contrast, the radial nerve is more ideal for localization by needle EMG since it gives off multiple motor branches at fairly regular and short intervals along its entire course.

2. *Fascicular nerve lesions.* Occasionally, partial peripheral nerve lesions spare one or two nerve fascicles resulting in muscles that escape denervation despite being located distal to the lesion site. This usually results in an erroneous localization that is more distal to the actual site of the lesion. The explanation for this phenomenon is based on the established findings that there is a high degree of somatotopic organization of nerve fibers into individual fascicles distally and close to the site of branch exit, but also on the recent evidence that, though fascicles intermingle more proximally to form a plexiform structure, the nerve fibers from a discrete distal fascicle would generally remain clustered despite crisscrossing from one fascicle to another. Examples of this fascicular involvement include sparing of ulnar muscles in the forearm (flexor carpi ulnaris and ulnar part of flexor digitorum profundus) following an axon loss ulnar nerve lesions at the elbow, and sparing the superficial peroneal innervated muscles (peroneus longus and brevis) following an axon loss common peroneal nerve lesion at the knee or fibular neck.

3. *Chronic nerve lesions.* The process of reinnervation includes proximodistal regeneration of nerve fibers from the site of the injury, collateral sprouting, or both (see below). Often with partial axon loss lesions that are mild or modest, proximodistal regeneration and reinnervation can be so efficient in proximally located muscles resulting in remodeling of the motor units. Hence, a needle EMG done several years after such lesions may only detect the neurogenic changes in the more distal muscles and result in mislocalizing the lesion more distally.

Timing of Electrodiagnostic Studies in Peripheral Nerve Injury

The ideal timing of the initial EDX study in a patient with peripheral nerve injury depends on the clinical situation. Treating physicians should be aware of the EDX limitations and know that the electrophysiologic abnormalities that are critical to the accurate interpretation of the location and severity of the lesion progressively appear during the first 2–3 weeks postinjury.

In patients with closed nerve trauma or severe limb trauma at several sites, where the exact site of injury may not be clear, early NCSs are very useful in attempting to identify conduction block across the site of the lesion. This should be done, if possible, very early and before 3–5 days from injury since the distal CMAP reaches its nadir after that time. Detecting conduction block with this early study is extremely useful in precise localization of the site of the lesion, though finding a conduction block cannot distinguish whether the lesion is due to axon loss, demyelination, or a mixture of both. A repeat study after allowing time for the completion of motor and sensory wallerian degeneration (i.e., after 10–11 days from injury) helps establish the pathophysiologic diagnosis and estimate the degree of injury and prognosis.

When NCSs are repeated, one of three scenarios may arise: (1) the conduction block does not change, hence the lesion is purely demyelinating (neurapraxia), (2) the distal CMAP drops to equal the proximal CMAP, hence the lesion is axon loss (axonotmesis or neurotmesis), and (3) the CMAP amplitude drops distally but there is a remaining drop proximally (i.e., the distal CMAP is low but significantly higher that the proximal CMAP), hence the lesion is mixed with evidence of demyelination and axon loss.

In axon loss lesions, waiting to obtain NCSs until after the completion of wallerian degeneration (after 10–11 days from injury) results in diffusely low-amplitude or absent CMAPs and SNAPs from all stimulation sites, which does not allow for precise localization of the injury site. This is accepted in circumstances where the site of lesion is clear and the lesion is likely axon loss (e.g., stab wound). Not infrequently, the patient presents to the specialist after the time expected for completion of wallerian degeneration (after 10–11 days postinjury). In these situations, localization will depend on the needle EMG, and the optimal timing of the EDX study would be 3–5 weeks after injury when fibrillation potentials are fully developed in all denervated muscles and reinnervation is barely apparent.

Determining Severity of Nerve Injury by Electrodiagnostic Studies

An important role of the EDX studies is to estimate the degree of nerve injury since this has a direct effect on prognosis and long-term disability. In demyelinating conduction block lesions, one can approximate the number of demyelinated motor axons by comparing the distal to the proximal CMAPs. For example in a patient with common radial nerve lesion across the spiral groove, a 6 mV response from extensor digitorum communis obtained from distal stimulation at the elbow and a 3 mV response from proximal stimulation above the spiral groove implies that about 50% of the axons are blocked (demyelinated) while the remaining 50% conduct normally.

In axon loss lesions, the CMAP amplitude is the best estimate of the degree of motor axon loss. In contrast, fibrillation potentials are the most sensitive indicator of motor axonal loss, since a loss of a single axon results in up to 200 denervated muscle fibers (depending on the innervation ratio of the innervated muscle). SNAP amplitude reflects the degree of sensory axon loss, though it has less implication on disability than CMAP amplitude. The changes seen on EDX studies with increasing severity of axon loss follow a certain pattern that is predictable and applies to most mixed sensorimotor nerve lesions examined after 3 weeks from injury. With *mild axon loss lesions*, there are usually only fibrillation potentials in affected muscles with normal or slightly reduced MUAP recruitment, and normal CMAP and SNAP amplitudes. With *moderate axon loss lesions*, fibrillation potentials and decreased recruitment are coupled with a low-amplitude or absent SNAP while the CMAP usually remains normal or is borderline in amplitude. Following *severe axon loss lesions*, the SNAP is absent and the CMAP is either very low in amplitude or absent. This is accompanied by profuse fibrillation potentials and marked reduction in MUAP recruitment.

The *sensitivity* exhibited by the various EDX parameters of axon loss is inversely related to the time these abnormalities become apparent after an acute lesion. For example, fibrillation potentials are most sensitive to axon loss but do not fully develop until 3–5 weeks, while the CMAP amplitude is the least sensitive, since it only decreases after significant axon loss and as early as 2–5 days from injury). Hence, it is important to always perform needle EMG about 3–5 weeks postinjury on all patients with suspected acute peripheral nerve trauma to look for fibrillation potentials and assess for the presence of axon loss.

In axon loss lesions, estimating the extent of motor axonal loss, after the completion of wallerian degeneration (more than 10–11 days), requires comparison of the distal CMAP to the same CMAP in the contralateral limb. Optimally, motor and sensory NCSs should be done bilaterally and compared, though there is up to 30% side-to-side variability in normal controls. Comparison to normal laboratory values may be necessary in bilateral lesions or when the contralateral limb cannot be studied (concomitant injury, amputation, etc.). In a complete nerve transection, there is absence of distal and proximal CMAPs. In a partial axonal lesion, the low distal CMAP amplitude reflects the number of axons lost. For example, in a patient with median nerve laceration in the forearm, a 2 mV response from abductor pollicis brevis obtained from distal stimulation at the wrist compared to a 10 mV response from the contralateral side implies that about 80% of axons were lost.

In mixed lesions, an estimate of the percentage of axons that are demyelinated versus those that underwent wallerian degeneration requires a combination of calculations that assess the degree of conduction block and axon loss which should be only done after the time of wallerian degeneration is completed. For example, in a patient with peroneal nerve lesion at the fibular neck, if a 3 mV response was obtained from the tibialis anterior following distal stimulation below the fibular neck and a 1.5 mV response from proximal stimulation above the fibular neck, coupled with a 5 mV response from distal stimulation on the contralateral side, one can approximate that 40% of the axons are lost while 30% are blocked (demyelinated) and the remaining 30% are intact.

Intraoperative Electrodiagnostic Studies

Intraoperative recording is pivotal in the surgical management of patients with severe nerve injuries. Surgery provides a unique opportunity for direct recordings of *compound nerve action potentials (CNAPs)* across the injured segment of the nerve. These studies are most helpful in nerve lesions associated with severe or total axonal injury that remains in continuity (second through fourth degree nerve injuries) since the clinical and routine EDX studies often cannot accurately classify the degree of nerve injury. In contrast, intraoperative studies are not useful in neurapraxia (first degree injury) since remyelination is expected and surgical intervention is rarely indicated, or in complete nerve transection (neurotmesis or fifth degree) since these studies will have no role in the choice of surgical intervention (reanastomosis or grafting).

The indication for surgical repair of a peripheral nerve lesion depends on the type and severity of the nerve lesion. With sharp nerve transection (such as with glass or knife injuries), primary (immediate) repair is often done at the time of the initial soft tissue repair. This may be delayed several weeks if infection is feared or complicates the wound, or when the nerve transection is blunt and the anatomy is distorted (such as with propeller blade or power saw injuries, or following compound fractures). When peripheral nerve lesions remain in continuity, the decision to operate is usually based on whether functional recovery and reinnervation has occurred after allowing several months for regeneration. If the nerve fails to regenerate or exhibits poor reinnervation, surgery is often indicated. Operative exploration of the site of injury allows visual inspection of the injured nerve which is useful in determining the extent of injury to the nerve, particularly to its supporting nerve structures. However, visual inspection only is notoriously inadequate in determining the severity of nerve injuries that are in continuity and cannot establish whether some axons have regenerated and bridged across the injured segment. Injured nerves may look good by inspection but show no evidence of regeneration due to endoneurial damage and fibrosis. In contrast, a nerve may look very bad at the time of exploration, with fibrosis and enlargement, yet with satisfactory regenerating axons.

Intraoperative recordings are performed by using two electrode pairs that hooks on the exposed nerve and are used for stimulating the nerve proximal to the lesion while recording distal to it. The purpose of this study is to try to record a CNAP across the lesion and to establish if some axons cross the injured segment, and if so, how many. If there is no distal CNAP, the recording electrode should be moved proximally until a CNAP is recorded. This indicates the distal end of conducting axons and is most important in evaluating a long lesion that extends a considerable distance, such as with extensive fibrosis due to hemorrhage, infection, or ischemia.

Electrodiagnostic Studies During the Recovery Phase

Once the diagnosis of the nerve injury is secure, the optimal timing of the repeat EDX studies depends mostly on the pathophysiology of the lesion, the nerve injured, and location of the nerve injury. Improvement following peripheral nerve injury depends on remyelination, reinnervation, or both. Reinnervation may follow collateral sprouting (in partial axon loss lesions only), proximodistal axon regeneration, or both. Recovery is quick and often complete with demyelinative conduction block lesions, while improvement is protracted and usually incomplete in axon loss lesions. In mixed lesions, the recovery is biphasic with an initial rapid improvement due to remyelination and a slower phase due to regeneration.

Remyelination

In patients with a neurapraxic nerve injury (first degree) that is due to segmental demyelination and manifests as conduction block, the process of remyelination is usually rapid and may take up to 2–3 months for completion, provided that the offending cause (such as compression by hematoma or bony structure) is removed. For example, a patient who develops a wrist drop due to a purely demyelinating radial nerve injury at the spiral groove often recovers completely in 2–3 months. Hence, if follow-up NCSs are done after that time, remyelination is confirmed by resolution of the conduction block and restoration of the proximal CMAP. During that phase and for a short period after the reversal of conduction block, NCSs may reveal focal slowing across the injured nerve segment which was not present on the initial EDX study. This is best explained by the presence of newly formed thin myelin that was laid out by the Schwann cells. As the myelin thickens with time, focal slowing also disappears.

Reinnervation by Collateral Sprouting

Collateral sprouting is a process in which the surviving (intact) motor axons send axon terminals (sprouts) to the denervated muscles in an attempt to reinnervate these muscle fibers and restore muscle power. This is a quick and effective method of reinnervation that applies only to partial axon loss lesions where some axons escape injury and wallerian degeneration. Collateral sprouting is clinically effective in restoring function when only a modest number of axons are injured. In practice, it is most effective when less than 80% of the axons are damaged. In very severe lesions, collateral sprouting may lead to little or no change of motor function.

Collateral sprouting in partial axon loss lesions starts as early as 1–2 days after injury. However, the early signs of reinnervation first become evident on needle EMG by one month, and are usually definite by 2–3 months postinjury. Immediately following nerve injury, there is a decrease in MUAP recruitment in affected muscles that is appropriate to the number of lost axons. In the first few weeks after injury, MUAPs of surviving axons retain their normal morphology. As collateral sprouting proceeds, muscle fibers become progressively incorporated to the territory of the motor unit.

Early on, the collateral axons (sprouts) have thin or incomplete myelin. Hence, action potentials along collateral sprouts conduct slowly. This is often reflected on needle EMG by MUAPs with *satellite potentials* (linked or parasite potentials), late spikes of the MUAP that are distinct and time-locked with the main potentials. The satellite potential trails the main MUAP because the newly formed nerve terminal may be long, or small and thinly myelinated, or both, resulting in slower conduction. When a satellite potential is suspected on needle EMG, it is useful to use a trigger line to demonstrate that this potential is time-locked to the main potential (Figure C1–7).

Reinnervation MUAPs, including satellite potentials, may be unstable (Figure C1–8). The MUAPs may show evidence of intermittent nerve conduction blocking or neuromuscular junction blocking due insecure action potential transmission at the sprout or endplate, respectively. This results in individual muscle fibers being either blocked or come to action potential at varying

intervals, leading to a MUAP that changes in configuration from impulse to impulse (amplitude or number of phases or both). Over time, the sprout matures and the conduction velocity increases and the satellite potential then fires more closely to the main potential, and ultimately fuses to become an additional phase or serration within the main MUAP complex (Figure C1–9). In general, MUAPs become more stable, more polyphasic, and longer in duration as collateral sprouting continues. In very chronic lesions, MUAPs are typically stable with long duration and high amplitude and little or no polyphasia, reflecting the maturity of all the nerve sprouts (Figure C1–10). Also, as reinnervation proceeds, there is a decline in the number of fibrillation potentials, since reinnervated muscle fibers will cease to generate this spontaneous activity.

On NCSs, the CMAP and SNAP amplitudes slowly increase in size with time as reinnervation continues. In mild to moderate nerve lesions, effective reinnervation may render the CMAP within normal values, and result in NCSs that do not clearly show evidence of a remote nerve injury. In these situations, however, needle EMG will continue to confirm the old injury by exhibiting large MUAPs that fire rapidly.

Reinnervation by Axon Regeneration

In complete or very severe axon loss peripheral nerve lesions, improvement is dependent solely or primarily on axonal regeneration that may occur spontaneously or following surgical repair. Unfortunately, in most cases of

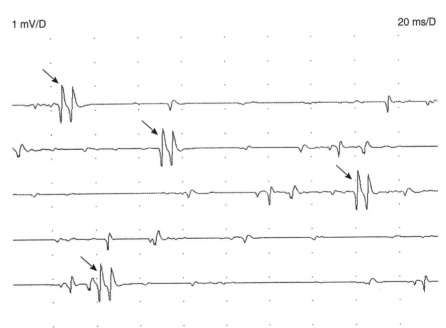

1 mV/D   20 ms/D

Figure C1–7. *A motor unit action potential with a satellite potential recorded in a raster mode (arrow). Note that the second potential is always linked to the first potential.*

0.2 mV/D   20 ms/D

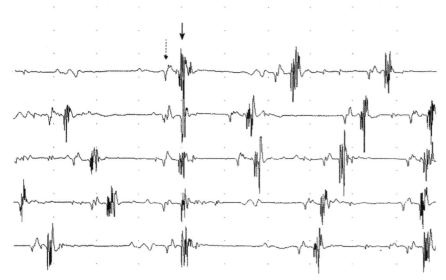

Figure C1–8. *Unstable motor unit action potential (arrow) preceded by a satellite potential that is also unstable (dashed arrow) from the brachioradialis muscle in a patient with severe radial nerve injury secondary to a compound humeral fracture, recorded four months postinjury. This complex potential is triggered upon using a trigger, delay line, and a raster mode. Note the extreme variation in the morphology of the unit and its satellite potential between subsequent discharges.*

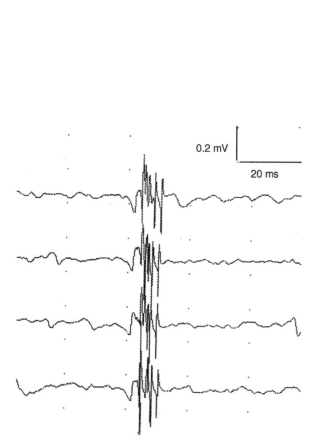

Figure C1–9. *Polyphasic and stable motor unit action potential with long duration recorded from the tibialis anterior, eight months after a severe axon loss peroneal nerve injury at the fibular neck. This complex potential is triggered upon using a trigger, delay line, and a raster mode. Note that all components of the units are present with every discharge.*

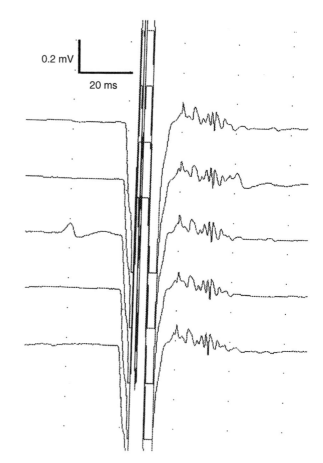

Figure C1–10. *Large (long-duration and high-amplitude) motor unit action potential from the abductor digiti minimi of a patient with a remote severe ulnar nerve laceration above the elbow. This complex potential is triggered upon using a trigger, delay line, and a raster mode. Note that the main potential is followed by several small polyphasic satellite potentials that trail the main component.*

nerve injury, regeneration is slow and incomplete. In more severe axon loss lesions, the regenerating axons may not find intact endoneurial tubes and sometimes form a neuroma with tangled axons at the site of injury. In such lesions as well as lesions with complete transection, surgical repair is often needed.

In humans, the axons have to first traverse the injured segment. This may be achieved in 8–15 days when the endoneurial tubes are intact (second degree nerve lesion). Once the axons cross successfully, they continue to regenerate at a slow rate averaging 1 to 2 mm/day (or about 1 inch/month). Based on this, the timing of repeat EDX studies in complete or severe axon loss lesions depends on the site of injury in relation to the most proximal muscle that is expected to be reinnervated first. For example, following a median nerve injury in the middle of the arm, the first muscle expected to show reinnervation is the pronator teres muscle with its branch arising from the nerve in the antecubital fossa. If the distance between this lesion and the muscle is 5 inches, then the repeat study should be done about five to six months after the injury. The timing of surgical intervention is based on the fact that muscles that do not reinnervate after 18–24 months will undergo atrophy and fibrosis and their muscle fibers will not be more viable. With more proximal severe or complete axon loss nerve lesions, such as those of the lower brachial plexus or sciatic nerve, the target muscles to be reinnervated (hand muscles or leg muscles respectively) are situated far from the site of injury so that early surgical intervention is often necessary.

On needle EMG, the early signs of regeneration can be confirmed by the appearance of small, complex, unstable MUAPs, sometimes referred to as *"nascent"* MUAPs, that precedes the onset of visible voluntary contraction. These units appear first in muscles nearest to the site of the injury and progress distally, and hence are useful in assessing the advancement of this proximodistal regeneration. Nascent MUAPs are very low in amplitude and extremely polyphasic, with normal or increased duration. These small nascent MUAPs mimic the MUAPs seen with necrotizing myopathies. Nascent MUAPs are often unstable due to conduction or neuromuscular junction blocking and are associated with decreased MUAP recruitment (Figure C1–11). As reinnervation proceeds, nascent MUAPs that are unstable become transformed into stable, long-duration, and polyphasic MUAPs, reflecting increased numbers of muscle fibers per motor unit, full myelination of the regenerating axons, and the maturity of the neuromuscular junctions. Similar to what is seen in reinnervation by collateral sprouting, there is also a decline in the number of fibrillation potentials and the progressive improvement of the SNAP and CMAP on NCS. However, in these severe or complete nerve lesions, it is common that the CMAP and

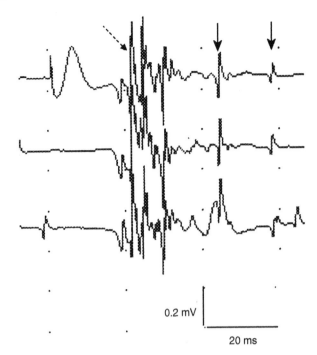

Figure C1–11. *Nascent motor unit action potentials from the quadriceps in a patient with severe femoral nerve injury following abdominal hysterectomy. This complex potential is triggered upon using a trigger, delay line, and a raster mode. Note the low-amplitude and highly polyphasic potential (dashed arrow), which is fairly stable and is followed by two distinct satellite potentials (arrows).*

SNAP never return to baseline values and there is often permanent slowing and dispersion of the CMAPs due to the extreme variability in the diameter and myelination of the regenerated axons that results in significant differential slowing of conduction velocities.

Aberrant Regeneration

Aberrant regeneration occurs when regenerating axons are misdirected into new end organs and is most common in axon loss nerve injuries that distort the endoneurial tubes (third degree or more) and in proximal peripheral nerve or root injuries. Misdirected fibers may not find endoneurial tubes and generate a neuroma at the site of the lesion. Regenerating motor axons in a mixed sensorimotor nerve may elongate into sensory nerves or vice versa. Motor axons may also get misdirected into the wrong muscles and result in co-contraction of muscles that can interfere with the intended function or cause abnormal movements.

The most common neurologic sequelae of aberrant reinnervation occur after facial nerve injury including after idiopathic Bell's palsy. Aberrant regeneration between motor axons results in facial synkinesis, mainly contraction

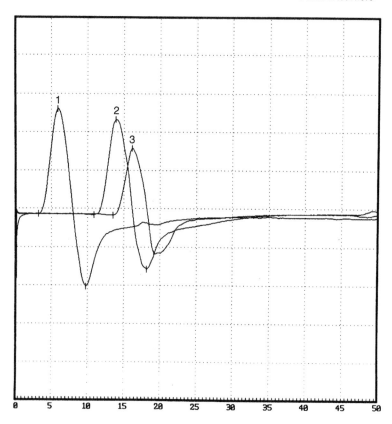

Figure C1–12. *Follow-up peroneal motor nerve conduction studies recording extensor digitorum brevis stimulating ankle (1), below fibular head (2), and knee (3). Note the significant improvement of CMAP amplitude and area stimulating at the knee (waveform 3) compared with the initial study done at presentation (compare with Figure C1–1). (Sensitivity: vertical scale = 2 mV.)*

of the lower facial muscles on the affected side whenever there is an eye blink or vice versa. Other much less common, yet more publicized, examples of abnormal regeneration patterns are the "crocodile tears," manifested as lacrimation of the ipsilateral eye during chewing, and the Marin-Amat syndrome, or "jaw-winking," manifested as closure of the ipsilateral eyelid when the jaw opens.

Another example of aberrant regeneration occurs following injury to the C5 spinal root. Motor axons destined to the diaphragm may get misdirected to one or more shoulder muscles (biceps, deltoid, or spinati) with the result that the shoulder muscles fire in time with the respiratory cycle (breathing arm). Similar phenomena were recently reported form obstetric brachial plexopathies involving the lower plexus and T1 cervical roots and resulting in aberrant reinnervation of hand muscles from axons destined into intercostal muscles (breathing hand).

FOLLOW-UP

On further questioning, it was determined that the patient was involved in a long meeting that lasted approximately 12 hours, during most of which he was seated around a table. He also admitted to frequent leg crossing. More importantly, he had been on an intensive weight loss program for 2 to 3 weeks and had lost 30 pounds (see Case 8 for further discussions). When he was seen 2 months later, he had no residual weakness and minimal numbness on the dorsum of the foot. Repeat nerve conduction studies showed significant improvement of proximal peroneal (knee) CMAP amplitude and area (Figure C1–12).

DIAGNOSIS

Acute common peroneal mononeuropathy, due to compression at the fibular head, manifested by significant conduction block (due to segmental demyelination) and minimal axonal loss, precipitated by weight loss and leg crossing.

ANSWERS

1. C; 2. C; 3. D; 4. C; 5. D.

SUGGESTED READINGS

Brushart TME. Central course of digital axons within the median nerve. J Comp Neurol 1991;311:197–209.

Chaudhry V, Cornblath DR. Wallerian degeneration in human nerves: serial electrophysiologic studies. Muscle Nerve 1992;15:687–693.

Cornblath DR et al. Conduction block in clinical practice. Muscle Nerve 1991;14:869–871.

Fowler CJ, Danta G, Gilliatt RW. Recovery of nerve conduction after a pneumatic tourniquet: observation on the hind-limb of the baboon. J Neurol Neurosurg Psychiatry 1972;35:638–647.

Gilliatt RW, Taylor JC. Electrical changes following section of the facial nerve. Proc R Soc Med 1959;52:1080.

Jabaley ME, Wallace WH, Heckler FR. Internal topography of major nerves of the forearm and hand: a current view. J Hand Surg [Am] 1980;5:1–18.

Katirji MB, Wilbourn AJ. Common peroneal mononeuropathy: a clinical and electrophysiologic study of 116 lesions. Neurology 1988;38:1723–1728.

Kimura J et al. Relation between size of compound sensory or muscle action potentials, and length of nerve segment. Neurology 1986;36:647–652.

Kline DG. Surgical repair of peripheral nerve injury. Muscle Nerve 1990;13:843–852.

Miller RG. Injury to peripheral motor nerves. Muscle Nerve 1987;10:698–710.

Oh SJ, Kim DE, Kuruoglu HR. What is the best diagnostic index of conduction block and temporal dispersion? Muscle Nerve 1994;17:489–493.

Rhee RK, England JD, Sumner AJ. Computer simulation of conduction block: effects produced by actual block versus interphase cancellation. Ann Neurol 1990;28:146–159.

Robinson LR. Traumatic injury to peripheral nerves. Muscle Nerve 2000;23:863–873.

Seddon H. Three types of nerve injury. Brain 1943;66:237–288.

Spinner RJ, Kline DG. Surgery for peripheral nerve and brachial plexus injuries or other nerve lesions. Muscle Nerve 2000;23:680–695.

Stewart JD. Peripheral nerve fascicles: anatomy and clinical relevance. Muscle Nerve 2003;28:525–541.

Sunderland S. The anatomy and physiology of nerve injury. Muscle Nerve 1990;13:771–784.

Sunderland S. Nerve injuries and their repair: a critical appraisal. Edinburgh: Churchill Livingstone, 1991.

Taylor PK. CMAP dispersion, amplitude decay and area decay in a normal population. Muscle Nerve 1993;16:1181–1187.

Wilbourn AJ. Nerve conduction studies: types, components, abnormalities and value in localization. Neurol Clin N Am 2002;20:305–338.

Case 2

HISTORY AND PHYSICAL EXAMINATION

Right buttock pain developed in a 67-year-old man, radiating to the lateral thigh and pretibial area. The pain worsened when he walked. Within a few weeks, he became aware of right foot weakness with partial footdrop. There had been no sensory symptoms. He did not respond to conservative therapy and was referred for an electrodiagnostic (EDX) examination. Past medical history was otherwise negative.

On neurological examination, the patient had moderate weakness of right foot and toe dorsiflexion, and ankle eversion and inversion (Medical Research Council [MRC] 4–/5) and severe weakness of right large toe dorsiflexion (MRC 3/5). Plantar flexion was minimally weak (MRC 5–/5). Deep tendon reflexes were normal except for trace ankle jerks bilaterally. Sensory examination revealed relative impairment of pain sensation over the dorsum of the foot. Straight leg raise was negative. The patient's gait was impaired by the partial right footdrop.

Please now review the Nerve Conduction Studies and Needle EMG tables.

QUESTIONS

1. The EMG findings are diagnostic of:
   A. A lumbosacral plexopathy.
   B. An L5 more than S1 radiculopathy due to a herniated disc at the L5–S1 space.
   C. An L5 more than S1 radiculopathy due to a herniated disc at the L4–L5 space.
   D. A sciatic neuropathy.
   E. An L5 more than S1 radiculopathy.

2. All of the following findings are consistent with an S1 radiculopathy *except:*
   A. Fibrillation potentials in the abductor hallucis.
   B. Fibrillation potentials in the medial head of the gastrocnemius.
   C. Fibrillation potentials in the flexor digitorum longus.
   D. Fibrillation potentials in the gluteus maximus.
   E. Absent sural sensory nerve action potentials (SNAPs).

3. In an L5 radiculopathy of about 6 months' duration, which muscle is likely to show the most amount of fibrillation potentials?
   A. Biceps femoris (short head).
   B. Extensor hallucis longus.
   C. Gluteus medius.
   D. Lumbar paraspinal muscles.
   E. Tensor fascia lata.

EDX FINDINGS AND INTERPRETATION OF DATA

Relevant EDX findings in this patient are:

1. Low-amplitude peroneal compound muscle action potentials (CMAPs), recording extensor digitorum brevis (EDB = L5, S1) and tibialis anterior (TA = L4, L5), at all points of stimulation, with no evidence of conduction block or focal slowing. The amplitudes are low when compared to normal values and, more importantly, to values in the contralateral asymptomatic limb. The mild slowing of peroneal motor distal latencies and conduction velocities, recording EDB and TA, is appropriate for the significant loss of CMAP amplitude and is best explained by the loss of large and fast-conducting axons.

Case 2: Nerve Conduction Studies

Nerve Stimulated	Stimulation Site	Recording Site	Amplitude (m = mV, s = μV)			Distal/Peak Latency (ms)			Conduction Velocity (m/s)			F Latency (ms)	
			Right	Left	Normal	Right	Left	Normal	Right	Left	Normal	Right	Left
Sural (s)	Calf	Ankle	8		≥3	3.5		≤4.6					
Super peron. (s)	Lateral leg	Ankle	6	5	≥3	3.6	3.8	≤4.6					
Peroneal (m)	Ankle	EDB	**0.8**	3.0	≥2.5	**6.9**	4.4	≤6.0				**NR**	49
Peroneal (m)	Bel. fibular head	EDB	**0.8**						38		≥40		
Peroneal (m)	Knee	EDB	**0.7**						39		≥40		
Peroneal (m)	Bel. fibular head	Tibialis anterior	**0.8**	4.5	≥3	**4.1**	2.6	≤4.0					
Peroneal (m)	Knee	Tibialis anterior	**0.8**						**35**		≥40		
Tibial (m)	Ankle	AH	8.0			5.1						53	
Tibial (m)	Knee	AH	6.0		≥4			≤6.0	45		≥40		
H reflex	Knee	Soleus	**NR**	2.0		**NR**	33						
M response	Knee	Soleus	6.0	7.0		5.8	5.7						

AH = abductor hallucis; Bel. fibular head = below fibular head; EDB = extensor digitorum brevis; m = motor; NR = no response; s = sensory; Super peron. = superficial peroneal. Data in bold type are abnormal.

Case 2: Needle EMG

| Muscle | Insertional Activity | Spontaneous Activity | | Voluntary Motor Action Potentials (MUAPs) | | | | | | | |
| | | | | Recruitment | | | | Configuration | | | Others |
		Fibs	Fasces	Normal	Activation	Reduced	Early	Duration	Amplitude	% Polyphasia	
R. tibialis anterior	↑↑	2+	0			↓↓↓		↑	Normal	Normal	3 MUPS
Medial gastrocnemius	↑	+/−	0			↓		↑	Normal	Normal	
Flexor digit longus	↑↑	3+	0			↓↓↓		↑↑	Normal	↑	1 MUP
Tibialis posterior	↑↑	3+	0			↓↓↓		↑↑	Normal	Normal	1 MUP
Extensor digit brevis	↓	0	0			↓↓		↑	Normal	Normal	
Extensor hallucis	↑	1+	0			↓↓↓		↑	Normal	↑	
Abductor hallucis	↑	1+	0	X				Normal	Normal	Normal	
Vastus lateralis	Normal	0	0	X				Normal	Normal	Normal	
Vastus intermedius	Normal	0	0	X		↓		↑	Normal	↑	
Gluteus medius	↑	+/−	0	−							
Upper lumbar paraspinal	Normal	0	0	−							
Middle lumbar paraspinal	↑	+/−	0	−							
Low lumbar paraspinal	↑	+/−	0	−							
Upper sacral paraspinal	↑	+/−	0	−							
L. tibialis anterior	Normal	0	0	X							
Tibialis posterior	Normal	0	0	X							

Extensor digit brevis = extensor digitorum brevis; Fascs = fasciculations; Fibs = fibrillations; Flexor digit longus = flexor digitorum longus; L. = left; MUP = motor unit potential; R. = right; ↑ = increased; ↓ = mildly reduced; ↓↓ = moderately reduced; ↓↓↓ = severely reduced.

2. Normal and symmetrical superficial peroneal sensory nerve action potentials (SNAPs).

   - Together, these two findings (1 and 2) are extremely helpful and suggest one of two possibilities: (1) a severe axon-loss, selective, deep peroneal nerve lesion (sparing the superficial branch), or (2) a severe L5 root lesion (i.e., a preganglionic L5 lesion) because both recording muscles (EDB and TA) get innervation via the L5 root. Axonal lesions of the common peroneal nerve, the sciatic nerve, or the lumbosacral plexus are extremely unlikely because they would result in absent or low-amplitude superficial peroneal SNAP and possibly the sural SNAP.

3. The H reflex is asymmetrically absent on the right, with normal response on the left. However, the right M response, recording soleus-gastrocnemius (S1), is normal and symmetrical when compared to the left.

4. The tibial motor study is normal.

5. The sural sensory study is normal.

   - The above three findings (3, 4, and 5), when interpreted together, suggest that the S1 root may be also involved in this patient with little or no significant axon loss since the M response, recording soleus-gastrocnemius (S1), and the tibial motor amplitude are normal. Although a tibial, sciatic, or sacral plexus lesion may also result in an absent H reflex, these conditions often result in an absent or low-amplitude sural SNAP.

6. The needle EMG confirms that the lesion is not restricted to the deep peroneal nerve because many muscles outside its innervation are affected. Of the muscles tested, the tibialis posterior and the flexor digitorum longus are the most relevant in this case because these muscles have a predominant L5 innervation but are innervated by the tibial nerve. Fibrillation potentials in the gluteus medius and paraspinal muscles are another supportive finding of an L5 lesion. The needle EMG examination also confirms slight S1 fibers' axonal loss, as evidenced by fibrillation potentials in the medial gastrocnemius (S1) and the abductor hallucis (S1, S2), both with no L5 representation. Finally, the needle EMG shows no evidence of a contralateral L5 or S1 involvement.

In *summary*, the findings in this case are consistent with a severe right L5 radiculopathy, with mild involvement of the right S1 root. The L5 lesion is severe and axonal, based mainly on low-amplitude CMAPs recording L5 innervated muscles (TA and EDB) and supported by fibrillation potentials and very few voluntary motor unit action potentials (MUAPs) in all distal L5-innervated muscles (tibialis anterior, extensor hallucis, tibialis posterior, flexor digitorum longus, and extensor digitorum brevis). However, the

S1 lesion is mild, with minimal axonal loss because the CMAP amplitudes recording S1 muscles (abductor hallucis and soleus) are normal, and many voluntary MUAPs are present.

DISCUSSION

Applied Anatomy

The dorsal root axons originate from the sensory neurons of the dorsal root ganglia (DRG), which lie outside the spinal canal within the intervertebral foramen (Figure C2–1), and immediately before the dorsal and ventral roots are joined. These sensory neurons are unique because they are unipolar. They have proximal projections through the dorsal root,

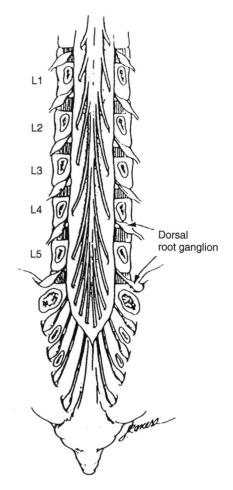

Figure C2–1. *Sagittal section of the lumbar spine, showing the location of the dorsal root ganglia in relation to the spinal canal. Note that the dorsal root ganglia are located in the distal cauda equina within the intervertebral foramen. (From Brown WF, Bolton CF. Clinical electromyography, 2nd ed. Boston, MA: Butterworth-Heinemann, 1993.)*

called the *preganglionic sensory fibers*, which extend to the dorsal horn and column of the spinal cord. The distal projections of these neurons, called the *postganglionic sensory fibers*, join the motor fibers in the ventral root to form the spinal nerve, and then pass through the corresponding peripheral nerve to reach their respective sensory endorgans. The ventral root axons are mainly motor, and originate from the anterior horn cells within the spinal cord. Passing through the spinal nerves and the peripheral nerve, these motor fibers terminate in the corresponding muscles. At each intervertebral foramen, a mixed spinal nerve is formed by the fusion of the dorsal (afferent, sensory) and ventral (efferent, motor, and sympathetic) roots. Nerve roots have no epineurium and less collagen than peripheral nerves, which result in increased susceptibility to compression, stretch, and infiltration.

Each spinal nerve divides as soon as it exits the intervertebral foramina into posterior and anterior rami. The small posterior ramus innervates the paravertebral skin and the deep paraspinal muscles of the neck, trunk, or back. The large anterior ramus innervates the skin and muscles of the remaining trunk or limbs.

In humans, there are 31 pairs of spinal nerve roots: 8 cervical, 12 thoracic, 5 lumbar, 5 sacral, and 1 coccygeal. In the cervical spine, each cervical root exits above the corresponding vertebra that shares the same numeric designation. For example, the C5 root exits above the C5 vertebra (i.e., between the C4 and C5 vertebrae). Because there are seven cervical vertebrae but eight cervical roots, the C8 root exits between the C7 and T1 vertebrae; subsequently, *all thoracic, lumbar, and sacral roots exit below their corresponding vertebrae* (Figure C2–2). For example, the L3 root exits below the L3 vertebra (i.e., between the L3 and L4 vertebrae).

In adults, the spinal cord ends at the L1 vertebra, resulting in a disparity between the lengths of the vertebral column and the spinal cord. Hence, spinal cord segments, mostly the thoracic and lumbar, are higher than the corresponding vertebras. This disparity is most pronounced in the lumbar region where there is a difference of approximately three segments, while there is usually a two-segment disparity in the thoracic region (see Figure C2–2). Since the cord terminates at L1 vertebra, the lumbosacral roots traverse relatively long intraspinal courses before exiting through their respective intervertebral foramina, thus forming the cauda equina. Due to the intricate anatomic relationships between the cauda equina and lumbar spinal column, a disc herniation at one level may injure different nerve roots and the vertebral level of a lumbosacral root compression does not always correlate with its exit level. For example, the S1 root is most often compressed by a posterolateral L5–S1 disc herniation (Figure C2–3). Also, the L5 root may be compressed by any disc herniation up to the level of conus medullaris at

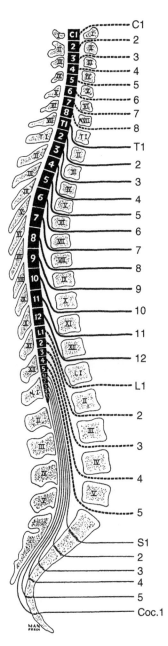

Figure C2–2. *Alignments of spinal segments and roots to vertebrae. The bodies and spinal processes of the vertebrae are indicated by Roman numerals, and the spinal segments and their respective roots by Arabic numerals. Note that the cervical roots (except C8) exit through the intervertebral foramina above their respective bodies, and that all other roots leave below these bodies. (From Haymaker W, Woodhall B. Peripheral nerve injuries: principles of diagnosis. Philadelphia, PA: WB Saunders, 1953, with permission.)*

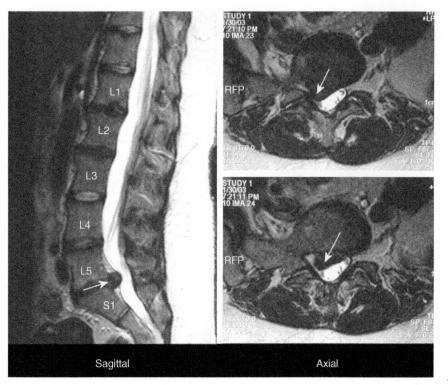

Sagittal   Axial

Figure C2–3. *A 42-year-old woman presented with a severe right buttock pain radiating to posterior thigh and calf for 2 months. Neurological examination reveals depressed right ankle jerk only. EDX study reveals fibrillation potentials in the gastrocnemius, biceps femoris, gluteus maximus, and low lumbar paraspinal muscles with normal MUAP recruitment and morphology and normal sural sensory SNAP. The H reflex was absent on the right. T2-weighted MRI of the lumbar spine reveals a large right posterolateral L5–S1 disc herniation (arrows). Note also that several discs (L1–2, L2–3, L4–5, and L5–S1) reveal decreased T2-weighted signal consistent with multilevel degeneration of nucleus pulposus. The patient had complete relief of pain after laminectomy and diskectomy with no further symptoms with a 4-year follow-up.*

or rostral to L5–S1 (see Figure C2–2), including a lateral L5–S1 disc herniation and a posterolateral L4–L5 disc herniation. Less often, the L4–L5 disc may protrudes laterally into the foramen at that level and compress the exiting L4 root. If large, the lateral disc may injure both the L4 and L5 roots. Finally, if the L4–L5 disc herniation is central, it may compress several roots on one or both sides of the cauda equina, often asymmetrically.

Clinical Features

Low back pain is an extremely common symptom, but only a relatively small number of patients with low back pain have root compression in the lumbar region. Lumbosacral radiculopathy may be due to a variety of causes (Table C2–1), but is often caused by disc herniation, spondylitic changes (especially at the facetal joints leading to foraminal stenosis), or calcification of the ligamentum flavum. When combined, these changes can result in acquired lumbar canal stenosis. Disc herniation is more common in patients younger than 50 years while degenerative and spondylotic changes are more common in patients older than 50 years.

Clinically, root compression often manifests by involvement of the sensory fibers, sensory and motor fibers, or rarely motor fibers only. Hence, the symptoms of lumbosacral radiculopathy include pain, tingling, numbness, or weakness. The pain and the sensory symptoms may be provoked by coughing, sneezing, or other Valsalva maneuvers, and often follow typical dermatomal distributions (radicular pain) that are useful in localization. Similarly, when weakness or reflex changes occur, they follow a corresponding segmental distribution.

Table C2–1. Causes of Lumbosacral Radiculopathy

Degenerative lumbar spine disease
    Lumbosacral disc herniation
    Lumbosacral spondylosis
    Lumbar canal stenosis
Neoplasms
    Epidural metastasis
    Vertebral metastasis
    Leptomeningeal carcinomatosus
    Primary schwannoma and meningioma
Infections
    Epidural abscess
    Lyme
    Herpes zoster
    Cytomeglovirus
    HIV
Others
    Epidural hematoma
    Epidural lipomatosis
    Spinal arachnoiditis
    Sarcoidosis
    Cyst
    Tethered cord
    Diabetes

Table C2–2 lists common findings in patients with the various lumbosacral radiculopathy. Straight leg raise test is a maneuver that causes stretching of the sciatic nerve, sacral plexus, and the L5 and S1 nerve roots. While the patient is supine, the pain is reproduced with passive straight leg raising or when the examiner flexes the leg at the hip and then extends it at the knee. The test is most reliable when it is positive between 30° and 70°. Reverse straight leg raise testing is performed by passive hip extension while the patient is prone and causes stretching of the femoral nerve, the lumbar plexus, and upper lumbar roots (L2, L3, or L4). Pain in the groin or anterior thigh is considered a positive test.

Lumbosacral root compression may involve a single root (monoradiculopathy) or multiple roots that are contiguous and may be bilateral (polyradiculopathy). Cauda equina lesions should be considered when more than two contiguous nerve roots are involved. *Midline cauda equina syndrome* results in early compression of sacral nerve roots, which lie medially within the cauda equina, leading to low back pain, sphincteric and sexual dysfunction, and paresthesias and sensory loss in sacral dermatomes ("saddle anesthesia"). When the lesion is large (such as with large midline L4–5 disc herniation), lumbosacral nerve roots may be involved resulting in leg weakness and sensory loss that may develop either early or later in the course, and sometimes result in paraplegia when multiple bilateral nerve roots are involved. Another clinically distinct cauda equina syndrome is the one caused by *lumbar canal stenosis* (Figure C2–4). This often presents with intermittent neurogenic claudication which is characterized by low back and leg pain, sometimes with paresthesias and weakness, brought on by standing and often worsened by walking. Typically, the symptoms are completely relieved several minutes after the patient sits down and are occasionally improved by bending at the waist. The symptoms are often bilateral but may be unilateral. The neurological examination in patients with lumbar canal stenosis may be entirely normal or show evidence of a single lumbosacral monoradiculopathy or patchy lumbosacral polyradiculopathy often involving the L4, L5, or S1 roots.

Electrodiagnosis

General Concepts

It is essential to appreciate certain general concepts before one can make such a diagnosis in the EMG laboratory.

1. *The SNAPs are normal in radiculopathy despite the presence of sensory loss.* Compression of the dorsal (sensory) root, from either disc herniation or spondylosis, usually occurs within the spinal canal proximal to the DRG and results in injury of the preganglionic sensory fibers, but leaves the postganglionic sensory fibers intact (Figure C2–5).
2. *Compression of the ventral (motor) root may cause demyelination or axon loss, or both.* As with focal lesions of peripheral nerves, this leads to different EDX findings:
   - With axon loss, wallerian degeneration occurs. Its effect is readily recognized by the presence of fibrillation potentials, long-duration and high-amplitude

Table C2–2. Common Clinical Presentations in Patients With Lumbosacral Radiculopathies

	Pain Radiation	Sensory Impairment	Provocative Test	Weakness	Hypo/Areflexia
L1	To groin	Inguinal region	None	None	None
L2	To groin and anterior thigh	Anterolateral thigh	Reversed straight leg test	Hip flexion	None
L3	To anterior thigh and knee	Groin and medial thigh	Reversed straight leg test	Hip flexion and adduction, and knee extension	Knee jerk
L4	To anterior thigh, knee, and medial foreleg	Anterior thigh and medial leg	Reversed straight leg test	Knee extension, hip adduction, and ankle dorsiflexion	Knee jerk
L5	To buttock, lateral thigh and leg, and dorsal foot	Lateral leg, dorsal foot, and big toe	Straight leg test	Toe and ankle dorsiflexion, inversion and eversion	None
S1	To buttock, posterior thigh and leg, and lateral foot	Posterior thigh, lateral foot, and little toe	Straight leg test	Plantar flexion, toe flexion	Ankle jerk

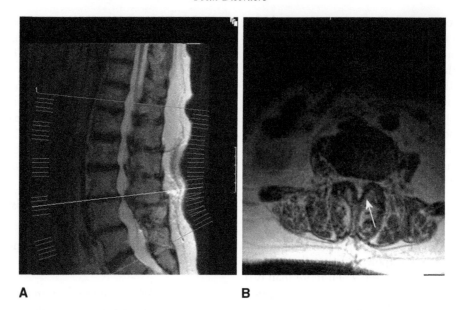

A   **B**

Figure C2–4. *A 75-year-old woman developed neurogenic claudication (pain in both posterior thigh and legs upon standing and walking relieved by rest) and had a normal neurological examination (except for absent ankle jerks bilaterally). EDX study showed chronic reinnervation changes without fibrillation potentials in the tibialis anterior, extensor hallucis, gastrocnemius, and biceps femoris bilaterally, with normal sural and superficial peroneal sensory responses and absent H reflexes consistent with chronic bilateral L5 and S1 radiculopathies. MRI of the lumbar spine reveals multilevel lumbar canal stenosis, worst at L3–4. (**A**) Sagittal T2-weighted image. (**B**) Axial T2-weighted image through L3–4 disc (as shown in **A**). Note the significant lumbar canal stenosis at L3–4 mostly due to ligamentum flavum thickening and bilateral facetal hypertrophy. The enlarged facet joints encroach on the posterolateral aspect of the spinal canal, creating a trefoil appearance on axial section (arrow). The patient responded very well to an L3–4 epidural block with steroids.*

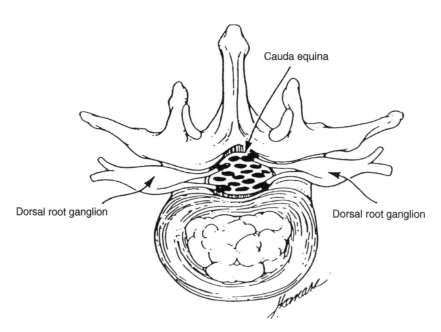

Figure C2–5. *Axial section through the lumbar region showing a common site of root compression. (From Brown WF, Bolton CF. Clinical electromyography, 2nd ed. Boston, MA: Butterworth-Heinemann, 1993.)*

MUAPs, and, when severe, low-amplitude CMAPs. *The needle EMG is the most sensitive electrodiagnostic test for the diagnosis of radiculopathy,* since it may diagnose mild axonal loss by detecting fibrillation potentials generated by the loss of only a few motor axons.

- With pure demyelination, there is either focal slowing or conduction block; both cannot be evaluated well because roots are not accessible to conduction studies (despite attempts to use magnetic or direct needle stimulation). Thus, apart from weakness (and reduced MUAP recruitment), EDX studies might be otherwise normal.

3. *The EMG examination determines the injured lumbosacral root(s), and not the vertebral level(s) of root compression or disc herniation.* In the lumbar region only, and due to the intricate anatomic relationships between the nerve roots and spinal column, the vertebral level of root compression or disc herniation does not always correlate with the involved root. This is because the spinal cord ends at the L1 vertebral level in adults, and the roots have to travel a relatively long distance before they exit at their respective intervertebral foramina, thereby forming the cauda equina (see Figure C2–2). Thus, in contrast to the cervical and thoracic regions, the EMG performed in the lumbar region has a suboptimal value in predicting the site of the vertebral compression.

4. *The needle EMG remains by far the most sensitive electrodiagnostic tool in patients with suspected radiculopathy.* Other electrophysiologic studies, including somatosensory evoked potentials, nerve conduction studies, late responses, and thermography, are much less sensitive and their use in practice is limited.

5. *By far, the most objective EMG finding in radiculopathy is the presence of fibrillation potentials.* Decrease recruitment and large or polyphasic MUAPs are useful findings but when these abnormalities are mild they are more difficult to analyze and may be subject to debate by different observers. Hence, the accuracies of these MUAP findings vary according to the electromyographer's experience.

6. *Fibrillation potentials seldom are found in the entire myotomal distribution of the compressed root.* This is best explained by one or more of the following reasons:
   - Root compression usually results in partial motor axon loss. Hence, some muscles innervated by the injured root may "escape" denervation and remain normal.
   - Proximal muscles innervated by the compressed root undergo more effective collateral sprouting and reinnervation than do distal muscles. This leads to

the disappearance of fibrillation potentials in proximal muscles. Hence, in chronic radiculopathy it is more likely to find fibrillation potentials in distal than proximal muscles, despite being innervated by the same root. For example, in L5 radiculopathy, it is more likely to detect fibrillation potentials in the tibialis posterior than in the gluteus medius; both have a preponderant innervation by the L5 root.
   - There is likely significant myotomal variability among individuals.

7. *F waves are rarely abnormal in radiculopathy.* Despite early enthusiasm about the utility of F waves, which test the integrity of the entire motor axon including the ventral roots, the F waves are not sensitive in the diagnosis of lumbosacral radiculopathies for the following reasons:
   - The recorded muscle frequently is innervated by more than one root. Thus, in a single-level radiculopathy, normal conduction through the intact neighboring root results in normal F wave minimal latency. For example, in L5 radiculopathy, the peroneal F wave recorded from the extensor digitorum brevis muscle (innervated by L5 and S1 roots) frequently is normal because the compression is concealed by a normal S1 root.
   - F wave latency is the most reproducible and clinically useful parameter. However, root compression resulting in significant motor axon loss can be associated with normal F wave latencies because the surviving axons are conducting normally.
   - If focal slowing occurs at the root segment of the motor axon, the delay in F wave latency may be obscured, because the latency becomes diluted by the relatively long motor axon.

Goals of the Electrodiagnostic Study

The EMG examination plays a pivotal role in the diagnosis, and sometimes the management, of lumbosacral radiculopathy. The diagnostic aims of the EMG examination in radiculopathy are to:

1. Exclude a more distal lesion (i.e., plexopathy or a mononeuropathy).
2. Confirm evidence of root compression.
3. Localize the compression to either a single or multiple roots.
4. Define the age and activity of the lesion.
5. Define the severity of the lesion.

Exclude a More Distal Nerve Lesion

Distinguishing a mononeuropathy from radiculopathy is relatively easy when the focal peripheral nerve lesion is associated with conduction block or focal slowing, such as in peroneal mononeuropathy at the fibular neck. Also, fibrillation potentials and MUAP denervation and reinnervation changes are limited to the muscles of the affected peripheral nerve in axon-loss mononeuropathy, while these abnormalities are widespread in radiculopathy and involve muscles that share a segmental innervation, irrespective of their peripheral nerves.

Distinguishing a lumbosacral plexus lesion from lumbosacral radiculopathy is clinically difficult because the same fibers are affected in both cases. Electrodiagnostically, the differential diagnosis depends mainly on two procedures: needle EMG of the paraspinal muscles and assessment of the SNAPs.

- The presence of fibrillation potentials in paraspinal muscles is not consistent with a lumbosacral plexus lesion because these muscles are innervated by the posterior primary rami that leave the spinal roots soon after the intervertebral foramina. Unfortunately, fibrillation potentials are not always present in the paraspinal muscles in chronic radiculopathy, presumably due to effective reinnervation of these muscles.

- SNAPs usually are abnormally low in amplitude or are absent in axon-loss lumbosacral plexopathy, because the lesion affects the postganglionic fibers. In contrast, these studies are normal in radiculopathy, in which compression involves the preganglionic fibers only (i.e., sensory fibers proximal to the DRG). The utility of the SNAP in the confirmation of lumbosacral radiculopathy has however several limitations:

  (a) The upper lumbar roots (L2 and L3) do not have a technically feasible SNAP.

  (b) The saphenous SNAP, which assesses the L4 root, may be difficult to evoke or absent in a large number of individuals, especially in the elderly, obese, and those with leg edema.

  (c) All the SNAPS of the lower extremities may be absent in the elderly, obese, and those with underlying polyneuropathy or leg edema.

  (d) The superficial peroneal SNAP is occasionally low in amplitude or absent in L5 radiculopathy. This is explained by an intraspinal location of the L5 DRG rendering the ganglion itself vulnerable to compression by disc herniation or foraminal spondylosis.

  (e) The SNAP amplitudes may be low or absent if the DRGs are involved by the pathological condition that may affect the DRG preferentially or extend from the intraspinal space through the neural foramen to the extraspinal space or vice versa. Examples include infiltrative malignancy such as lymphoma, infection such as herpes zoster, tumor such as schwannoma or meningioma, or autoimmune attack on DRG such as in Sjogren syndrome or with small-cell lung cancer.

Confirm Evidence of Root Compression

Two criteria are necessary to establish the diagnosis of radiculopathy:

1. *Denervation in a segmental myotomal distribution* (i.e., in muscles innervated by the same roots via more than one peripheral nerve), with or without denervation of the paraspinal muscles. At least two muscles, and preferably more, should reveal evidence of denervation (fibrillation potentials and/or reinnervation MUAP changes and reduced recruitment). Fibrillation potentials in the paraspinal muscles are strong evidence of a root lesion within the spinal canal. However, they may be absent particularly in chronic radiculopathies, likely due to effective reinnervation.

2. *Normal SNAP of the corresponding dermatome.* Once myotomal denervation is detected by needle EMG, the lesion must be confirmed as preganglionic (i.e., within the spinal canal) and not postganglionic (i.e., due to a lumbosacral plexus injury). This can be achieved by recording one or more dermatomal SNAPs, appropriate for the myotome involved, and then establishing SNAP normality. For example, in a suspected S1 radiculopathy, the sural SNAP should be performed, sometimes bilaterally for comparison. Table C2–3 lists technically feasible SNAPs with their corresponding roots that are helpful in confirming the diagnosis of lumbosacral radiculopathy. Note again that no SNAP has been devised to assess the L2 or L3 fibers, the saphenous SNAP is technically not reliable in assessment of the L4 fibers, and the superficial peroneal SNAP is occasionally low or absent in L5 radiculopathy. Also, all the lower extremity SNAPs frequently are often unevokable bilaterally in elderly or obese patients. These SNAP limitations result in difficulty to differentiate a preganglionic lesion (i.e., lumbosacral radiculopathy) from a postganglionic lesion (i.e., lumbosacral plexopathy), unless fibrillation potentials are evident in the paraspinal muscles.

Table C2–3. Lower Extremity Sensory Nerve Action Potentials (SNAPs) and their Segmental Representation

Root	SNAP
S1	Sural
L5	Superficial peroneal
L4	Saphenous*

*Saphenous SNAP is not always technically reliable especially in the elderly.

Localize the Compression to One or Multiple Roots

This requires meticulous knowledge of the segmental innervation of limb muscles (myotomes). Many myotomal charts have been devised, with significant variability; this may lead to confusion and disagreement between the EMG and the level of root compression as seen by imaging techniques or during surgery. EMG-derived charts also are very helpful and have had anatomic verification (see Tsao et al.). Figure C2–6 shows a common and most useful EMG-extracted myotomal chart.

A minimal "root search" should be performed in all patients with suspected lumbosacral radiculopathy to

Table C2–4. Suggested Muscles to be Sampled in Suspected Lumbosacral Radiculopathy

Muscle	Root Innervation*
Tibialis anterior	**L4**, **L5**
Medial gastrocnemius	**S1**, S2
Flexor digitorum longus and tibialis posterior	**L5**, S1
Extensor digitorum brevis	**L5**, **S1**
Vastus lateralis and medialis	**L2**, **L3**, **L4**
Biceps femoris (short or long head)	L5, **S1**
Gluteus medius and tensor fascia lata	**L5**, S1
Mid: lumbar paraspinal	
Low: lumbar paraspinal	

*Roots in bold type represent the major innervation.

ensure that a radiculopathy either is confirmed or excluded. In other words, certain muscles of strategic value in EMG, because of their segmental innervation, should be sampled in these patients (Table C2–4). When abnormalities are found or when the clinical manifestations suggest a specific root compression, more muscles must be sampled, after being selected based on their innervation (see Figure C2–6), to verify the diagnosis and to establish the exact root(s) compressed. In contrast to limb muscles, fibrillation potentials in the paraspinal muscles are not useful in the diagnosis of the specific compressed root, though they often confirm that the lesion is intraspinal. This is due to observations that each primary posterior ramus has a highly variable segmental innervation that may extend up to 6 segments beyond the vertebral level of its root exit.

Define the Age and Activity of the Radiculopathy

Changes seen on needle EMG help to determine the age of the lesion in an axon loss radiculopathy. As with many processes wherein motor axon loss occurs, increased insertional activity is the first abnormality seen and, when isolated, suggests that the process may be only 1–2 weeks old. Fibrillation potentials, which are spontaneous action potentials generated by denervated muscle fibers, develop soon after and become full after 3 weeks from acute motor axonal loss. These potentials often appear first in the lumbar paraspinal muscles, then in proximal muscles, and lastly in distal muscles. They also disappear after reinnervation or following muscle fiber fatty degeneration.

As time elapses, collateral sprouting from intact axons results in MUAPs with polyphasia and satellite potentials. These MUAPs, usually seen after 2 to 3 months from acute injury, are often unstable by showing moment-to-moment

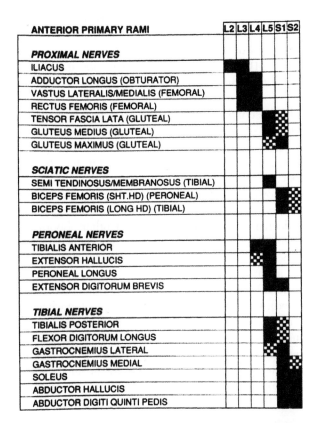

Figure C2–6. *Chart of lower extremity muscles useful in the needle electromyographic recognition of lumbosacral radiculopathy. Solid squares indicate muscles that most often contain abnormalities, and checkered squares indicate muscles that are abnormal less frequently. (From Brown WF, Bolton CF. Clinical electromyography, 2nd ed. Boston, MA: Butterworth-Heinemann, 1993.)*

variation in morphology. With further time, MUAPs with high amplitude and long duration dominate, reflecting a more complete reinnervation and the chronicity of the root compression.

In assessing a patient with possible lumbosacral radiculopathy, it is often important to comment on whether the root compression is chronic or ongoing (active). This is easy when one encounters large and stable MUAPs, reflecting chronicity, along with fibrillation potentials, reflecting ongoing (active) denervation. In contrast, when fibrillation potentials are absent, it is presumed that the findings are chronic and remote, such as in a patient with a prior history of a severe lumbosacral radiculopathy. This simplistic differentiation has, however, several limitations:

- It is not uncommon that the electromyographer cannot distinguish with certainty between a patient with chronic ongoing root compression (such as with spondylosis) from one with chronic remote (old) root compression (such as with a prior disc herniation). In situations where the rate of motor axon loss is slow, reinnervation may keep pace with denervation that no or minimal fibrillation potentials are seen on needle EMG. Some electromyographers may erroneously use the absence of fibrillation potentials as absolute evidence against ongoing root compression. A correlation with the clinical history, the neurological findings and the imaging is warranted.
- A contrasting situation arises in patients with remote radiculopathy that has resulted in severe axon loss. In these inactive cases, some muscle fibers never fully reinnervate, especially in distal muscles located farthest from the injury site. In these radicular lesions, fibrillation potentials may continue to be seen in distal muscles, mistakenly suggesting that there is an ongoing axon loss process.
- The postoperative EDX evaluation of patients with lumbosacral radiculopathy is challenging particularly when there was no preoperative EDX study. Since fibrillation potentials may persist for several months despite successive surgery, their presence does not mean a failed surgical procedure. Additionally, fibrillation potentials may be present in the paraspinal muscles after lumbar spine surgery because of muscle denervation during surgical exposure. Because of this, many electromyographers, including the author, will not sample the paraspinal muscles if a patient has a history of lumbar spine surgery. These postoperative EDX studies are often not satisfying to the electromyographer or clinician, since they cannot exclude or confirm persistent root compression.

Define the severity of the radiculopathy

In assessing the severity of a radiculopathy, one tends to rely on the degree of abnormalities seen on needle EMG, namely decreased recruitment ("neurogenic" MUAP firing pattern), fibrillation potentials, and MUAP configuration. Using these parameters in assessing severity of lesion (i.e., extent of axon loss) is suboptimal for the following caveats:

1. Although there is a correlation between the degree of reduced MUAP recruitment and the degree of weakness, decreased recruitment is not necessarily due to axon loss but may be due to conduction block (due to segmental demyelination) at the root level. The latter has a very good prognosis for rapid recovery.
2. Although the presence of fibrillation potentials is consistent with motor axon loss, measuring the number of fibrillation potentials in a muscle is subjective and does not correlate with the degree of axon loss. Fibrillation potentials denote a recent axon loss but cannot assess its severity.
3. MUAP reinnervation changes are permanent. However, reinnervation may be quite robust so that weakness may not be or only minimally detected. Hence, finding very large MUAPs (giant MUAPs) does not always reflect severity or prognosis.

The best indicator of motor axon loss is the *CMAP amplitude* (or area) recorded during routine motor nerve conduction studies of the lower extremity. Although these studies are performed distally and do not include the roots, a root lesion causing demyelinative conduction block (or focal slowing), with little or no accompanying axonal degeneration, may result in weakness, but does not lead to any decrease n CMAP amplitude or other abnormalities on motor conduction studies. Only when significant axonal loss occurs at the root level does the CMAP recording from an involved muscle become low in amplitude (or occasionally absent when multiple adjacent roots are compressed). In acute lesions, this is only detected when sufficient time has elapsed for wallerian degeneration to occur (usually 7–10 days). For example, only in moderate or severe L5 radiculopathy is the peroneal CMAP, recording from extensor digitorum brevis (L5, S1) or tibialis anterior (L4, L5), borderline or low in amplitude at least after 10 days from onset of acute symptoms.

Electrodiagnostic Findings in Lumbosacral Radiculopathies

In patients with unilateral lumbosacral radiculopathy on needle EMG, signs of denervation are frequently present in a contralateral root, usually of the same myotome, and despite the lack of clinical manifestations. This is caused by the unique anatomy of the cauda equina (not present in the cervical and thoracic regions), in which more than one root can be compressed by a single disc herniation. Thus, it is essential to sample a few contralateral muscles, at least of the same affected myotome, in patients with severe lumbosacral radiculopathy.

L2, L3, L4 Radiculopathies

These radiculopathies are less common than the L5 and S1 radiculopathies, probably because of their relatively short course within the cauda equina, which makes them less susceptible to compression. The electrodiagnostic confirmation of an upper lumbar radiculopathy is the most challenging among all lumbosacral radiculopathies because of the following limitations:

- It is often difficult to identify the exact compressed root among these upper lumbar roots because of the limited number of muscles innervated by these roots and the marked overlap in innervation. These muscles include the quadriceps, thigh adductors, the iliacus, and the tibialis anterior (see Figure C2–6). Since not every segmental muscle must be abnormal in radiculopathy, the limited myotomal representation of these roots results in the suboptimal localization power of EMG in these situations. For example, fibrillation potentials in the quadriceps (L2, L3, and L4) and tibialis anterior (L4 and L5) muscles is consistent with an L4 radiculopathy, but does not negate the coexistence of L2 and L3 radiculopathy, even if the iliacus (L2 and L3) is normal. Using the same logic, fibrillation potentials in the quadriceps (L2, L3, and L4) and thigh adductors (L2 and L3) muscles is consistent with compression of the L2 and/or L3 root(s), but it does not rule out a concomitant L4 radiculopathy, even if the tibialis anterior is normal.
- The myotomal representation of these lumbar roots are in proximally situated muscles, mostly above the knee (except for the tibialis anterior). Thus, because of effective sprouting, fibrillation potentials tend to disappear relatively early, resulting in many false-negative EMG results in patients with chronic static upper lumbar root compression.
- There is a lack of available SNAPs for confirming that the upper lumbar lesion is preganglionic. Only a saphenous

SNAP (L4 dermatome) is possible, although difficult to obtain, especially in the elderly. Thus, it is sometimes difficult to separate these upper lumbar radiculopathies from lumbar plexopathy, especially in chronic situations in which fibrillation potentials are less common in the paraspinal muscles. The upper lumbar radiculopathies must also be distinguished from femoral neuropathy (Table C2–5).

L5 Radiculopathy

L5 radiculopathy is the most common radiculopathy seen in the EMG laboratory in general, and in the lower extremity in particular. L5 and S1 root compressions are common because of their long course within the cauda equina (making them susceptible to compression at several intraspinal levels).

L5 radiculopathy is relatively easy to diagnose in the EMG laboratory because L5 muscles are numerous and span the entire lower extremity, both proximally and distally. Because of more effective sprouting in proximal muscles, fibrillation potentials are most prevalent in the L5-innervated muscles located below the knee. Usually, a few or all of the common peroneal muscles (such as the tibialis anterior, the extensor hallucis, the extensor digitorum brevis, and the peroneus longus) are abnormal; however, denervation in the tibial L5-innervated muscles (such as the flexor digitorum longus and the tibialis posterior) is essential for confirmation. Active denervation in proximal muscles, such as the gluteus medius or the tensor fascia lata, is less common, but is very useful when present. Also, fibrillation potentials in the paraspinal muscles, although not always present, are strong supportive evidence for a root lesion.

It is not unusual for patients with severe L5 radiculopathy, in whom significant motor axon loss has occurred, to present with footdrop. In cases associated with motor axon loss, motor nerve conduction studies reveal low-amplitude peroneal CMAPs, recording extensor digitorum brevis and/or tibialis anterior. This mimics a peroneal mononeuropathy,

Table C2–5. Differential Electrodiagnosis of Upper Lumbar Radiculopathy

	Upper Lumbar Radiculopathy (L2, L4, L5)	**Femoral Mononeuropathy**	**Lumbar Plexopathy**
Thigh adductors	Denervation	Normal	Denervation
Tibialis anterior	Denervation*	Normal	Denervation*
Saphenous SNAP†	Normal	Low or absent†	Low or absent†
Paraspinal fibrillations	Usually present	Absent	Absent

*Abnormal in L4 radiculopathy/plexopathy only.
†May be technically difficult, particularly in elderly patients, or if there is leg edema.
‡Normal in purely demyelinating lesions.

especially of the deep branch. In these situations, denervation in the tibialis posterior and/or the flexor digitorum longus excludes a selective peroneal lesion because these are tibial innervated muscles (Table C2–6). Thus, *needle EMG of the tibialis posterior and/or the flexor digitorum longus is essential in all patients presenting with footdrop.*

Finally, to confirm that the compressive lesion is in the intraspinal canal (i.e., preganglionic), the superficial peroneal SNAP (L5 dermatome) should be normal. The superficial peroneal SNAP is occasionally asymmetrically low in amplitude or absent in L5 radiculopathy. This is explained by an intraspinal location of the L5 DRG rendering the ganglion itself vulnerable to compression by disc herniation or foraminal spondylosis.

S1, S2 Radiculopathy

S1 radiculopathy is common and often due to posterolateral disc herniation (see Figure C2–3). It is difficult to distinguish S1 from S2 radiculopathy (though the latter is rare), because their myotomal representations overlap almost completely. As with the L5 root, the segmental distribution of the S1 root is diffuse, with both proximal and distal muscle representation. Again, here distal muscles (below the knee), such as the medial and lateral heads of the gastrocnemius, soleus, or abductor hallucis, are more likely to reveal fibrillation potentials. Unfortunately, these S1/S2 muscles are all of tibial innervation, and fibrillation potentials must be found in other nerve distributions. The extensor digitorum brevis is the only distal peroneal muscle with substantial S1 innervation, but this muscle is subject to atrophy and chronic denervation, probably from local trauma. Proximal muscles such as the biceps femoris

or gluteus maximus can be useful, but these are more subject to sprouting, which abolishes fibrillation potentials.

In S1 radiculopathy, the sural SNAP (S1 dermatomal SNAP) should be normal. Also, fibrillation potentials in the paraspinal muscles, although not always present, are strong evidence for a radiculopathy.

It is generally accepted that the H reflex is helpful in the diagnosis of S1 radiculopathy. The tibial H reflex is the clinical counterpart of the ankle jerk; it tests the integrity of the entire S1 reflex arc, including the Ia afferent fibers, the spinal cord S1 segment, and the alpha motor efferent fibers (see Chapter 3). It is the only test available within the routine EDX test that includes the preganglionic segment of the sensory fibers of the S1 root. The amplitude of the tibial H wave correlates well with the magnitude of the ankle jerk. Controversy continues regarding whether the amplitude or the latency asymmetry is more valuable in S1 radiculopathy. Although a unilaterally absent or abnormally low amplitude or slow latency is common in S1 radiculopathy, certain limitations exist:

- An abnormal H reflex does not localize the lesion to the S1 root because any pathologic process along its long arc may result in an abnormal H reflex.
- A normal H reflex does not exclude an S1 radiculopathy because the H reflex is not always abnormal in definite cases of S1 radiculopathy.
- The H reflex is commonly absent bilaterally in elderly patients and in patients with polyneuropathy.

As with other lumbosacral radiculopathies, bilateral S1/S2 radiculopathies are relatively common, and most are chronic. Because the symptoms usually are bilateral and involve the feet predominantly, these cases may imitate a peripheral

Table C2–6. Electrophysiological Differentiation Between L5 Radiculopathy and Peroneal Mononeuropathy

	L5 Radiculopathy	**Peroneal Mononeuropathy**
Nerve Conduction Studies		
Peroneal CMAP recording extensor digitorum brevis	Normal or low amplitude	Conduction block at fibular head or low amplitude or both
Peroneal CMAP recording tibialis anterior	Normal or low amplitude	Conduction block at fibular head or low amplitude or both
Superficial peroneal SNAP	Frequently normal	Low/absent; normal in deep peroneal or purely demyelinating lesions
Needle EMG		
Tibialis anterior	Abnormal	Abnormal
Extensor digitorum brevis	Abnormal	Abnormal
Extensor hallucis	Abnormal	Abnormal
Peroneus longus	Abnormal	Abnormal; normal in selective deep peroneal lesions
Tibialis posterior	Abnormal	Normal
Flexor digitorum longus	Abnormal	Normal
Gluteus medius	May be normal	Normal
Tensor fascia lata	May be normal	Normal
Lumbar paraspinals	May be normal	Normal

Table C2–7. Electrophysiological Differentiation of Chronic S1/S2 Radiculopathy

	Chronic S1/S2 Radiculopathy	Tarsal Tunnel Syndrome	Peripheral Polyneuropathy
Nerve Conduction Studies			
Sural sensory study	Normal	Normal	Abnormal
Peroneal motor study	Normal or low amplitude	Normal	Abnormal
Tibial motor study	Normal or low amplitude	Low amplitude and/or slow latency	Low amplitude and/or slow latency
Motor conduction velocities	Normal or slowed	Normal	Slowed
Plantar studies	Normal	Slow latency or absent	Slow latency or absent
H reflex	Abnormal	Normal	Abnormal
Upper extremity conductions	Normal	Normal	Can be abnormal
Needle EMG			
AH/ADQP	Denervated	Denervated	Denervated
EDB	Denervated	Normal	Denervated
Medial gastrocnemius	Denervated	Normal	Denervated
Tibialis anterior	Normal	Normal	Denervated
Paraspinal muscles	Normal or fibs	Normal	Normal or fibs
Symmetry of Findings (When Bilateral)			
	Asymmetrical	Asymmetrical	Symmetrical

ADQP = abductor digiti quinti pedis, AH = abductor hallucis, EDB = extensor digitorum brevis.

polyneuropathy or bilateral tarsal syndromes. Differentiating these three entities requires meticulous EDX examination and is often difficult, especially in elderly patients (Table C2–7). In elderly patients, the sural SNAPs and H reflexes are frequently absent bilaterally, and the foot muscles may show denervational changes of unclear etiology.

Lumbar Canal Stenosis

The EDX findings in lumbar canal stenosis are extremely variable due to the variable level and degree of root(s) compression (see Figure C2–4). The abnormalities seen on EDX testing often mirror the variable clinical presentations in these patients which may vary from neurogenic claudication with normal neurologic examination, to severe disability with weakness, reflex changes, and sensory loss. The EDX findings in lumbar canal stenosis may manifest as one of the following scenarios:

- An entirely normal EMG.
- Absent H reflex only, unilaterally or bilaterally.
- Denervation in a single root distribution (single radiculopathy), unilaterally or bilaterally and asymmetrically. Among the roots that can be affected, those with the longest paths in the cauda equina (S2, S1, L5) tend to be the most likely, because of their potential compression at multiple levels. The EMG findings are chronic, with some fibrillation potentials, mostly in the distal muscles.

- Bilateral and asymmetrical lumbosacral radiculopathies, affecting the L5, S1, and S2 roots predominantly, but sometimes extending into the upper lumbar roots (L2, L3, or L4); the changes are chronic with some fibrillation potentials, mainly distally, below the knees. At times, the motor axon loss may be so severe that the tibial CMAPs, recording abductor hallucis, and the peroneal CMAPs, recording extensor digitorum brevis, are low in amplitude, or even absent. These common EDX findings associated with lumbar canal stenosis findings may also mimic a severe peripheral polyneuropathy and a detailed EMG is often required for correct diagnosis (see Table C2–7).

Could an EMG Be Normal in a Patient With Definite Lumbosacral Radiculopathy?

This is a question commonly asked by clinicians and reflects the limitations of the EDX test in the evaluation of lumbosacral radiculopathy. The general rule is *"a normal EMG does not exclude a root compression."* An EMG study may be normal in a lumbosacral radiculopathy with the following circumstances:

1. *If only the dorsal root is compressed and the ventral root is not compromised.* This occurs in significant numbers of patients whose symptoms are limited to pain and/or paresthesias with or without reflex changes. However, because of the lack of ventral root

involvement, the sensory and motor nerve conduction studies, F wave latencies, and needle EMG are normal. The H reflex might be the sole abnormality in cases of S1 radiculopathy.

2. *If the ventral root compression has caused demyelination only (leading to conduction block) with no axonal loss.* In this situation, no fibrillation potentials or large or polyphasic MUAPs are seen. The expected reduced recruitment may also be masked, particularly when the ventral root compression is partial, by normal adjacent root since all muscles have two or three segmental innervations.

3. *If the root compression is acute.* Here, no fibrillation potentials are seen because these potentials appear 3 weeks after axonal injury and become maximal at 4 to 6 weeks. Also, the MUAPs are normal because sprouting starts at least 4 to 6 weeks after axonal injury.

4. *If the injured root lacks of adequate myotomal representation.* Examples include the L1 or L2 root, which are difficult to assess by EMG.

FOLLOW-UP

The patient underwent magnetic resonance imaging of the lumbar spine and a computed tomography/myelography (Figure C2–7). This revealed a large L4–L5 posterolateral disc herniation, with compression and displacement of the right L5 and S1 roots, and secondary canal stenosis at that level. The patient underwent an L4–L5 laminectomy and diskectomy. Four months later, he demonstrated significant improvement in the footdrop and did not require an ankle brace anymore. When seen 6 years later, he was completely asymptomatic.

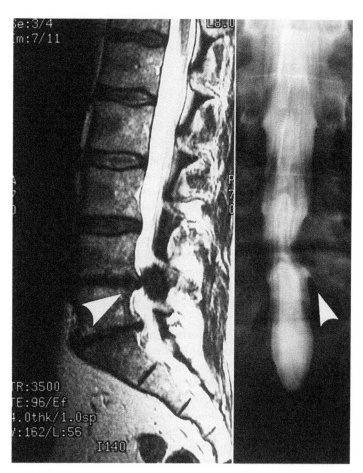

A **B**

Figure C2–7. *Sagittal T2-weighted magnetic resonance image of the lumbar spine (**A**) and lumbar myelography (**B**), revealing a large L4–L5 posterolateral disc herniation with compression, and displacement of the right L5 and S1 roots.*

DIAGNOSIS

Severe right L5 radiculopathy due to disc herniation/canal stenosis at the L4–L5 interspace.

ANSWERS

1. E; 2. E; 3. B.

SUGGESTED READINGS

Aminoff MJ et al. Electrophysiological evaluation of lumbosacral radiculopathies: electromyography, late responses and somatosensory evoked potentials. Neurology 1985;35: 1514–1518.

Chu J. Lumbosacral radicular symptoms: Importance of bilateral electrodiagnostic studies. Arch Phys Med Rehabil 1981;62:522.

Hardy RW, ed. Lumbar disc disease, 2nd ed. New York: Raven Press, 1992.

Katirji B, Weissman JD. The ankle jerk and the tibial H-reflex: a clinical and electrophysiological correlation. Electromyogr Clin Neurophysiol 1994;34:331–334.

Lajoie WV. Nerve root compression: correlation of electromyographic, myelographic and surgical findings. Arch Phys Med Rehabil 1972;53:390–392.

Levin KH. L5 radiculopathy with reduced superficial peroneal sensory responses: intraspinal and extraspinal causes. Muscle Nerve 1998;21:3–7.

Levin KH. Electrodiagnostic approach to the patient with suspected radiculopathy. Neurol Clin N Am 2002;20: 397–421.

Nishada T et al. H reflex in S-1 radiculopathy: latency versus amplitude controversy revisited. Muscle Nerve 1996;19: 915–917.

Phillips LH, Parks TS. Electrophysiologic mapping of the segmental anatomy of the muscles of the lower extremity. Muscle Nerve 1991;14:1213–1218.

Sunderland S. Nerves and nerve injuries, 2nd ed. New York: Churchill Livingstone, 1978.

Tonzola RF et al. Usefulness of electrophysiological studies in the diagnosis of lumbosacral root disease. Ann Neurol 1981;9:305–308.

Tsao B, Levin KH, Bodner R. Comparison of surgical and electrodiagnostic findings in single root lumbosacral radiculopathies. Muscle Nerve 2003;27:60–64.

Wilbourn AJ, Aminoff MJ. The electrophysiologic examination in patients with radiculopathies. Muscle Nerve 1988;11: 1099–1114.

Case 3

HISTORY AND PHYSICAL EXAMINATION

Acute, severe left foot pain and weakness, coincident with an intramuscular gluteal injection of meperidine (Demerol®) developed in a 46-year-old woman, with recurrent cluster headaches since 15 years of age. She was otherwise in good health. Her foot pain worsened and she developed extreme sensitivity to touch. Two months later, she was referred to the electromyography (EMG) laboratory.

On examination, the left foot was warmer than the right. There were no skin or nail dystrophic changes, but there was allodynia over the dorsum of the foot. There was moderate weakness of the left foot and toe dorsiflexion (Medical Research Council [MRC] 4/5), with mild weakness of toe flexion (5–/5) but intact ankle plantar flexion. Eversion of the ankle was much weaker than inversion (4/5 versus 5–/5). Left ankle jerk was depressed compared to the right. Knee flexion and extension and hip functions were normal.

An electrodiagnostic (EDX) examination was performed. Please now review the Nerve Conduction Studies and Needle EMG tables.

QUESTIONS

1. The clinical and EMG examinations are consistent with:
   A. A common peroneal mononeuropathy.
   B. A sciatic mononeuropathy.
   C. An L5 radiculopathy.
   D. A lumbosacral plexopathy.
   E. A deep peroneal mononeuropathy.
2. The two most commonly reported causes of this lesion are:
   A. Gluteal injection and thigh hematoma.
   B. Vasculitis and nerve tumor.
   C. Hip replacement and coma.
   D. Gunshot wound and diabetes.
3. All of the following are factors that more often result in peroneal than tibial nerve injury in sciatic lesions *except:*
   A. The tibial nerve has more fascicles than the peroneal nerve in the thigh.
   B. There is more supporting structure within the tibial than the peroneal nerve.
   C. The peroneal nerve is taut between the fibular head and the hip.
   D. The tibial nerve is located lateroposteriorly.

EDX FINDINGS AND INTERPRETATION OF DATA

Pertinent EDX findings include:

1. Absent left superficial peroneal sensory nerve action potential (SNAP).
2. Low-amplitude left sural SNAP when compared with the right (7 µV versus 20 µV).
3. Low-amplitude left peroneal compound muscle action potential (CMAP), recording extensor digitorum brevis (EDB) and tibialis anterior. There is also diffuse mild slowing of peroneal motor conduction velocities (32 m/s and 38 m/s) consistent with significant axonal loss.
4. Low-amplitude left tibial CMAP, particularly when compared with the right (6 mV versus 10 mV) with normal distal latencies and conduction velocities.
5. Asymmetrical H responses (lower in amplitude on the left), with possible low-amplitude left M response when compared with the right (18 mV versus 24 mV).
6. Fibrillation potentials and neurogenic recruitment with long-duration and, sometimes, polyphasic motor unit action potentials (MUAPs) in all common peroneal innervated muscles, including the short head of the

Case 3: Nerve Conduction Studies

Nerve Stimulated	Stimulation Site	Recording Site	Amplitude (m = mV, s = µV)			Distal/Peak Latency (ms)			Conduction Velocity (m/s)			F Latency (ms)	
			Right	Left	Normal	Right	Left	Normal	Right	Left	Normal	Right	Left
Sural (s)	Calf	Ankle	20	**7**	≥5	3.7	4.0	≤4.5	44	40	≥40		
Sup. peroneal (s)	Lateral leg	Ankle	13	**NR**	≥5	2.7	**NR**	≤4.5					
Peroneal (m)	Ankle	EDB	3.5	**0.24**	≥3	5.4	5.2	≤5.5					
Peroneal (m)	Knee	EDB	3.0	**0.16**					45	32	≥40	47	**NR**
Peroneal (m)	Bel. fibular head	Tibialis anterior	4.5	**2.5**	≥4	2.2	3.1	≤4.0					
Peroneal (m)	Knee	Tibialis anterior	4.0	**2.2**					43	38	≥40		
Tibial (m)	Ankle	AH	10	**6**	≥8	5.6	5.1	≤6.0					
Tibial (m)	Knee	AH	8.5	**4.2**					46	44	≥40	46	49
H reflex	Knee	Soleus	1.7	**0.7**		32.4	34.0						
M response	Knee	Soleus	24	18		5.6	5.6						

AH = abductor hallucis; Bel. fibular head = below fibular head; EDB = extensor digitorum brevis; m = motor; NR = no response; s = sensory; Sup. peroneal = superficial peroneal. Data in bold type are abnormal.

Case 3: Needle EMG

Muscle	Insertional Activity	Spontaneous Activity Fibs	Fascs	Recruitment Normal	Activation	Reduced	Early	Voluntary Motor Unit Action Potentials (MUAPs) Configuration Duration	Amplitude	% Polyphasia	Others
L. tibialis anterior	↑	2+	0			↓		↑	Normal	↑	↑
Medial gastrocnemius	↑	Few	0	X				↑	Normal	Normal	
Flexor digitorum longus	↑	1+	0			↓		↑	Normal	Normal	
Extensor hallucis	↑	2+	0			↓↓		↑	Normal	Normal	
Abductor hallucis	↑	1+	0			↓↓		↑	Normal	Normal	
Extensor dig. brevis	↑	2+	0			↓↓↓		↑	Normal	Normal	
Peroneus longus	↑	1+	0			↓↓		↑	Normal	↑	
Biceps fem. (short head)	↑	Few	0			↓		↑	Normal	↑	
Biceps fem. (long head)	Normal	0	0	X				Normal	Normal	Normal	
Vastus lateralis	Normal	0	0	X				Normal	Normal	Normal	
Gluteus medius	Normal	0	0	X				Normal	Normal	Normal	
Gluteus maximus	Normal	0	0	X				Normal	Normal	Normal	
Midlumbar paraspinal	Normal	0	0	–							
Low lumbar paraspinal	Normal	0	0	–							

Biceps fem. = biceps femoris; Extensor dig. brevis = extensor digitorum brevis; Fascs = fasciculations; Fibs = fibrillations; L. = left; ↑ = increased; ↓ = mildly reduced; ↓↓ = moderately reduced; ↓↓↓ = severely reduced.

biceps femoris. Similar, but less prominent MUAP changes are also seen in the distal tibial innervated muscles. However, the glutei and lumbar paraspinal muscles are normal.

This is consistent with a high sciatic mononeuropathy, proximal to the hamstring innervation, that affects the peroneal division predominantly and is axonal in nature.

DISCUSSION

Applied Anatomy

Originating from the L4, L5, S1, and S2 roots, the sciatic nerve is composed of lateral and medial divisions. The lateral division is named the common peroneal nerve or the lateral popliteal nerve, and the medial division is named the tibial nerve or the medial popliteal nerve. Although both divisions are enclosed in a common sheath, these two nerves are separate from the outset and do not exchange any fascicles.

The sciatic nerve (Figure C3–1) leaves the pelvis via the sciatic notch and then passes, usually, under the piriformis muscle, which is covered by the gluteus maximus. In healthy individuals, the sciatic nerve passes underneath the piriformis muscle in 85 to 90% of cases, while in the rest, the peroneal division only passes above or through the muscle. Rarely (1 to 2% of persons), the entire sciatic nerve pierces the piriformis muscle.

The superior gluteal nerve, which innervates the gluteus medius and minimus and tensor fascia lata, branches off the sciatic trunk before the piriformis. However, the inferior gluteal nerve, which innervates the gluteus maximus, passes under the muscle (Figure C3–2). In the thigh, the tibial nerve innervates most hamstring muscles (semitendinosus, semimembranosus, and the long head of the biceps femoris), except the short head of the biceps femoris; the latter is the only hamstring muscle innervated by the common peroneal nerve. Also, the tibial nerve contributes, with the obturator nerve, to innervation of the adductor magnus muscle.

Lesions of the proximal sciatic nerve at the hip or in the upper thigh affect usually the lateral division (common peroneal nerve) more severely than the medial division (tibial nerve). The greater vulnerability of the peroneal division is caused by the following:

- *The difference in both the fascicular pattern and the cushioning effect of the epineurium between the two divisions.* The tibial nerve has many fascicles that are distributed throughout elastic epineural tissue while the peroneal nerve is composed of fewer fascicles and has limited supportive tissue.

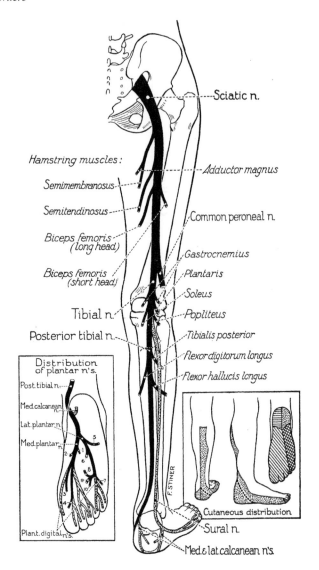

Figure C3–1. *The sciatic nerve and its main branches. (Reprinted with permission from Haymaker W, Woodhall B. Peripheral nerve injuries: principles of diagnosis. Philadelphia, PA: WB Saunders, 1953.)*

- *The difference in anatomic course between the two nerves.* The tibial nerve is loosely fixed posteriorly while the peroneal nerve is taut and is secured at the sciatic notch proximally and the fibular neck distally. Consequently, traction of the sciatic nerve results in more damage to the peroneal than the tibial nerve in the thigh.

The sciatic nerve divides into its two terminal branches near the midthigh, although this is extremely variable and the separation may be as low as the popliteal fossa. In the popliteal fossa and before it winds around the fibular neck, the common peroneal nerve gives off first the *lateral cutaneous nerve of the calf*, which innervates the skin over the

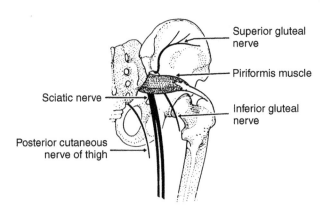

Figure C3–2. *The nerve of the sciatic notch and the piriformis muscle. (Reprinted from Stewart JD. Focal peripheral neuropathies, 2nd ed. New York: Raven Press, 1993, with permission.)*

upper third of the lateral aspect of the leg. At the fibular neck, the common peroneal nerve lies in close contact with the bone, and passes through a tendinous tunnel, sometimes referred to as the fibular tunnel, which is formed between the edge of the peroneus longus muscle and the fibula. Near that point, the common peroneal nerve divides into superficial and deep branches (see Figure C8–3, Case 8). The superficial peroneal nerve innervates the peroneus longus and brevis, as well as the skin of the lower two-thirds of the lateral aspect of the leg and the dorsum of the foot. The deep peroneal nerve is primarily a motor nerve; it innervates the ankle and toe extensors (the tibialis anterior, extensor hallucis, extensor digitorum longus, and brevis) and the peroneus tertius, in addition to a small area of skin in the web space between the first and second toes.

In the popliteal fossa, the tibial nerve gives off the sural nerve, a purely sensory nerve that innervates the lateral aspect of the lower leg and foot, including the little toe. In 40 to 80% of individuals, there is a communication between the common peroneal nerve and the sural nerve in the popliteal fossa. This nerve is referred to as the *sural communicating nerve* but also is called the *lateral sural nerve* (with the main sural trunk being the medial sural nerve). This nerve may play role in preserving sensation in the lateral foot and little toe in proximal tibial nerve lesions, and causing sensory loss in this distribution following a common peroneal or proximal deep peroneal lesion.

While in the calf, the tibial nerve innervates the gastrocnemius, soleus, tibialis posterior, flexor digitorum profundus, and flexor hallucis longus. At the medial aspect of the ankle, the tibial nerve passes through the tarsal tunnel and divides at, or slightly distal to, the tunnel into its three terminal branches (see inset of Figure C3–1): (1) the calcaneal branch, a purely sensory nerve that innervates the skin of the sole of the heel; (2) the *medial plantar nerve*, which innervates the abductor hallucis, the flexor digitorum

brevis, and the flexor hallucis brevis, in addition to the skin of the medial sole and, at least, the medial three toes; and (3) the *lateral plantar nerve*, which innervates the abductor digiti quinti pedis, the flexor digiti quinti pedis, the adductor hallucis, and the interossei, in addition to the skin of the lateral sole and two lateral toes.

Clinical Features

Sciatic ononeuropathy is the second most common lower extremity mononeuropathy, following common peroneal mononeuropathy. The sciatic nerve is predisposed to injury by its proximity to the hip joint and its relatively long course from the sciatic notch to the popliteal fossa.

Table C3–1 lists the common causes of sciatic mononeuropathy. *Total hip joint replacement* is currently a leading cause of such lesions, and sciatic nerve injury is the most common neurologic complication of total hip arthroplasty, particularly with revisions or procedures requiring limb lengthening, and in patients with congenital hip dislocation or dysplasia. The estimated incidence of sciatic nerve lesion following total hip replacement is about 1–3%, although EDX studies may detect subclinical signs of sciatic nerve damage in as many as 70% of patients. The sciatic nerve lesion is due to direct intraoperative stretch injury, but occasionally is caused by hemorrhage, prosthetic dislocation, migrating trochanteric wire, or leaking cement (methylmethacrylate) used in the arthroplasty. The manifestations of the sciatic nerve injury are acute and often noted in the immediate postoperative period. Occasionally, the onset of symptoms is delayed for several years, and the injury is due to prosthetic dislocation, osseous formation, or migrating trochanteric wire. Hip fracture or dislocation, or femur fracture may also result in sciatic nerve injury, which may also occur during closed reduction or internal fixation. *External compression* of the sciatic nerve is the second common cause of sciatic nerve

Table C3–1. Common Causes of Sciatic Mononeuropathy (Listed in Descending Order of Frequency)

Hip replacement, hip fracture/dislocation, or femur fracture

Acute compression (coma or prolonged sitting)

Gunshot or knife wound

Infarction (vasculitis, iliac artery occlusion, arterial bypass surgery)

Gluteal contusion or compartmental syndrome (e.g., during anticoagulation)

Gluteal intramuscular injection

Endometriosis (catamenial sciatica)

"Piriformis syndrome"

lesions at the hip. This usually occurs in the setting of unattended coma (such as with drug overdose), but occasionally follows operative positioning in the sitting position (such as with craniotomy), poor positioning of unconscious patient (such as in the intensive care unit), or prolonged sitting ("toilet seat" and "lotus" neuropathies). Mass lesions in the buttock or thigh, such as malignant or benign tumors, persistent sciatic artery, or enlargement of the lesser trochanter (possibly from frequent sitting on hard benches), may compress the sciatic nerve. *Open injuries* of the sciatic nerve are usually caused by gunshot wounds, knives, or other sharp objects. Hemorrhage within the gluteal compartment is sometimes associated with sciatic nerve lesions. This may occur during anticoagulant therapy, in hemophiliacs, or following rupture of an iliac artery aneurysm or hip surgery. *Intramuscular gluteal injections*, not administered properly in the upper outer quadrant of the buttock particularly in thin patients or children, may damage the sciatic nerve or its peroneal component exclusively. This often occurs soon after the injection of a large quantity of a neurotoxic drug but may be delayed following repeated injections or due to fibrosis. Menstruating women with *endometriosis* may have cyclic radicular pain (i.e., sciatica) or overt sciatic mononeuropathy. Typically, the symptoms start few days before menstruation and stop after menses end. With progression of disease, the manifestations of endometriosis become more constant, though often worse during menses. *Ischemia* resulting in sciatic nerve injuries may be due to vasculitis involving the vasa nervorum, or occlusion of the iliac or femoral artery such as during intra-aortic balloon pump therapy with a catheter placed through the ipsilateral femoral artery. Occasionally, a slowly progressive sciatic mononeuropathy is *idiopathic* and no identifiable cause is identified despite imaging studies and surgical exploration.

Severe or complete sciatic nerve lesion is associated with weakness of all the muscles below the knee and the hamstrings with sensory loss below the knee that spans both the peroneal and tibial distributions but spares the saphenous nerve distribution (the medial leg). In contrast, a partial sciatic nerve lesion usually affects the peroneal more than the tibial division, and mimics a common peroneal nerve lesion at the fibular neck. It usually presents with foot drop and sensory loss mostly in common peroneal nerve distribution. This lesion may be difficult to differentiate from peroneal mononeuropathy, lumbosacral radiculopathy, and lumbosacral plexopathy. Table C3–2 lists some clinical hints that cast doubt on a peroneal nerve lesion at the fibular head in patients presenting with footdrop, while Table C3–3 (A) lists the differential diagnoses of patients with footdrop. Note that dysesthetic, sometimes disabling, pain is common in sciatic mononeuropathy but is rare in peroneal nerve lesions around the fibular neck.

Table C3–2. Helpful Clues Suggesting That Footdrop is Not Caused by an Isolated Peroneal Nerve Lesion

Severe dysesthetic foot pain

Radicular pain ("sciatica")

Positive straight leg test

Absent or depressed ankle jerk

Weakness of toe flexion and/or ankle inversion, hamstrings, or gastrocnemius

Sensory loss in upper third of lateral leg (lateral cutaneous of calf distribution) or sole (tibial distribution)

Electrodiagnostic Studies

The electrodiagnostic (EDX) findings in sciatic mononeuropathy parallel the clinical manifestations. Complete and severe lesions are easy to diagnose since both the tibial and peroneal motor nerve conduction studies (NCS) as well as the sural and the superficial peroneal sensory studies are low in amplitudes or absent with normal or slightly slowed distal latencies and conduction velocities. The needle EMG reveals denervation in all muscles below the knee, in addition to all the hamstring muscles. In contrast, the anterior and medial thigh muscles (quadriceps, thigh adductors, and iliacus) and the glutei and tensor fascia lata as well as the saphenous sensory and femoral motor NCSs, if studied, are normal.

A partial sciatic nerve lesion poses more of a diagnostic challenge because it often affects the peroneal nerve predominantly. The EDX study is essential in confirming the presence of sciatic nerve injury and excluding a more distal peroneal nerve lesion resulting from compression around the fibular neck. The NCS, especially the motor ones, might suggest that the lesion is an axonal common peroneal mononeuropathy because the peroneal nerve is usually affected more severely than the tibial nerve. In most situations, the EDX studies unveil involvement of the tibial nerve that may have gone undetected on the neurological examination. Helpful diagnostic clues on NCS include abnormal findings that points to additional pathology of the tibial nerve: (1) an asymmetrically abnormal H reflex, (2) a low-amplitude or absent sural SNAP, and/or (3) a low-amplitude tibial motor CMAP, recording abductor hallucis. Thus, it is highly recommended that the contralateral H reflex be assessed, and that sural sensory and tibial motor nerve conduction studies be done in all patients with footdrop, especially when peroneal nerve lesion is in doubt.

Since the sural nerve receives a major contribution from the common peroneal nerve in the popliteal fossa in 40 to 80% of individuals, this communication may contribute to the antidromic sural SNAP, stimulating at the calf and

Table C3–3. Differential Diagnosis of Common Causes of Footdrop

	Peroneal Neuropathy at the Fibular Head	L5 Radiculopathy	Lumbar Plexopathy (Lumbosacral Trunk)	Sciatic Neuropathy (Mainly Peroneal)
(A) Clinical				
Common causes	Compression (weight loss, perioperative), trauma	Disc herniation, spinal stenosis	Pelvic surgery, hematoma, prolonged labor	Hip surgery, injection injury, coma
Ankle inversion	Normal	Weak	Weak	Normal or mildly weak
Toe flexion	Normal	Weak	Weak	Normal or mildly weak
Plantar flexion	Normal	Normal	Normal	Normal or mildly weak
Ankle jerk	Normal	Normal (unless with S1)	Normal (unless with S1)	Normal or depressed
Sensory loss distribution	Peroneal distribution only	Poorly demarcated, predominantly big toe	Well demarcated to L5 dermatome	Peroneal distribution plus lateral cutaneous of calf and sole (tibial)
Pain	Rare, deep	Common, radicular	Common, can be radicular	Can be severe
(B) Electrodiagnosis				
Peroneal motor study to EDB and/or Tib Ant	Low in amplitude or conduction block across fibular head or both	Usually normal but can be low in amplitude	Low in amplitude	Low in amplitude
Superficial peroneal sensory study	Low or absent*	Normal	Low or absent	Low or absent
Sural sensory study	Normal	Normal	Normal or low amp	Normal or low amp
Peroneal muscles†	Abnormal	Abnormal	Abnormal	Abnormal
Tibial L5 muscles‡	Normal	Usually abnormal	Usually abnormal	Normal or abnormal
Other L5 muscles¶	Normal	Normal or abnormal	Normal or abnormal	Normal
Biceps femoris (short head)	Normal	Usually normal	Usually normal	Abnormal
Paraspinal muscles fibrillations	Absent	May be absent	Absent	Absent

*Can be normal in purely demyelinating lesions or lesion of the deep peroneal nerve only.
†Below knee (tibialis anterior (Tib Ant), extensor digitorum longus, extensor digitorum brevis (EDB), extensor hallucis, +/– peroneus longus).
‡Tibialis posterior and flexor digitorum longus.
¶Gluteus medius and tensor fascia lata.

recording at the ankle. *Hence, an abnormally low amplitude sural SNAP does not automatically indicate involvement of the tibial nerve.*

A detailed needle EMG examination is frequently necessary to confirm that the cause of footdrop is a sciatic nerve lesion rather than a peroneal. The tibial-innervated muscles below the knee are most useful in detecting fibrillation potentials, especially in a mild to moderate lesion that is relatively chronic where the hamstring muscles may have reinnervated well. Among these muscles, the flexor digitorum longus, tibialis posterior, the gastrocnemius (medial and lateral heads), and the abductor hallucis are most helpful, and these muscles should be sampled in all patients with footdrop. Fibrillation potentials, decreased recruitment, and neurogenic MUAP changes are seen in all of these muscles, as well as in the hamstring muscles innervated by the tibial nerve (semitendinosus, semimembranosus, and the long head of the biceps femoris).

The short head of the biceps femoris is innervated by the peroneal nerve proper and is frequently much more seriously affected than the other hamstrings. Occasionally and particularly in severe sciatic nerve injury, neurogenic MUAP changes are detected in the thigh adductors, because the adductor magnus receives dual innervation from the sciatic and obturator nerves. The needle EMG examination is not complete unless the glutei and lumbar paraspinal muscles are sampled and show no abnormalities to exclude a lumbosacral plexopathy or radiculopathy.

Sciatic nerve lesions, particularly when partial and mild to moderate, must be distinguished from peroneal neuropathy, lumbar plexopathy, and lumbosacral radiculopathy. Table C3–3(B) lists the electrodiagnostic features of common causes of footdrop.

On rare occasions, the common peroneal component of the sciatic nerve is the only one injured, both clinically and electrophysiologically. When this occurs, the H reflex, tibial motor NCS, and all tibial innervated muscles above and below the knee are normal. These cases are purely axonal and mimic a peroneal mononeuropathy at the fibular head. Thus, *sampling the short head of the biceps femoris is mandatory in all patients with peroneal mononeuropathy*, especially those due to axon loss that cannot be localized by NCS because of the lack of conduction block (or focal slowing). On clinical examination, this muscle cannot be evaluated satisfactorily in isolation. Even when it is denervated completely, its lack of function during hamstring strength testing is concealed by the normal contractions of the other three hamstring muscles, all of which are innervated by the tibial nerve.

The Piriformis Syndrome

The piriformis syndrome is a nebulous and controversial entrapment neuropathy. Based on the close relation between the sciatic nerve and the piriformis muscle, it is proposed that leg pain ("sciatica") may be caused by compression of the sciatic nerve (and sometimes the inferior gluteal nerve also) at the pelvic outlet by the piriformis muscle.

The piriformis syndrome was first described by Yeoman in 1928 and subsequently refined by Freiberg in 1937. He described a triad of symptoms: tenderness at the sciatic notch, positive Lasègue sign and improvement with conservative therapy. Later, in 1947, Robinson coined the term "pyriformis syndrome" and set six criteria for diagnosis (Table C3–4). The syndrome became less popular after the description of nerve root compression by herniated nucleus pulposus as a common cause of sciatica. This was enhanced by the development of imaging techniques, including myelography, CT, and MRI, that could demonstrate these disc herniations and other spondylotic spine changes that encroaches on spinal roots in the lumbar canal. However, there is a recent resurgence of increasing interest in the piriformis syndrome in an attempt to explain the cause of sciatica and buttock pain in patients with no demonstrable nerve root compression on imaging studies.

The piriformis syndrome, according to its *proponents*, is more common in women than men (women/men ratio = 6/1). Often, the patient complains of buttock pain and tenderness that may radiate to the thigh and lower leg. The pain is worse with prolonged sitting particularly on hard surfaces (such as a toilet seat or a bicycle seat), during bending at the waist, or during activity that require hip adduction and internal rotation (such as cross-country skiing). It is often much relieved with standing or walking. Dyspareunia in women or pain with bowel movements are not uncommon symptoms. Back pain is usually absent or minimal. Paresthesias of the buttock and/or in a patchy sciatic nerve distribution are not uncommon. A detailed

Table C3–4. Diagnosis of Piriformis Syndrome

Robinson Initial Diagnostic Criteria (1947)
History of trauma to the buttock
Pain in the buttock extending to the leg
Worsening of pain by stooping or lifting
Palpable and tender sausage-shaped mass over the piriformis muscle
Positive Lasègue sign
Possible gluteal atrophy

Accepted Diagnostic Criteria
Usually a woman
History of trivial trauma to the buttock
Pain in buttock radiating to posterior thigh and leg
Pain is worst when sitting and best when standing
Exquisite buttock tenderness near the sciatic notch
Pain with passive AIF (abduction, internal rotation, and flexion) of hip
Normal neurological examination*
Normal electrodiagnostic studies or mild axon loss sciatic mononeuropathy*
Normal imaging of lumbar spine
Normal imaging of pelvis and hip regions†
Positive response to nerve block near the piriformis muscle

*Occasionally gluteal atrophy with inferior gluteal mononeuropathy.
†Occasionally anomalous vessel or fibrous band close to the sciatic nerve.

history often unveils a history of buttock trauma which may be trivial that predated the onset of symptoms by weeks or months.

On *examination*, there are either no findings or subtle abnormalities. Tenderness in the buttock that is usually maximal near the sciatic notch is common. Straight leg raise test, and internal rotation or abduction and external rotation of the hip often triggers the pain. Occasionally, the leg is externally rotated when the patient is rested in a supine position (positive piriformis sign). Similarly, when patient walks the leg may be also externally rotated. When there is concomitant entrapment of the inferior gluteal nerve, there may be mild weakness or wasting of the gluteus maximus, or a positive Trendelenburg test (the buttock of the unsupported foot falls rather than rise when the patient stand on the asymptomatic leg). Apart from these findings, there is usually no other weakness, sensory loss, or reflex changes.

Many proponents of the piriformis syndrome rely on the presence of bedside test maneuvers in the diagnosis of the piriformis syndrome. These signs involve either passive stretching or active contraction of the piriformis muscle. Pain in the affected buttock or thigh renders the maneuver positive.

- *Freiberg test*. Passive forceful internal rotation of the extended thigh at the hip, while the patient is lying, reproduces the pain. Unfortunately, this test may be positive in other disorders around the hip joint and buttock.

- *Pace test.* Resisted abduction of the thigh, while the patient is in the sitting position, induces the pain. However, this may be difficult to interpret since most patients have pain when sitting.
- *Beatty test.* The patient lies on the asymptomatic side with the painful leg semiflexed at the hip and the knee resting on the table. Pain is reproduced when the patient lifts (abducts) the thigh and holds the knee several inches off the table. However, this maneuver may induce pain in herniated lumbar disc and hip joint abnormalities.
- *Adduction, internal rotation and flexion (AIF) test.* This is the most useful and specific test for the piriformis muscle. The patient lies on the unaffected side, bend the knee of the affected leg to a 90° angle and catching the foot behind the calf of the affected leg, swing the affected leg over the healthy one until the knee touches the examining table (Figure C3–3). This reproduces the buttock pain and sciatica.

The *diagnosis* of the piriformis syndrome is a clinical one with the EDX and imaging studies playing an important role, mostly in excluding lumbar spine disease, hip pathology, or mass lesions compressing the sciatic nerve. In almost all cases of piriformis syndrome, the *EDX studies* (NCS and needle EMG) are normal. Rarely, there are mild chronic denervation and reinnervation changes on needle EMG, often with normal sensory and motor NCS which renders these changes difficult to distinguish from lumbosacral radiculopathy. In these cases, the pattern of denervation is useful; the gluteus medius and tensor fascia lata, both innervated by the superior gluteal nerve, which branches from the sciatic trunk before the piriformis muscle, are normal. However, the sciatic-innervated muscles (particularly the hamstrings, gastrocnemius, and peroneal-innervated muscles) and, sometimes, the gluteus maximus (innervated by the inferior gluteal nerve) are abnormal because these nerves usually pass under the piriformis muscle (see Figure C3–2). A single study of the H reflexes done at rest and during the AIF maneuver reported an asymmetrical delay of the H reflex latency during such a

• Flexion   • Adduction   • Internal rotation

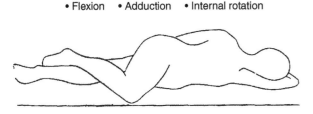

Figure C3–3. *Adduction, internal rotation, and flexion (AIF) test in the diagnosis of piriformis syndrome.*

procedure in patients with the piriformis syndrome. *Imaging* of the sciatic notch may reveal hypertrophy of the piriformis or help in identifying abnormal vessels or bands in the region of the piriformis muscle. However, these findings are also common on the asymptomatic side of patient with sciatica and in control subjects. Relief of symptoms by a CT-guided *nerve block* in the region of the sciatic notch is considered a diagnostic confirmation of the piriformis syndrome.

Treatment of the piriformis syndrome should always start with a conservative approach. Physical therapy that concentrates on prolonged stretching exercises of the piriformis muscle by flexion, adduction, and internal rotation of the hip is often helpful. Injection into the piriformis muscle is advocated with long acting corticosteroids alone or in combination with an anesthetic agent, and preferably done under imaging guidance via the sciatic notch, the perineum, or vagina. This often alleviates the symptoms temporarily and serves also as a diagnostic test. Surgical exploration of the sciatic nerve in the region of the piriformis muscle should be a last resort in cases resistant to conservative therapy. Section of the piriformis muscle is the most popular advocated procedure, and abnormal bands or vessels constricting the sciatic nerve in the buttock should also be removed.

The *prognosis* of patients with the piriformis syndrome is unknown, since most series are small. Good outcome seems to correlate with patients with abnormal EMG findings and those with compressive bands or vessels.

Despite its increasing popularity, mostly among surgeons and anesthesiologists, there are many *opponents* to the existence of this syndrome. These physicians argue that (1) the symptoms of the piriformis syndrome are seldom substantiated by clinical or electrophysiologic findings, (2) the pain relief from corticosteroid injection is not a proof that the sciatic nerve is compressed by the piriformis muscle, since patients with distal sciatic nerve or proximal root lesions (such as lumbosacral radiculopathies) often get pain relief by sciatic nerve blocks, and (3) when denervation in the sciatic nerve distribution is detected (as in the few cases reported), aberrant fascial bands, rather than piriformis muscle, was found to be the cause of sciatic nerve compression. Finally, many opponents believe that most patients with this alleged syndrome have either a lumbosacral radiculopathy that cannot be detected by current imaging techniques or, at best, a myofascial syndrome rather than true nerve compression.

FOLLOW-UP

Although the patient's foot weakness improved over time, she developed severe allodynia, with trophic skin changes of the foot. She responded temporarily to sympathetic block.

During the next 2 years, the pain was controlled partially by a combination of a tricyclic, an anticonvulsant, and relaxation therapy.

DIAGNOSIS

Acute partial axonal sciatic mononeuropathy in the gluteal region, affecting the peroneal component predominantly, due to inadvertent gluteal injection.

ANSWERS

1. B; 2. C; 3. D.

SUGGESTED READINGS

Barton PM. Piriformis syndrome: a rational approach to management. Pain 1991;47:345–351.

Fishman LM, Zybert PA. Electrophysiologic evidence of piriformis syndrome. Arch Phys Med Rehabil 1992;73:359–364.

Freiberg AH, Vinke TH. Sciatica and the sacro-iliac joint. J Bone Joint Surg 1934;16:126–136.

Hughes SS et al. Extrapelvic compression of the sciatic nerve. J Bone Joint Surg 1992;74A:1533–1559.

Katirji MB, Wilbourn AJ. High sciatic lesions mimicking peroneal neuropathy at the fibular head. J Neurol Sci 1994;121:172–175.

Parziale JR, Hudgins TH, Fishman LM. The piriformis syndrome. Am J Orth 1996;25:819–823.

Rodrigue T, Hardy RW. Diagnosis and treatment of piriformis syndrome. Neurosurg Clin N Am 2001;12:311–319.

Schmalzried TP, Amstutz HC, Dorey FJ. Nerve palsy associated with total hip replacement. Risk factors and prognosis. J Bone Joint Surg (Am) 1991;73:1074–1080.

Stookey B. Gunshot wounds of peripheral nerves. Surg Gynecol Obstet 1916;23:639–656.

Sunderland S. The relative susceptibility to injury of the medial and lateral popliteal divisions of the sciatic nerve. Br J Surg 1953;41:300–302.

Sunderland S. Nerves and nerve injuries. Baltimore, MD: Williams & Wilkins, 1968.

Synek VM. The piriformis syndrome: review and case presentation. Clin Exp Neurol 1987;23:31–37.

Weber ER, Daube JR, Coventry MB. Peripheral neuropathies associated with total hip arthroplasty. J Bone Joint Surg (Am) 1976;58:66–69.

Yeoman W. The relation of arthritis of the sacro-iliac joint to sciatica, with analysis of 100 cases. Lancet 1928;2:1119–1122.

Yuen EC, Olney RK, So YT. Sciatic neuropathy: clinical and prognostic features in 73 patients. Neurology 1994;44:1669–1674.

Yuen EC, So YT, Olney RK. The electrophysiologic features of sciatic neuropathy in 100 patients. Muscle Nerve 1995;18:414–420.

Case 4

HISTORY AND PHYSICAL EXAMINATION

A 49-year-old woman with ulcerative colitis, status post total abdominal colectomy, underwent a proctectomy, using a combined abdominal and perineal approach, for persistent proctitis in the retained rectal stump. When she awoke from general anesthesia, she became aware of right leg weakness, and numbness in the anterior thigh and leg.

Examination revealed severe weakness of the right quadriceps (Medical Research Council [MRC] 2/5) and iliopsoas (MRC 4–/5), with normal thigh adduction and ankle dorsiflexion. The right knee jerk was absent. There was sensory loss in the right anterior thigh and medial leg.

The clinical diagnosis of a right femoral neuropathy was made. The patient had been in a lithotomy position during surgery. Three weeks postoperatively, and because of persistent weakness, the electromyographer was asked to confirm, localize, and prognosticate.

Please now review the Nerve Conduction Studies and Needle EMG tables.

QUESTIONS

1. A normal femoral compound muscle action potential (CMAP) amplitude in this patient is consistent with:
   A. Axon-loss femoral mononeuropathy.
   B. Axon-loss lumbar plexopathy.
   C. Axon-loss lumbar polyradiculopathy (L3 and L4).
   D. Demyelinating femoral mononeuropathy.

2. The clinical and EDX findings in this patient are the result of:
   A. A femoral nerve lesion at the inguinal ligament.
   B. A lumbar plexus lesion.
   C. A saphenous nerve lesion.
   D. A femoral nerve lesion in the pelvis.

3. The neurologic complications of pelvic surgery include:
   A. Compression of the femoral nerve by a retracting blade.
   B. Compression of the femoral nerve by an iliacus hematoma or lumbar plexus by a psoas hematoma.
   C. Inadvertent femoral or obturator nerve transection.
   D. Compression of the femoral nerve at the inguinal ligament during lithotomy positioning.
   E. All of the above.

EDX FINDINGS AND INTERPRETATION OF DATA

The pertinent electrodiagnostic (EDX) findings in this case include:

1. Absent right saphenous sensory nerve action potential (SNAP) with a normal left saphenous SNAP. This excludes an L4 root lesion within the intraspinal canal.
2. Normal right femoral CMAP, symmetrical to the left (6.0 mV versus 5.5 mV), without significant difference in distal latencies.
3. Fibrillations and neurogenic recruitment in the quadriceps and iliacus muscles, with normal thigh adductors and tibialis anterior.

A lumbar plexus lesion is excluded by documenting normal thigh adductor muscles. Involvement of the iliacus muscle confirms that the femoral lesion is within the pelvis (i.e., proximal to the takeoff of the motor branch to the iliacus muscle), and is not the result of compression of the femoral nerve at the inguinal ligament which may follow a lithotomy positioning.

The prognosis for recovery is good because the distal femoral CMAP amplitude is normal, consistent with a

Case 4: Nerve Conduction Studies

Nerve Stimulated	Stimulation Site	Recording Site	Amplitude (m = mV, s = μV)			Distal/Peak Latency (ms)			Conduction Velocity (m/s)			F Latency (ms)	
			Right	Left	Normal	Right	Left	Normal	Right	Left	Normal	Right	Left
Sural (s)	Calf	Leg	12		≥5	3.7		≤4.5	42		≥40		
Saphenous (s)	Leg	Ankle	**NR**	6	≥4	**NR**	2.8	≤4.5					
Peroneal (m)	Ankle	EDB	6.0		≥3	4.8		≤5.5	46		≥40	55	
Peroneal (m)	Knee	EDB	5.0										
Tibial (m)	Ankle	AH	11.0		≥8	5.0		≤6.0	46		≥40	44	
Tibial (m)	Knee	AH	9.0										
Femoral (m)	Groin	Rectus femoris	6.1	5.5	≥4	6.0	5.7	≤6.5					

AH = abductor hallucis; EDB = extensor digitorum brevis; m = motor; NR = no response; s = sensory.
Data in bold type are abnormal.

Case 4: Needle EMG

| Muscle | Insertional Activity | Spontaneous Activity | | Voluntary Motor Unit Action Potentials (MUAPs) | | | | | | | |
| | | | | Recruitment | | | | Configuration | | | |
		Fibs	Fascs	Normal	Activation	Reduced	Early	Duration	Amplitude	% Polyphasia	Others
R. vastus lateralis	↑	3+	0			↓↓↓		Normal	Normal	Normal	
Vastus intermedius	↑	3+	0			↓↓↓		Normal	Normal	Normal	
Iliacus	↑	3+	0			↓↓		Normal	Normal	↑	
Thigh adductors	Normal	0	0	X				Normal	Normal	Normal	
Tibialis anterior	Normal	0	0	X				Normal	Normal	Normal	
Medial gastrocnemius	Normal	0	0	X				Normal	Normal	Normal	
Middle lumbar paraspinal	Normal	0	0	–							
Lower lumbar paraspinal	Normal	0	0	–							

Fascs = fasciculations; Fibs = fibrillations; R. = right; ↑ = increased; ↓↓ = moderately reduced; ↓↓↓ = severely reduced.

predominant proximal demyelination. Note that the femoral nerve may be stimulated only at the inguinal canal distal to the location of the pelvic lesion. Some axonal loss obviously has occurred, based on the fibrillations and the absent saphenous SNAP, but these findings have no prognostic value for the outcome of motor function.

This intraoperative and intrapelvic femoral nerve lesion is most likely due to compression by the surgical retractor against the pelvic wall. A retroperitoneal hematoma also is possible and must be ruled out urgently. An inadvertent femoral nerve transection is unlikely since it results in axonal loss and not segmental demyelination.

DISCUSSION

Applied Anatomy

The femoral nerve (also called the anterior crural nerve) is formed by the combination of the posterior divisions of the ventral rami of the L2, L3, and L4 spinal roots (the anterior divisions of the same roots form the obturator nerve). It immediately gives branches to the psoas muscle which receives additional branches from the L3 and L4 roots directly. Then, the femoral nerve passes between the psoas and iliacus muscles and is covered by a tight iliac fascia which forms the roof of the iliacus compartment. The iliacus muscle and femoral nerve are the main constituents of this compartment.

The femoral nerve emerges from the iliacus compartment after passing underneath the rigid inguinal ligament in the groin. About 4–5 cm before crossing the inguinal ligament, it innervates the iliacus muscle. Soon after passing under the inguinal ligament (lateral to the femoral vein and artery), the femoral nerve branches widely into (1) terminal motor branches to all four heads of the quadriceps (rectus femoris, vastus lateralis, vastus intermedius, and vastus lateralis) and sartorius muscles, and (2) three terminal sensory branches, the medial and intermediate cutaneous nerve of the thigh which innervate the skin of the anterior thigh, and the saphenous sensory nerve (Figure C4–1).

The saphenous nerve travels the thigh, lateral to the femoral artery, by passing posteromedially from the femoral triangle through the subsartorial (Hunter or adductor) canal. It gives off the infrapatellar branch that innervates the skin over the anterior surface of the patella. About 10 cm proximal and medial to the knee, the saphenous nerve becomes subcutaneous by piercing the fascia between the sartorius and gracilis muscles. Then, it crosses a bursa at the upper medial end of the tibia (pes anserinus bursa). In the lower third of the leg, it divides into two terminal branches to innervate the skin of the medial surface

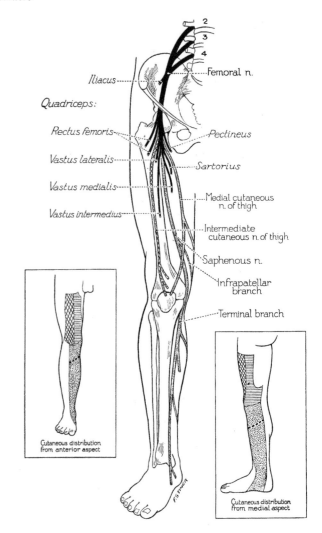

Figure C4–1. *The femoral nerve and its terminal motor and sensory branches including the saphenous nerve. (From Haymaker W and Woodhall B. Peripheral nerve injuries: principles of diagnosis. Philadelphia, PA: WB Saunders, 1953, with permission.)*

of the knee, medial leg, medial malleolus, and a small area of the medial arch of the foot.

Clinical Features

The femoral nerve is a relatively short nerve. Its main trunk can be compressed at the inguinal ligament or in the retroperitoneal pelvic space. Most femoral mononeuropathies are iatrogenic, occurring during intra-abdominal, intrapelvic, inguinal, or hip surgical or diagnostic procedures. The nerve injury often results from direct nerve trauma or poor leg positioning during one of these procedures but may be due to a compressive hematoma or rarely due to inadvertent nerve laceration, suturing or stapling.

Table C4–1 lists the various causes of femoral mononeuropathy grouped according to the site of injury.

By far the most commonly reported causes of femoral mononeuropathies are those related to *pelvic surgery.* This includes abdominal hysterectomy, radical prostatectomy, renal transplantation, colectomy, proctectomy, inguinal herniorrhaphy, lumbar sympathectomy, appendectomy, tubal ligation, abdominal aortic repair, and a variety of other intra-abdominal vascular, urologic, or gynecologic operations. During these surgical procedures, the femoral nerve becomes compressed between the retractor blade and the pelvic wall. This occurs more often with the use of self-retracting blades than with handheld blades.

Acute hemorrhage within the iliacus compartment in the retroperitoneal space and, less commonly, the psoas muscle can lead to a compartmental syndrome. This usually results in severe femoral nerve injury; however, the hematoma is sometimes large and extends into the retroperitoneal space, leading to extensive injury of either the lumbar plexus or, rarely, the entire lumbosacral plexus. The hematoma may be a complication of anticoagulant therapy (heparin or warfarin), hemophilia or other blood dyscrasias, ruptured abdominal aortic aneurysm, pelvic operations, traumatic rupture of the iliopsoas muscle, or femoral artery (and less commonly femoral vein) catheterization for coronary, cerebral, and aortic angiography. In patients with acute femoral neuropathy and severe pain, particularly in the setting of anticoagulation or coagulopathy, a spontaneous iliacus hematoma should be considered and ruled out urgently by computed tomography (CT)

scan or magnetic resonance imaging (MRI) of the pelvis. Controversy continues regarding the indication and timing of surgical evacuation of the hematoma once the femoral nerve lesion is clinically apparent.

Compression of the femoral nerve may follow *lithotomy positioning* for vaginal delivery, vaginal hysterectomy, prostatectomy, or laparoscopy is not uncommon. The femoral nerve is kinked and becomes compressed underneath the inguinal ligament usually following prolonged lithotomy positioning, particularly with extreme hip flexion and external rotation. This type of femoral nerve injury is frequently reversible, and is likely underestimated. To prevent compression at the inguinal ligament, prolonged lithotomy positioning with extreme hip flexion and external rotation should be avoided.

Femoral nerve injury during *surgical procedures of the hip joint* occurs mostly after total hip replacement. It is due to misplacement of the anterior acetabular retractors during the procedure, and is highest in revisions and complicated reconstructions.

Although the literature published in the 1950s and 1960s led many to believe that diabetes mellitus is associated with selective *"diabetic femoral neuropathy,"* it is now clear that this is a misnomer. Diabetic patients actually have more extensive peripheral nerve disease that involves the lumbar plexus and roots, and is better known as diabetic amyotrophy, diabetic proximal neuropathy, or diabetic radiculoplexopathy (see Case 7). Although the brunt of weakness in these patients often falls on the quadriceps muscle, mimicking selective femoral nerve injuries, careful clinical and needle EMG examinations reveal more widespread involvement of thigh adductors and sometimes foot dorsiflexors, muscles not innervated by the femoral nerve.

The clinical presentation of femoral mononeuropathy often is acute, with thigh weakness and numbness. Patients frequently complain that their legs buckle underneath them, leading to many falls. Except with iliacus hematoma, groin or thigh pain is usually mild. Neurologic examination reveals weakness of the quadriceps muscle (knee extension), with absent or depressed knee jerk. Thigh adduction is, however, normal. The iliopsoas muscle (hip flexion) usually is weak when the lesion is intrapelvic (such as during pelvic surgery), but is spared when the lesion is at the inguinal region (such as during lithotomy positioning). Hypesthesia over the anterior thigh and medial calf is common.

Femoral mononeuropathy should be differentiated from L2, L3, and L4 radiculopathy, and from lumbar plexopathy. *Weakness of the thigh adductors, which are innervated by the obturator nerve, excludes a selective femoral lesion.* Positive reversed straight leg test is common in lumbar radiculopathy, but it may occur with plexopathy and femoral nerve lesion caused by iliacus hematoma.

Table C4–1. Common Causes of Femoral Mononeuropathy

1. Compression in the pelvis
   - by retractor blade during pelvic surgery (iatrogenic): abdominal hysterectomy, radical prostatectomy, renal transplantation, etc.
   - by iliacus or psoas retroperitoneal hematoma (anticoagulation [systemic or subcutaneous abdominal heparin], hemophilia, coagulopathy, ruptured abdominal aneurysm, femoral artery catheterization)
   - by pelvic mass (lymphadenopathy, tumor, abscess, cyst, aortic or iliac aneurysm)
2. Compression in the inguinal region
   - by inguinal ligament during lithotomy position (vaginal delivery, laparoscopy, vaginal hysterectomy, urologic procedures)
   - by inguinal hematoma (femoral artery catheterization, such as for coronary angiography)
   - during total hip replacement
   - by inguinal mass (e.g., lymphadenopathy)
3. Stretch injury (hyperextension, dancing, yoga)
4. Others (radiation, laceration, misplaced injection, ?diabetes)

In plexopathy or L4 radiculopathy, weakness of ankle dorsiflexion (tibialis anterior) is common.

Except for iliacus or retroperitoneal hematoma, which might require surgical intervention, most other patients with femoral mononeuropathy are treated conservatively, allowing for spontaneous remyelination or reinnervation. A knee brace is helpful in preventing falls for patients with severe weakness of the quadriceps.

Electrodiagnosis

The role of electrodiagnostic testing in femoral mononeuropathy is threefold.

The first role is to *confirm* the presence of a selective femoral nerve injury. This is particularly important when the neurologic examination is difficult to perform because of pain, recent pelvic surgery, or vaginal delivery. A femoral mononeuropathy may mimic a lumbar plexopathy and upper lumbar (L2, L3, or L4) radiculopathy (Table C4–2). The saphenous SNAP, which evaluates the postganglionic L4 sensory fibers, is often absent in femoral mononeuropathy and lumbar plexopathy but normal in L4 radiculopathy since the root lesion is intraspinal, i.e., proximal to the dorsal root ganglion. Rarely, the saphenous SNAP is normal in "purely" demyelinating femoral mononeuropathies where there is no wallerian degeneration which is usually complete in 10–11 days in sensory fibers. The saphenous SNAPs should be studied bilaterally for comparison, since these potentials may be difficult to obtain in the elderly and obese patients and in patients with leg edema. On needle EMG, fibrillation potentials and decreased recruitment of large and polyphasic MUAPs are seen in the quadriceps in all three entities (femoral mononeuropathy, lumbar plexopathy, or radiculopathy). However, these changes are also present in the thigh adductors (L2/L3/L4 obturator nerve) in patients with upper lumbar radiculopathy or plexopathy. Also, in L4 radiculopathy, similar changes may be present in the tibialis anterior (L4/L5 common peroneal nerve).

The second role of EDX study is to *localize* the site of the femoral nerve lesion. Since the branch to the iliacus muscle originates 4–5 cm above the inguinal ligament, needle EMG of this muscle is crucial to help determining whether the femoral nerve lesion is distal (i.e., around the inguinal ligament) or proximal (i.e., intrapelvic). When the iliacus is denervated, the lesion is in the pelvis and when spared, the lesion is distal, such as at the inguinal ligament. This is particularly important when clinical examination of the iliopsoas (hip flexion) is difficult because of groin pain, recent pelvic surgery, or vaginal delivery. Also, weakness of hip flexion could be attributed falsely to involvement of the iliopsoas muscle when the quadriceps is flaccid because the latter assists in hip flexion.

A third and important role of the EDX study is to *prognosticate* the recovery of motor function in acute femoral nerve lesions. A femoral CMAP amplitude and/or area is the most useful semiquantitative measure of the extent of femoral motor axonal loss. The femoral nerve could only be stimulated at the groin and, hence, lesions at the inguinal ligament or pelvis cannot be bracketed by two stimulation sites as done in many other peripheral nerve motor conduction studies. Femoral nerve stimulation at the groin is usually distal to the site of the lesion, and allows evaluation of a distal CMAP only. Care should be taken in accounting for the time for wallerian degeneration: the CMAP amplitude reaches its nadir in 4 to 5 days while the decrease in SNAP amplitudes lags behind and is completed in 8 to 11 days (Figure C4–2). Hence, the femoral CMAP must be obtained bilaterally for comparison at least after 4 to 5 days from injury before any conclusion could be made regarding the primary pathophysiologic process or prognosis. In contrast to the CMAP, fibrillation potentials are a poor quantitative measure of the extent of axonal loss since they are identified whenever axonal loss occurs, even if minimal. In other words, fibrillation potentials are extremely sensitive for the presence of any recent axonal loss, but do quantitate its degree, and are therefore, by themselves, poor indicators of the extent of peripheral nerve injury. Based on the above, the primary

Table C4–2. Differential Electrodiagnosis of Femoral Neuropathy

	Femoral Neuropathy	Lumbar Plexopathy	Lumbar Radiculopathy
Thigh adductors	Normal	Denervation	Denervation
Tibialis anterior	Normal	Denervation*	Denervation*
Saphenous SNAP[†]	Low or absent[‡]	Low or absent[‡]	Normal
Paraspinal fibrillations	Absent	Absent	Usually present

*Abnormal in L4 radiculopathy/plexopathy only.
[†]May be technically difficult, particularly in the elderly patients or if there is leg edema.
[‡]Normal in purely demyelinating lesions.

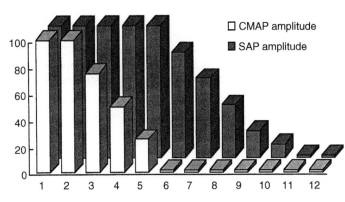

Figure C4–2. *A diagrammatic representation of the decline of distal compound motor action potential (CMAP) and sensory nerve action potential (SNAP) amplitudes, due to wallerian degeneration.*

pathophysiologic process and prognosis of a unilateral femoral nerve lesion are assessed according to the following:

1. If the femoral CMAP amplitude and/or area are normal despite significant reduction of MUAP recruitment, the lesion is primarily demyelinating and the prognosis is very good, because outcome is dependent on remyelination. Almost all patients with such findings recover in about 2 months.

2. If the femoral CMAP amplitude and/or area are low or absent, in the presence of moderate or severe decrease in MUAP recruitment, the lesion is primarily axonal, and the prognosis is relatively protracted because improvement depends on sprouting and reinnervation. In general, patients with femoral CMAP amplitude more than 50% of the contralateral side significantly improve within 1 year, while fewer than half the patients with a CMAP less than 50% of the contralateral side have a meaningful improvement at one year. In spite of this, the long-term prognosis of axon-loss femoral nerve injury is better than other axon-loss peripheral nerve lesions, since the nerve is relatively short and the target muscle (quadriceps) is proximal and close to the site of injury, resulting in optimal conditions for sprouting and reinnervation.

FOLLOW-UP

Urgent CT scan of the pelvis did not reveal an iliacus hematoma. As was predicted by the EDX study, the patient's right leg weakness improved significantly over the next 2 months. At that time, the quadriceps and iliacus weakness were mild (MRC 4+/5) and the right knee jerk returned, although it remained depressed. Hypesthesia in the anterior thigh was much better, but it was unchanged in the medial leg.

ANSWERS

1. D; 2. D; 3. E.

SUGGESTED READINGS

Al Hakim M, Katirji MB. Femoral mononeuropathy induced by the lithotomy position: a report of 5 cases and a review of the literature. Muscle Nerve 1993;16:891–895.

Calverley JR, Mulder DW. Femoral neuropathy. Neurology 1960;10:963–967.

Chaudhry V, Cornblath DR. Wallerian degeneration in human nerves: serial electrophysiologic studies. Muscle Nerve 1992;15:687–693.

Jog MS, Turley JE, Berry H. Femoral neuropathy in renal transplantation. Can J Neurol Sci 1994;21:38–42.

Katirji MB, Lanska DJ. Femoral mononeuropathy after radical prostatectomy. Urology 1990;36:539–540.

Kent KC, Moscussi M, Gallagher SG et al. Neuropathy after cardiac catheterization: incidence, clinical patterns and long term outcome. J Vasc Surg 1994;19:1008–1012.

Kent KC, Moscucci M, Mansour KA et al. Retroperitoneal hematoma after cardiac catheterization: prevalence, risk factors, and optimal management. J Vasc Surg 1994;20:905–910.

Kim DH, Kline DG. Surgical outcome for intra- and extrapelvic femoral nerve lesions. J Neurosurg 1995;83:783–790.

Kuntzer T, Van Melle G, Regli F. Clinical and prognostic features in unilateral femoral neuropathies. Muscle Nerve 1997;20: 205–211.

Kvist-Poulsen H, Borel J. Iatrogenic femoral neuropathy subsequent to abdominal hysterectomy: incidence and prevention. Obstet Gynecol 1982;60:516–520.

Simmons C Jr., Izant TH, Rothman RH et al. Femoral neuropathy following total hip arthroplasty. Anatomic study, case reports, and literature review. J Arthroplasty 1991;6:S57–66.

Vargo MM, Robinson LR, Nicholas JJ et al. Postpartum femoral neuropathy: relic of an earlier era? Arch Phys Med Rehabil 1990;71:591–596.

Weber ER, Daube JR, Coventry MB. Peripheral neuropathies associated with total hip arthroplasty. J Bone Joint Surg (Am) 1976;58A:66–69.

Young MR, Norris JW. Femoral neuropathy during anticoagulant therapy. Neurology 1976;26:1173–1175.

Case 5

HISTORY AND PHYSICAL EXAMINATION

A 34-year-old women, gravida 3, para 2 at 40 weeks' gestation, was admitted for irregular uterine contractions and induction of labor. The pregnancy was complicated by gestational diabetes and thrombophlebitis of the left leg, treated with subcutaneous heparin. Previous pregnancies were uneventful vaginal deliveries that resulted in 9 lb 6 oz (4252 g) and 11 lb 11 oz (5301 g) baby girls. After she was infused intravenously with pitocin, the patient's contractions became strong, and the cervix effaced to 10 cm 2 hours later. During labor, she noticed intermittent numbness of the right foot. After 2½ hours of active labor, with the baby in a persistent vertex position, forceps delivery was attempted but was unsuccessful. Failure to progress was diagnosed and the patient underwent a low transverse cesarean section under general anesthesia. A 12 lb 2 oz (5500 g) baby boy was delivered.

On the first attempt to get out of bed 6 hours after delivery, the patient noticed complete right footdrop and numbness of the entire foot and the lateral aspect of the leg. She had mild pain in the right buttock with no back pain, radicular symptoms, or bruising. On examination by her obstetrician, she had no detectable function of right ankle dorsiflexion, eversion and inversion, and dorsiflexion of the toes. Plantar flexion was normal. Deep tendon reflexes, including ankle jerks, were normal. There was decreased sensation in the right lateral leg and the dorsum of the foot, with minimal involvement of the sole. Computed tomography (CT) scan of the pelvis and abdomen and magnetic resonance imaging (MRI) of the lumbar spine were normal. Plantar numbness improved over the next few days, and the patient was discharged using an ankle–foot orthosis.

On neurological examination 1 month later, the patient was a 5 ft 7 in (167.5 cm) tall woman who was still unable to dorsiflex, invert, or evert the ankle, or dorsiflex the toes (Medical Research Council [MRC] scale 0/5). Plantar flexion was normal, but toe flexion was weak (MRC 4/5). Right hip abduction was weak (MRC 4–/5), as were hip extension and knee flexion (MRC 4/5). Knee extension and hip flexion were, however, normal. Both straight and reverse-straight leg raise tests were negative. Knee and ankle jerks were normal and symmetrical. There was an area of hypesthesia to touch, and pain over the lateral aspect of the right leg and the dorsum of the foot. Sensation on the plantar surface of the foot had normalized.

An electrodiagnostic (EDX) examination was requested.

Please now review the Nerve Conduction Studies and Needle EMG tables.

QUESTIONS

1. The EDX findings are most consistent with:
   A. L5 radiculopathy.
   B. Sciatic mononeuropathy.
   C. Peroneal mononeuropathy at the fibular neck.
   D. Lumbosacral plexopathy.

2. Differentiating a lumbosacral trunk lesion from L5 radiculopathy is dependent on:
   A. Gluteus medius denervation.
   B. Absent/low superficial peroneal sensory nerve action potentials (SNAPs).
   C. Flexor digitorum longus denervation.
   D. Tibialis anterior denervation.

3. Common causes of lumbosacral trunk lesions include all of the following *except:*
   A. Labor.
   B. Pelvic fracture.
   C. Pelvic mass.
   D. Total hip revision.

Case 5: Nerve Conduction Studies

Nerve Stimulated	Stimulation Site	Recording Site	Amplitude (m = mV, s = µV)			Distal/Peak Latency (ms)			Conduction Velocity (m/s)			F Latency (ms)	
			Right	Left	Normal	Right	Left	Normal	Right	Left	Normal	Right	Left
Sural (s)	Calf	Ankle	10	20	≥5	4.4	4.0	≤4.5					
Super. peron. (s)	Lateral leg	Ankle	**14**	25	≥5	3.2	2.7	≤4.5					
Peroneal (m)	Ankle	EDB	**1.8**	2.5	≥3	**6.1**	5.2	≤5.5	46	49	≥40	44	42
Peroneal (m)	Bel. fibular head	EDB	**1.8**	2.5									
Peroneal (m)	Knee	EDB	**1.7**	2.5					46	53	≥40		
Peroneal (m)	Bel. fibular head	Tibialis anterior	**1.2**	4.5	≥4	2.4	2.5	≤4.0					
Perongeal (m)	Knee		**1.0**	4.0					50	56	≥40		
Tibial (m)	Ankle	AH	10.0	14.5	≥8	5.1	4.6	≤6.0	43	52	≥40	46	48
Tibial (m)	Knee	AH	8.0	11.5									
H reflex	Knee	Soleus	7	7		30	31						
M response	Knee	Soleus	10	10		5.2	5.6						

AH = abductor hallucis; Bel. fibular head = below fibular head; EDB = extensor digitorum brevis; m = motor; s = sensory; Super. peron. = superficial peroneal. Data in bold type are abnormal.

Case 5: Needle EMG

Muscle	Insertional Activity	Spontaneous Activity		Recruitment				Configuration			Others
		Fibs	Fascs	Normal	Activation	Reduced	Early	Duration	Amplitude	% Polyphasia	
R. tibialis anterior	↑	1+	0	None fired							
Medial gastrocnemius	↑	+/–	0	X				Normal	Normal	Normal	
Flexor digitorum longus	↑	2+	0	None fired							
Extensor hallucis	↑	2+	0	None fired							
Abductor hallucis	↑	0	0			↓		Normal	Normal	Normal	
Extensor dig. brevis	↑	1+	0			↓↓↓		Normal	Normal	Normal	
Tibialis posterior	↑	2+	0	None fired							
Biceps fem. (short head)	↑	1+	0			↓		Normal	Normal	Normal	
Biceps fem. (long head)	↑	0	0	X				Normal	Normal	Normal	
Vastus lateralis	Normal	0	0	X				Normal	Normal	Normal	
Gluteus medius	↑	2+	0			↓↓↓		Normal	Normal	Normal	
Gluteus maximus	Normal	1+	0			↓		Normal	Normal	Normal	
Midlumbar paraspinal	Normal	0	0	–							
Lower lumbar paraspinal	Normal	0	0	–							
L. tibialis anterior	Normal	0	0	X							

Biceps fem. = biceps femoris; Extensor dig. brevis = extensor digitorum brevis; Fascs = fasciculations; Fibs = fibrillations; R. = right; ↑ = increased; ↓ = mildly reduced; ↓↓↓ = severely reduced.

EDX FINDINGS AND INTERPRETATION OF DATA

The relevant electrodiagnostic findings in this case are the followings:

1. The superficial peroneal and sural sensory nerve action potentials (SNAPs) were lower in amplitudes on the affected limb when compared with the asymptomatic limb. This excludes root(s) lesions because it places the lesion distal to the dorsal root ganglia, as seen with either a plexus or peripheral nerve lesions.
2. The peroneal compound muscle action potentials (CMAPs) were borderline to low in amplitude following all stimulation sites (ankle, below fibula neck, and knee) without evidence of focal slowing or conduction block. Also, the peroneal CMAPs, recording the tibialis anterior, were more affected than when recording the extensor digitorum brevis. In contrast, tibial CMAPs, H reflexes, and M responses were normal and symmetrical.
3. All conduction velocities, distal latencies, H reflexes, and F wave latencies were normal.
4. Needle muscle examination showed significant decrease in recruitment of motor unit action potentials (MUAPs) and variable fibrillation potentials in all L5-innervated muscles, with normal paraspinal muscles.

In summary, this case revealed L5 (with minimal S1) denervation associated with low superficial peroneal and sural SNAPs and normal paraspinal muscles. This is consistent with a lumbosacral trunk (cord) lesion, which is formed mainly by the L5 root (with some L4 contribution), as seen with intrapartum lumbosacral plexopathy. Recording a peroneal CMAP from tibialis anterior combined with absent voluntary MUAPs from tibialis anterior suggests that a significant number of fibers are blocked (demyelinated) proximally. This points to a relatively good prognosis.

DISCUSSION

Applied Anatomy

The lumbosacral plexus is divided anatomically into the lumbar plexus and the sacral plexus with a connecting nerve trunk, the lumbosacral trunk (Figure C5–1).

- The *lumbar plexus* is formed from the ventral rami of L1, L2, L3, and most of the L4 roots. These rami divide near the vertebral column into dorsal and ventral branches. The dorsal branches of L2, L3, and L4 roots combine to form the femoral nerve, while the ventral branches of these same roots join to form the obturator nerve. The lumbar plexus gives also rise to direct motor branches to the underlying iliacus and psoas muscles, and to the ilioinguinal, iliohypogastric, genitofemoral, and lateral femoral cutaneous nerves.
- The *lumbosacral trunk* (also called the lumbosacral cord) is formed primarily by the L5 root, with a contributing branch from the L4 root (see Figure C5–1). It then travels a relatively long distance in close contact with the ala of the sacrum, which is adjacent to the sacroiliac joint. It is covered throughout its course by the psoas muscle, except at its terminal portion near the bony pelvic rim, where it is joined by the S1 root. Many fibers within the lumbosacral trunk are destined to reach the common peroneal nerve, and they terminate primarily in muscles of the lateral compartment of the leg.
- The *sacral plexus* is formed by the fusion of the lumbosacral trunk with the ventral rami of S1, S2, and S3 and with a branch from the S4 roots (see Figure C5–1). It overlies the lateral sacrum and the posterolateral pelvic wall. Its main branches are the sciatic nerve (L4, L5, S1, S2, S3), the superior gluteal nerve (which innervates the gluteus medius and the gluteus minimus), and the inferior gluteal nerve (which innervates the gluteus maximus). Other nerves that arise directly from the

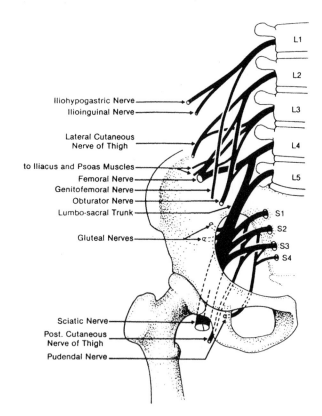

Figure C5–1. *The lumbosacral plexus, its important anatomic features, and the nerves that derive from it. (From Stewart JD. Focal peripheral neuropathies, 2nd ed. New York: Raven Press, 1993, with permission.)*

sacral plexus are the posterior cutaneous nerve of the thigh and pudendal nerves.

Clinical Features

Lumbosacral plexus lesions are much less common than brachial plexopathies. A detailed examination of hip girdle muscles, particularly the gluteal muscles, thigh adductors, and iliopsoas, is helpful in accurate diagnosis because these muscles often are abnormal in lumbosacral plexus lesions but usually are normal in peripheral nerve lesions, such as those involving the sciatic or femoral nerves.

- A lumbar plexus lesion may cause symptoms in the territories of the iliohypogastric, genitofemoral, ilioinguinal, femoral, and obturator nerves. This may result in weakness of hip flexion, knee extension, and thigh adduction with sensory loss in the lower abdomen, inguinal region, and over the entire medial, lateral, and anterior surfaces of the thigh and the medial lower leg.

The knee jerk may be decreased or absent. A lumbar plexus lesion often mimic a femoral neuropathy or an L4 radiculopathy because all present with anterior thigh pain or numbness or quadriceps weakness.

- A lumbosacral trunk injury frequently poses a diagnostic challenge because such a lesion results predominantly in footdrop and imitates a common peroneal mononeuropathy or an L5 radiculopathy (Table C5–1). Lesions of the lumbosacral trunk present with footdrop, with variable buttock pain and numbness in the lateral leg and the dorsum of the foot. Neurologic findings include not only weakness of ankle and toe dorsiflexion and ankle eversion, but also ankle inversion and toe flexion. There also is variable weakness of the glutei and hamstring muscles. Plantar flexion and ankle jerk usually are normal. Sensory loss is in the L5 dermatomal distribution. Detecting weakness in ankle inversion (tibialis posterior) or toe flexion (flexor digitorum longus), eliminates a peroneal neuropathy. It is more difficult to separate

Table C5–1. Differential Diagnosis of a Lumbosacral Trunk Lesion Causing Footdrop

	Peroneal Neuropathy at the Fibular Head	L5 Radiculopathy	Lumbar Plexopathy (Lumbosacral Trunk)	Sciatic Neuropathy (Mainly Peroneal)
(A) Clinical				
Common causes	Compression (weight loss, perioperative), trauma	Disc herniation, spinal stenosis	Pelvic surgery, hematoma, prolonged labor	Hip surgery, injection injury, coma
Ankle inversion	Normal	Weak	Weak	Normal or mildly weak
Toe flexion	Normal	Weak	Weak	Normal or mildly weak
Plantar flexion	Normal	Normal	Normal	Normal or mildly weak
Ankle jerk	Normal	Normal (unless with S1)	Normal (unless with S1)	Normal or depressed
Sensory loss distribution	Peroneal only	Poorly demarcated, predominantly big toe	Well demarcated to L5 dermatome	Peroneal and lateral cutaneous of calf
Pain	Rare, deep	Common, radicular	Common, can be radicular	Can be severe
(B) Electrodiagnosis				
Peroneal motor study to EDB and/or Tib Ant	Low in amplitude or conduction block across fibular head or both	Usually normal but can be low in amplitude	Low in amplitude	Low in amplitude
Superficial peroneal sensory study	Low or absent*	Normal	Low or absent	Low or absent
Sural sensory study	Normal	Normal	Normal or low amp	Normal or low amp
Peroneal muscles†	Abnormal	Abnormal	Abnormal	Abnormal
Tibial L5muscles‡	Normal	Usually abnormal	Usually abnormal	Normal or abnormal
Other L5 muscles¶	Normal	Normal or abnormal	Normal or abnormal	Normal
Biceps femoris (short head)	Normal	Usually normal	Usually normal	Abnormal
Paraspinal muscles fibrillations	Absent	May be absent	Absent	Absent

*Can be normal in purely demyelinating lesions or lesion of the deep peroneal nerve only.
†Below knee (tibialis anterior (Tib Ant), extensor digitorum longus, extensor digitorum brevis (EDB), extensor hallucis, +/– peroneus longus).
‡Tibialis posterior and flexor digitorum longus.
¶Gluteus medius and tensor fascia lata.

lumbosacral trunk lesions from L5 radiculopathy because the weakness, in both conditions, involves the L5 myotome. Often, this will depends on a detailed electrodiagnostic studies and other ancillary studies such as CT scan and MRI of the plexus and lumbar spine.

• A sacral plexus lesion may cause manifestations in the distributions of the gluteal, sciatic, tibial, and peroneal nerves. This manifests in weakness of the hip extensors, hip abductors, knee flexors, and all foot and toe functions. Diminished sensation may involve the posterior aspect of the thigh, anterolateral and posterior aspect of the leg below the knee and almost the entire foot. The ankle jerk may be diminished or absent. A sacral plexus lesion most often mimics a sciatic nerve lesion, except that the gluteal muscles often are involved in plexus injury only.

Causes of lumbosacral plexopathy are shown in Table C5–2, but the following entities are the most common. Diabetic amyotophy is discussed in details in Case 7.

Acute hemorrhage in the retroperitoneal space may be limited to the iliacus muscle and, less commonly it may be more extensive within the psoas muscle. The limited hemorrhage into the iliacus muscle usually leads to an iliacus compartmental syndrome, which may result in severe femoral nerve injury. When the hematoma is into the psoas muscle, it is often large and extends widely through the retroperitoneal space, leading to a more extensive injury of the lumbar plexus, and occasionally, to the entire lumbosacral plexus. Most cases of hemorrhage occur in the setting of anticoagulation or coagulopathy, and their clinical presentation is unique. There is usually an acute severe pain in the lower abdomen, groin, and thigh followed by weakness and sensory loss. Patients frequently keep the hip flexed to minimize pain because hip extension (such as occurs with reversed-straight leg test) is extremely painful. In cases of iliacus hematoma, the neurologic deficit is restricted to the femoral nerve with weakness of hip flexion and knee extension and sensory loss in the anterior

Table C5–2. Common Causes of Lumbosacral Plexopathy

Iliacus hematoma (only femoral nerve)

Psoas (retroperitoneal) hematoma

Intrapartum maternal

Pelvic mass

    Malignant neoplasms (lymphoma; ovarian, colorectal, and uterine cancer)

    Retroperitoneal lymphadenopathy

    Abscess

Pelvic fracture

Radiation injury

Diabetes (diabetic amyotrophy, diabetic proximal neuropathy)

Idiopathic lumbosacral plexitis

thigh and medial leg. A more extensive psoas hematoma may result in damage to the lumbar plexus, and occasionally the entire lumbosacral plexus. The neurologic findings include weakness in the femoral as well as the obturator nerve distributions (hip flexion, knee extension and thigh adduction), and often in the lumbosacral trunk distribution (ankle dorsiflexion). In these cases, there may be also an abrupt reduction in the hematocrit which may be the only sign of retroperitoneal hemorrhage. *The diagnosis should be confirmed promptly by a CT scan or an MRI of the pelvis.* Controversy continues regarding the indications and timing of surgical evacuation of hematoma once the plexus or femoral nerve lesion is clinically apparent.

Intrapartum maternal lumbosacral plexopathy is a disorder caused by compression of the lumbosacral trunk by the descending fetal head during labor. The disorder is also known by a variety of names including postpartum footdrop, maternal birth palsy, maternal obstetric sciatic paralysis, traumatic neuritis of the puerperium, maternal obstetric paralysis, traumatic maternal birth palsy, obstetric neurapraxia, and obstetric lumbosacral plexus injury. The lumbosacral trunk is a long structure is most susceptible to pressure from the fetal presenting part at the pelvic rim, where it is unprotected by the psoas muscle (Figure C5–2). Incriminating risk factors for the development of intrapartum maternal lumbosacral plexopathy include short maternal stature, the birth of a large infant, or both. This leads to cephalopelvic disproportion and potential compression of the lumbosacral trunk by the fetal head against the pelvic rim. The labor is either prolonged or arrested and delivery is often accomplished by a caesarean section. The patient usually presents as a postpartum footdrop. However, sensory symptoms or pain referred to the symptomatic leg may be noted by some patients during active labor, because neural compression develops during fetal descent into the pelvis. However, these symptoms may be completely masked by epidural anesthesia for pain control, or dismissed by the treating physicians and nurses who may consider them part of labor pain. As delivery is completed by a cesarean section in many of these patients, using epidural or general anesthesia, foot drop was not detected until the immediate postpartum period. The clinical findings mimic a severe L-5 radiculopathy since the L-5 root fibers travel exclusively through the lumbosacral trunk. In contrast to L5 radiculopathy, however, these patients have always a foot drop since the tibialis anterior, the main ankle dorsiflexor, receives all its innervation (L5 and L4 fibers) via the lumbosacral trunk, while ankle dorsiflexion is often only modestly weak in selective L5 radiculopathy since the tibialis anterior has usually a dual L5 and L4 segmental innervation. Most patients recover in weeks to months, suggesting that the primary pathologic process is demyelination.

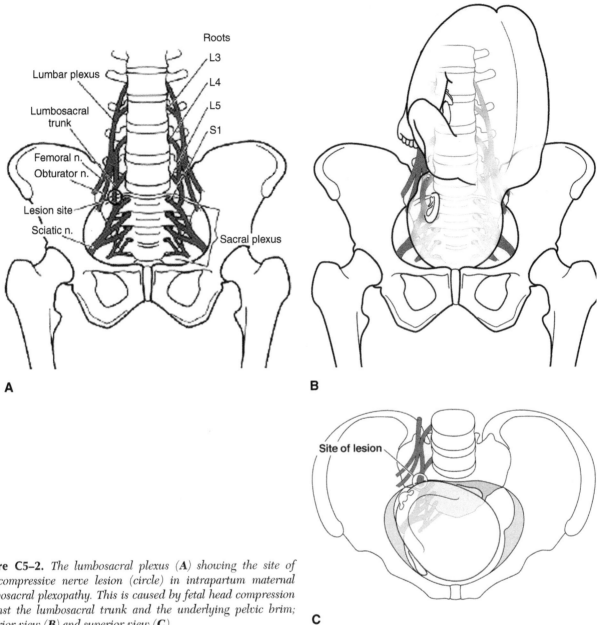

Figure C5–2. *The lumbosacral plexus* (**A**) *showing the site of the compressive nerve lesion (circle) in intrapartum maternal lumbosacral plexopathy. This is caused by fetal head compression against the lumbosacral trunk and the underlying pelvic brim; anterior view* (**B**) *and superior view* (**C**).

Idiopathic lumbosacral plexitis is the leg counterpart of neuralgic amyotrophy in the arm (acute brachial neuritis, Parsonage-Turner syndrome), although it is much less common. This disorder is somehow similar to diabetic amyotrophy, but it occurs in nondiabetics. Onset is acute or subacute and is heralded by severe leg pain followed by weakness that usually ensues several days to weeks after the onset of pain. Sensory symptoms are less prominent. The neurological findings may predominantly affect fibers of either the lumbar or sacral plexus. An elevated sedimentation rate may be present. The prognosis is good, but recovery of pain or weakness may be protracted, and recurrence is rare.

Electrodiagnosis

The roles of electrodiagnosis are to confirm the site of the lesion and to distinguish between lumbosacral plexopathy, lumbosacral radiculopathy, and lower limb mononeuropathy. In order to accurately identify a lumbosacral plexopathy, multiple sensory and motor nerve conduction studies in the symptomatic and the opposite limb, and extensive needle EMG are often necessary.

Differentiating a lumbosacral plexus lesion from lumbosacral radiculopathy is clinically difficult because the same fibers are affected at either location. Electrodiagnostically,

Table C5–3. Differential Diagnosis of Lumbar Plexopathy

	Lumbar Plexopathy	Femoral Mononeuropathy	Lumbar Radiculopathy
Thigh adductors	Denervation	Normal	Denervation
Tibialis anterior	Denervation*	Normal	Denervation*
Saphenous SNAP[†]	Low or absent[‡]	Low or absent[‡]	Normal
Paraspinal fibrillations	Absent	Absent	Usually present

*Abnormal in L4 radiculopathy/plexopathy only.
[†]May be technically difficult, particularly in elderly patients, or if there is leg edema.
[‡]Normal in purely demyelinating lesions.

this is accomplished mainly with needle EMG of the paraspinal muscles and the SNAPs:

- The presence of fibrillation potentials in paraspinal muscles is not consistent with a lumbosacral plexus lesion because these muscles are innervated by the posterior primary rami, before formation of the plexus. Unfortunately, fibrillation potentials of t he paraspinal muscles are not always present in radiculopathy, presumably due to rapid and effective reinnervation.

- In axon-loss lumbosacral plexopathy, the SNAPs usually are abnormally low in amplitude or absent because the lesion affects the postganglionic fibers. In contrast, these studies are normal in radiculopathy because compression occurs against the preganglionic fibers only (i.e., sensory fibers proximal to the dorsal root ganglion). Unfortunately, some of the sensory nerves that would be very helpful to evaluate the lumbar roots (L2, L3, and L4) are, for technical reasons, not possible to study (such as the iliohypogastric and ilioinguinal nerves) or difficult to evoke in normal subjects (such as the lateral femoral cutaneous and saphenous nerves).

A lumbar plexus lesion may imitate an L4 radiculopathy or a femoral mononeuropathy (Table C5–3). The differential diagnosis may be difficult because the saphenous SNAP may be unelicitable in elderly, obese patients, or in patients with leg edema or associated peripheral polyneuropathy (as in diabetics). In contrast, the differential diagnosis of a lumbosacral trunk lesion includes an L5 radiculopathy or a peroneal mononeuropathy and is less difficult to confirm (Table C5–1). Finally, differentiating a sciatic mononeuropathy from a sacral plexopathy depends solely on the establishment of denervation in the gluteal muscles, and possibly in the external anal sphincter.

FOLLOW-UP

Two months after delivery, there was a dramatic improvement in ankle dorsiflexion (MRC 4+/5) and near resolution of sensory symptoms. When seen a year later, the patient was totally asymptomatic.

DIAGNOSIS

Intrapartum maternal lumbosacral plexopathy, mixed (demyelinative and axonal) causing a selective lumbosacral trunk lesion, caused by cephalopelvic disproportion related to delivery of a large baby.

ANSWERS

1. D; 2. B; 3. D.

SUGGESTED READINGS

Asbury AK. Proximal diabetic neuropathy. Ann Neurol 1977; 2:179–180.

Barohn RJ et al. The Bruns-Garland syndrome (diabetic amyotrophy). Revisited 100 years later. Arch Neurol 1991;48:1130–1135.

Feasby TE, Burton SR, Hahn AF. Obstetrical lumbosacral plexus injury. Muscle Nerve 1992;15:937–940.

Katirji B, Wilbourn AJ, Scarberry SL et al. Intrapartum maternal lumbosacral plexopathy. Muscle Nerve 2002;26:340–347.

Stewart JD. Focal peripheral neuropathies, 2nd ed. New York: Raven Press, 1993.

Subramony SH, Wilbourn AJ. Diabetic proximal neuropathy. J Neurol Sci 1982;53:293–304.

Whittaker WG. Injuries to the sacral plexus in obstetrics. Can Med Assoc J 1958;79:622–636.

Young MR, Norris JW. Femoral neuropathy during anticoagulant therapy. Neurology 1976;26:1173–1175.

Case 6

HISTORY AND PHYSICAL EXAMINATION

Pain and numbness developed in the left big toe of a 28-year-old white man with rheumatoid arthritis. Symptoms were worse upon standing or walking. He had no leg weakness and experienced no similar symptoms in the hands or right leg. He denied any history of ankle trauma. He had been treated with oral methotrexate and chloroquine and was referred to the electromyography (EMG) laboratory.

On examination, the patient had slight swelling of the left ankle compared with the right. There was hypesthesia, most pronounced over the plantar surfaces of the big and second toes. There was possible weakness of left big toe flexion. Plantar flexion and dorsiflexion of left ankle were normal. He had a Tinel sign on percussion of the left tibial nerve over the flexor retinaculum. There was no sensory impairment or weakness in the right foot or hands. Deep tendon reflexes were normal and symmetrical.

An electrodiagnostic (EDX) examination was performed. Please now review the Nerve Conduction Studies and Needle EMG tables.

QUESTIONS

1. The findings are consistent with:
   A. Sensorimotor peripheral polyneuropathy.
   B. Right tarsal tunnel syndrome.
   C. Right S1/S2 radiculopathy.
   D. Right proximal tibial mononeuropathy.
2. Difficulties in establishing the diagnosis of this entity, especially in the elderly, are due to all of the following except:
   A. When bilateral, it can mimic early sensorimotor polyneuropathy.
   B. Chronic denervation changes in intrinsic muscles of the foot are common.
   C. Percutaneous plantar mixed nerve conduction studies are technically difficult.
   D. When axonal and not associated with focal slowing, it can mimic S1/S2 radiculopathy.
   E. It is a common entrapment neuropathy in the lower extremity.
3. Common underlying factors include all of the following except:
   A. Rheumatoid arthritis.
   B. Tenosynovitis.
   C. Ankle trauma.
   D. Recent anesthesia and surgery.
   E. Lipoma.

EDX FINDINGS AND INTERPRETATION OF DATA

Pertinent EDX studies include the following:

1. Low-amplitude left tibial compound muscle action potentials (CMAPs) with delayed distal latencies, recording abductor hallucis (AH) and abductor digiti quinti pedis (ADQP), with normal tibial proximal motor conduction velocities. This is evident when compared to normal values and to the asymptomatic right side. Note that the tibial study, recording AH, assesses the medial plantar terminal nerve, while the tibial study, recording ADQP, evaluates the lateral plantar nerve.
2. Delayed left medial and lateral plantar mixed nerve latencies across the ankle. These mixed responses assess both sensory and motor fibers in the corresponding nerves.
3. Chronic denervation restricted to the tibial-innervated muscles of the left foot.

Case 6: Nerve Conduction Studies

Nerve Stimulated	Stimulation Site	Recording Site	Amplitude (m = mV, s = μV)			Distal/Peak Latency (ms)			Conduction Velocity (m/s)			F Latency (ms)	
			Right	Left	Normal	Right	Left	Normal	Right	Left	Normal	Right	Left
Sural (s)	Calf	Leg	20		≥5		3.8	≤4.5		43	≥40		
Peroneal (m)*	Ankle	EDB		4	≥3		4.3	≤5.5					
Peroneal (m)	Knee	EDB		4						48	≥40		50
Tibial (m)	Ankle	AH	10.0	4	≥8	5.5	**6.1**	≤6.0		49	≥40		
Tibial (m)	Knee	AH	8.2	3					47				52
Tibial (m)	Ankle	ADQP	4.0	**2.5**	≥4	5.0	**6.8**	≤6.0		46	≥40		
Tibial (m)	Knee	ADQP	2.5	**1.8**					48				
Medial plantar	Sole	Ankle*	7	8		3.7	**4.8**	≤3.8					
Lateral plantar	Sole	Ankle*	12	10		3.4	**5.5**	≤3.8					
H reflex	Knee	Soleus	1.5	2.0		6.7	6.9						
M response	Knee	Soleus	11.5	12.0		30.1	29.9						

ADQP = abductor digiti quinti pedis; AH = abductor hallucis; EDB = extensor digitorum brevis; m = motor; s = sensory.
Data in bold type are abnormal.
*Above flexor retinaculum.

Case 6: Needle EMG

Muscle	Insertional Activity	Spontaneous Activity		Recruitment				Configuration			Others
		Fibs	Fascs	Normal	Activation	Reduced	Early	Duration	Amplitude	% Polyphasia	
L. abductor hallucis	Normal	0	0			↓↓		↑↑	↑↑	↑	
Abductor dig. quinti ped.	Normal	0	0			↓		↑	↑	Normal	
Extensor dig. brevis	Normal	0	0	X				Normal	Normal	Normal	
Medial gastrocnemius	Normal	0	0	X				Normal	Normal	Normal	
Flexor digitorum longus	Normal	0	0	X				Normal	Normal	Normal	
Tibialis anterior	Normal	0	0	X				Normal	Normal	Normal	
Gluteus maximus	Normal	0	0	X				Normal	Normal	Normal	
Midlumbar paraspinal	Normal	0	0	–							
Low lumbar paraspinal	Normal	0	0	–							
R. abductor hallucis	Normal	0	0	X				Normal	Normal	Normal	
Abductor dig. quinti ped.	Normal	0	0	X				Normal	Normal	Normal	
Extensor dig. brevis	Normal	0	0	X				Normal	Normal	Normal	

Voluntary Motor Unit Action Potentials (MUAPs)

Abductor dig. quinti ped. = abductor digiti quinti pedis; Extensor dig. brevis = extensor digitorum brevis; Fascs = fasciculations; Fibs = fibrillations; L. = left; R. = right; ↑ = increased; ↓ = mildly reduced; ↓↓ = moderately reduced; ↑↑ = significantly increased.

These findings are consistent with a right tibial mononeuropathy at, or distal to, the ankle, affecting both terminal branches (medial and lateral plantar nerves), and compatible with a left tarsal tunnel syndrome (TTS). The study is not consistent with an S1 radiculopathy due to the normal H reflex and lack of denervation in other S1-innervated muscles (medial gastrocnemius, flexor digitorum longus, extensor digitorum brevis, gluteus maximus, and lumbar paraspinal muscles). A sensorimotor polyneuropathy is unlikely because of the lack of denervation in the contralateral foot and normal H reflexes, right sural sensory nerve action potential (SNAP), and left peroneal and right tibial motor distal latencies and conduction velocities.

DISCUSSION

Applied Anatomy

After innervating the gastrocnemius, soleus, tibialis posterior, flexor digitorum profundus, and flexor hallucis longus in the calf, the tibial nerve passes through the *tarsal tunnel* at the medial aspect of the ankle. There, the tibial nerve is accompanied by the tibial artery and the tendons of the flexor digitorum longus, flexor hallucis longus, and tibialis posterior muscles. This tunnel's roof is composed of a thin fascia, the *laciniate ligament (flexor retinaculum)*, which connects the medial malleolus to the calcaneus.

The tibial nerve bifurcates into its two terminal branches within 1 cm of the malleolocalcaneal axis in 90% of patients (Figure C6–1). Its terminal branches are: (1) the *calcaneal branch*, a purely sensory nerve, which has a variable takeoff in relation to the flexor retinaculum and explain its involvement or its lack of in nerve entrapments at that site (Figure C6–2); (2) the *medial plantar nerve*, which innervates the abductor hallucis, flexor digitorum brevis, and flexor hallucis brevis, in addition to the skin of the medial sole and, at least, the medial three toes; and (3) *the lateral plantar nerve*, which innervates the abductor digiti quinti pedis, flexor digiti quinti pedis, adductor hallucis, and the interossei, in addition to the skin of the lateral sole and two lateral toes. The innervation of the skin of the sole of the foot is provided primarily through the three terminal branches of the tibial nerves, with minimal contribution from the saphenous and sural nerves (Figure C6–3).

Clinical Features

Tarsal tunnel syndrome (TTS) is caused by compression of the tibial nerve or any of its three terminal branches under the flexor retinaculum. It was first described by

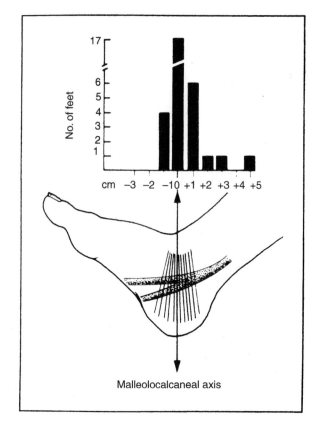

Figure C6–1. *The distribution of location of the tibial nerve along the malleolocalcaneal axis and the flexor retinaculum. (From Dellon AL, Mackinnon SE. Tibial nerve branching in the tarsal tunnel. Arch Neurol 1984;41:645–646, with permission from the American Medical Association.)*

Keck in 1962. Its true incidence is unknown, though it is an uncommon entrapment mononeuropathy. TTS is sometimes referred to as the medial tarsal tunnel syndrome, to distinguish it from the anterior tarsal tunnel syndrome which is an entrapment of the terminal segment of the deep peroneal nerve under the extensor retinaculum in the dorsum of the foot.

The disorder is insidious in onset, more common in women and is usually unilateral. Bilateral TTS is rare accounting for 10–20% of cases. Most cases of TTS are idiopathic but remote ankle trauma, particularly sprains and fractures, is common. Runners, joggers, and dancers are particularly at high risk for developing TTS. Other causes include arthritis or tenosynovitis of the ankle with or without rheumatoid arthritis, hypertrophic or anomalous muscles, biomechanical factors (such as ill-fitting foot wear or heel varus and valgus deformity), or a mass lesion within the tunnel (ganglion, lipoma, schwannoma, or varicose vein).

The most common symptom of TTS is burning foot pain, which often worsens after prolonged standing

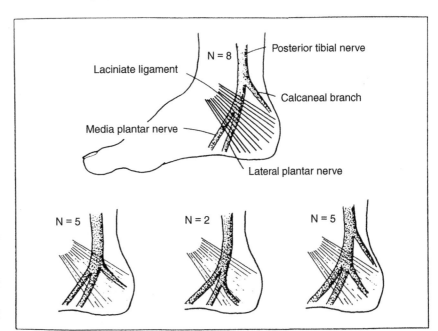

Figure C6–2. *Patterns of origin of the medial calcaneal branch from the tibial nerve in 20 patients. (From Dellon AL, Mackinnon SE. Tibial nerve branching in the tarsal tunnel. Arch Neurol 1984;41:645–646, with permission from the American Medical Association.)*

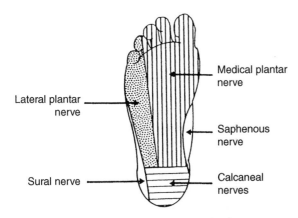

Figure C6–3. *The cutaneous innervation of the sole of the foot. (From Dyck PJ, Thomas PK. Peripheral neuropathy, 3rd ed. Philadelphia, PA: WB Saunders, 1993, with permission from the American Medical Association.)*

or walking. Sometimes, the pain radiates proximally to the calf. Paresthesia in the sole is common, but weakness or imbalance is extremely rare. The neurologic examination shows sensory impairment in the sole in the distribution of one or more of the three terminal tibial branches (medial plantar, lateral plantar, or calcaneal). In 40% of patients, the medial and lateral plantar nerves are involved while the heel is spared. In 25% of patients, the sensory loss involves all three terminal branches territory, and in another 25%, the sensory loss is only in the medial plantar nerve distribution, while selective entrapment of the lateral plantar nerve is only present in 10% of the cases. The sensory symptoms may be triggered or exaggeration by foot eversion. Tinel sign, induced by percussion of the tibial nerve at the flexor retinaculum, is a useful sign and is present in the majority of patients. Muscle atrophy in one sole is rarely encountered. Weakness is rare because the long toe flexors are intact. Ankle jerk and sensation of the dorsum of the foot are normal.

True TTS is likely a clinical rarity, despite that some podiatrists and orthopedists consider it to be a common disorder. A variety of more common orthopedic, rheumatologic, and neurologic conditions may result in foot pain and may be misdiagnosed as TTS (Table C6–1). The diagnosis of TTS is particularly difficult in patients with a history of foot or ankle trauma. Careful evaluation of the ankle and foot, including x-rays, bone scan, tomogram, magnetic resonance imaging, and EMG, is often necessary before a correct diagnosis is made. Of the neurologic disorders that mimic TTS, proximal tibial mononeuropathy, caused by nerve compression by the tendinous arch of the soleus muscle or due to a nerve sheath tumor, may present with indolent symptoms that are very similar to those of TTS. These rare lesions manifest with foot pain and numbness, but they are usually associated with calf weakness or atrophy and absent or depressed ankle jerk, findings not consistent with TTS. An S1 or S2 radiculopathy, in isolation or as a component of lumbar spinal canal stenosis, may result in foot numbness or pain which

Table C6–1. Differential Diagnosis of Tarsal Tunnel Syndrome

Plantar fasciitis

Stress fracture

Arthritis

Bursitis

Reflex sympathetic dystrophy

Medial plantar neuropathy in the foot*

Joplin neuroma (injury to the medial plantar proper digital nerve to the great toe)*

High tibial or sciatic neuropathy

Sacral radiculopathy (S1 or S2)

Peripheral polyneuropathy (when bilateral)

*Due to trauma, bunion surgery, foot deformities, or ill-fitted shoes.

is often worse with walking or standing. However, there is usually low back and posterior thigh pain ("sciatica"), depressed or absent ankle jerk or weakness of gastrocnemius, hamstrings, or glutei muscles. A particularly troublesome task is distinguishing patients with TTS from those with early sensory peripheral polyneuropathy, particularly in the elderly. A useful feature is that TTS is rarely bilateral while peripheral polyneuropathy often affects both feet. Also, the sensory loss in polyneuropathy usually involves both the sole and dorsum of the foot and is rarely associated with a Tinel sign at the flexor retinaculum.

Conservative treatment of TTS should be provided first to all patients. Sources of pressure, such as ill-fitting shoes, should be identified and eliminated. Other helpful measures include minimization of ankle edema through elevation, the use of special stockings or a medial arch orthotic support, bracing of the foot with a light orthosis, administration of anti-inflammatory agents, or local injection with long-acting corticosteroids. Only a small proportion of patients require surgical decompression with variable results. Good outcome can be achieved by selecting either patients with documented entrapment who have failed conservative treatment or those with an identifiable mass. Although most patients improve without any sequelae, in some, especially those who experienced ankle trauma, chronic pain and features of complex regional pain syndrome (reflex sympathetic dystrophy) may develop.

Electrodiagnosis

Electrodiagnostic confirmation of TTS relies on techniques studying nerve fibers that traverse either the medial or the lateral plantar nerves. The following are the most commonly utilized EDX studies in patients with suspected TTS:

1. Tibial *motor NCSs recording from the abductor hallucis (medial plantar motor NCS) and the abductor digiti*

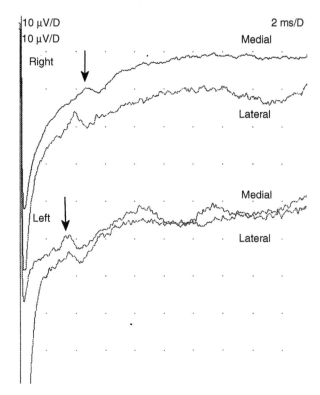

Figure C6–4. *Medial and lateral mixed plantar responses in a 45-year-old woman with a right tarsal tunnel syndrome. Note that the medial and, to a lesser extent, the lateral plantar mixed responses (arrows) were significantly delayed on the right when compared to the left (right medial and lateral plantar latencies were 4.7 ms and 4.0 ms respectively, while both latencies on the left were 3.5 ms).*

quinti pedis (lateral plantar motor NCS). These are the first NCSs described to diagnose TTS and consist of performing tibial motor NCSs while recording from the abductor hallucis (AH) and the abductor digiti quinti pedis (ADQP) muscles. A prolonged medial and/or lateral plantar motor distal latencies, using absolute values or by comparing to the contralateral asymptomatic limb, is considered diagnostic. Absolute value greater than approximately 4.8 ms or side-to-side difference greater than approximately 2 ms are diagnostic values. These motor studies are easy to perform, but are not sensitive since they only assess tibial motor fibers. They are diagnostic in only about half of symptomatic limbs.

2. *Medial and lateral plantar mixed NCSs.* These are the most widely employed studies for the evaluation of TTS. These are mixed nerve action potentials of the medial and lateral plantar nerves that evaluate the sensory and motor fibers. They are obtained by percutaneous (surface) stimulation of the medial and lateral plantar nerves on the sole of the foot, while recording

orthodromically with surface electrodes over the tibial nerve posterior to the medial malleolus. These studies are the counterparts of the median and ulnar palmar mixed studies performed for the evaluation of carpal tunnel syndrome, except that they are less reliable and sometimes not reproducible. Asymmetrical delay of latency of the medial or lateral (or both) mixed nerve action potentials is considered abnormal (Figure C6–4). Another likely significant, though poorly localizing, abnormality is absent mixed plantar responses on the symptomatic side. This test is more sensitive than the tibial motor distal latencies since it is abnormal in about 2/3 of symptomatic limbs. However, it may be technically difficult to elicit these potentials in subjects with foot calluses, foot or ankle edema, foot deformities, or even in normal adults over 45 years of age. Hence, absent bilateral plantar responses cannot be considered a definite supportive abnormality.

3. *Medial and lateral plantar sensory NCSs.* NCS techniques for assessing solely the sensory fibers of the medial and lateral plantar nerves are reported. The orthodromic techniques consist of stimulating the first and fifth toes, while recording from the tibial nerve proximal to the flexor retinaculum. Antidromic studies stimulating the ankle and recording the toes are also possible. A variation of the orthodromic sensory NCS technique includes recording via needle electrode placed close to the tibial nerve and proximal to the flexor retinaculum. Unfortunately, with any of these NCS procedures, the elicited SNAPs are extremely low in amplitude in normal subjects and require signal averaging. Moreover, in some healthy individuals, the responses cannot be evoked. As with the other plantar NCS techniques, prolonged latencies are sought. A possibly significant finding is absent SNAPs on the symptomatic side only. This particular procedure has not gained wide popularity, even though on theoretical grounds it should be the most sensitive technique (thought to be abnormal in over 90% of symptomatic limbs).

4. *Needle examination of the muscles of the sole (such as AH and ADQP)* may be abnormal with TTS if axon loss has occurred. Also, MUAPs loss, chronic neurogenic MUAP changes, and fibrillation potentials in various combinations may be found. A complicating factor is that these muscles are painful, difficult to activate, and may show denervation changes in asymptomatic patients, especially in the older age group.

In practical terms, tibial motor NCS, recording AH and ADQP, and medial and lateral plantar mixed NCS should be performed bilaterally for comparison. These should be followed by needle EMG sampling of the AH and ADQP muscles bilaterally for comparison. In a classical case of unilateral TTS, the motor amplitudes are low with delayed

Table C6–2. Electrophysiological Differentiation of Tarsal Tunnel Syndrome

	Tarsal Tunnel Syndrome	**Chronic S1/S2 Radiculopathy**	**Peripheral Polyneuropathy**
Nerve Conduction Studies			
Sural sensory study	Normal	Normal	Abnormal
Peroneal motor study	Normal	Normal or low amplitude	Abnormal
Tibial motor study	Low amplitude and/or slow latency	Normal or low amplitude	Low amplitude and/or slow latency
Motor conduction velocities	Normal	Normal or slowed	Slowed
Plantar mixed studies	Slow latency or absent	Normal	Slow latency or absent
H reflex	Normal	Abnormal	Abnormal
Upper extremity conductions	Normal	Normal	May be abnormal
Needle EMG			
AH/ADQP	Denervated	Denervated	Denervated
EDB	Normal	Denervated	Denervated
Medial gastrocnemius	Normal	Denervated	Denervated
Tibialis anterior	Normal	Normal	Denervated
Paraspinal muscles	Normal	Normal or fibs	Normal or fibs
Symmetry of Findings (When Bilateral)			
	Asymmetrical	Asymmetrical	Symmetrical

ADQP = abductor digiti quinti pedis; AH = abductor hallucis; EDB = extensor digitorum brevis; fibs = fibrillation potentials.

distal latencies and the mixed plantar studies are delayed or absent on the affected side only. Needle EMG shows fibrillation potentials in the AH and ADQP muscles with chronic neurogenic MUAP changes on the symptomatic side only. Findings restricted to the medial or lateral plantar nerves do also occur. In these situations, all the NCS and needle EMG abnormalities point to the compressed terminal nerve only. Unfortunately, it has been the experience of many physicians that the lesion is far more likely to be manifested as axon loss only without focal demyelinating slowing. In these situations, none of the above NCS techniques used to diagnose TTS is effective. Instead, the EDX study is nonlocalizing, since the NCS will demonstrate low amplitude or unelicitable responses without slowing, and the needle EMG will confirm the axonal nature by showing neurogenic MUAP changes.

An important task of the EDX study is to differentiate TTS from a peripheral polyneuropathy and S1/S2 radiculopathy. All three disorders have foot numbness and result in abnormal tibial motor conduction studies and denervation of intrinsic muscles of foot. Table C6–2 lists an EDX guide to help in differentiating TTS from these two neurologic disorders. It should be pointed out that distinguishing these three illnesses from one another sometimes is very difficult, especially in elderly patients in whom the sural SNAPs and H reflexes may be absent.

FOLLOW-UP

Following EDX confirmation of TTS, and failure of conservative therapy (corticosteroids and orthotic device), the patient underwent surgical release of the tibial nerve under the flexor retinaculum. Four months postoperatively, he had no pain but experienced mild residual numbness that was confirmed by sensory examination.

DIAGNOSIS

Left tibial mononeuropathy at, or distal to, the ankle, compatible with a left tarsal tunnel syndrome, affecting both the medial and lateral plantar nerves, chronic without active (ongoing) denervation.

ANSWERS

1. B; 2. E; 3. D.

SUGGESTED READINGS

Baba H, Wada M, Annen S et al. The tarsal tunnel syndrome: evaluation of surgical results using multivariate analysis. Int Orthop 1997;21:67–71.

Dawson DM, Hallett M, Wilbourn AJ. Entrapment neuropathies, 3rd ed. Boston, MA: Lippincott, Williams & Wilkins, 1999.

DeLisa JA, Saeed MA. The tarsal tunnel syndrome. Muscle Nerve 1983;6:664–670.

Dellon AL, Mackinnon SE. Tibial nerve branching in the tarsal tunnel. Arch Neurol 1984;41:645–646.

Galardi G et al. Electrophysiologic studies of tarsal tunnel syndrome: diagnostic reliability of motor distal latency, mixed nerve and sensory nerve conduction studies. Am J Phys Med Rehab 1994;73:193–198.

Keck C. The tarsal tunnel syndrome. J Bone Joint Surg 1962; 44A:180–182.

Oh SH, Meyer RD. Entrapment neuropathies of the tibial (posterior tibial) nerve. Neurol Clin 1999;17:593–615.

Oh SJ, Sarala PK, Kuba T et al. Tarsal tunnel syndrome: electrophysiological study. Ann Neurol 1979;5:327–530.

Pfeiffer WH, Cracchiolo A III. Clinical results after tarsal tunnel decompression. J Bone Joint Surg 1994;76A:1222–1230.

Stewart JD. Focal peripheral neuropathies, 3rd ed. New York: Lippincott, Williams & Wilkins, 2000.

Case 7

HISTORY AND PHYSICAL EXAMINATION

In a 72-year-old woman, pain developed in the right anterior thigh and knee, became severe over 2 to 3 weeks, and did not respond to steroid injection into the knee joint. The pain was maximal at night and did not worsen with standing or walking. Within 1 month, she noticed that her right leg was weak because the knee frequently would buckle from underneath her. She had fallen many times. She denied any symptoms in the left leg. She denied numbness in the legs or hands. She had mild low back pain. Her medical history was significant for diabetes mellitus, hypertension, and hypercholesterolemia. She was taking glyburide and diltiazem.

On physical examination, the patient was in modest discomfort because of right leg pain. Mental status and cranial nerve examinations were normal. Straight and reversed straight leg testing were negative bilaterally. Motor examination revealed mild atrophy of the right quadriceps muscle. There were no fasciculations. Muscle tone was normal. Manual muscle examination revealed severe weakness of right knee extension (Medical Research Council (MRC) 4–/5), thigh adduction (MRC 4–/5), and hip flexion (MRC 4/5). All other muscle groups were normal. Deep tendon reflexes revealed were normal in the upper extremities. In the lower extremities, the left knee jerk was normal, but the right knee jerk was absent and both ankle jerks were trace. Sensory examination was normal, both distally and in the anterior thighs. Gait was impaired by the right leg weakness. Romberg test was negative.

The patient was referred to the electromyography (EMG) laboratory.

Please now review the Nerve Conduction Studies and Needle EMG tables.

QUESTIONS

1. The root most likely to be affected in this disorder is:
   A. L4.
   B. L5.
   C. S1.
2. Which electrodiagnostic (EDX) study is most useful in differentiating lumbar radiculopathy from lumbar plexopathy?
   A. Saphenous sensory nerve action potential (SNAP).
   B. Needle EMG of the iliacus muscle.
   C. Femoral compound muscle action potential (CMAP).
   D. Needle EMG of the tibialis anterior.
3. This subacute disorder is characterized by all of the following *except*:
   A. It is commonly associated with distal sensorimotor polyneuropathy.
   B. It is usually painless.
   C. It results in weakness that is often maximal in the anterior thigh muscles.
   D. It is often confused with upper lumbar radiculopathy.
   E. It may be unilateral or bilateral.

EDX FINDINGS AND INTERPRETATION OF DATA

Relevant EDX findings in this case include:

1. Diffuse and mild slowing of sensory and motor distal latencies, conduction velocities, and F wave latencies in the upper and lower extremities, with absent H reflexes bilaterally.
2. Asymmetrically low-amplitude right femoral CMAP.

Case 7: Nerve Conduction Studies

Nerve Stimulated	Stimulation Site	Recording Site	Amplitude (m = mV, s = μV)			Distal/Peak Latency (ms)			Conduction Velocity (m/s)			F Latency (ms)	
			Right	Left	Normal	Right	Left	Normal	Right	Left	Normal	Right	Left
Sural (s)	Calf	Ankle	10		≥3	4.8		≤4.6	35		≥39		
Saphenous (s)	Medial leg	Ankle	**NR**	**NR**	≥3	**NR**	**NR**	≤4.6					
Peroneal (m)	Ankle	EDB	**2.0**		≥2.5	**6.3**		≤6.0					
Peroneal (m)	Knee	EDB	1.8						37		≥39	**50.8**	
Tibial (m)	Ankle	AH	**5.0**		≥4	**6.5**		≤6.0					
Tibial (m)	Knee	AH	2.9						38		≥39	**52**	
Femoral (m)	Groin	Rectus femoris	**0.5**	3.5	≥3	**7.6**	5.5	≤6.5					
H reflex	Knee	Soleus	**NR**	**NR**		**NR**	**NR**						
M response	Knee	Soleus	4.5	6.5		5.7	5.6						
Median (s)	Wrist	Index	**10**		≥10	**4.6**		≤3.8					
Median (s)	Elbow	Index	5						45		≥49		
Ulnar (s)	Wrist	Little finger	18		≥5	**3.6**		≤3.2					
Radial (s)	Distal forearm	Dorsum of hand	16		≥10	**3.1**		2.8					
Medial (m)	Wrist	APB	**7.0**		≥5	**4.2**		4.0					
Medial (m)	Elbow	APB	6.0						**45**		≥49	**35.0**	
Ulnar (m)	Wrist	ADM	9.0		≥7	3.3		3.1					
Ulnar (m)	Elbow	ADM	8.0						48		≥49	**32.5**	

ADM = abductor digiti minimi; AH = abductor hallucis; APB = abductor pollicis brevis; EDB = extensor digitorum brevis; m = motor; NR = no response; s = sensory. Data in bold type are abnormal.

Case 7: Needle EMG

| Muscle | Insertional Activity | Spontaneous Activity | | Voluntary Motor Unit Action Potentials (MUAPs) | | | | | | | |
| | | Fibs | Fascs | Recruitment | | | | Configuration | | | Others |
				Normal	Activation	Reduced	Early	Duration	Amplitude	% Polyphasia	
R. abductor hallucis	↑	+/−	0			↓		↑	↑	Normal	
Extensor digitorum brevis	↑	+/−	0			↓		↑	↑	Normal	
Flexor digitorum longus	Normal	0	0	Normal				↑	Normal	Normal	
Tibialis anterior	↑	+/−	0			↓		↑	Normal	↑	
Medial gastrocnemius	Normal	0	0	Normal				↑	Normal	Normal	
Vastus lateralis	↑	3+	0			↓↓↓		↑	Normal	↑	
Vastus intermedius	↑	3+	0			↓↓↓		↑	Normal	↑	
Thigh adductors	↑	2+	0			↓↓		↑	Normal	↑	
Iliacus	↑	2+	0			↓↓		↑	Normal	↑	
Gluteus medius	Normal	0	0	Normal							
Upper lumbar paraspinal	↑	2+	0	−							
Midlumbar paraspinal	↑	2+	0	−							
Lower lumbar paraspinal	↑	2+	0	−							
Upper sacral paraspinal	↑	1+	0	−							
L. abductor hallucis	↑	+/−	0			↓		↑	↑	Normal	
Tibialis anterior	Normal	0	0	Normal				Normal	Normal	Normal	
Vastus lateralis	Normal	0	0	Normal				↑	Normal	Normal	
Midlumbar paraspinal	↑	+/−	0	−							
R. first dorsal interosseous	Normal	0	0		Normal			↑	Normal	Normal	

Fasces = fasciculations; Fibs = fibrillations; L. = left; R. = right; ↑ = increased; ↓ = mildly reduced; ↓↓ = moderately reduced; ↓↓↓ = severely reduced.

3. Absent saphenous SNAPs bilaterally. This bilateral finding is not uncommon, particularly in elderly or obese patients or those with leg swelling or diabetes, and thus is of no diagnostic value in this case.

4. Profuse fibrillation potentials in the right quadriceps, thigh adductors, and iliacus, with minimal fibrillation potentials in the tibialis anterior. These muscles revealed decreased recruitment of motor unit action potentials (MUAPs) that correlated fairly with the quantity of fibrillation potentials. There were also signs of reinnervation (polyphasic and long duration MUAPs). Additionally, the right lumbar paraspinal muscles showed profuse fibrillation potentials at several levels.

5. There are subtle reinnervation MUAP changes without fibrillation potentials in the left quadriceps, and minimal fibrillations in the left lumbar paraspinal muscles.

6. There is mild distal denervation as evidenced by reinnervation MUAPs in both feet and hand muscles and minimal number of fibrillation potentials.

These findings are consistent with a subacute severe right lumbar polyradiculopathy, affecting the L2–L4 roots, combined with mild chronic sensorimotor peripheral polyneuropathy. With unevokable saphenous SNAPs bilaterally in this patient with diabetes, the lesion could be anatomically a lumbar plexopathy, a lumbar radiculopathy, or more likely, a radiculoplexopathy. This case is compatible with the EMG findings seen in diabetic amyotrophy (diabetic proximal neuropathy). It is also common to find minor denervation in the contralateral limb, even when asymptomatic.

DISCUSSION

Definition and Classification

Diabetes mellitus is a common disorder of two types. Type 1 is characterized by a severe or complete absence of insulin and is due to an autoimmune attack on the islets of Langerhans in the pancreas. Type 2 is more common accounting for about 90% of diabetics in the United States, and is characterized by insulin resistance and influenced by many factors including obesity, diet, physical activity, and inheritance.

Diabetes mellitus has a propensity to cause microvascular disease, nephropathy, retinopathy, and peripheral neuropathy. Because of the heterogeneity of diabetic peripheral nervous complications, there is a lack of agreement among clinicians regarding the definition of *diabetic neuropathy*. An accepted definition of diabetic neuropathy is *the presence of a clinical or subclinical diffuse disorder*

Table C7–1. Classification of Diabetic Neuropathy

1. Distal symmetrical polyneuropathy
   A. Mixed sensory-motor-autonomic
   B. Predominantly sensory
      1. Small fiber (including autonomic)
      2. Large fiber
      3. Mixed large and small fiber
   C. Predominantly motor
2. Asymmetrical polyradiculoneuropathy
   A. Proximal asymmetrical motor neuropathy (amyotrophy)
   B. Thoracic (truncal) radiculopathy
3. Cranial mononeuropathy
   A. Oculomotor (third)
   B. Trochlear (fourth)
   C. Abducens (sixth)
   D. Facial (seventh, Bell's palsy)*
4. Entrapment mononeuropathy*
   A. Median mononeuropathy at the wrist (carpal tunnel syndrome)
   B. Ulnar mononeuropathy at the elbow
   C. Peroneal mononeuropathy at the fibular head
5. Combination of the above (1, 2, 3, and 4)

*Common mononeuropathies with increased incidence in diabetics.

of somatic and/or autonomic parts of the peripheral nervous system in the setting of diabetes mellitus and in the absence of other causes of peripheral neuropathy.

The classification of diabetic neuropathies cannot be rigid because many overlap syndromes may be seen. A practical categorization, based on clinical presentation rather than precise etiology, divides these neuropathies into distal symmetrical polyneuropathy (the commonest), asymmetrical polyradiculoneuropathy, cranial mononeuropathy, and entrapment mononeuropathy (Table C7–1). Detailed discussions of all these syndromes are beyond the scope of this section and have been summarized in recent reviews (see Bird and Brown 2002; Brown and Asbury1984; Harati 1987; Wilbourn 1993).

Clinical Features

Diabetic Sensorimotor Autonomic Polyneuropathy

Diabetic neuropathies are by far the most prevalent peripheral neuropathies encountered in clinical practice. Among all diabetic neuropathies, the mixed sensory-motor-autonomic peripheral polyneuropathy is by far the most common, and is usually related to the duration and severity of hyperglycemia. However, this form may occasionally be the presenting symptom of occult diabetes mellitus. The exact incidence of this diabetic polyneuropathy is not

Table C7–2. Available Measures That May Be Used to Assess for Diabetic Peripheral Polyneuropathy

History

Neurological examination

Electrodiagnostic testing
  Nerve conduction studies
  Late responses
  Needle EMG examination

Autonomic testing
  Cardiac response to deep breathing (R-R interval)
  Cardiac response to Valsalva maneuver
  Tilt table testing
  Quantitative sudomotor axon reflex test (QSART)
  Sympathetic skin response

Quantitative sensory test (QST)

Biopsy
  Nerve
  Muscle
  Skin

known; this is, in part, because of its diverse clinical presentations and different measurements used to define the presence or absence of neuropathy (Table C7–2). The reported incidence of diabetic neuropathy in general is extremely variable, ranging from 5 to 50%. In a large cohort study followed for 25 years, it was estimated that 8% of diabetics have neuropathy at the time of diagnosis, and neuropathy develops in 50% of patients within 25 years of diagnosis (see Pirart 1978).

The clinical manifestations of mixed diabetic polyneuropathy are due to an axonopathy and follow a length-dependent pattern, with the longest axons involved first distally. The sensory manifestations often begin in the toes and progress slowly cephalad to the distal legs. They generally do reach the fingertips or hands when the lower limb symptoms are at around the level of the knees. Sensory symptoms due to loss of small fibers usually appear first, as paresthesias and neuropathic pain (deep aching or throbbing and superficial burning or stabbing). Pain and temperature sensation are usually blunted on examination. Impaired leg proprioception and vibration sense and diminution of ankle jerks, manifestations of large fiber loss, occur later in the course of the illness.

Motor fiber involvement in mixed diabetic polyneuropathy is minimal in the early stages of the disease. This is typically confined to weakness and atrophy of the intrinsic foot muscles and weakness of toe flexors and extensors. However, when weakness worsens, it follows also a distal to proximal gradient resulting in progressive foot weakness sometimes leading to bilateral flail foot, and hand weakness and atrophy occasionally causing bilateral clawed hands.

Manifestations of autonomic dysfunction become increasingly important as the neuropathy progresses, and occasionally they dominate the clinical picture. This includes impotence due to impaired dysfunction, abdominal pain, diarrhea, and constipation due to impaired gastrointestinal motility, distal anhidrosis due to sudomotor dysfunction, and orthostatic intolerance due to vasomotor denervation. More advanced dysautonomia may manifest as recurrent syncope due to orthostatic hypotension or neurogenic bladder resulting in reduced sensation of bladder fullness and incomplete emptying. Loss of hypoglycemia warnings results from the combination of adrenal gland denervation (leading to blunted catecholamines excretion), sudomotor denervation (leading to loss of sweating), and cardiac denervation (leading to the loss of reactive tachycardia). Finally, acrodystrophic changes of skin, nails, and joints may dominate due to small fiber sensory loss, with accompanying foot ulcerations and neuropathic arthropathy (Charcot joint) of the ankle and foot.

Diabetic Amyotrophy

Diabetic amyotrophy is a much less common neuropathy than the chronic mixed sensorimotor diabetic polyneuropathy. The term was first coined in 1953 by Garland and Taverner. They first called this syndrome "diabetic myelopathy," because they presumed that the pathology was in the spinal cord, particularly in the anterior horn cell column. This disorder has been surrounded by controversy primarily because of lack of understanding of the exact site and nature of the pathology, which has been attributed to lesions of the anterior horn cells, lumbar roots, lumbar plexus, and femoral nerve. Authors have thus ascribed many terminologies to this disorder, based on their own theory of the nature of the illness (Table C7–3). Although many have

Table C7–3. Common Synonyms of Diabetic Amyotrophy

Bruns-Garland syndrome

Diabetic amyotrophy

Diabetic anterior neuropathy

Diabetic asymmetrical proximal neuropathy

Diabetic lumbar plexopathy

Diabetic lumbosacral plexus neuropathy

Diabetic lumbosacral radiculoplexus neuropathy

Diabetic polyradiculopathy

Diabetic polyradiculoplexopathy

Diabetic proximal motor neuropathy

Diabetic proximal neuropathy

Garland syndrome

Subacute diabetic proximal diabetic neuropathy

Adapted with revisions from Wilbourn AJ. The diabetic neuropathies. In: Brown WF, Bolton CF, eds. Clinical electromyography, 2nd ed. Boston, MA: Butterworth-Heinemann, 1993.

suggested that the name "diabetic amyotrophy" be abandoned because of its ambiguity, the term continues to be the most commonly used for this disorder in neurologic practice. Another popular designation is *"subacute diabetic proximal neuropathy."*

Diabetic amyotrophy affects primarily the L2, L3, and L4 roots/plexus. This may be a unilateral, bilaterally asymmetrical, or bilaterally symmetrical condition. Sometimes, additional adjoining roots become involved, such as the lower thoracic roots (leading to diabetic thoracic radiculopathy), or the L5 and S1 roots (resulting in so-called diabetic footdrop).

The typical patient is a type 2 diabetic adult, usually older than 50 years of age, in whom a subacute unilateral proximal leg weakness develops that evolves over several weeks to months. Thigh pain is extremely common; it usually is deep and worse at night, but it can be burning and severe. At times, it involves the buttock and back. Weakness invariably involves the quadriceps, iliopsoas, and thigh adductor muscles but may extend into the tibialis anterior, glutei, hamstrings, and, rarely, the gastrocnemius. Knee jerk is depressed or absent. Not infrequently, there is clinical or only electrophysiologic evidence of contralateral involvement, usually milder in degree. Also, the contralateral leg may become affected later, while the initial ipsilateral weakness is improving.

The site of the lesion and the exact pathophysiology of diabetic amyotrophy are not well known, partially because of the lack of adequate pathologic studies. An inflammatory vasculopathy (vasculitis or perivasculitis) causing ischemic nerve infarction is the most popular theory and is supported by a single autopsy (see Raff et al. 1968) and several nerve biopsy series injury (see Said et al. 1994, 1997). Some observers distinguish between diabetic patients with proximal neuropathy in whom an asymmetrical neuropathy rapidly develops and those with more gradually progressive symmetrical neuropathy. These authors have proposed that the former syndrome is ischemic (vascular) in nature, and the latter metabolic. In practice, many patients fit into a spectrum between these two extremes, making the distinction difficult and two separate mechanisms unlikely.

The following are *frequently asked questions* regarding diabetic amyotrophy:

1. *What is the status of glycemic control in diabetic amyotrophy?* Although earlier reports suggested that most patients with this syndrome are brittle (i.e., difficult to control) or poorly controlled, many patients have fair blood glucose control at the time of onset of this disorder. In fact, some have very mild diabetes and in others diabetic amyotrophy is the first manifestation of diabetes mellitus or follows a recent change in treatment or control of hypoglycemia. Also, it appears that the rate of recovery is not influenced by the initiation of insulin therapy or subsequent glycemic control in these patients.

2. *Is weight loss a feature of diabetic amyotrophy?* Weight loss is a frequent, but not a universal, association. Weight loss, which may evolve over 1 or more years, usually is associated with anorexia and averages 15–20 kg.

3. *How often is a diabetic distal symmetrical polyneuropathy associated with diabetic amyotrophy?* Almost two-thirds of patients with subacute diabetic proximal neuropathy have an associated chronic, distal, predominantly sensory, peripheral polyneuropathy. This may be clinically apparent, or it may be seen only on electrodiagnostic studies.

4. *What is the prognosis and recurrence rate in diabetic amyotrophy?* Diabetic amyotrophy carries a good prognosis for spontaneous and near-complete recovery. Pain is the first manifestation to improve, as early as a few weeks, but little beyond 12 months. Weakness starts to improve within 3 to 4 months but may take up to 3 years depending on severity. Most patients resume normal walking, while some severely affected patients continue to ambulate with an aid, or are occasionally wheelchair bound. Recurrent episodes may occur in up to 20% of patients.

The primary differential diagnosis of diabetic amyotrophy is an L2–L4 radiculopathy due compressive spinal lesion. Night pain and allodynia favor diabetic amyotrophy. Imaging of the spine is often necessary for confirmation. When quadriceps weakness is severe, spinal compressive disease must include at least two lumbar roots. Other considerations involve other causes of lumbar plexopathy, femoral neuropathy, and motor neuron disease.

Electrodiagnosis

Diabetic Sensorimotor Autonomic Polyneuropathy

Electrodiagnostic (EDX) studies are valuable in confirming the presence of chronic axon loss peripheral polyneuropathy. During the early stages of the disorder and in a small percentage of patients whose manifestations are restricted to the toes or small fiber symptomatology, the NCS and needle EMG examination, which assess only the large myelinated nerve fibers, may be normal. In these situations, other modalities such as quantitative sudomotor axon reflex test, quantitative sensory testing, or skin biopsy may be necessary to show involvement of small unmyelinated fibers. When large fibers undergo axonal degeneration, the EDX abnormalities are initially found only in the lower extremities. These typically consist of one or more of these NCS abnormalities: absent H reflexes, low-amplitude or absent sural and superficial peroneal SNAPs, low-amplitude tibial and peroneal CMAPs, and mild slowing of peroneal and tibial motor distal latencies and conduction velocities (Figure C7–1). The needle EMG often shows long-duration and high-amplitude MUAPs with or without fibrillation potentials in the intrinsic foot muscles. With more advanced disease, the neurogenic MUAP changes worsen in the leg and ascend that abnormalities are found in the upper limbs. Initially, this usually presents as reduction of the median, ulnar, and radial SNAP amplitudes with mild slowing, low, or borderline median and ulnar CMAPs with mild sensory and motor conduction slowing, with long-duration and high-amplitude MUAPs with or without fibrillation potentials in the intrinsic hand muscles. In severe polyneuropathy there is often complete absence of all routine sensory and motor conduction studies in the legs and hands, with long-duration, high-amplitude and rapidly recruited MUAPs with or without fibrillation potentials in all the leg and arm muscles, which are worse distally.

The EDX features of diabetic sensorimotor peripheral polyneuropathy are characteristic of a primarily axon loss polyneuropathy. However, the abnormalities are not specific for diabetes mellitus and are encountered with a wide variety of other metabolic or toxic etiologies. The EDX are most useful when the cause of the neuropathy is unclear, and the EDX studies become essential in looking for demyelinating features, which would suggest another diagnosis, such as an acquired or familial demyelinating polyneuropathies. The EDX studies are also very useful in diabetic patients with disproportionately upper extremity symptoms in order to exclude entrapment neuropathies such as the carpal tunnel syndromes.

Diabetic Amyotrophy

Routine sensory and motor nerve conduction studies are abnormal, particularly in the legs, in a majority of patients with diabetic amyotrophy because there usually is a concomitant diabetic sensorimotor peripheral polyneuropathy. Based on electrophysiologic criteria, two-thirds of patients with diabetic amyotrophy have an associated distal peripheral polyneuropathy. In addition to the peroneal and tibial motor NCS, the femoral CMAP should be obtained in all patients with suspected diabetic amyotrophy. Although this study adds little to the diagnosis, it is very useful in assessing the degree of axonal loss. In diabetic amyotrophy, it is frequently low in amplitude, unilaterally or bilaterally, which is consistent with the

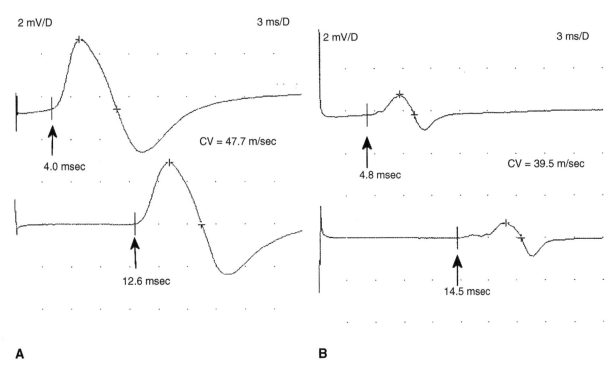

Figure C7–1. *Peroneal motor nerve conduction study recording extensor digitorum brevis in a 50-year-old patient with a 7-year history of type 2 diabetes mellitus and chronic distal peripheral polyneuropathy (**B**), compared to an age-matched control (**A**). Note that the distal CMAP amplitude is significantly lower in the diabetic patient than the control (3.8 mV versus 10.0 mV) while the distal latencies and conduction velocities are only marginally slowed, consistent with an axonopathy (axon-loss peripheral polyneuropathy).*

axonal nature of the lesion. Slowing is, however, minimal. The saphenous SNAPs also should be done bilaterally, although they often are unelicitable in both legs in these patients because of age, obesity, or concomitant distal sensorimotor peripheral polyneuropathy.

Needle EMG findings in diabetic amyotrophy reflects the consequences of axonal loss, but are heterogeneous in distribution and chronicity. Most commonly, the needle examination reveals fibrillation potentials, decreased recruitment, and large and polyphasic MUAPs in an L2 through L4 roots distribution. The muscles that are usually most involved include the quadriceps (L2–L3–L4), the thigh adductors (L2–L3–L4), and the iliacus (L2–L3), with less prominent changes noted in the tibialis anterior (L4–L5). In patients with an overlapping distal diabetic chronic polyneuropathy, there often is distal denervation also, particularly in the abductor hallucis, extensor digitorum brevis, extensor hallucis, and flexor digitorum longus. Thus, when needle EMG is being performed on patients with diabetic amyotrophy, starting distally in the foot and proceeding proximally, fibrillation potentials and loss of MUAPs are often noted in the foot muscles and the anterior thigh muscles but not in the leg muscles. This creates a typical "skip region," which includes the medial gastrocnemius and sometimes the tibialis anterior also. This region is surrounded by the abnormal muscles; the denervation in the intrinsic foot and distal leg muscles is caused by the distal polyneuropathy, while the denervation in the quadriceps, thigh adductors, and iliacus proximally is caused by the diabetic amyotrophy.

In some patients, the subacute denervation of diabetic amyotrophy extends caudally into the L5 root. In these patients, fibrillation potentials with loss of MUAPs are also prominent in the tibialis anterior, the extensor hallucis (resulting in so-called *diabetic footdrop*), the tibialis posterior, the flexor digitorum longus, and, occasionally, the hamstrings and glutei. In severe cases, the denervation may become so diffuse in the lower extremity that few muscles escape the condition. Among these, the medial head of the gastrocnemius (S1–S2) is the most likely to be free of fibrillation potentials; however, it might harbor chronic neurogenic changes when an overlapping chronic distal diabetic polyneuropathy coexists.

Regardless of the clinical picture (unilateral or bilateral), it is common to find abnormalities on needle EMG in the contralateral muscles of many patients with diabetic amyotrophy. Even in patients with symmetrical weakness at the time of the EMG examination, the neurogenic changes on needle EMG are often different, suggesting a different time course of the processes in both legs. Typical needle EMG findings include profuse fibrillation with highly polyphasic MUAPs in one thigh, consistent with a subacute process, and rare fibrillations with many polyphasic

MUAPs of increased duration and amplitudes in the contralateral thigh, consistent with a more chronic disorder.

Based on the aforementioned findings, an extensive needle EMG is often required in patients with suspected diabetic amyotrophy. Sampling the quadriceps (preferably at least two heads), the thigh adductors, the iliacus, the tibialis anterior, and the lumbar paraspinal muscles is essential. Because the disorder is often bilateral, testing the same muscles on the contralateral side in symptomatic limbs or, at least, the quadriceps and iliacus in asymptomatic limbs is recommended. Finally, sampling more distal muscles is essential when there is possible concomitant distal polyneuropathy.

It is often necessary to perform imaging studies, such as MRI, on the lumbar spine to exclude a compressive lesion within the lumbar intraspinal canal, because differentiating diabetic amyotrophy from L2–L4 intraspinal lesions is difficult, even for the seasoned electromyographer, for several reasons:

1. Saphenous SNAPs frequently are absent in patients with diabetic amyotrophy. In the ideal situation, the saphenous SNAP, a predominantly L4 dermatomal SNAP, should help to distinguish an L4 root lesion from an L4 plexus lesion; the SNAP is normal in root lesions because the dorsal root ganglion and its peripheral sensory axons remain intact and excitable. However, it is low in amplitude or absent in plexus lesions (or peripheral nerve lesions) as a result of axon loss, because the peripheral sensory axons are involved in the pathologic process. Unfortunately, the saphenous SNAP often is absent bilaterally in patients with diabetic amyotrophy owing to other factors, such as age, obesity, or a concomitant diabetic distal sensorimotor peripheral polyneuropathy. This precludes exclusion of a preganglionic lesion, as is seen in compressive root disease.

2. Fibrillation potentials are typically prominent in the upper or mid lumbar paraspinal muscles in patients with diabetic amyotrophy. This reinforces the theory that this debilitating disorder is a multifocal vasculopathy that simultaneously involve the roots (primarily L2, L3, and L4), the plexus (primarily lumbar) and peripheral nerves (femoral and obturator). Hence, the name diabetic lumbosacral radiculoplexus neuropathy.

3. Fibrillation potentials in the paraspinal muscles are commonly encountered diffusely in patients with diabetes. These muscles are innervated by the posterior primary rami of the spinal nerves. They often reveal fibrillation potentials in root lesions but are normal in plexus (or peripheral nerve) lesions. Unfortunately, fibrillation potentials are seen in a high proportion of patients with diabetes without diabetic amyotrophy. Thus, identifying them in the paraspinal muscles in

patients with possible diabetic amyotrophy does not necessarily indicate compressive root disease.

Until recently, it was widely accepted that isolated femoral mononeuropathy is a complication of diabetes mellitus. However, it is now clear that this is a misnomer. It is likely that most reported cases, published more than 30 years ago, actually involved mislabeled patients with diabetic amyotrophy; this occurred because many physicians and electromyographers did not assess other muscles thoroughly, in particular the thigh adductors. Although the brunt of weakness in many patients with diabetic amyotrophy often falls on the quadriceps muscle mimicking selective femoral nerve lesions, careful clinical and needle EMG examinations reveal more widespread involvement of thigh adductors and sometimes foot dorsiflexors, muscles not innervated by the femoral nerve. Despite the current knowledge, the term diabetic femoral neuropathy, unfortunately, has not completely vanished (see Coppack and Watkins 1991).

DIAGNOSIS

Diabetic proximal neuropathy (diabetic amyotrophy), with mild diabetic distal sensorimotor peripheral polyneuropathy.

ANSWERS

1. A; 2. A; 3. B.

SUGGESTED READINGS

Al Hakim M, Katirji MB. Femoral mononeuropathy induced by the lithotomy position: a report of 5 cases and a review of the literature. Muscle Nerve 1993;16:891–895.

Asbury AK. Proximal diabetic neuropathy. Ann Neurol 1977; 2:179–180.

Barohn RJ et al. The Bruns-Garland syndrome (diabetic amyotrophy). Revisited 100 years later. Arch Neurol 1991;48: 1130–1135.

Bird SJ, Brown MJ. Diabetic neuropathies. In: Katirji B, Kaminski HJ, Preston DC, Ruff RL, Shapiro EB, eds. Neuromuscular disorders in clinical practice. Boston, MA: Butterworth-Heinemann, 2002, pp. 598–621.

Brown MJ, Asbury AK. Diabetic neuropathy. Ann Neurol 1984;15:2–12.

Chokroverty S et al. The syndrome of diabetic amyotrophy. Ann Neurol 1977;2:181–194.

Coppack SW, Watkins PJ. The natural history of diabetic amyotrophy, QJM 1991;79:307–325.

Dyck PJ et al. Diabetic neuropathy. Philadelphia, PA: WB Saunders, 1987.

Garland H. Diabetic amyotrophy. Br Med J 1955;2:181–194.

Garland H. Diabetic amyotrophy. Br J Clin Pract 1961;15:9–13.

Garland H, Taverner D. Diabetic myelopathy. Br Med J 1953;1:1405–1408.

Harati Y. Diabetic peripheral neuropathies. Ann Intern Med 1987;107:546–559.

Pirart J. Diabetes mellitus and its degenerative complications: a prospective study of 4,400 patients observed between 1947 and 1973. Diabetes Care 1978;1:168–252.

Raff MC, Sangalang V, Asbury AK. Ischemic mononeuropathy multiplex associated with diabetes mellitus. Arch Neurol 1968;18:487–499.

Said G, Elgrably F, Lacroix C et al. Painful proximal diabetic neuropathy: inflammatory nerve lesions and spontaneous favorable outcome. Ann Neurol 1997;41:762–770.

Said G, Goulon-Goeau C, Lacroix C et al. Nerve biopsy findings in different patterns of proximal diabetic neuropathy. Ann Neurol 1994;35:559–569.

Subramony SH, Wilbourn AJ. Diabetic proximal neuropathy. J Neurol Sci 1982;53:293–304.

Wilbourn AJ. The diabetic neuropathies. In: Brown WF, Bolton CF, eds. Clinical electromyography, 2nd ed. Boston, MA: Butterworth-Heinemann, 1993.

Case 8

HISTORY AND PHYSICAL EXAMINATION

A 36-year-old man underwent mitral valve replacement for rheumatic heart disease. On awakening from general anesthesia, he noted weakness of the right foot and numbness of the dorsum of the foot. He had no pain. His footdrop did not improve, and he was referred to the electromyography (EMG) laboratory 5 weeks after the onset of footdrop.

On examination, there was a near-complete right foot and toes drop (Medical Research Council [MRC] strength 1/5). Foot eversion was markedly weak (3/5), but inversion and plantar flexion were normal. Deep tendon reflexes, including ankle jerk, were normal. There was sensory impairment to touch, and pin sensation over the dorsum of the right foot. Tinel sign was negative on percussion of the right peroneal nerve at the fibular neck. The rest of the neurologic examination was normal.

Please now review the Nerve Conduction Studies (NCS) and Needle EMG tables.

QUESTIONS

1. Based on the nerve conduction studies only, the lesion is likely:
   A. Axonal.
   B. Demyelinating.
   C. Mixed, demyelinating and axonal.
   D. Undetermined until the needle EMG is completed.
2. The most common precipitating factor for this type injury, when acute, is:
   A. Leg crossing.
   B. Weight loss.
   C. Diabetes mellitus.
   D. Recent general anesthesia and surgery.
   E. Underlying peripheral polyneuropathy.

3. The most common precipitating factors for this type of injury, when subacute or chronic, are:
   A. Weight loss.
   B. Diabetes mellitus.
   C. Diabetes mellitus and underlying peripheral polyneuropathy.
   D. Recent prolonged hospitalization.
4. The prognosis for recovery of footdrop in this patient is:
   A. Poor because of prominent fibrillation potentials.
   B. Poor because of the near absence of voluntary motor unit potentials.
   C. Favorable and biphasic, with anticipated early rapid improvement and some delayed recovery.
   D. Poor, because of very low proximal peroneal compound motor action potential (CMAP) amplitudes recording tibialis anterior and the extensor digitorum brevis.

EDX FINDINGS AND INTERPRETATION OF DATA

Relevant electrodiagnostic (EDX) findings in this case include the following:

1. Low-amplitude right superficial peroneal sensory nerve action potential (SNAP), compared with the left (5 µV versus 20 µV).
2. Low-amplitude right peroneal CMAP stimulating at the ankle, while recording extensor digitorum brevis (1.9 mV on the right versus 8.0 mV on the left). In addition, there is a conduction block in the peroneal nerve segment between below the fibular head and knee stimulation sites (1.7 mV to 0.8 mV, respectively). The loss in CMAP amplitude (i.e., block) measures 53% across both sites and is supported by a 48% drop in CMAP area (Figure C8–1). Finally, there is a concomitant focal slowing of the conducting fibers across the fibular head

Case 8: Nerve Conduction Studies

Nerve Stimulated	Stimulation Site	Recording Site	Amplitude (m = mV, s = µV)			Distal/Peak Latency (ms)			Conduction Velocity (m/s)			F Latency (ms)	
			Right	Left	Normal	Right	Left	Normal	Right	Left	Normal	Right	Left
Sup peroneal (s)	Leg	Ankle	5	20	≥5.0	2.4	2.2	≤4.5	48		≥40		
Sural (s)	Calf	Ankle	18		≥0.5	3.2		≤4.5			≥40		
Peroneal (m)*	Ankle	EDB	**1.9**	8.0	≥3.0	4.6	4.5	≤5.5	45	44	≥40	**46.0**	41.3
Peroneal (m)*	Bel fibular head	EDB	**1.7**	7.0									
Peroneal (m)*	Knee	EDB	**0.8**	6.5					30	45	≥40		
Peroneal (m)	Bel fibular head	Tibialis anterior	**3.2**	5.5	≥4.0	2.7	2.8	≤4.0					
Peroneal (m)	Knee	Tibialis anterior	**0.4**	5.0					**20**	43	≥40		
Tibial (m)	Ankle	AH	15		≥8.0	4.6		≤6.0	46		≥40	49.0	
Tibial (m)	Knee	AH	13										
H reflex	Knee	Soleus	1.5	1.3		29.3	28.5						
M response	Knee	Soleus	12.5	14.5		4.8	4.8						

AH = abductor hallucis; Bel fibular head = below fibular head; EDB = extensor digitorum brevis; m = motor; s = sensory; Sup peroneal = superficial peroneal.
Data in bold type are abnormal.
*See Figure C8–1.

Case 8: Needle EMG

Muscle	Insertional Activity	Spontaneous Activity		Voluntary Motor Unit Action Potentials (MUAPs)							
		Fibs	Fascs	Recruitment				Configuration			
				Normal	Activation	Reduced	Early	Duration	Amplitude	% Polyphasia	Others
R. tibialis anterior	↑	1+	0			↓↓		↑	Normal	↑	
Extensor hallucis	↑	1+	0			↓↓↓		↑	Normal	Normal	
Extensor digitorum brevis	↑	1+	0			↓↓↓		↑	Normal	Normal	
Peroneus longus	↑	+/−	0			↓↓		↑	Normal	↑	
Tibialis posterior	Normal	0	0	X				Normal	Normal	Normal	
Flexor digitorum longus	Normal	0	0	X				Normal	Normal	Normal	
Media gastrocnemius	Normal	0	0	X				Normal	Normal	Normal	
Vastus lateralis	Normal	0	0	X				Normal	Normal	Normal	
Biceps femoris (short h.)	Normal	0	0	X				Normal	Normal	Normal	
Gluteus medius	Normal	0	0	X				Normal	Normal	Normal	
Midlumbar paraspinal	Normal	0	0	−							
Low lumbar paraspinal	Normal	0	0	−							

Fascs = fasciculations; fibs = fibrillations; R. = right; short h. = short head; ↑ = increased; ↓↓ = moderately reduced; ↓↓↓ = severely reduced.

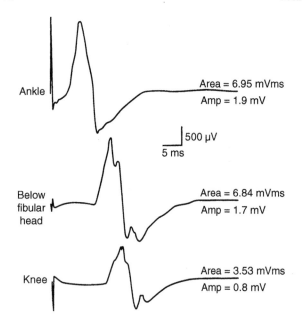

Ankle   Area = 6.95 mVms
         Amp = 1.9 mV

500 µV
5 ms

Below
fibular   Area = 6.84 mVms
head   Amp = 1.7 mV

Knee   Area = 3.53 mVms
         Amp = 0.8 mV

Figure C8–1. *Right peroneal motor conduction studies recording extensor digitorum brevis. The distal compound muscle action potential (CMAP) amplitude is low (1.9 mV compared to 8.0 mV on the left), consistent with axon loss. In addition, there is evidence of conduction block across the fibular head, manifested by a significant drop in CMAP amplitude (53%) and area (48%) with stimulation below the fibular head and knee.*

(conduction velocity of 30 m/s proximally versus 45 m/s distally).

3. The peroneal CMAP, recording tibialis anterior, is similarly, low in amplitude with distal stimulation (below the fibular head: 3.2 mV on the right versus 5.5 mV on the left). Also, there is significant conduction block across the fibular head (3.2 mV from below the fibular head and 0.4 mV from the knee). This is equivalent to an 87.5% amplitude loss and is supported by a significant decrease in CMAP area (not shown). There is also slowing of the conducting fibers (20 m/s on the right versus 43 m/s on the left).

4. The right sural sensory and tibial motor conduction studies as well as the bilateral H reflexes are normal.

5. The needle examination confirms that all common peroneal innervated muscles, except the short head of the biceps femoris, are abnormal, as evidenced by the presence of fibrillation potentials, decreased recruitment, and the increased duration and polyphasic motor unit action potentials. In contrast, all sampled tibial-innervated muscles (tibialis posterior, flexor digitorum longus, medial gastrocnemius), as well as all other muscles innervated by the L5 root (tibialis posterior, flexor digitorum longus, gluteus medius) and the lumbar paraspinal muscles, are normal.

This is consistent with a common peroneal mononeuropathy across the fibular head, manifested by segmental demyelination and axonal loss.

• Segmental demyelination in this case is confirmed by the identification of peroneal motor conduction block (recording tibialis anterior and extensor digitorum brevis [EDB]) across the fibular head 5 weeks after the onset of this acute lesion. It also is supported by the presence of focal slowing of the conducting fibers in the same segment of the peroneal nerve.

• Motor axonal loss is verified by the low peroneal CMAP amplitudes (recording tibialis anterior and EDB), stimulating distal to the lesion (i.e., at the ankle and below the fibular head, respectively). Sensory axonal loss also is confirmed by a low amplitude superficial peroneal SNAP, which is studied distal to the lesion. The presence of fibrillation potentials is another proof of motor fiber axonal loss, but this is a poorly quantitative measurement since it is seen in mild acute or subacute lesions and is absent in chronic lesions.

The prognosis for this patient should be relatively good and is likely to be biphasic. The initial phase of recovery would be dependent on remyelination and should be relatively rapid, occurring within 2 to 3 months. The second phase is slower and more protracted because it is dependent on sprouting and reinnervation. Sprouting should be relatively productive in this patient because the lesion is partial, and reinnervation is likely to be effective because several of the affected muscles, such as the tibialis anterior and peroneus longus, are located relatively close the site of injury.

DISCUSSION

Applied Anatomy

The common peroneal nerve (also called the lateral popliteal nerve) shares a common sheath with the tibial nerve (also called the medial popliteal nerve) to form the sciatic nerve. The common peroneal nerve innervates the short head of biceps femoris only, via a motor branch that exits the nerve close to the gluteal fold. All the other hamstring muscles (long head of biceps femoris, semitendinosus and semimembranosus) are innervated by the tibial nerve. The complete separation of the common peroneal nerve from the tibial nerve is variable, but is usually at the popliteal crease or up to 10 cm above it (Figure C8–2).

Soon after separating from the tibial nerve in the popliteal fossa, the common peroneal nerve gives off first the *lateral cutaneous nerve of the calf*, which innervates the skin over the upper third of the lateral aspect of the leg (Figure C8–3, top inset). It also gives the peroneal communicating nerve which joins the sural nerve in midcalf.

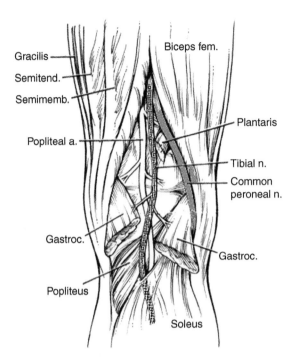

Figure C8–2. *Anatomy of the common peroneal and tibial nerves in the popliteal fossa.*

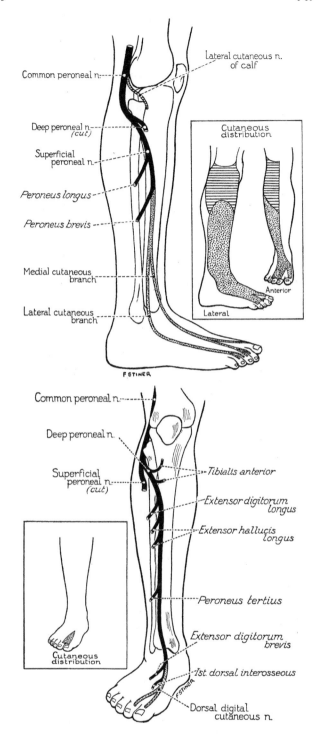

Figure C8–3. *The common peroneal nerve, with its superficial branch* (top) *and deep branch* (bottom), *showing its relation to the fibular head and its terminal branches. (From Haymaker W, Woodhall B. Peripheral nerve injuries: principles of diagnosis. Philadelphia, PA: WB Saunders, 1953, with permission.)*

Then, the common peroneal nerve winds around the fibular neck, where it lies in close contact with it, and passes through a tendinous tunnel between the edge of the peroneus longus muscle and the fibula, sometimes referred to as the *fibular tunnel.*

The common peroneal nerve divides into superficial and deep terminal branches usually near the fibular neck but sometimes more proximally (Figure C8–4). The common peroneal nerve around the fibular neck has a topographical arrangement where the fibers to the superficial branch are placed laterally while those destined to the deep peroneal nerve are located medially in close contact with the fibular bone. This renders the deep peroneal nerve more susceptible to compression at the fibular neck than the superficial nerve.

The superficial peroneal nerve innervates the peroneus longus and brevis and the skin of the lower two thirds of the lateral aspect of the leg and the dorsum of the foot (see Figure C8–3, top). The deep peroneal nerve is primarily motor; it innervates all ankle and toe extensors (the tibialis anterior, the extensor hallucis, and the extensor digitorum longus and brevis) and the peroneus tertius, in addition to the skin of the web space between the first and second toes (see Figure C8–3, bottom).

The accessory deep peroneal nerve is a common anomaly of the peroneal nerve. It is present in about 20% of the

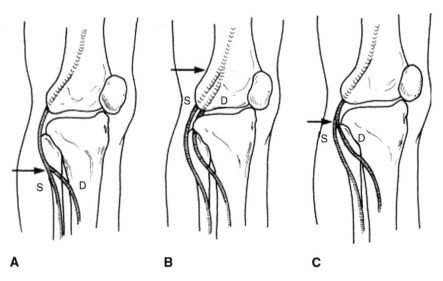

Figure C8–4. *Locations of the division of the common peroneal nerve into its terminal branches, the deep (D) and superficial (S) peroneal nerves. (**A**) Most common site close to the fibular neck. Less common variations with more proximal divisions close to the knee joint line (**C**) or in the distal part of the popliteal fossa (**B**).*

population and sometimes bilaterally. The nerve arises as a motor branch of the superficial peroneal nerve, usually a continuation of the muscular branch that innervates the peroneus brevis muscle. The accessory deep peroneal nerve traverses along the posterior aspect of the peroneus brevis muscle, and then, accompanied by peroneus brevis tendon, passes behind the lateral malleolus near the sural nerve to reach the foot. There, it sends branches to the lateral part of extensor digitorum brevis, ankle joint, and ligaments (Figure C8–5).

Clinical Features

Peroneal mononeuropathy usually presents with a *foot drop*, defined as severe weakness of ankle dorsiflexion (extension) with intact plantar flexion. Foot drop should be distinguished from *flail foot* which, in contrast, is characterized by no or minimal ankle and foot movements in all directions, including severe weakness of ankle dorsiflexion, plantar flexion, and intrinsic foot muscles. Voluntary movement at or distal to the ankle occur in foot drop due to intact plantar flexion and intrinsic foot muscles, but are absent in flail foot. Table C8–1 lists the common causes of unilateral and bilateral footdrop, starting caudally and progressing cephalad along the neuraxis.

Peroneal mononeuropathy is the most common compressive mononeuropathy in the lower extremity. All age groups are equally affected but the disorder is almost three times more common in men. Most peroneal nerve lesions are unilateral, and affect the right and the left side equally.

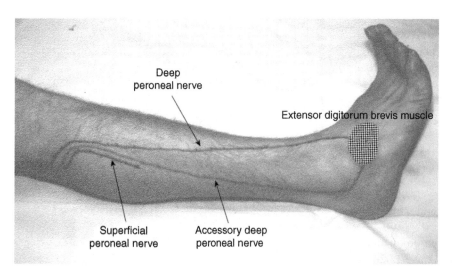

Figure C8–5. *The accessory deep peroneal nerve anomaly. (Adapted with revisions from Preston DC, Shapiro BE. Electromyography and neuromuscular disorders. Boston MA: Elsevier/Butterworth-Heinemann, 2005, with permission.)*

Table C8–1. Causes of Unilateral and Bilateral Footdrop

Unilateral footdrop
    Deep peroneal mononeuropathy
    Common peroneal mononeuropathy
    Anterior compartmental syndrome of the leg
    Sciatic mononeuropathy
    Lumbosacral plexopathy (lumbosacral trunk)
    L5 radiculopathy
    L4 radiculopathy
    Multifocal motor neuropathy
    Hereditary neuropathy with liability to pressure palsy
    Amyotrophic lateral sclerosis
    Poliomyelitis and post-poliomyelitis syndrome
    Cortical or subcortical parasagittal cerebral lesion
Bilateral footdrop
    Myopathies
        Distal myopathies*
        Facioscapulohumeral muscular dystrophy
        Myotonic dystrophy
    Neuropathies
        Multifocal motor neuropathy
        Chronic inflammatory demyelinating polyneuropathy
        Bilateral peroneal neuropathies
        Bilateral sciatic neuropathies
        Bilateral lumbosacral plexopathies
    Radiculopathies
        Bilateral L5 radiculopathies
        Conus medullaris lesion
    Anterior horn cell disorders
        Amyotrophic lateral sclerosis
        Poliomyelitis and the post-poliomyelitis syndrome
    Cerebral lesions
        Bilateral cortical or subcortical parasagittal lesions

*Including the Markesburry-Udd, Welander, Nonaka, and Liang types.

Bilateral lesions constitute about 10% of cases. In most cases, it results from prolonged compression of the peroneal nerve at the fibular neck between an external object and the rigid bone. Table C8–2 lists the causes of peroneal mononeuropathy at the fibular head.

Most cases of peroneal mononeuropathy present with acute footdrop. However, footdrop develops in some patients subacutely over days or even weeks. The precipitating factors vary according to the mode of onset (acute versus nonacute). Figure C8–6 shows the relative frequency of the precipitating factors in relation to the mode of onset. Perioperative compression and trauma are the two most common causes of acute peroneal mononeuropathy at the fibular head. However, weight loss and prolonged hospitalization are the two major precipitating factors for peroneal nerve lesions with subacute or gradual onset. Extrinsic masses (osteomas, ganglia, lipomas, Baker cysts), or intrinsic nerve sheath tumors usually present with a slowly progressive footdrop.

Table C8–2. Causes of Peroneal Nerve Lesions at the Fibular Neck

Compression
    During anesthesia
    Weight loss
    Habitual leg crossing*
    Prolonged hospitalization*
    Prolonged bed rest*
    Anorexia nervosa*
    Coma
    Diabetes mellitus
    Peripheral polyneuropathy
    Prolonged squatting
        Yoga
        Crop harvesting, "strawberry pickers"
        Childbirth
    Iatrogenic
        Above or below knee cast
        Ankle-foot orthosis (brace)
        Pneumatic compression device
        Antithrombotic stocking
        Bandage
        Strap
            Lithotomy position with stirrups
        Intrauterine (with breech presentation)
Trauma
    Blunt
        Fibular fracture
        Ligamental knee joint rupture
        Knee dislocation
        Tibiofibular joint dislocation
            Ankle sprain
    Open
        Laceration
        Gunshot wound
        Animal bite
    Iatrogenic
        Conventional knee surgery
        Knee joint replacement
        Arthroscopic knee surgery
Mass lesion
    Extrinsic
        Osteochondroma
        Baker cyst
        Ganglion cyst
        Hematoma
        Pseudoaneurysm
    Intrinsic
        Schwannoma
        Neurofibroma
        Neurogenic sarcoma
Infection
    Leprosy

*Usually with weight loss.
Adapted with revision from Katirji B. Compressive and entrapment mononeuropathies of the lower extremity. In: Katirji B, Kaminski HJ, Preston DC, Ruff RL, Shapiro BE, eds. Neuromuscular disorders in clinical practice. Boston, MA: Butterworth-Heinemann, 2002.

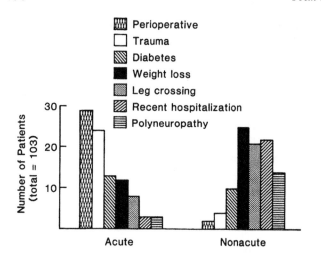

Figure C8–6. *Precipitating factors in peroneal mononeuropathies. Note the difference between lesions of acute versus nonacute onset. (From Katirji MB, Wilbourn AJ. Common peroneal mononeuropathy: a clinical and electrophysiologic study of 116 lesions. Neurology 1988;38:1723–1728, with permission.)*

Although the deep peroneal nerve is more frequently affected than the superficial nerve (as in this patient), selective deep peroneal nerve involvement is not uncommon. Peroneal neuropathies in the thigh (i.e., sciatic nerve lesions affecting the common peroneal nerve exclusively) are rare, accounting for less than 5% of all peroneal mononeuropathies. Table C8–3(A) reveals the most helpful clinical distinctions between peroneal mononeuropathy, lumbar plexopathy, L5 radiculopathy, and sciatic mononeuropathy. In short, weakness of ankle inversion, toe flexion, or plantar flexion, and absent or depressed ankle jerk are findings that are not consistent with a selective peroneal nerve lesion.

In the management of acute compressive lesions, patients should be treated in a way that allows for improvement by either remyelination or reinnervation. As can be seen in this patient, conduction block lesions (due to segmental demyelination) recover spontaneously within 2 to 3 months as long as further compression is prevented. Proper padding of beds, prevention of leg crossing, and

Table C8–3. Differential Diagnosis of Common Causes of Footdrop

	Peroneal Neuropathy at the Fibular Head	L5 Radiculopathy	Lumbar Plexopathy (Lumbosacral Trunk)	Sciatic Neuropathy (Mainly Peroneal)
(A) Clinical				
Common causes	Compression (weight loss, perioperative), trauma	Disc herniation, spinal stenosis	Pelvic surgery, hematoma, prolonged labor	Hip surgery, injection injury, coma
Ankle inversion	Normal	Weak	Weak	Normal or mildly weak
Toe flexion	Normal	Weak	Weak	Normal or mildly weak
Plantar flexion	Normal	Normal	Normal	Normal or mildly weak
Ankle jerk	Normal	Normal (unless with S1)	Normal (unless with S1)	Normal or depressed
Sensory loss distribution	Peroneal only	Poorly demarcated, predominantly big toe	Well demarcated to L5 dermatome	Peroneal and lateral cutaneous of calf
Pain	Rare, deep	Common, radicular	Common, can be radicular	Can be severe
(B) Electrodiagnosis				
Peroneal motor study to EDB and/or Tib Ant	Low in amplitude or conduction block across fibular head or both	Usually normal but can be low in amplitude	Low in amplitude	Low in amplitude
Superficial peroneal sensory study	Low or absent	Normal	Low or absent	Low or absent
Sural sensory study	Normal	Normal	Normal or low amp	Normal or low amp
Peroneal muscles*	Abnormal	Abnormal	Abnormal	Abnormal
Tibial L5 muscles[†]	Normal	Usually abnormal	Usually abnormal	Normal or abnormal
Other L5 muscles[‡]	Normal	Normal or abnormal	Normal or abnormal	Normal
Biceps femoris (short head)	Normal	Usually normal	Usually normal	Abnormal
Paraspinal muscles fibrillations	Absent	May be absent	Absent	Absent

Can be normal in purely demyelinating lesions or lesion of the deep peroneal nerve only.
*Below knee (tibialis anterior (Tib Ant), extensor digitorum longus, extensor digitorum brevis (EDB), extensor hallucis, +/− peroneus longus).
[†]Tibialis posterior and flexor digitorum longus.
[‡]Gluteus medius and tensor fascia lata.

attempts to arrest or reverse weight loss should be initiated promptly. Ankle bracing is important when the footdrop is profound, to prevent ankle contractures and sprains. Surgical intervention is indicated (1) when the nerve is lacerated; (2) when clinical and/or EMG evidence for reinnervation cannot be established in the anterior compartment muscles (the tibialis anterior and the peroneus longus) 4 to 6 months after injury; and (3) in slowly progressive peroneal mononeuropathies.

Electrodiagnosis

The electrodiagnostic studies in peroneal mononeuropathies help to (1) confirm the site of the lesion (e.g., fibular head, upper thigh, or deep branch); (2) estimate the extent of injury (based on nerve conduction studies data); (3) judge its pathophysiologic nature (demyelinating versus axonal versus mixed); and (4) predict the prognosis and expected course of recovery (weeks or months). Sequential studies are helpful in following the progress of recovery (remyelination, reinnervation, or both).

Electrodiagnostic Strategy

The electrodiagnostic evaluation of patients with foot drop and suspected peroneal mononeuropathy is among the most fulfilling studies in the EMG laboratory. This is due the anatomy of the peroneal nerve and its accessibility to multiple nerve conduction studies and the needle EMG. The following are important electrodiagnostic strategies for use in patients presenting with footdrop, or in those suspected of having a peroneal mononeuropathy:

1. In addition to the common practice of recording the EDB, the peroneal motor study recording tibialis anterior must be included, for two reasons:
   - The tibialis anterior is the principal ankle dorsiflexor. Hence, establishing whether the disorder is demyelinating or axonal and prognosticating the outcome of foot drop are more pertinent while recording the tibialis anterior than the EDB.
   - The EDB is not uncommonly atrophic (presumably because of the use of tight shoes), resulting in an erroneous conclusion that the lesion is axonal or severe.
2. Peroneal motor (recording tibialis anterior and EDB) and superficial peroneal sensory conduction studies should be obtained bilaterally for comparison. This is particularly helpful in unilateral lesions in order to estimate the extent of axonal loss by comparing the distal peroneal CMAPs and the SNAPs.
3. At least two deep peroneal innervated muscles (such as the tibialis anterior, the extensor hallucis, and the extensor digitorum brevis) and one superficial peroneal innervated muscle (such as the peroneus longus) should

be sampled. In "pure" axonal peroneal mononeuropathies, which are unlocalizable by nerve conduction studies, sampling the short head of the biceps femoris is necessary to rule out a high peroneal lesion (sciatic neuropathy affecting the peroneal nerve, predominantly or exclusively).

4. Sampling nonperoneal muscles such as the tibialis posterior, the flexor digitorum longus, or the gluteus medius is also essential. These muscles are normal in peroneal lesions, but abnormal in L5 radiculopathy and lumbosacral plexopathy. Table C8–3(B) lists the distinguishing electrodiagnostic features.

A technical pitfall may arise during peroneal motor NCS recording EDB if there is an associated accessory deep peroneal nerve anomaly. The peroneal CMAP amplitude is larger stimulating proximally than distally since the anomalous fibers are not present at the ankle. This anomaly can be confirmed by stimulating behind the lateral malleolus (Figure C8–7). This yields a CMAP (not present in normal situations) that, when added to the distal CMAP, is approximately equal or higher than the CMAP obtained with proximal peroneal nerve stimulations.

Electrodiagnostic Findings in Peroneal Mononeuropathies

The findings on nerve conduction studies in peroneal mononeuropathies are extremely helpful in establishing a correct diagnosis and excluding other causes of foot drop, particularly L5 radiculopathy or sciatic mononeuropathy (see Table C8–3(B)). The EDX findings in peroneal mononeuropathies can be divided into several patterns (Figure C8–8 and Table C8–4):

1. *"Pure" conduction block across the fibular neck (partial or complete)* (see Figure C8–8B and B[1]). These cases represent 20–30% of all peroneal nerve lesions. In this situation, the distal peroneal CMAPs (recording EDB and tibialis anterior) and the superficial peroneal SNAP are normal and symmetrical to the asymptomatic limb in unilateral lesions. However, there is complete or partial conduction block (i.e., >20–50% decrease in amplitude and/or area) across the fibular head. Sometimes, the pathology is fascicular and the conduction block affects only fibers destined to either the EDB, or more commonly TA (Figure C8–9).

   Conduction block lesions are due to segmental demyelination and carry excellent prognosis with expected recovery in two to three months provided the cause of compression is eliminated. In contrast to carpal tunnel syndrome and ulnar neuropathy across the elbow, peroneal motor conduction velocities are usually normal and focal slowing across the fibular head is not a common feature of

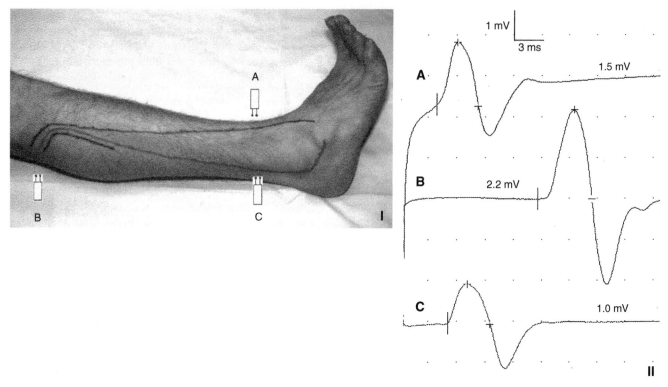

Figure C8–7. *Stimulation sites in a situation associated with the accessory deep peroneal nerve anomaly while performing a peroneal motor conduction study recording extensor digitorum brevis. (**I**) Peroneal nerve anatomy revealing the course of the accessory deep peroneal nerve anomaly and the stimulation sites. (**II**) Electrodiagnostic findings in accessory deep peroneal nerve anomaly is shown. The distal stimulation of the deep peroneal nerve at the ankle (**A**) results in a CMAP that is lower in amplitude that the proximal response following knee stimulation (**B**). Stimulation behind the lateral malleolus over the accessory deep peroneal nerve yielded a CMAP (**C**). (**I** is adapted with revisions from Preston DC, Shapiro BE. Electromyography and neuromuscular disorders. Philadelphia, PA: Elsevier Butterworth-Heinemann, 2005, with permission.)*

peroneal mononeuropathy. When present, it is always associated with a localizing conduction block, and it may be seen during the recovery phase of these lesions.

Before establishing the diagnosis of conduction block due to segmental demyelination, the time required for wallerian degeneration should be considered. Axon loss lesions will manifest as conduction block on NCS when performed soon after the onset of symptoms. In these axon loss lesions, the distal peroneal CMAP amplitudes decline to reach nadir in 5–6 days while the distal superficial peroneal SNAP takes 10–11 days to plateau.

2. *"Pure" axonal loss (partial or complete)* (see Figure C8–8D and D[1]). These lesions constitute about 45–50% of all peroneal neuropathies. On NCS, the distal and proximal peroneal CMAPs, recording EDB and tibialis anterior, are low in amplitude or absent. The superficial peroneal SNAP is usually absent. The conduction velocities are normal in mild or moderate lesions but can be slightly decreased diffusely in

severe lesions. Focal slowing does not accompany these types of lesions. These axon loss injuries are slow to improve because recovery is dependent on reinnervation. In general, the weakness in partial lesions improves faster as a result of local sprouting. Based on the needle EMG, these cases are localized to one of two sites:

- *At or above the fibular neck, i.e., at or above the peroneal nerve bifuraction.* The lesion cannot be localized accurately due the absence of both conduction block and focal slowing. When the short head of the biceps femoris is normal, this axon loss lesion is likely at the fibular head, but may be between the gluteal fold (the take off of the branch to short head of the biceps femoris) and the fibular neck, or even more proximally in fascicular lesions that may spare the fibers to the short head of the biceps femoris.
- *Proximal to the gluteal fold.* These are technically sciatic nerve lesions affecting the peroneal nerves exclusively. They are relatively rare lesions, accounting

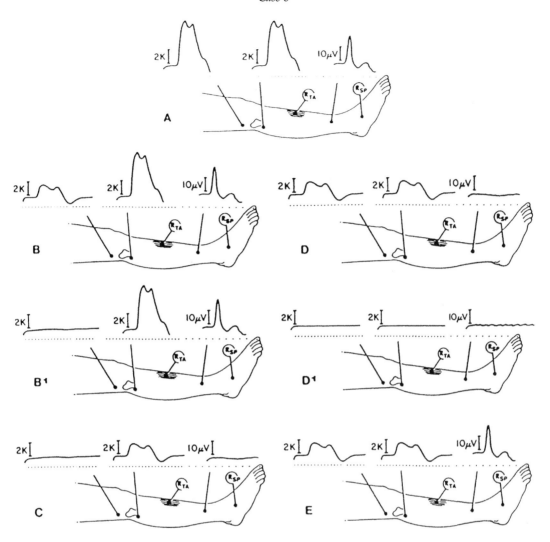

Figure C8–8. *Diagrams of the nerve conduction studies in peroneal mononeuropathy. (RTA = peroneal CMAP, recording tibialis anterior; RSP = recording site of the superficial peroneal SNAP.)* (**A**) *Normal.* (**B**) *and* (**B¹**) *"Pure" conduction block, partial and complete.* (**D**) *and* (**D¹**) *"Pure" axonal loss, partial and complete.* (**C**) *Mixed.* (**E**) *Deep peroneal. (Proximal latencies are not shown to scale.) (From Katirji MB, Wilbourn AJ. Common peroneal mononeuropathy: a clinical and electrophysiologic study of 116 lesions. Neurology 1988;38:1723–1728, with permission.)*

for less than 5% of all peroneal mononeuropathies. More often, the tibial component of the sciatic nerve is affected slightly, as evidenced by an abnormal H reflex, a low-amplitude or absent sural SNAP on NCS, or mild denervation in the tibial-innervated muscles (such as the medial gastrocnemius, the flexor digitorum longus, the tibialis posterior, or the abductor hallucis) on needle EMG.

3. *Mixed lesions (conduction block across the fibular neck with axonal loss)* (see Figure C8–8C). These lesions constitute 25–30% of peroneal nerve lesions. In these lesions, the distal peroneal CMAPs, recording EDB and tibialis

anterior, are low in amplitude and/or area, but there also is additional partial or complete conduction block across the fibular head. The superficial peroneal SNAP is low in amplitude or absent. Conduction velocities usually are normal, although occasionally there is an accompanying focal slowing. Recovery usually is biphasic; the first phase is relatively rapid, occurring over 2 to 3 months and is due to remyelination; the second phase is slower because it depends on reinnervation and sprouting.

In mixed common peroneal nerve lesions at the fibular head, it is not uncommon to find low-amplitude peroneal CMAP, recording EDB, without conduction block, along

Table C8–4. Electrophysiological Patterns of Peroneal Mononeuropathies

Pattern	Site of Lesion	Frequency	Superficial Peroneal SNAP	Distal Peroneal CMAPs*	Conduction Block at Fibular Head	Focal Slowing Across the Fibular Head	Needle EMG of Peroneus Longus	Needle EMG of Biceps Femoris (Short Head)	Prognosis for Recovery
Conduction block	Fibular head	20–30%	Normal	Normal	Present	Rare	Abnormal	Normal	Excellent
Axonal loss	Midthigh and fibular head†	45–50%	Usually absent	Low amplitude or absent	Absent	Absent	Abnormal	Normal	Protracted
Axonal loss	Deep peroneal	5%	Normal	Low amplitude or absent	Absent	Absent	Normal	Normal	Fair
Axonal loss	Proximal‡	<5%	Usually absent	Low amplitude or absent	Absent	Absent	Abnormal	Abnormal	Very poor
Mixed	Fibular Head	25–30%	Low amplitude or absent	Low amplitude	Present	Rare	Abnormal	Normal	Biphasic

*Recording tibialis anterior and extensor digitorum brevis.
†Usually around the fibular head.
‡High, proximal to the gluteal fold.
From Katirji B. Peroneal neuropathy. Neurol Clin 1999;17:567–591, with permission.

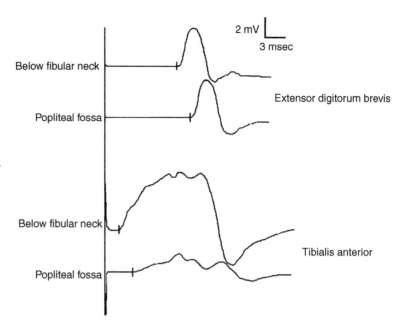

Figure C8–9. *Fascicular demyelinating peroneal nerve lesion at the fibular neck. This case shows a nerve conduction pattern that is not uncommon in peroneal mononeuropathy and emphasizes the importance of peroneal motor nerve conduction study recording tibialis anterior. Note that the motor conduction study recording extensor digitorum brevis is normal with no conduction block. In contrast, a significant conduction block (>50% drop in CMAP amplitude and area) is detected across the fibular neck recording tibialis anterior. (From Preston DC, Shapiro BE. Electromyography and neuromuscular disorders. Philadelphia, PA: Elsevier Butterworth-Heinemann, 2005, with permission.)*

with a definite conduction block across the fibular head, while recording tibialis anterior. This is extremely helpful prognostically, since conduction block due to segmental demyelination carries an excellent prognosis for recovery, while axonal lesions require much longer time for reinnervation.

4. *Deep peroneal axonal loss lesions* (see Figure C8–8E). The deep peroneal branch is often more severely affected than the superficial branch in most cases of common peroneal mononeuropathy at the fibular head. This is related to the topographic arrangement of the common peroneal nerve around the fibular head, where the exiting fascicles that form the superficial branch are placed laterally, and do not directly contact the fibular bone. However, selective deep peroneal mononeuropathies are less common and constitute about 5% of all peroneal nerve lesions. In these cases, the distal peroneal CMAPs, recording EDB and tibialis anterior, are low in amplitude and/or area, with normal superficial peroneal SNAP. The peroneus longus and brevis are normal. Motor conduction velocities are normal or borderline without focal slowing. The pattern on NCSs is identical to that seen in patients with moderate or severe L5 radiculopathy. Thus, sampling other L5-innervated muscles such as the flexor digitorum longus, the tibialis posterior, or the gluteus medius, as well as the lumbar paraspinal muscles, is important for distinguishing a deep peroneal lesion from an L5 radiculopathy.

In general, axon-loss peripheral nerve lesions are common encounters in the EMG laboratory. The peroneal nerve takes no exception for the following reasons:

- *Fibrillation potentials are seen in all weak muscles,* when examined by needle EMG at least 3 weeks after the onset of footdrop. These are found in "pure" axonal as well as demyelinating lesions (conduction block). In "purely" demyelinating lesions, the occurrence of fibrillation potentials is best explained by the loss of a few clinically irrelevant axons in the midst of significant demyelination.

- *Significant axonal loss is common in most peroneal nerve lesions.* This is based on low distal peroneal CMAPs with or without low superficial peroneal SNAPs, and is present in about 80% of peroneal nerve lesions (alone or mixed with conduction block due to segmental demyelination).

- *Significant axonal loss is common in all types of peroneal nerve lesions.* Axonal loss is evident (based on low distal peroneal CMAPs) independent of the mode of onset of foot drop (acute, subacute, or undetermined) or the cause of peroneal nerve lesion (perioperative compression, trauma, etc.). This applies to all compressive peroneal lesions including the perioperative cases, such as following anesthesia for coronary bypass surgery or craniotomy. This finding is in contrast to the common belief that patients with acute perioperative compressive peroneal lesions are due to neurapraxia (i.e., segmental demyelination) and should recover rapidly. This is incorrect since 80% of patients have evidence of significant axonal loss. It is only after a detailed EMG that the primary pathophysiologic process is determined and the prognosis is predicted.

FOLLOW-UP

The patient was treated with an ankle brace and physical therapy. Two months later, he had modest improvement of footdrop, as evidenced by neurologic examination findings, which revealed residual mild right foot dorsiflexion and eversion weakness (MRC 4/5), but greater weakness of toe extensors (MRC 4–/5). Sensation had improved with relative hypesthesia over the dorsum of the foot. When the patient was seen 1 year later, there were no residual findings.

DIAGNOSIS

Acute right common peroneal mononeuropathy at the fibular head, caused by intraoperative compression, manifested by segmental demyelination and axonal loss.

ANSWERS

1. C; 2. D; 3. A; 4. C.

SUGGESTED READINGS

Aprile I, Caliandro P, Giannini F et al. Italian multicentre study of peroneal mononeuropathy at the fibular head: study design and preliminary results. Acta Neurochir Suppl 2005;92:63–68.

Berry H, Richardson PM. Common peroneal nerve palsy: a clinical and electrophysiological review. J Neurol Neurosurg Psychiatry 1976;39:1162–1171.

Devi S, Lovelace RE, Duarte N. Proximal peroneal nerve conduction velocity: recording from anterior tibial and peroneus brevis muscle. Ann Neurol 1977;2:116–119.

Jabre JF. The superficial peroneal nerve revisited. Arch Neurol 1981;38:666–667.

Katirji B. Peroneal neuropathy. Neurol Clin N Am 1999;17: 567–591.

Katirji MB, Wilbourn AJ. Common peroneal mononeuropathy: a clinical and electrophysiologic study of 116 lesions. Neurology 1988;38:1723–1728.

Katirji MB, Wilbourn AJ. High sciatic lesions mimicking peroneal neuropathy at the fibular head. J Neurol Sci 1994;121: 172–175.

Marciniak C, Armon C, Wilson J et al. Practice parameter: utility of electrodiagnostic techniques in evaluating patients with suspected peroneal neuropathy: an evidence-based review. Muscle Nerve 2005;31:520–527.

Pickett JB. Localizing peroneal nerve lesions to the knee by motor conduction studies. Arch Neurol 1984;41:192–195.

Sourkes M, Stewart JD. Common peroneal neuropathy: a study of selective motor and sensory involvement. Neurology 1991; 41:1029–1033.

Upper Extremity

Case 9

HISTORY AND PHYSICAL EXAMINATION

Right hand weakness and atrophy, without numbness or pain, developed over several months in a 38-year-old man. A prior electromyography (EMG) suggested cervical radiculopathy. The patient then had a cervical magnetic resonance imaging (MRI) scan, a cervical myelogram/computed tomography, MRI of the right brachial plexus, and MRI and magnetic resonance angiography of the brain. All were normal. His hand weakness worsened. He was suspected to have early motor neuron disease and was referred to the EMG laboratory.

On examination, he had right hand "ulnar" clawing, positive Froment sign with severe weakness, and atrophy of all interossei. The strength and bulk of the thenar and hypothenar muscles were normal. No other weakness was detected and deep tendon reflexes were normal. The patient complained of mild, deep, boring pain in the palm near the hypothenar eminence and had some tenderness over the hypothenar eminence to deep pressure.

Electrodiagnostic (EDX) examination was performed.

Please now review the Nerve Conduction Studies and Needle EMG tables.

QUESTIONS

1. Results of the EDX studies are most consistent with:
   A. Ulnar mononeuropathy across the elbow.
   B. C8/T1 radiculopathy.
   C. Lower trunk brachial plexopathy.
   D. Ulnar mononeuropathy at the wrist or palm.
   E. Medial cord brachial plexopathy.
2. The most common cause of this lesion at this site is:
   A. Fracture.
   B. Ganglion.
   C. Acute compression.
   D. Aberrant muscle.
3. The lesion is:
   A. In the forearm, proximal to the dorsal ulnar branch.
   B. At Guyon canal, proximal to the takeoff of the superficial ulnar cutaneous branch.
   C. At Guyon canal, distal to the takeoff of the superficial ulnar cutaneous branch.
   D. At the cubital tunnel.

EDX FINDINGS AND INTERPRETATION OF DATA

Pertinent EDX findings include:

1. Absent ulnar compound muscle action potential (CMAP), recording first dorsal interosseus (DI) in the setting of borderline-low ulnar CMAP, recording abductor digiti minimi (ADM; 5 mV on the affected side versus 9 mV on normal side). The latter had a borderline distal latency (3.1 ms) and normal proximal conduction velocities in the forearm and across the elbow (55 ms and 54 ms, respectively).
2. Normal ulnar and dorsal ulnar sensory nerve action potentials (SNAPs).
3. Normal median motor conduction study (CMAP amplitude, distal latency, and conduction velocity).
4. Prominent active denervation and loss of motor unit action potentials (MUAPs) in all dorsal interossei and the adductor pollicis in the setting of minimal neurogenic changes in the ADM.
5. Normal median and radial C8/T1-innervated muscles (abductor pollicis brevis, flexor pollicis longus, and extensor indicis).

This is consistent with ulnar mononeuropathy at the wrist, affecting the motor branch exclusively, distal to the main branch to the hypothenar muscles, but proximal to the branch to the fourth dorsal interosseus (i.e., at the

Case 9: Nerve Conduction Studies

Nerve Stimulated	Stimulation Site	Recording Site	Amplitude (m = mV, s = µV)			Distal/Peak Latency (ms)			Conduction Velocity (m/s)			F Latency (ms)	
			Right	Left	Normal	Right	Left	Normal	Right	Left	Normal	Right	Left
Ulnar (s)	Wrist	Little finger	13	14	≥12	2.7	2.8	≤3.1					
Ulnar (s)	Elbow	Little finger	6						65		≥50		
Median (s)	Wrist	Index finger	24	22	≥20	2.8	2.5	≤3.4					
Radial (s)	Distal forearm	Thumb base	20		≥18	2.4		≤2.7					
Median (m)	Wrist	APB	10.0		≥6	3.8		≤3.9				28	
Median (m)	Elbow	APB	9.0						60		≥50		
Ulnar (m)	Wrist	ADM	**5.0**	9.0	≥7	**3.1**	2.8	≤3.1				28	
Ulnar (m)	Below elbow	ADM	**4.5**						55		≥50		
Ulnar (m)	Above elbow	ADM	**4.5**						54		≥50		
Ulnar (m)	Wrist	First DI	**NR**	13.0	≥7	**NR**	3.8	≤4.3	**NR**		≥50	**NR**	
Ulnar (m)	Below elbow	First DI	**NR**						**NR**		≥50		
Ulnar (m)	Above elbow	First DI	**NR**										
Dorsal ulnar (s)	Wrist	Dorsum of hand	14	15	≥12	2.4	2.2	≤3.1					

ADM = abductor digiti minimi; APB = abductor pollicis brevis; First DI = first dorsal interosseus; m = motor; NR = no response; s = sensory. Data in bold type are abnormal.

Case 9: Needle EMG

Muscle	Insertional Activity	Spontaneous Activity Fibs	Fascs	Recruitment Normal	Activation	Reduced	Early	Duration	Amplitude	% Polyphasia	Others
R. first dorsal interosseous	↑	3+	0			No MUAPs					
Adductor pollicis	↑	3+	0			No MUAPs					
Second dorsal interosseous	↑	3+	0			No MUAPs					
Third dorsal interosseous	↑	3+	0			↓↓↓		↑	Normal	↑	
Fourth dorsal interosseous	↑	3+	0			↓↓↓		↑	Normal	↑	
Abductor digiti minimi	Normal	0	0			↓		↑	Normal	↑	
Abductor pollicis brevis	Normal	0	0	X				Normal	Normal	Normal	
Flexor pollicis brevis	Normal	0	0	X				Normal	Normal	Normal	
Extensor indicis	Normal	0	0	X				Normal	Normal	Normal	
Pronator teres	Normal	0	0	X				Normal	Normal	Normal	
Biceps	Normal	0	0	X				Normal	Normal	Normal	
Triceps	Normal	0	0	X				Normal	Normal	Normal	
Deltoid	Normal	0	0	X				Normal	Normal	Normal	
Middle cervical paraspinal	Normal	0	0	–							
Lower cervical paraspinal	Normal	0	0	–							
L. first dorsal interosseous	Normal	0	0	X				Normal	Normal	Normal	
Abductor digiti minimi	Normal	0	0	X				Normal	Normal	Normal	
Biceps	Normal	0	0	X				Normal	Normal	Normal	

Voluntary Motor Unit Action Potentials (MUAPs) — Recruitment, Configuration

Fascs = fasciculations; Fibs = fibrillations; L. = left; MUP = motor unit potential; R. = right; ↑ = increased; ↓ = mildly reduced; ↓↓↓ = severely reduced.

pisohamate hiatus [PHH]). The normal ulnar sensory study rules out a proximal ulnar nerve, or a lower brachial plexus lesion. This case is not due to C8/T1 radiculopathy is because the median CMAP is preserved, and there is no denervation seen in other C8/T1-innervated muscles.

DISCUSSION

Applied Anatomy

The ulnar nerve gives off the *dorsal ulnar cutaneous branch* 6 to 8 cm proximal to the ulnar styloid, to innervate the skin over the ulnar side of the dorsum of the hand and the dorsal aspect of digit V and half of digit IV. Then, the ulnar nerve enters Guyon canal (distal ulnar tunnel) at the level of the distal wrist crease where it divides into superficial (primarily sensory) and deep (pure motor) palmar branches. The deep branch enters the hand through the pisohamate hiatus while the superficial branch travels subcutaneously passing over the hypothenar muscles.

Guyon canal is formed proximally by the pisiform bone and distally by the hook of the hamate. Its floor is formed by the triquetrum and hamate bones along with the thick transverse carpal ligament, while its roof is composed of a loose connective tissue (Figure C9–1). In the distal portion of Guyon canal lies the *pisohamate hiatus* (PHH). This aperture is bounded anteriorly by a fibrous arch formed by the two musculotendinous attachments of the flexor brevis digiti minimi (or quinti), a hypothenar muscle, to the hook of hamate and the pisiform bone (Figure C9–2). The posterior boundary of the PHH, is formed by a thick pisohamate ligament which extends from the pisiform bone to the hook of the hamate. The origin of the major motor branch to the ADM is proximal to this hiatus in the majority of hands.

The *deep palmar motor branch* innervates the hypothenar muscles (the ADM, flexor brevis digiti minimi, and opponens digiti minimi) while in Guyon canal and often gives these muscles an additional branch after it enter the PHH. Then, the deep palmar motor branch travels through the palm and innervates all four dorsal and three palmar interossei, the third and fourth lumbricals, the adductor pollicis, and the deep head of the flexor pollicis brevis. The *superficial cutaneous branch* innervates the palmaris brevis muscle, as well as the ulnar side of the palm and palmar aspect of digit V and half of digit IV.

Clinical Features

Patients with ulnar neuropathy at the wrist often presents with painless unilateral hand atrophy. These ulnar nerve

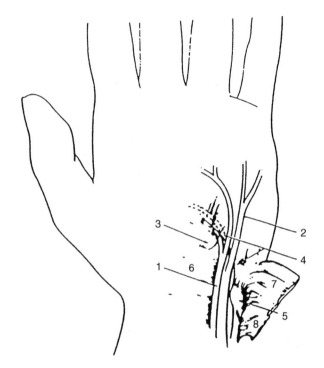

Figure C9–1. *Anatomy of the ulnar nerve within Guyon canal at the wrist. 1 = ulnar artery, 2 = superficial branch of the ulnar nerve, 3 = hamulus, 4 = fibrous arch of the hypothenar muscles (see also Figure C9–2), 5 = pisiform, 6 = transverse carpal ligament, 7 = palmaris brevis, 8 = palmar carpal ligament. (From Gross MS, Gelberman RH. The anatomy of the distal ulnar tunnel. Clin Orthop 1985;196:238–247, with permission.)*

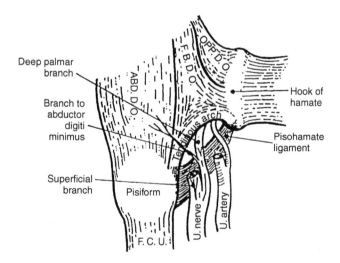

Figure C9–2. *The pisohamate hiatus (PHH) in the distal portion of Guyon canal. ABD.D.Q. = abductor digiti quinti (or minimi), F.B.D.Q. = flexor brevis digiti quinti (or minimi), F.C.U. = flexor carpi ulnaris, Opp.D.Q. = opponens digiti quinti, U. = ulnar. (Modified from Uriburu IJF, Morchio FJ, Marin JC. Compression syndrome of the deep motor branch of the ulnar nerve [pisohamate hiatus syndrome]. J Bone Joint Surg 1976;58A:145–147, with permission.)*

Table C9–1. Causes of Unilateral Atrophy and Weakness of Intrinsic Hand Muscles

All intrinsic hand muscles
    Combined ulnar mononeuropathy and carpal tunnel syndrome
    Lower brachial plexopathy (including neurogenic thoracic outlet syndrome)
    C8/T1 radiculopathy
    Motor neuron disease
    Monomelic amyotrophy (Focal motor neuron disease)
    Cervical syringomyelia
    Cervical cord compression around the foramen magnum
All intrinsic muscles, excluding the thenar muscles
    Ulnar mononeuropathy at the elbow
    Ulnar mononeuropathy at Guyon canal
All intrinsic muscles, excluding the thenar and hypothenar muscles
    Ulnar mononeuropathy at the pisohamate hiatus
Thenar muscles only
    Carpal tunnel syndrome
    High median mononeuropathy (including pronator syndrome)
    Neurogenic thoracic outlet syndrome
    T1 radiculopathy

lesions pose a diagnostic challenge, particularly when the weakness is not associated with sensory loss. It is useful in sorting out the cause of hand weakness or atrophy to distinguish between atrophy of all intrinsic hand muscles from atrophy that is restricted to the thenar or hypothenar muscles. Table C9–1 lists the various causes of wasting and weakness of the hand.

The signs and symptoms of distal ulnar lesions vary with the site of compression. In all types of ulnar mononeuropathy at the wrist, sensation over the dorsal medial hand and the dorsal aspect of the fifth and ring fingers, a territory of the dorsal ulnar cutaneous branch, is normal. The terminal branches of the ulnar nerve (deep palmar motor and superficial cutaneous) may be compressed at Guyon canal, but only the deep palmar motor branch is potentially compressed at the PHH.

Several classifications of ulnar mononeuropathy at the wrist have been proposed; most separate the lesions into four types. Table C9–2 lists the common types of ulnar mononeuropathy at the wrist and hand, with their corresponding sites of lesion and clinical presentation. In ulnar neuropathy at the wrist, selective compression of the deep palmar motor branch, with normal superficial sensory branch functions, is the most common type accounting for 39 to 75% of distal ulnar nerve lesions depending on published series.

Table C9–3 lists the common causes of ulnar mononeuropathy at the wrist. A ganglion is the most common cause accounting for 28 to 45% of cases depending on reported series. The second most common cause is entrapment of the motor branch at the pisohamate hiatus, which may be spontaneous or as an occupational or recreational hazard (such as after prolonged bicycling, use of hand tools, etc.). Compression at this anatomic hiatus explains the selective involvement of the deep motor branch at the wrist with complete or relative sparing of the hypothenar muscles and the normal superficial sensory functions.

Imaging should be considered in patients with ulnar neuropathy at the wrist who have a history of progressive worsening and who do not have clearly identified occupational or recreational risk factors. MRI imaging of the wrist is helpful in identifying structural lesions within Guyon canal, including ganglion cyst and nerve sheath tumor.

Decisions regarding the management of these lesions are made on the basis of their etiologies, presentations, and clinical courses. In patients with fractures, ganglia, or mass lesions, surgical intervention is necessary. However, in patients with ulnar neuropathy at the wrist who do not

Table C9–2. Various Types of Distal Ulnar Mononeuropathy

Lesion Site	Nerve Affected	Clinical Presentation
Proximal Guyon canal	Main trunk of ulnar nerve *or*	Ulnar palmar sensory loss and weakness of all ulnar intrinsic hand muscles *or*
	Ulnar cutaneous branch	Ulnar palmar sensory loss only
Distal Guyon canal	Deep palmar branch (proximal to branch to the abductor digiti minimi)	Weakness of all ulnar intrinsic hand muscles (interossei, ulnar lumbricals, and hypothenars) without sensory loss
Pisohamate hiatus	Deep palmar branch (distal to branch to the abductor digiti minimi)	Weakness of ulnar intrinsic hand muscles with sparing of the hypothenar muscles and without sensory loss
Palm (rare)	Deep palmar branch (distal to hypothenars)	Weakness of adductor pollicis, 1st, 2nd, and possibly the 3rd interossei only, usually sparing 4th interossei and without sensory loss

Table C9–3. Common Causes of Ulnar Mononeuropathy at the Wrist

Ganglion
Compression at the pisohamate hiatus (distal to Guyon canal)
  – Associated with occupational or recreational risks (e.g., use of hand tools, bicycling, etc.)
  – Associated with acute closed injury (e.g., fall on hand, carpal fracture)
  – Idiopathic (entrapment)
Carpal bone fracture
Other space-occupying lesions (neuroma, lipoma, cyst, calcification, false aneurysm, giant cell tumor)

harbor an obvious mass or fracture and have a predominantly demyelinating lesion, careful review of the history for any occupational or recreational trauma should be initiated; if found, sources of the trauma should be eliminated. Then, the patient should be followed clinically and by serial EDX studies. If recovery is not evident, surgical exploration of Guyon canal extending into the PHH should be done. The prognosis for patients with this disorder is usually good after surgical decompression because the lesion is distal and reinnervation to the target hand muscles is efficient.

Electrodiagnosis

An important purpose of the EDX study is to localize the ulnar nerve lesion to the wrist or to the elbow and to differentiate ulnar mononeuropathy from a lower brachial plexopathy affecting the lower trunk or medial cord, and from a C8/T1 radiculopathy. In addition to the routine NCSs done that include ulnar sensory NCS recording little finger and ulnar motor NCS recording ADM, several other strategic EDX studies are extremely important to assure a correct and precise diagnosis of the ulnar nerve lesion. These include the following:

1. *Ulnar motor nerve conduction study recording first DI.* This study is essential in the accurate diagnosis of ulnar nerve lesions at the wrist due to the fact that many lesions, such as those at the PHH or in the palm, spares the hypothenar muscles and result in normal ulnar NCS recording ADM. In most cases, the ulnar CMAP recording first DI is low in amplitude stimulating at the wrist, and the distal latency is either borderline or slightly delayed. Slowing of the distal latency should also interpreted cautiously since it may be slowed in any axon-loss ulnar nerve lesion, including at the elbow, due to the loss of large fibers. In cases of ulnar neuropathy at the wrist, the addition of more stimulation site(s) distal to Guyon canal, while recording first DI, is

technically feasible with minimal interference by shock artifact. This could be achieved using one of both of the following techniques:

- *Palm stimulation recording first DI.* Adding a single palm stimulation site to the routine wrist, below-elbow and above-elbow sites, often confirm that the lesion is at the wrist by showing conduction block in the majority of patients (Figure C9–3). Even in patients with a seemingly axon-loss ulnar neuropathy and uniformly low CMAP amplitudes stimulating wrist, below elbow and above elbow, palm stimulation often shows that there is a component of segmental demyelination manifesting by a partial conduction block (i.e., more than 20–50% drop in CMAP amplitude and/or area). This finding is very specific since it localizes the lesion to the wrist.

- *Short segment stimulation across the wrist recording first DI.* During ulnar motor NCS, inclusion of the unaffected segments in distal latency calculation may dilute the effect of focal slowing at the injured site and decreases the sensitivity of the test. Segmental stimulation in short increments of 1 cm across the nerve segment helps localize a focal abnormality that might otherwise escape detection. "*Inching*" the stimulus in short increments of 1 cm along the course of the nerve is very specific and often shows a precise site of compression. However, it is more technically challenging and time consuming than the single palm stimulation. Though this study is technically more demanding and subject to inherent measurement errors (due multiple stimulations in short increments), detecting an abrupt drop in amplitude (>20%) or increase in latency difference (>0.5 ms) compensates for these shortcomings (Figure C9–4).

2. *Dorsal ulnar SNAP.* This study is useful since an absent or low-amplitude response exclude a lesion at the wrist or hand. The study should be performed bilaterally for comparison purposes since interpreting the result of the dorsal ulnar SNAP may be misleading due to two caveats:

- A fascicular involvement of the ulnar nerve at the elbow may totally or partially spare the dorsal ulnar nerve resulting in normal SNAP.

- There is a considerable overlap, in some individuals, between the territories of the dorsal ulnar cutaneous nerve and that of the superficial radial cutaneous nerve. Hence, this may result in a low-amplitude, or occasionally absent, dorsal ulnar SNAP when the radial sensory nerve dominates the innervation of the dorsum of the hand. In these situations, radial sensory nerve stimulation while recording the ulnar side of the dorsum of the hand will yield a well-defined SNAP.

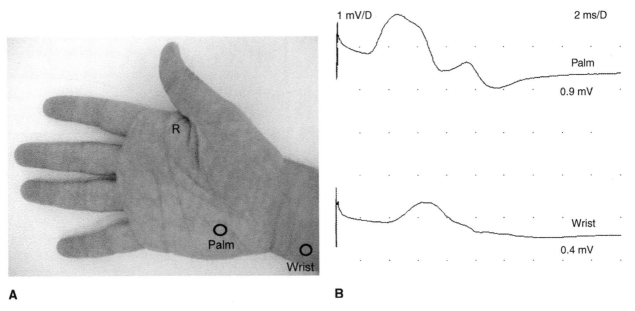

Figure C9–3. *Palm and wrist stimulations recording first dorsal interosseous muscle. This 37-year-old woman developed subacute painless weakness of left hand. Neurological examination reveals severe weakness of all ulnar-innervated muscles in the hand with a positive Froment sign. There was no sensory loss. Tinel signs were negative at the wrist and elbow. Routine EDX studies revealed findings compatible with an axon loss ulnar mononeuropathy at the distal portion of Guyon canal (see Table C9–4). (A) The stimulation points at the palm and wrist (circles) while recording first DI (R). (B) Note that both wrist and palm stimulations result in low ulnar CMAPs, but there is a localizing partial conduction across both stimulation points (>50% drop in amplitude).*

3. *Second lumbrical-interosseous motor distal latencies comparison.* This study is most often used in the diagnosis of carpal tunnel syndrome where the median motor distal latency recording second lumbrical muscle is usually prolonged in carpal tunnel syndrome when compared to the ulnar motor distal latency recording second interossei (palmar and dorsal). Since the ulnar second interossei are innervated by the deep palmar motor branch, this test is also useful in identifying focal ulnar slowing at the wrist or palm in ulnar nerve lesions at Guyon canal or deep palmar motor branch lesions at the PHH. A motor distal latency difference greater than 0.5 ms suggests focal slowing across the wrist; the median is relatively slowed compared to the ulnar in carpal tunnel syndrome while the findings are reversed in ulnar nerve lesion at the wrist (Figure C9–5). Obviously, this study is not useful when there is a coexisting carpal tunnel syndrome. Similar to the ulnar motor distal latency stimulating at the wrist and recording the first DI, this study also should be interpreted cautiously since it may be slowed in any axon-loss ulnar nerve lesion, including at the elbow, due to the loss of fast conducting fibers.

4. *Medial antebrachial SNAP.* The medial antebrachial cutaneous nerve is a pure sensory nerve that originates

from the medial cord of the brachial plexus and innervates the skin of the medial forearm. In cases of ulnar neuropathies in general, a normal medial antebrachial SNAP is useful in excluding the possibility of a lower brachial plexopathy as a cause of hand weakness and medial hand sensory loss. The medial brachial SNAP serves similar purposes but it is technically more difficult to evoke particularly in elderly and obese patients.

5. *Needle EMG of hand intrinsics.* In suspected ulnar nerve lesion at the wrist, needle EMG of at least the ADM and first DI should be done to look for disparity between the findings of these two muscles. It is also preferable to needle few other hand intrinsics that are innervated by the deep palmar branch such as the fourth DI, a muscle with a branch that originate immediately after the nerve passes under the PHH, and the adductor pollicis, one of the most distal muscle innervated by the ulnar nerve and its deep palmar branch. In lesions of the deep palmar branch at the PHH, an abrupt change from a normal (or minimally abnormal) ADM to markedly denervated fourth and third interosseous is often evident. The flexor digitorum profundus (ulnar part) and the flexor carpi ulnaris, both forearm muscles innervated by the ulnar nerve are normal in ulnar mononeuropathy at the wrist and

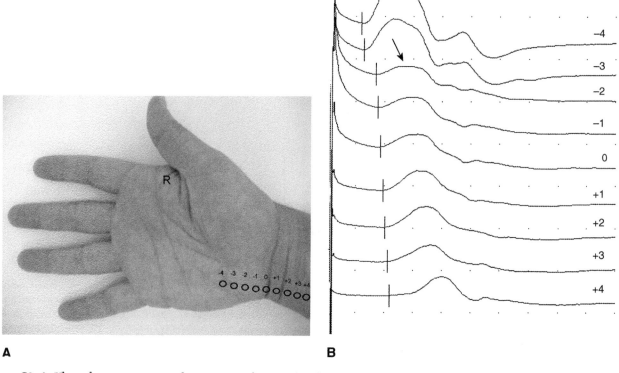

A   **B**

Figure C9-4. *Ulnar short segment stimulations across the wrist ("inching") recording first dorsal interosseous muscle. (**A**) Nine sites of stimulation (circles) in 1 cm increments along the length of the ulnar nerve while recording first DI (R): 0 level is at the distal crease of the wrist, while negative sites are progressively distal points and positive sites are proximal. (**B**) Same patient as Figure C9-3. Note that the most distal response, stimulating the palm at point -4, is low (0.9 mV), consistent with axon loss. However, there is also a localizing partial conduction block between points -3 and -2 (arrow), consistent with additional segmental demyelination. This is evidenced by a drop in CMAP amplitude from 0.7 mV at point -3 to 0.2 mV at point -2 (70% amplitude decay). There is also focal slowing at the same segment (between points -3 and -2) as evidenced by a larger increase in latency between the same two points resulting in a latency difference of 0.9 ms. This is contrasted to 0.1 to 0.2 ms latency differences at all other sites.*

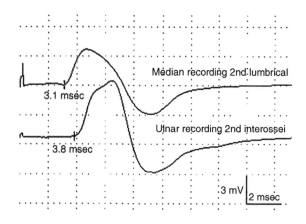

Figure C9-5. *Second lumbrical-interosseous motor distal latencies comparison in a patient with ulnar mononeuropathy at the wrist. Note that the ulnar motor distal latency recording second interossei (dorsal and palmar) is significantly prolonged when compared to the median motor distal latency recording second lumbrical (0.7 ms difference).*

useful in confirming the diagnosis. Finally, median and radial C8–T1 muscles (such as abductor pollicis brevis, flexor pollicis longus and extensor indicis proprius) and the lower cervical paraspinals muscles must be sampled to exclude a cervical root or motor neuron lesion.

The EDX findings in ulnar mononeuropathy at the wrist parallel the clinical manifestations and vary with the site of the lesion (Table C9–4). In addition to try to localize the lesions accurately within Guyon canal, at the PHH or in the palm, the EDX study play a pivotal role in excluding an ulnar neuropathy at the elbow, a common entrapment neuropathy. Several features on the EDX examination are not consistent with an ulnar neuropathy at the wrist:

1. Low-amplitude or absent dorsal ulnar SNAP, excluding the anatomical variability where the territory of the superficial radial cutaneous nerve overrides that of the dorsal ulnar cutaneous nerve.

Table C9–4. Electrodiagnostic Findings in Ulnar Neuropathies

Location of Ulnar Nerve Lesion	Dorsal Ulnar SNAP Amplitude Recording Dorsum of Hand	Ulnar SNAP Amplitude Recording Fifth Digit	Ulnar CMAP Distal Amplitude Recording ADM	Ulnar CMAP Distal Amplitude Recording First DI	Active Denervation and/or Reinnervation of Ulnar-innervated Muscles
Across the elbow	Absent or low*	Absent or low[†]	Low[†]	Low[†]	All, in hand and, sometimes, forearm
At proximal Guyon canal	Normal	Absent or low	Low	Low[‡]	All, in hand only
At distal Guyon canal	Normal	Normal	Low	Low[‡]	All, in hand only
At pisohamate hiatus	Normal	Normal	Normal[¶]	Low[‡]	All, in hand only except ADM[¶]
Palm (rare)	Normal	Normal	Normal	Low	Most distal in hand only[§]

SNAP = sensory nerve action potential; ADM = abductor digiti minim; CMAP = compound muscle action potential; first DI = first dorsal interosseus.

*May be normal in fascicular lesions that spare the dorsal ulnar fascicle and nerve or in purely demyelinating lesion.

[†]May be normal or borderline in purely demyelinating lesion manifesting only with conduction block and/or focal slowing and/or differential slowing across the elbow and without axon loss.

[‡]There is often a conduction block across the wrist following palm stimulation and an abrupt focal latency shift and conduction block on short segment incremental study across the wrist.

[¶]Ulnar CMAP amplitude recording ADM may be borderline and ADM may reveal minimal denervation.

[§]Adductor pollicis and first and second dorsal and first palmar interossei are always abnormal while there is a variable involvement of the third dorsal and palmar interossei and the third lumbrical muscles, while the fourth dorsal and third palmar interossei and fourth lumbrical muscles are spared.

2. Focal slowing, conduction block, or differential slowing across the elbow is not compatible with a lesion at the wrist. Note that in a significant number of ulnar nerve lesions at the elbow, especially those resulting in axonal loss, there is no focal slowing, and, if slowing is present, it is diffuse due to the loss of fast conducting fibers, and evident in all segments of the ulnar nerve.

3. Denervation of the flexor carpi ulnaris or the flexor digitorum profundus (ulnar portion) is not compatible with a lesion at the wrist. Note that these muscles are denervated in only a proportion of patients with ulnar mononeuropathy around the elbow.

Among all ulnar mononeuropathies at the wrist, selective lesion of the deep motor branch at the PHH, sparing the hypothenar muscles completely or partially, is the most common. This entrapment is suspected when a patient presents with wasting and weakness of all intrinsic muscles of the hand except the thenar and hypothenar muscles, and without sensory manifestations. Table C9–5 lists the pathognomonic EDX features of such a lesion.

FOLLOW-UP

On further questioning, the patient recalled that a month before the onset of symptoms, he had spent an entire weekend vigorously chopping wood. Because the patient demonstrated no improvement, a surgical exploration of the proximal portion of Guyon canal was performed, which revealed normal structures. Despite this, there was no evidence of clinical or electrophysiologic improvement over the ensuing 6 months. A second operation was performed that achieved more distal exploration of the deep palmar branch into the PHH. This revealed a fibrous band constricting the deep motor branch at the PHH,

Table C9–5. Pathognomonic Electrodiagnostic Features of Deep Palmar Ulnar Neuropathy at the Pisohamate Hiatus

Normal ulnar SNAP, dorsal ulnar SNAP, and medial antebrachial SNAP

Normal to borderline ulnar CMAP amplitude recording the ADM

Low ulnar CMAP amplitude recording the first DI with conduction block with or without slowing across the wrist*

Normal ADM or with minimal chronic neurogenic changes

Prominent loss of motor units with fibrillation potentials in the adductor pollicis, all four dorsal and three palmar interossei, third and fourth lumbricals

ADM = abductor digiti minimi; CMAP = compound motor action potential; DI = dorsal interosseus; SNAPs = sensory nerve action potentials.

*Following palm stimulation and short segment stimulations.

Table C9–6. Ulnar Nerve Motor Conduction Studies at Diagnosis and 12 Months After Release at the Pisohamate Hiatus

	Ulnar/First DI		Ulnar/ADM	
	Amplitude	**Distal Latency**	**Amplitude**	**Distal Latency**
Preoperative	NR	NR	5	3.1
Postoperative (12 months)	2	4.8	8.8	2.5
Normal values	>7.0	<4.5	>7.0	<3.1

ADM = abductor digiti minimi; DI = dorsal interosseus; NR = no response.

which was resected. The patient had significant and gradual improvement of strength and experienced reversal of atrophy over the next year. Twelve months after the second decompression, the ulnar CMAP amplitude, which recorded the first DI and the ADM, showed significant improvement (Table C9–6). Needle EMG of the first and fourth DI showed significant reinnervation and a decline in fibrillation potentials.

DIAGNOSIS

Subacute deep palmar ulnar mononeuropathy, at the pisohamate hiatus, manifested by axonal loss.

ANSWERS

1. D; 2. B; 3.C.

SUGGESTED READINGS

Cowdery SR, Preston DC, Herrmann DN et al. Electrodiagnosis of ulnar neuropathy at the wrist: conduction block versus traditional tests. Neurology 2002;59:420–427.

Ebling P, Gilliatt RW, Thomas PK. A clinical and electrical study of ulnar nerve lesions in the hand. J Neurol Neurosurg Psychiatry 1960;23:1–9.

Gross MS, Gelberman RH. The anatomy of the distal ulnar tunnel. Clin Orthop 1985;196:238–247.

Katirji B, Dokko Y. Electrodiagnosis of deep palmar ulnar neuropathy at the pisohamate hiatus. Eur J Neurol 1996; 3:389–394.

Kothari MJ, Preston DC, Logigian EL. Lumbrical and interossei recordings localize ulnar neuropathy at the wrist. Muscle Nerve 1996;19:170–174.

Jabley ME, Wallace WH, Heckler FR. Internal topography of the major nerves of the forearm and hand. J Hand Surg 1980; 5:1–21.

McIntosh KA, Preston DC, Logigian EL. Short segment incremental studies to localize ulnar entrapments at the wrist. Neurology 1998;50:303–306.

Olney RK, Wilbourn AJ. Ulnar nerve conduction study of the first dorsal interosseus muscle. Arch Phys Med Rehabil 1985;66:16–18.

Peterson AR et al. Variations in dorsomedial hand innervation. Electrodiagnostic implications. Arch Neurol 1992;49:870–873.

Shea JD, McClain EJ. Ulnar nerve compression syndromes at or below the wrist. J Bone Joint Surg 1969;51A:1095–1103.

Stewart JD. The variable clinical manifestations of ulnar neuropathies at the elbow. J Neurol Neurosurg Psychiatry 1987;3:429–432.

Streib EW et al. Distal ulnar neuropathy: clinical and electrophysiologic aspects. Surg Neurol 1985;23:281.

Uriburu IJF, Morchio FJ, Marin JC. Compression syndrome of the deep motor branch of the ulnar nerve (pisohamate-hamate hiatus syndrome). J Bone Joint Surg 1976;58A:145–147.

Ventakesh S, Kothari MJ, Preston DC. The limitations of the dorsal ulnar cutaneous sensory response in patients with ulnar neuropathy at the elbow. Muscle Nerve 1995;18:345–347.

Wu JS, Morris JD, Hogan GR. Ulnar neuropathy at the wrist: case report and review of the literature. Arch Phys Med Rehabil 1985;66:19–21.

Case 10

HISTORY AND PHYSICAL EXAMINATION

An 82-year-old woman tripped and fell on her right shoulder. An anterior dislocation of the right shoulder was reduced on the same day; however, she continued to have pain and weakness in the right shoulder. Arthrography and magnetic resonance imaging (MRI) of the shoulder failed to reveal rotator cuff tear. She denied any numbness. She was otherwise in excellent health.

On examination 6 weeks later, she had significant restriction of passive range of movement of the right shoulder to approximately 90°. This movement was associated with pain. There was atrophy of the right deltoid and possibly the spinati. Motor examination of all shoulder girdle muscles, including assessment of active shoulder abduction, was limited by pain. However, the biceps, triceps, and brachioradialis seemed normal in strength. All forearm and hand muscle movements also were determined to be normal, as was sensation. Deep tendon reflexes were normal and the sensory examination revealed no clear abnormalities. The patient was referred to the electromyography (EMG) laboratory to explore the possibility of an injury of the brachial plexus or the axillary nerve.

Please now review the Nerve Conduction Studies and Needle EMG tables.

QUESTIONS

1. In addition to the deltoid muscle, the axillary nerve innervates the:
   A. Teres major muscle.
   B. Teres minor muscle.
   C. Rhomboideus major muscle.
   D. Subscapularis muscle.
   E. Brachialis muscle.

2. Most fibers within the affected nerve originate from:
   A. The C5 and C6 roots via the upper trunk and the lateral cord.
   B. The C6 and C7 roots via the upper and middle trunks and the posterior cord.
   C. The C5 and C6 roots via the upper trunk and posterior cord.
   D. The C6 and C7 roots via the upper and middle trunks and the lateral cord.

3. Common causes of this nerve palsy include all of the following except:
   A. Shoulder dislocation.
   B. Mid-humeral fracture.
   C. Neuralgic amyotrophy.
   D. Misplaced injection.

EDX FINDINGS AND INTERPRETATION OF DATA

Pertinent electrodiagnostic (EDX) findings include:

1. Very low-amplitude axillary compound muscle action potential (CMAP) on the right (0.88 mV versus 6.2 mV on the left) with slow distal latency (5.8 ms on the right versus 2.6 ms on the left).
2. Normal musculocutaneous CMAP.
3. Normal median sensory nerve action potentials (SNAPs), recording thumb, index, and middle fingers; radial SNAP; and lateral cutaneous forearm (lateral antebrachial) SNAP.
4. Fibrillation potentials and no voluntary motor unit action potentials in the right deltoid muscle only, without involvement of other upper plexus innervated muscles (supraspinatus, infraspinatus, biceps, brachioradialis, and pronator teres), posterior cord innervated muscles

Case 10: Nerve Conduction Studies

Nerve Stimulated	Stimulation Site	Recording Site	Amplitude (m = mV, s = µV)			Distal/Peak Latency(ms)			Conduction Velocity (m/s)			F Latency (ms)	
			Right	Left	Normal	Right	Left	Normal	Right	Left	Normal	Right	Left
Axillary (m)	Erb point	Deltoid	**0.88**	6.2	3	**5.8**	2.6	≤5.0					
Musculocut (m)	Axilla	Biceps	6.0	5.8	≥3	2.8	2.9	≤4.0	53	55	≥50		
Musculocut (m)	Erb point	Biceps	5.0	5.0									
Median (s)	Wrist	Thumb	18	19	≥10	3.6	3.5	≤3.8					
Median (s)	Wrist	Index finger	19	20	≥10	3.6	3.6	≤3.8					
Median (s)	Wrist	Middle finger	25	22	≥10	3.6	3.7	≤3.8					
Lat cut fore (s)	Elbow	Forearm	30	28	≥10	2.5	2.6	≤2.8					
Ulnar (s)	Wrist	Little finger	11		≥5	3.0		≤3.2					
Radial (s)	Forearm	Dorsum of hand	30		>10	2.7		≤2.8					
Median (m)	Wrist	APB	9.0		>5	3.4		≤4.0				27.6	
Median (m)	Elbow	APB	8.7						58		≥50		
Ulnar (m)	Wrist	ADM	10.0		>7	3.1		≤3.1				27.2	
Ulnar (m)	Above elbow	ADM	9.4						56		≥50		
Ulnar (m)	Axilla	ADM	9.0						58		≥50		

ADM = abductor digiti minimi; APB = abductor pollicis brevis; Lat cut fore = lateral cutaneous of forearm (lateral antebrachial cutaneous); m = motor; Musculocut = musculocutaneous; s = sensory.
Data in bold type are abnormal.

Case 10: Needle EMG

Muscle	Insertional Activity	Spontaneous Activity Fibs	Spontaneous Activity Fascs	Voluntary Motor Unit Action Potentials (MUAPs) Recruitment Normal	Recruitment Activation	Recruitment Reduced	Recruitment Early	Configuration Duration	Configuration Amplitude	Configuration % Polyphasia	Others
R. deltoid	↑	4+	0	No voluntary	MUAPs			Normal	Normal	Normal	
Biceps	Normal	0	0	X				Normal	Normal	Normal	
Brachioradialis	Normal	0	0	X				Normal	Normal	Normal	
Triceps	Normal	0	0	X				Normal	Normal	Normal	
Pronator teres	Normal	0	0	X				Normal	Normal	Normal	
Flexor pollicis longus	Normal	0	0	X				Normal	Normal	Normal	
First dorsal interosseous	Normal	0	0	X				Normal	Normal	Normal	
Extensor indicis proprius	Normal	0	0	X				Normal	Normal	Normal	
Supraspinatus	Normal	0	0	X				Normal	Normal	Normal	
Infraspinatus	Normal	0	0	X				Normal	Normal	Normal	
Midcervical paraspinal	Normal	0	0	–							
Low cervical paraspinal	Normal	0	0	–							

Fascs = fasciculations; Fibs = fibrillations; R. = right; ↑ = increased.

(triceps, brachioradialis, and extensor indicis), or cervical paraspinal muscles.

These findings are consistent with an isolated severe injury to the right axillary nerve with no involvement of the upper trunk or posterior cord of the brachial plexus.

DISCUSSION

Applied Anatomy

The axillary nerve (also called the circumflex nerve) arises from the posterior cord of the brachial plexus near the shoulder joint. Its fibers originate from the C5 and C6 roots and travel through the upper trunk to the posterior cord. The nerve has a very short path. It courses posteriorly, inferior to the shoulder joint where it traverses the quadrilateral space, bounded superiorly by the teres minor muscle, inferiorly by the teres major muscle, medially by the long head of the triceps muscle, and laterally by the humeral neck. At this point, the axillary nerve gives branches to the teres minor muscle and then it curves around the neck of the humerus, under the deltoid muscle. There, it terminates into two branches, one posterior and the other, anterior; both innervate the deltoid muscle. The upper lateral cutaneous nerve of the arm, which innervates the skin overlying the deltoid muscle (Figure C10–1), originates from the posterior branch.

Clinical Features

Injury of the axillary nerve is associated most often with shoulder trauma or surgery around the shoulder joint; or, it may be a component of idiopathic brachial plexitis (Table C10–1). Axillary mononeuropathy is a common complication of shoulder dislocation, especially among the elderly. Also, the axillary nerve may be injured individually during an episode of acute brachial plexitis (neuralgic amyotrophy); alternatively, this may occur with the suprascapular, long thoracic, or anterior interosseous nerve (refer to Case 16).

Axillary nerve lesion causes weakness of shoulder abduction and extension, and a patch of sensory loss and paresthesias over the lateral deltoid (see Figure C10–1). Deltoid atrophy becomes predominant later resulting in flattening of the shoulder. Weakness of the teres minor is seldom clinically significant since the supraspinatus muscle performs similar functions.

Axillary mononeuropathy may mimic C5 or C6 radiculopathies, but biceps and brachioradialis muscle weakness and depressed reflexes are common findings in C5 and C6 radiculopathies. Lesions of the upper trunk or posterior

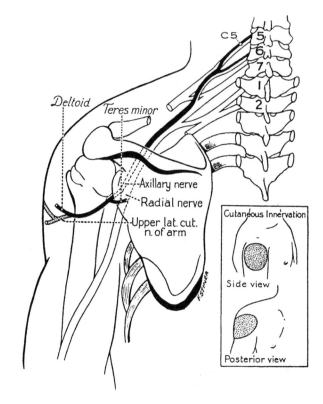

Figure C10–1. *The axillary nerve, a terminal branch of the posterior cord. (From Haymaker W and Woodhall B. Peripheral nerve injuries: principles of diagnosis. Philadelphia, PA: WB Saunders, 1953, with permission.)*

cord of the brachial plexus result also in weakness of the deltoid muscle. However, there is weakness of the biceps and brachioradialis muscles in upper trunk lesions and with posterior cord lesion there is often associated weakness of radial innervated muscles including the triceps and wrist and finger extensors. Musculoskeletal conditions such as rotator cuff tear, adhesive capsulitis of the shoulder, and rupture of deltoid muscle tendon may present with apparent weakness of the deltoid muscle, but are associated with significant shoulder pain and restriction of passive shoulder abduction.

Table C10–1. Common Causes of Axillary Nerve Injury

Trauma
  1. Shoulder dislocation
  2. Fractures of neck of humerus
  3. Blunt trauma
Iatrogenic
  4. During shoulder joint surgery
  5. Injection injury
Idiopathic
  6. Brachial plexitis (neuralgic amyotrophy)

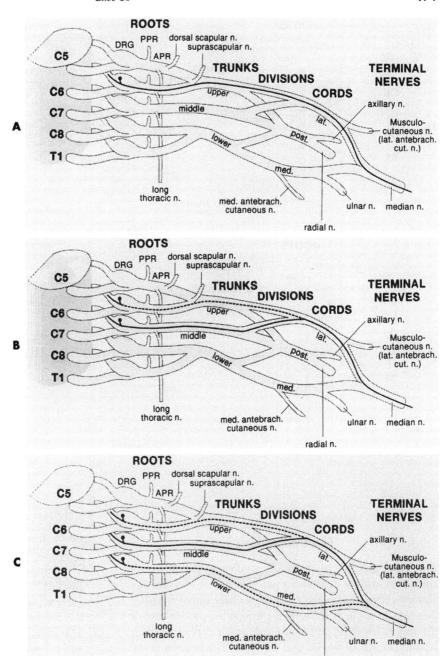

Figure C10–2. *Brachial plexus pathways for the sensory fibers, assessed by median sensory nerve action potential (SNAP) (to thumb (**A**), and index (**B**) and middle (**C**) fingers), radial SNAP (**D**), and lateral antebrachial SNAP (**E**). Solid lines represent predominant pathways and dashed lines represent possible additional pathways. (From Ferrante MA and Wilbourn AJ. The utility of various sensory nerve conduction responses in assessing brachial plexopathies. Muscle Nerve 1995;18:879, with permission.)*

In general, the prognosis for axillary nerve lesions is relatively good because of the short distance required for reinnervation to the target muscle (deltoid). Unfortunately, adhesive capsulitis of the shoulder develop in many patients, which, by itself, has a negative effect on final functional outcome. Thus, an aggressive stretching and range-of-motion program should be initiated as soon after diagnosis as possible.

The *quadrilateral space syndrome* is a rare pain syndrome that implicates entrapment of the axillary nerve and accompanying posterior humeral circumflex artery as they pass this space. The reported patients have been young athletes such as professional volleyball players. The onset of symptoms is insidious and characterized by pain in the shoulder which worsens with shoulder abduction, external rotation, and flexion. Weakness of the deltoid is uncommon but can be difficult to examine in the presence of severe pain in the shoulder.

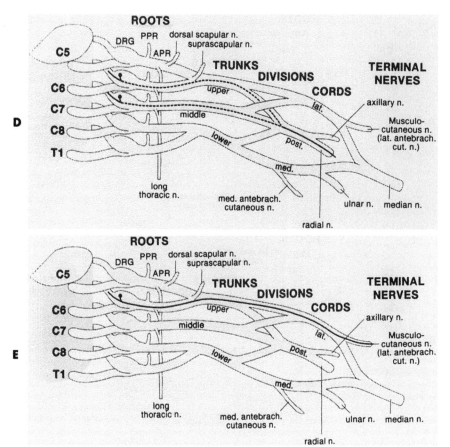

Figure C10–2, cont'd.

Electrodiagnosis

The main purpose of the EDX studies in patients with suspected axillary mononeuropathy is to confirm that the abnormalities are restricted to the axillary nerve distribution and to exclude a brachial plexopathy, particularly of the upper trunk or posterior cord, and a cervical radiculopathy, mostly of the C5 and C6 roots. The *sensory nerve conduction studies* are extremely useful in these cases because they usually are abnormal in relatively mild plexus lesions, assisting in the diagnosis of brachial plexopathy that sometimes could not be detected on clinical evaluation. Among various studies in the upper extremity, the following SNAPs should be normal in isolated axillary nerve lesions (Figure C10–2):

1. The median SNAP recording all three median innervated fingers. The thumb SNAP is innervated by C6 through the upper trunk, the index finger by C6 and C7 through the upper and middle trunks, and the middle finger by C7 through the middle trunk. All three SNAP fibers traverse the lateral cord to reach the median nerve (see Figure C10–2A,B,C).
2. The lateral antebrachial cutaneous SNAP is similar to the median SNAP to the thumb fibers that originate in C6 and pass through the upper trunk and lateral cord to the musculocutaneous nerve (see Figure C10–2E).
3. The radial SNAP with fibers that originate from the C6 and C7 roots and reach the posterior cord via the upper and middle trunks (see Figure C10–2D).

In cases of suspected axillary nerve lesions, the role of *motor nerve conduction studies* is twofold. First, they confirm what is seen on the needle EMG, such as normal musculocutaneous CMAP with normal needle EMG of the biceps muscle. The second, and perhaps more important, role is prognostic; the CMAP amplitude is the best semiquantitative and objective measure of axonal loss. Thus theoretically, and extrapolating from other proximal nerves for which only a single site of stimulation is possible (such as the femoral or facial nerve), a low axillary CMAP, stimulating Erb point and recording the deltoid muscle,

Table C10–2. Needle EMG Findings and Differentials in Upper Trunk Brachial Plexopathy, C5 or C6 Radiculopathy and Axillary Mononeuropathy

Muscle	Upper Trunk Brachial Plexopathy	C5 or C6 Radiculopathy	Axillary Mononeuropathy
Deltoid	Abnormal	Abnormal	Abnormal
Biceps	Abnormal	Abnormal	Normal
Brachioradialis	Abnormal	Abnormal	Normal
Infraspinatus	Abnormal	Abnormal	Normal
Rhomboid	Normal	Abnormal	Normal
Serratus anterior	Normal	Abnormal	Normal

is consistent with a severe axonal loss lesion and a protracted recovery. However, Erb point stimulation is supraclavicular and is likely to result in widespread stimulation of the brachial plexus, including the posterior cord and the proximal axillary nerve. Hence, it is conceivable that a demyelinative axillary nerve lesion around the head of the humerus (i.e., distal to the stimulation point) may result in distal conduction block, thus leading to a low axillary CMAP. Therefore, caution should be used when making definitive prognostication in cases of axillary nerve lesion.

On needle EMG, certain muscles are essential for accurate localization of the lesion (Table C10–2). These muscles are listed in order of their importance:

1. The *brachioradialis* muscle. This muscle shares roots (C5 and C6), trunk (upper), and cord (posterior) with the deltoid muscle; thus it is useful muscle that helps differentiate an isolated axillary mononeuropathy from posterior cord, upper trunk, or C5–C6 root lesions.
2. The *biceps* muscle. This muscle shares roots (C5 and C6) and trunk (upper) with the deltoid muscle, but its nerve fibers are directed into the lateral cord toward the musculocutaneous nerve (rather than into the posterior cord as are the deltoid fibers). Thus it can be used to differentiate an isolated axillary mononeuropathy from upper trunk, or C5–C6 root lesions.
3. The *infraspinatus and supraspinatus* muscles. These muscles are both innervated by the suprascapular nerve, which is frequently injured, along with the axillary nerve, in injuries near the shoulder joint and girdle. They are also abnormal in upper trunk plexopathy and C5–C6 root lesions.
4. The *rhomboid and serratus anterior muscles.* These two muscles are innervated by nerves that arise very proximally, the dorsal scapular nerve (C5 root) and the long thoracic nerve (C5, C6, and C7 roots). When one or both of these muscles are abnormal, it is highly likely that the findings are due to cervical radiculopathy and not to a selective lesion of the upper trunk of the brachial plexus.

FOLLOW-UP

Weakness of the deltoid muscle improved very gradually. With the use of aggressive physical therapy, including passive range of movement and active therapy, deltoid strength improved. Six months later, there was no pain. Deltoid strength was 4–/5. Passive range of movement of the shoulder joint was much better, reaching 160°.

DIAGNOSIS

Severe axon-loss axillary mononeuropathy, caused by shoulder dislocation, with secondary adhesive capsulitis of the shoulder joints.

ANSWERS

1. B; 2. C; 3. B.

SUGGESTED READINGS

Berry H, Bril V. Axillary nerve palsy following blunt trauma to the shoulder region: a clinical and electrophysiological review. J Neurol Neurosurg Psychiatry 1982;45:1027–1032.

Blom S, Dahlback LO. Nerve injuries in dislocations of the shoulder joint and fractures of the neck of the humerus. J Bone Joint Surg 1965;47B:9–22.

Cahill BR, Palmer RE. Quadrilateral space syndrome. J hand Surg 1983;8:65.

Ferrante MA, Wilbourn AJ. The utility of various sensory nerve conduction responses in assessing brachial plexopathies. Muscle Nerve 1995;18:879–889.

Francel TJ, Dellon AL, Campbell JN. Quadrilateral space syndrome: diagnosis and operative decompression technique. Plast Reconstr Surg 1991;87:911–916.

Liveson JA. Nerve lesions associated with shoulder dislocation: an electrodiagnostic study of 11 cases. J Neurol Neurosurg Psychiatry 1984;47:742–744.

Paladini D, Dellantonio R, Cinti A et al. Axillary neuropathy in volleyball players: Report of two cases and literature review. J Neurol Neurosurg Psychiatry 1996;60:345–347.

Case 11

HISTORY AND PHYSICAL EXAMINATION

A 30-year-old right-handed man developed neck and left parascapular pain over 2 weeks. Two days before presentation, his pain worsened and he had a radiating pain to the posterior aspect of the arm and numbness of the hand, particularly the index and middle fingers. He became aware of weakness of the left arm. His pain was exacerbated by coughing and neck movement. He denied any history of trauma. He had a history of left parascapular pain that occurred 2 years earlier, which responded to nonsteroidal anti-inflammatory agents. Otherwise, he had been in excellent health.

On examination, the range of neck movements was restricted in all directions. Lateral neck flexion to the left reproduced the left parascapular and arm pain. There was no atrophy or fasciculations. He had moderate weakness of the left triceps muscle (Medical Research Council [MRC] grade 4/5) and very mild weakness of the left wrist extensors (MRC grade 5–/5). All other muscles were normal. The left triceps reflex was trace. All other reflexes were 2/4. Sensory examination revealed no objective sensory impairment. Examination of the right upper and both lower extremities revealed no abnormalities.

Cervical spine x-rays showed reversal of the normal cervical lordosis with normal disk interspaces. Initially, the patient was treated conservatively with cervical traction, nonsteroidal anti-inflammatory agents, and analgesia. Ten days later, there was no improvement.

An electromyography (EMG) examination was then performed.

Please now review the Nerve Conduction Studies and Needle EMG tables.

QUESTIONS

1. The clinical and EMG findings are consistent with:
   A. C8 radiculopathy.
   B. C5 radiculopathy.
   C. C5 and C6 radiculopathy.
   D. C7 radiculopathy.
   E. C8 and T1 radiculopathy.
2. The most common cervical radiculopathy is:
   A. C6 radiculopathy.
   B. C5 radiculopathy.
   C. C7 radiculopathy.
   D. C4 radiculopathy.
   E. C8 radiculopathy.
3. Neurologic findings most suggestive of C6 radiculopathy include:
   A. Weakness of the hand intrinsics.
   B. Weakness of the triceps muscle with sensory loss of the ring finger.
   C. Depressed triceps reflex with sensory loss of the middle finger.
   D. Weakness of the brachioradialis and depressed biceps reflex.

EDX FINDINGS AND INTERPRETATION OF DATA

Pertinent electrodiagnostic (EDX) findings in this case include:

1. Normal sensory nerve action potentials (SNAPs), particularly those pertinent to C6 and C7 dermatomes (median SNAP recording thumb, index, and middle fingers, and radial SNAP).
2. Variably increased insertional activity, fibrillation potentials, and decrease in recruitment in the pronator teres (C6, C7), flexor carpi radialis (C6, C7), triceps (C6, C7, C8), and extensor carpi radialis (C6, C7), with normal biceps (C5, C6), brachioradialis (C5, C6), and deltoid (C5, C6). The abnormal muscles are innervated by two different nerves (median and radial), but they all share C7 root innervation. Also, muscles that share C6 but not C7 myotomes are normal.

Case 11: Nerve Conduction Studies

Nerve Stimulated	Stimulation Site	Recording Site	Amplitude (m = mV, s = µV)			Distal/Peak Latency (ms)			Conduction Velocity (m/s)			F Latency (ms)	
			Right	Left	Normal	Right	Left	Normal	Right	Left	Normal	Right	Left
Median (s)	Wrist	Thumb	24	25	≥20	3.0	3.1	≤3.3					
Median (s)	Wrist	Index finger	30	36	≥20	3.1	3.3	≤3.3					
Median (s)	Wrist	Middle finger	28	33	≥20	3.2	3.1	≤3.3					
Ulnar (s)	Wrist	Little finger		22	≥18		2.8	≤3.0					
Radial (s)	Distal forearm	Dorsum of hand	27	25	≥18	2.5	2.4	≤2.7					
Median (m)	Wrist	APB		12.5	≥6		2.7	≤3.9					
Median (m)	Elbow	APB		12.0						58	≥50		28.4
Ulnar (m)	Wrist	ADM		9.5	≥8		2.4	≤3.0					
Ulnar (m)	Elbow	ADM		8.5						56	≥50		30.4

ADM = abductor digiti minimi; APB = abductor pollicis brevis; m = motor; s = sensory.

Case 11: Needle EMG

Voluntary Motor Unit Action Potentials (MUAPs)

Muscle	Insertional Activity	Spontaneous Activity Fibs	Fascs	Recruitment Normal	Activation	Reduced	Early	Configuration Duration	Amplitude	% Polyphasia	Others
L. first dorsal interosseous	Normal	0	0	X				Normal	Normal	Normal	
Flexor pollicis brevis	Normal	0	0	X				Normal	Normal	Normal	
Extensor indicis propius	Normal	0	0	X				Normal	Normal	Normal	
Pronator teres	↑	1+	0			↓		Normal	Normal	Normal	
Flexor carpi radialis	↑	1+	0			↓↓		Normal	Normal	↑	
Extensor carpi radialis	Normal	0	0			↓		Normal	Normal	Normal	
Brachioradialis	Normal	0	0	X				Normal	Normal	Normal	
Biceps	Normal	0	0	X				Normal	Normal	Normal	
Triceps	↑	1+	0			↓↓		↑	Normal	Normal	
Deltoid	Normal	0	0	X				Normal	Normal	Normal	
Midcervical paraspinal	Normal	0	0	–							
Low cervical paraspinal	↑	Few	0	–							

Fascs = fasciculations; Fibs = fibrillations; L. = left; ↑ = increased; ↓ = mildly reduced; ↓↓ = moderately reduced.

3. Decreased recruitment of motor unit action potential (MUAP), and minimal reinnervation changes of the MUAPs are findings consistent with a subacute disorder.
4. Fibrillation potentials in the low cervical paraspinal region.

These findings are compatible with a subacute left C7 radiculopathy with active denervation. Normal SNAPs and fibrillation potentials in the cervical paraspinal muscles confirm that the lesion is proximal to the dorsal root ganglion (DRG), i.e., within the intraspinal canal.

DISCUSSION

Applied Anatomy

The dorsal root axons originate from the sensory neurons of the DRG, which lie outside the spinal canal, within the intervertebral foramen, immediately before the junction of the dorsal and ventral roots (Figure C11–1). These sensory neurons are unique because they are unipolar. They have proximal projections through the dorsal root, called the *preganglionic sensory fibers*, to the dorsal horn and column of the spinal cord. The distal projections of these neurons, called the *postganglionic peripheral sensory fibers*, pass through the spinal nerve to their respective sensory endorgans. The ventral root axons, however, are mainly motor (some are sympathetic, with origins from the anterolateral horn of the cord). The motor axons originate from the anterior horn cells within the spinal cord. Passing through the spinal nerves and the peripheral nerve, these motor fibers terminate in the corresponding muscles.

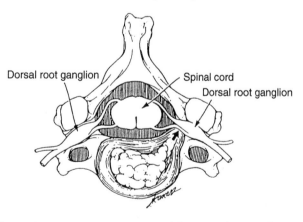

Figure C11–1. *Transverse section of the cervical spine, showing the usual site of root injury in cervical radiculopathy due to disc herniation (arrow). Note that the sensory fibers are injured proximal to the dorsal root ganglion, which is located within the intervertebral foramen. (From Brown WF, Bolton CF. Clinical electromyography, 2nd ed. Boston, MA: Butterworth-Heinemann, 1993, with permission.)*

The spinal nerves terminate as soon as they exit the intervertebral foramina, by branching into posterior and anterior rami. The small posterior rami innervate the paravertebral skin and deep paraspinal muscles of the neck, trunk, and back; the large anterior rami innervate the skin and muscles of the trunk and limbs.

In humans, there are 31 pairs of spinal nerve roots: 8 cervical, 12 thoracic, 5 lumbar, 5 sacral, and 1 coccygeal. In the cervical spine, each cervical root exits *above* the corresponding vertebra that shares the same numeric designation (Figure C11–2). For example, the C5 root exits above the C5 vertebra (i.e., between the C4 and C5 vertebrae). Because there are seven cervical vertebrae but eight cervical roots, the C8 root exits between the C7 and T1 vertebrae; subsequently, all thoracic, lumbar, and sacral roots exit *below* their corresponding vertebrae. For example, the L3 root exits below the L3 vertebra (i.e., between the L3 and L4 vertebrae).

Clinical Features

Cervical radiculopathy frequently is the result of a herniated intervertebral disc, or osteophytic spondylitic changes that result in mechanical compression of the cervical root. The symptoms may be acute, subacute, or chronic. Neck pain radiating to the parascapular area and upper extremity, made worse by certain neck positions, is common. The pain radiation tends to follow the dermatomal innervation of the compressed root. Subjective paresthesias within the involved dermatome is more common than objective sensory findings. The diminution of deep tendon reflexes helps in localizing the lesion to one or two roots. Weakness is uncommon; when present, it involves muscles innervated by the compressed root.

The classic study by Yoss et al., published in 1957, remains the best available clinicoanatomic study of cervical root compression. This detailed study analyzed the symptoms and signs of 100 patients with surgically proven single cervical lesions. C7 radiculopathy was the most common cervical radiculopathy, accounting for almost two thirds of patients (Figure C11–3). Figure C11–4 shows the common sensory symptoms and signs observed in these patients, while Figure C11–5 shows the weakened muscles caused by cervical radiculopathy. This study revealed the extreme variability of sensory manifestations in patients with cervical radiculopathy. Also, no single muscle was exclusively diagnostic of a specific root compression. However, based on the data, certain clinical conclusions can be made:

1. When sensory manifestations occur in C7 radiculopathy, the index or middle finger is always involved.
2. When sensory manifestations occur in C8 radiculopathy, the little or ring finger is always involved.

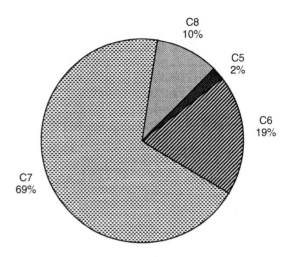

Figure C11–3. *Incidence of cervical root involvement in a series of 100 patients with surgically proven single-level lesions. (Data adapted from Yoss RE et al. Significance of symptoms and signs in localization of involved root in cervical disc protrusion. Neurology 1957;7:673–683, with permission.)*

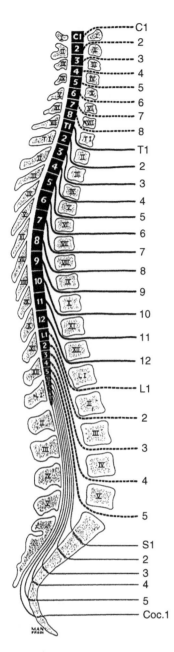

Figure C11–2. *Alignments of spinal segments and roots to vertebrae. The bodies and spinal processes of the vertebrae are indicated by Roman numerals, and the spinal segments and their respective roots by Arabic numerals. Note that the cervical roots (except C8) exit through intervertebral foramina above their respective bodies and that all other roots leave below these bodies. (From Haymaker W, Woodhall B. Peripheral nerve injuries: principles of diagnosis. Philadelphia, PA: WB Saunders, 1953, with permission.)*

3. The thumb is never involved exclusively in C7 radiculopathy.
4. Significant triceps weakness is seen only in C7 radiculopathy.

5. Significant supraspinatus and infraspinatus weakness is seen only in C5 radiculopathy.
6. Significant interossei and hand intrinsics weakness is seen only in C8 radiculopathy.

However, despite the variability in sensory and motor presentations of cervical radiculopathies, certain classical symptoms and signs exist and are extremely helpful in localizing the compressed root. Table C11–1 reveals the common presentations of cervical radiculopathies.

Electrodiagnosis

General Concepts
Certain general concepts are essential to appreciate before one makes a diagnosis of a cervical radiculopathy in the EMG laboratory.

1. *The SNAPs are normal in radiculopathy despite the presence of sensory loss.* Compression of the dorsal (sensory) root, from either disc herniation or spondylosis, usually occurs within the spinal canal proximal to the DRG and results in injury of the preganglionic sensory fibers, but leaves the postganglionic sensory fibers intact (see Figure C11–1).
2. *Compression of the ventral (motor) root may cause demyelination or axon loss, or both.* As with focal lesions of peripheral nerves, this leads to different EDX findings:
   - With axon loss, wallerian degeneration occurs. Its effect is readily recognized after 2–3 weeks by the

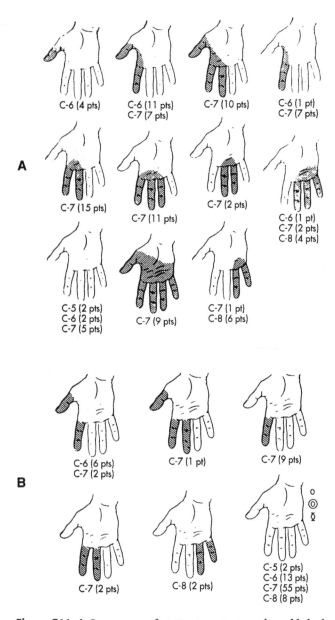

Figure C11–4. *Sensory manifestation in patients with established single cervical root lesions (C5–C8). (**A**) patterns of paresthesias in 91 patients and (**B**) objective sensory impairment in 23 of the same patients. (From Yoss RE et al. Significance of symptoms and signs in localization of involved root in cervical disc protrusion. Neurology 1957;7:673–683, with permission.)*

presence of fibrillation potentials, long-duration and high-amplitude MUAPs, and, when severe, low-amplitude CMAPs.

- With pure demyelination, there is either focal slowing or conduction block; both cannot be evaluated well because roots are not accessible to conduction studies (despite attempts to use magnetic or direct needle stimulation). Thus, apart from weakness (and

reduced MUAP recruitment), EDX studies might be otherwise normal.

3. *The EMG examination determines the injured cervical root(s), as well as the vertebral level(s) of root compression or disc herniation.* This advantage is in contrast to lumbosacral radiculopathies where the vertebral level of root compression or disc herniation does not always correlate with the involved root (see Case 2).

4. *The needle EMG remains the most sensitive electrodiagnostic tool in patients with suspected radiculopathy.* Other electrophysiologic studies, including somatosensory evoked potentials, nerve conduction studies, late responses and thermography, are much less sensitive and their use in practice is limited.

5. *The most objective EMG finding in radiculopathy is the presence of fibrillation potentials.* Decrease recruitment and large or polyphasic MUAPs are useful findings but when these abnormalities are mild they are more difficult to analyze and may be subject to debate by different observers. Hence, the accuracies of these MUAP findings vary according to the electromyographer's experience.

6. *Fibrillation potentials are seldom found in the entire myotomal distribution of the compressed root.* This is best explained by one or more of the following reasons:
   - Root compression usually results in partial motor axon loss. Hence, some muscles innervated by the injured root may "escape" denervation and remain normal.
   - Proximal muscles innervated by the compressed root undergo more effective collateral sprouting and reinnervation than do distal muscles. This leads to the disappearance of fibrillation potentials in proximal muscles. Hence, in a chronic radiculopathy it is more likely to find fibrillation potentials in distal than proximal muscles, despite being innervated by the same root. For example, in C5 or C6 radiculopathy, it is more likely to detect fibrillation potentials in the brachioradialis than in the infraspinatus; both have a preponderant innervation by the C5 and C6 roots.
   - There likely is significant myotomal variability among individuals.

7. *F waves are rarely abnormal in radiculopathy.* Despite early enthusiasm about the utility of F waves, which test the integrity of the entire motor axon including the ventral roots, the F waves are not sensitive in the diagnosis of cervical radiculopathies for the following reasons:
   - The recorded muscle frequently is innervated by more than one root. Thus, in a single-level radiculopathy, normal conduction through the intact neighboring root results in normal F wave minimal latency. For example, in C8 radiculopathy, the ulnar F wave recorded from the abductor digiti minimi muscle (innervated by C8 and T1 roots) frequently is normal

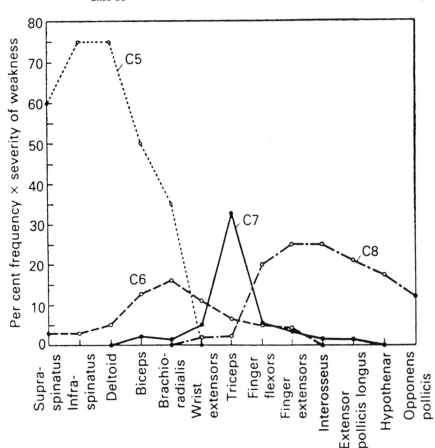

Figure C11–5. *Incidence and severity of weakness of muscles or groups of muscles in cervical radiculopathy (C5–C8). (From Yoss RE et al. Significance of symptoms and signs in localization of involved root in cervical disc protrusion. Neurology 1957;7:673–683, with permission.)*

because the compression is concealed by a normal T1 root.

- F wave latency is the most reproducible and clinically useful parameter. However, root compression resulting in significant motor axon loss can be associated with normal F wave latencies because the surviving axons are conducting normallys.

- If focal slowing occurs at the root segment of the motor axon, the delay in F wave latency may be obscured, because the latency becomes diluted by the relatively long motor axons.
- The median and ulnar F waves, recording abductor pollicis brevis, adductor pollicis or first dorsal interosseous, are the only upper extremity F waves

Table C11–1. Common Clinical Presentations in Patients With Cervical Radiculopathies

	Pain Radiation	Sensory Impairment	Weakness	Hypo/Areflexia
C5	To parascapular area, shoulder, and upper arm	Upper arm	Scapular fixators, shoulder abduction, and elbow flexion	Biceps and/or brachioradialis reflexes
C6	To shoulder, arm, forearm, and thumb/index finger	Lateral arm, forearm, and thumb and/or index fingers	Shoulder abduction, elbow flexion, and forearm pronation	Biceps and/or brachioradialis reflexes
C7	To posterior arm, forearm, and index/middle fingers	Index and/or middle fingers	Elbow extension, wrist and fingers extension, and forearm pronation	Triceps jerk
C8	To medial arm, forearm, and little/ring fingers	Medial forearm, and little finger	Hand intrinsics, and long flexors and extensors of fingers	None
T1	To axilla, medial arm and forearm	Axilla, medial arm and forearm	Thenar muscles	None

studied in clinical practice. These F waves evaluate the C8 and T1 roots since these three muscles are innervated solely by the C8 and T1 roots. Hence, upper extremity F waves that are used in clinical practice do not assess the more common C7, C6, and C5 radiculopathies.

Goals of the Electrodiagnostic Study

The EDX examination plays a pivotal role in the diagnosis, and sometimes the management, of cervical radiculopathy. The diagnostic aims of the EDX examination in radiculopathy are to:

1. Exclude a more distal lesion (i.e., plexopathy or a mononeuropathy).
2. Confirm evidence of root compression.
3. Localize the compression to either a single or multiple roots.
4. Define the age and activity of the lesion.
5. Define the severity of the lesion.

Exclude a More Distal Nerve Lesion

Differentiating a mononeuropathy from radiculopathy is relatively easy when the focal peripheral nerve lesion is associated with conduction block or focal slowing, such as in carpal tunnel syndrome or ulnar mononeuropathy at the elbow. Also, in mononeuropathy, fibrillation potentials and MUAP reinnervation changes are limited to muscles innervated by the involved peripheral nerve. However, these abnormalities in radiculopathy are more widespread and involve muscles that share the same root innervation, regardless of their peripheral nerve.

Differentiating a brachial plexus lesion from cervical radiculopathy involves mostly evaluating the SNAPs and needle EMG of the cervical paraspinal muscles as well as very proximal muscles.

- The presence of fibrillation potentials in paraspinal muscles is not consistent with a brachial plexus lesion because these muscles are innervated by the dorsal rami before the formation of the plexus. Unfortunately, fibrillation potentials in paraspinal muscles are not always present in radiculopathy, presumably due to of effective reinnervation of these very proximal muscles.
- Detecting signs of denervation and reinnervation in muscles innervated by peripheral nerves arising before the formation of the brachial plexus is a strong support for the diagnosis of cervical radiculopathy. These muscles are the rhomboids (C5 root via the thoracodorsal nerve) and serratus anterior (C6, C7, C8 roots via the long thoracic nerve) (see Figure C13–2 in Case 13). One caveat is that these nerves may be selectively injured along with the brachial plexus during shoulder trauma or with a bout of neuralgic amyotrophy (see Case 16).

- In brachial plexopathy, the SNAPs usually are abnormally low in amplitude, or they are absent, because the lesion affects the postganglionic fibers. In contrast, these studies are normal in cervical radiculopathy, in which compression involves the preganglionic fibers only (i.e., sensory fibers proximal to the DRG). However, the utility of the SNAP in the confirmation of cervical radiculopathy has few limitations:
  (a) The C5 cervical root does not have a technically feasible SNAP.
  (b) The medial brachial SNAP, which assesses the T1 root, may be difficult to evoke or is absent bilaterally in a significant number of individuals, especially in the elderly, obese, and those with limb edema.
  (c) The SNAP amplitudes may be low or absent if the DRGs are involved by the pathological condition that may affect the DRG preferentially or extend from the intraspinal space through the neural foramen to the extraspinal space or vice versa. Examples include infiltrative malignancy such as lymphoma, infection such as herpes zoster, tumor such as schwannoma or meningioma, or autoimmune attack on DRG such as in Sjogren syndrome or with small-cell lung cancer.

Confirm Evidence of Root Compression

Two criteria are necessary to establish the diagnosis of cervical radiculopathy.

1. *Denervation in a segmental myotomal distribution* (i.e., in muscles innervated by the same roots via more than one peripheral nerve), with or without denervation of the cervical paraspinal muscles. At least two muscles, and preferably more, should reveal evidence of denervation (fibrillation potentials and/or reinnervation MUAP changes and reduced recruitment). Fibrillation potentials in the paraspinal muscles are strong evidence of a root lesion within the spinal canal. However, they may be absent particularly in chronic radiculopathies, likely due to effective reinnervation.
2. *Normal SNAP of the corresponding dermatome*. Once myotomal denervation is detected by needle EMG, the lesion must be confirmed as preganglionic (i.e., within the spinal canal) and not postganglionic (i.e., due to a brachial plexus injury). This can be achieved by recording one or more dermatomal SNAPs, appropriate for the myotome involved, and then establishing SNAP normality. For example, in a suspected C7 radiculopathy, the median SNAP recording middle finger should be performed, preferably bilaterally for comparison. Table C11–2 lists technically feasible SNAPs with their corresponding roots that are helpful in confirming the diagnosis of cervical radiculopathy. Note that no SNAP has been devised to assess the C5 fibers, and the medial brachial SNAP is not

Table C11–2. Upper Extremity Sensory Nerve Action Potentials (SNAPs) and Their Segmental Representation

Root	SNAP
C6	Lateral antebrachial (Lateral cutaneous of forearm)
	Median recording thumb
	Median recording index
	Radial recording dorsum of hand
C7	Median recording index
	Median recording middle finger
	Radial recording dorsum of hand
C8	Ulnar recording little finger
	Medial antebrachial (Medial cutaneous of forearm)
T1	Medial brachial (Medial cutaneous of arm)

always technically reliable in assessing the T1 fibers. These SNAP limitations, though much less significant than the lower extremity SNAPs, result in occasional difficulties in distinguishing a preganglionic lesion (i.e., cervical radiculopathy) from a postganglionic lesion (i.e., brachial plexopathy), unless fibrillation potentials are evident in the cervical paraspinal or very proximally innervated muscles (serratus anterior or rhomboids).

Localize the Compression to One or Multiple Roots

This requires meticulous knowledge of the segmental innervation of both limb muscles (myotomes) and skin (dermatomes). Many myotomal charts have been devised, with significant variability; this may lead to confusion and disagreement between the needle EMG and the level of root compression as seen by imaging techniques or during surgery. EMG-derived charts are also helpful and have had anatomic confirmation (see Levin et al. and Katirji et al.). Figure C11–6 reveals a common and most useful EMG-extracted myotomal chart.

A minimal "root search" should be performed in all patients with suspected cervical radiculopathy to ensure that a radiculopathy is either confirmed or excluded. In other words, certain muscles of strategic value in EMG because of their segmental innervation should be sampled (Table C11–3). When abnormalities are found or when the clinical manifestations suggest a specific root compression, more muscles must be sampled after being selected based on their innervation (see Figure C11–6), to verify the diagnosis and establish the exact compressed root(s).

Once myotomal denervation is detected by needle EMG, it is essential to confirm that the lesion is preganglionic (i.e., within the spinal canal) and not postganglionic

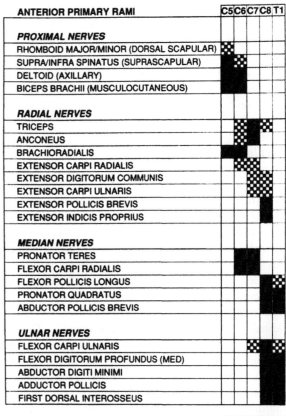

Figure C11–6. *Chart of upper extremity muscles useful in the electromyographic recognition of cervical radiculopathy. Solid squares indicate muscles that most often contain abnormalities, and checkered squares indicate muscles that are abnormal less frequently. (From Brown WF, Bolton CF. Clinical electromyography, 2nd ed. Boston, MA: Butterworth-Heinemann, 1993, with permission.)*

Table C11–3. Suggested Muscles to be Sampled in Patients With Suspected Cervical Radiculopathy*

Muscle	Roots
First dorsal interosseous	**C8**, T1
Flexor pollicis longus	**C8**, T1
Pronator teres	**C6, C7**
Biceps	**C5, C6**
Triceps	C6, **C7**, C8
Deltoid	**C5, C6**
Mid-cervical paraspinal	C5, C6
Low-cervical paraspinal	C7, C8

*Roots in bold type represent the major innervation.

(i.e., due to a brachial plexus injury). This can be achieved by recording one or more SNAPs appropriate for the myotome involved, and then establishing normality of SNAPs. For example, in a suspected C6 radiculopathy, the antidromic (or orthodromic) median SNAPs, recording the thumb and index, should be performed, preferably bilaterally for comparison (see Table C11–2).

Define the Age and Activity of the Radiculopathy

Changes seen on needle EMG help to determine the age of the lesion in an axon-loss cervical radiculopathy. As with many processes wherein motor axon loss occurs, increased insertional activity is the first abnormality seen and, when isolated, suggests that the process may be only 1–2 weeks old. Fibrillation potentials, which are spontaneous action potentials generated by denervated muscle fibers, develop soon after and become full after 3 weeks from acute motor axonal loss. These potentials often appear first in the cervical paraspinal muscles, then in proximal muscles, and lastly in distal muscles. They also disappear after reinnervation or following muscle fiber fatty degeneration. As time elapses, collateral sprouting from intact axons results in MUAPs with polyphasia and satellites potentials. These MUAPs, usually seen after 2 to 3 months from acute injury, are often unstable by showing moment-to-moment variation in morphology. With further time, MUAPs with high amplitude and long duration dominate, reflecting a more complete reinnervation and the chronicity of the root compression.

In assessing a patient with possible cervical radiculopathy, it is often important to comment on whether the root compression is chronic or ongoing (active). This is easy when one encounters large and stable MUAPs, reflecting chronicity, along with fibrillation potentials, reflecting ongoing (active) denervation. In contrast, when fibrillation potentials are absent, it is presumed that the findings are chronic and remote, such as in patients with a prior history of a severe cervical radiculopathy. This simplistic differentiation has, however, several limitations:

- It is not uncommon that the electromyographer cannot distinguish with certainty between a patient with chronic ongoing root compression (such as with spondylosis) from one with chronic remote (old) root compression (such as with a prior disc herniation). In situations where the rate of motor axon loss is slow, reinnervation may keep pace with denervation that no or minimal fibrillation potentials are seen on needle EMG. Some electromyographers may use erroneously the absence of fibrillation potentials as absolute evidence against ongoing root compression. A correlation with the clinical history, the neurological findings, and the imaging is warranted.

- A contrast situation rise in patients with remote radiculopathy that had resulted in severe axon loss. In these clinically inactive cases, some muscle fibers never fully reinnervate, especially in distal muscles located farthest from the injury site. In these radicular lesions, fibrillation potentials may continue to be seen in distal muscles, mistakenly suggesting that there is an ongoing root compression and axon loss process.

- The postoperative EDX evaluation of patients with cervical radiculopathy is challenging particularly when there was no preoperative EDX study. Since fibrillation potentials may persist for several months despite successive surgery, their presence does not mean a failed surgical procedure. Additionally, fibrillation potentials may be present in the paraspinal muscles after posterior cervical spine surgery because of muscle denervation during surgical exposure. Because of this, many electromyographers, including the author, will not sample the paraspinal muscles if a patient has a history of posterior cervical spine surgery. These postoperative EDX studies are often not satisfying to the electromyographer or clinician, since they cannot exclude or confirm persistent root compression.

Define the Severity of the Radiculopathy

In assessing the severity of a radiculopathy, one erroneously tends to rely on the degree of abnormalities seen on needle EMG, namely decreased recruitment ("neurogenic" MUAP firing pattern), fibrillation potentials, and MUAP configuration. Using these parameters in assessing severity of lesion (i.e., extent of axon loss) is suboptimal for the following caveats:

1. Although there is a correlation between the degree of reduced MUAP recruitment and the degree of weakness, decreased recruitment is not necessarily due to axon loss but may be due conduction block (segmental demyelination) at the root level. The latter has a very good prognosis for rapid recovery.
2. Although the presence of fibrillation potentials is consistent with motor axon loss, measuring the number of fibrillation potentials in a muscle is subjective and does not correlate with the degree of axon loss. Fibrillation potentials denote a recent axon loss but cannot assess its severity.
3. MUAP reinnervation changes are permanent. However, reinnervation may be quite robust that weakness may not or be minimally detected. Hence, finding very large MUAPs (giant MUAPs) does not always reflect severity or prognosis.

The best indicator of motor axon loss is the CMAP amplitude (or area) recorded during routine motor nerve conduction studies of the upper extremity. Although these studies are performed distally and do not include the roots, a root lesion causing demyelinative conduction block (or focal slowing), with little or no accompanying axonal degeneration, may result in weakness, but does not lead to any decrease in CMAP amplitude or other abnormalities on motor conduction studies. Only when significant axonal loss occurs at the root level does the CMAP recording from an involved muscle become low in amplitude (or occasionally absent when multiple adjacent roots are compressed). In acute lesions, this is only detected when sufficient time has elapsed for wallerian degeneration to occur (usually 7–10 days). For example, only in moderate or severe C8 radiculopathy is the ulnar CMAP, recording from abductor digiti minimi (C8, T1), borderline or low in amplitude at least after 10 days from onset of acute symptoms.

Electrodiagnostic Findings in Cervical Radiculopathies

The EMG findings in isolated cervical radiculopathy are dependent on the myotomal innervation of the upper limb. It should be emphasized that multiple cervical radiculopathies are not uncommon, especially in elderly people with cervical spondylosis. Spondylosis can frequently result in compression of more than one root, usually but not necessarily adjacent to each other. A contralateral root may also be affected frequently, although this occurs more often in lumbosacral radiculopathies.

C5/C6 Radiculopathies

It is difficult, both clinically and by EMG, to separate lesions of C5 roots from those of C6 roots because of the significant overlap of their corresponding myotomes. Muscles that share both C5 and C6 segmental innervation, with about equal frequency, include the supraspinatus, infraspinatus, deltoid, biceps, and brachioradialis. However, the following muscles can help, when involved, to distinguish lesions of these roots:

1. Pronator teres and/or flexor carpi radialis are innervated by the C6 and C7 roots and are never involved in C5 radiculopathy. Hence, the compromised root is the C6 if one or both muscles are abnormal along with some or all of the aforementioned muscles.
2. Rhomboid major is innervated by the C5 root exclusively. Hence, the C5 root is the compressed root when this muscle is abnormal.

Although the identification of denervation in the pronator teres/flexor carpi radialis or rhomboid muscles is beneficial in localizing the compressed root to C6 or C5 roots respectively, the lack of these findings does not exclude compression of the neighboring root because it is not necessary for all muscles innervated by the compressed root to reveal evidence of denervation.

Differentiating C5 or C6 radiculopathy from upper trunk brachial plexopathy is also sometimes difficult because the C5 dermatome has no clearly defined SNAP. Thus, in isolated C5 radiculopathy, finding fibrillation potentials in the cervical paraspinal muscles and/or in the rhomboid major is practically the only way to confirm a root lesion and rule out an upper plexus lesion. In C6 radiculopathy, however, the additional findings of normal median SNAPs, recording thumb (C6) and index (C6, C7), and of a lateral antebrachial cutaneous SNAP (C6) are supportive findings against an upper trunk or lateral cord lesion.

C7 Radiculopathy

C7 radiculopathy is the most common cervical radiculopathy encountered in clinical practice. The EMG findings in C7 radiculopathy typically are mostly restricted to radial and median innervated muscles via the C7 root. The triceps, anconeus, flexor carpi radialis, and pronator teres have a prominent C7 root innervation and are by far the most common muscles affected in C7 radiculopathy. Other supplementary muscles include the extensor carpi radialis (radial nerve) and the latissimus dorsi (thoracodorsal nerve).

C6 radiculopathy may sometimes be difficult to differentiate from C7 radiculopathy because of some EMG overlap between C6 and C7 myotomes, which is not as prominent as the overlap between the C6 from C5 myotomes. The C7 root is often the compressed one when the pronator teres (C6, C7) and triceps (C6, C7, C8) are the only abnormal muscles. However, making the distinction between C6 and C7 radiculopathy becomes easy when the "traditional" C6 innervated muscles (supraspinatus, infraspinatus, deltoid, biceps, and brachioradialis) are normal.

C7 radiculopathy can be differentiated from isolated middle trunk brachial plexopathy, which is extremely rare, by confirming that the median SNAPs to the middle finger (C7) and the index finger (C6, C7), and the radial SNAP (C6, C7) are normal. Also, fibrillation potentials in the cervical paraspinal muscles, when present, are strong evidence against plexopathy.

C8/T1 Radiculopathies

As in the C5 and C6 situation, distinguishing C8 from T1 lesions is difficult because of significant myotomal overlap. The myotomal representation of the C8/T1 root involves the three major nerves in the upper extremity: the median, radial, and ulnar nerves. Muscles affected include the first dorsal interosseous and abductor digiti minimi (ulnar), the abductor pollicis brevis and flexor pollicis longus (median), and the extensor indicis proprius and extensor pollicis brevis (radial). The triceps muscle seldom is affected, but when also denervated, it is strong evidence of a C8 radiculopathy.

The ulnar SNAP, recording the little finger, and medial antebrachial SNAP are essential in the final diagnosis of C8/T1 radiculopathy. These studies are normal in C8/T1 radiculopathies, but usually abnormal in lower trunk/medial cord plexopathies. Finally, as with all radiculopathies, fibrillation potentials in the cervical paraspinal muscles, when present, are strong evidence against a brachial plexopathy.

Although all C8 muscles of the hand have T1 contributions, the abductor pollicis brevis muscle appears to be the only muscle with predominately T1 innervation. On rare occasions, the only abnormalities in selective T1 radiculopathy are low amplitude median CMAP and fibrillation potentials and reinnervation changes in the abductor pollicis brevis muscle.

Could an EMG be Normal in a Patient With Definite Cervical Radiculopathy?

This is a question commonly asked by clinicians and reflects the limitations of the EDX test in the evaluation of cervical radiculopathy. The general rule is *"a normal EMG does not exclude a root compression."* An EMG study may be normal in a cervical radiculopathy in the following circumstances:

1. *If only the dorsal root is compressed and the ventral root is not compromised.* This occurs in significant numbers of patients whose symptoms are limited to pain and/or paresthesias with or without reflex changes. However, because of the lack of ventral root involvement, the sensory and motor nerve conduction studies, F-wave latencies, and needle EMG are normal.

2. *If the ventral root compression has caused demyelination only (leading to conduction block) with no axonal loss.* In this situation, no fibrillation potentials or large or polyphasic MUAPs are seen. The expected reduced recruitment may also be masked, particularly when the ventral root compression is partial, by normal adjacent root since all muscles have two or three segmental innervations.

3. *If the root compression is acute.* Here, no fibrillation potentials are seen because these potentials appear 3 weeks after axonal injury and become maximal at 4 to 6 weeks. Also, the MUAPs are normal because sprouting starts at least 4 to 6 weeks after axonal injury.

4. *If the injured root lacks of adequate myotomal representation.* Examples include the C3 or C4 roots which are not possible to assess by EMG.

FOLLOW-UP

Magnetic resonance imaging of the cervical spine showed a large focal posterolateral disc herniation at the C6–C7 interspace, with impingement of the left C7 root and slight flattening of the cervical cord (Figure C11–7). The patient

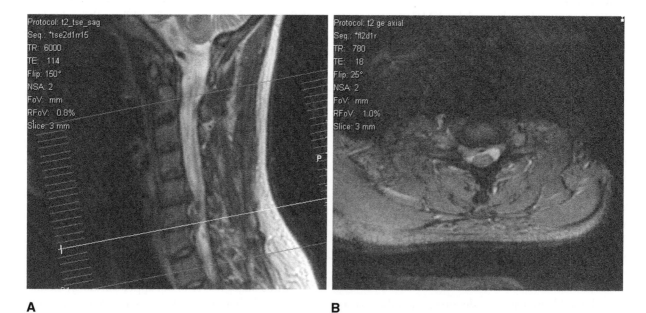

A   **B**

Figure C11–7. *Sagittal T2-weighted (**A**) and axial T1-weighted (**B**) magnetic resonance images of the cervical spine, revealing C6–C7 lateroposterior disc herniation to the left, with compression of the left C7 root. Note that there is also a C5–C6 disc herniation.*

underwent an anterior cervical diskectomy at C6–C7. Intraoperatively, a large subligamentous disc herniation was observed to be compressing the left C7 root. Arm and neck pain began resolving in a few days and disappeared within 2 months. Strength improved steadily and, on reexamination 6 months later, the patient demonstrated normal triceps strength and reflex.

DIAGNOSIS

Subacute left C7 radiculopathy due to left postero-lateral C6–C7 disc herniation.

ANSWERS

1. D; 2. C; 3. D.

SUGGESTED READINGS

Benecke R, Conrad B. The distal sensory nerve action potential as a diagnostic tool for the differentiation of lesions in dorsal roots and peripheral nerves. J Neurol 1980;223:231–239.

Bonney G, Gilliatt RW. Sensory nerve conduction after traction lesion of the brachial plexus. Proc R Soc Med (Clin Sec) 1958;51:365–367.

Katirji MB, Agrawal R, Kantra TA. The human cervical myotomes: an anatomical correlation between electromyography and CT/myelography. Muscle Nerve 1988;11:1070–1073.

Levin K. Cervical radiculopathies. In: Katirji B, Kaminski HJ, Preston DC, Ruff RL, Shapiro EB, eds. Neuromuscular disorders in clinical practice. Boston, MA: Butterworth-Heinemann, 2002, pp. 838–858.

Levin K, Maggiano HJ, Wilbourn AJ. Cervical radiculopathies: comparison of surgical and EMG localization of single-root lesions. Neurology 1996;46:1022–1025.

Wilbourn AJ, Aminoff MJ. The electrophysiologic examination in patients with radiculopathies. Muscle Nerve 1988;11:1099–1114.

Yoss RE et al. Significance of symptoms and signs in localization of involved root in cervical disc protrusion. Neurology 1957;7:673–683.

Case 12

HISTORY AND PHYSICAL EXAMINATION

During an automobile repair, the right arm of a 23-year-old man was pinned under a car for 2 to 3 minutes when the jack came off accidentally. Immediately, he noticed a right wristdrop. There were no lacerations or bruises. Radiographs of the right arm and forearm were normal. The wristdrop improved slightly over the next few weeks. He was referred to the electromyography (EMG) laboratory 5 weeks after the incident.

On examination, there was severe weakness of the right wrist extensors, all finger extensors, and the brachioradialis (Medical Research Council [MRC] 2/5), with intact finger and wrist flexors, biceps, triceps, and deltoid muscles. He had impairment of pain and touch sensation over the dorsum of the hand. The right brachioradialis reflex was absent. All other deep tendon reflexes were normal. The rest of the neurological examination was normal.

EMG examination was done 5 weeks postinjury.

Please now review the Nerve Conduction Studies (NCS) and Needle EMG tables.

QUESTIONS

1. The clinical and electrodiagnostic (EDX) findings are consistent with:
   A. Lower cervical radiculopathy.
   B. Posterior cord brachial plexopathy.
   C. Posterior interosseous mononeuropathy.
   D. Radial mononeuropathy in the arm.
2. All the following muscles are innervated by the posterior interosseous nerve *except:*
   A. Extensor digitorum profundus.
   B. Extensor indicis proprius.
   C. Extensor carpi ulnaris.
   D. Abductor pollicis longus.
   E. Extensor carpi radialis longus.

3. Common causes of this injury include all of the following *except:*
   A. Midhumeral fracture.
   B. "Saturday night palsy."
   C. Occupational use with repetitive wrist movements.
   D. Strenuous muscular effort.

EDX FINDINGS AND INTERPRETATION OF DATA

Abnormal EDX findings include:

1. A partial right radial motor conduction block across the spiral groove, as evidenced by a drop in amplitude of the compound muscle action potential (CMAP) from 5.6 mV, stimulating below the spiral groove, to 2.0 mV, stimulating above the spiral groove (Figure C12–1). This 64% amplitude decay is supported by the lack of significant CMAP dispersion and the concomitant decrease in negative CMAP area from 25.5 mV/ms to 5.65 mV/ms, respectively (78% area loss). Also, there is relative and mild focal slowing of the conducting radial motor fibers within the spiral groove (when the right radial motor nerve conduction velocity of 57 m/s is compared to the distal velocity of 66 m/s, and to the left radial motor velocities of 69 m/s proximally and 68 m/s distally). The presence of partial conduction block with relative mild focal slowing across the spiral groove is consistent with segmental demyelination at that site.
2. The distal radial CMAP is relatively low in amplitude on the right (5.8 mV) compared to the left (7.5 mV) and to the lower limit of normal value (6.0 mV). This is consistent with partial motor axonal loss distal to the site of the lesion (wallerian degeneration).
3. The right radial sensory nerve action potential (SNAP) is low in amplitude when compared with the left (10 μV versus 20 μV). This is consistent with partial sensory

Case 12: Nerve Conduction Studies

Nerve Stimulated	Stimulation Site	Recording Site	Amplitude (m = mV, s = µV)			Distal/Peak Latency (ms)			Conduction Velocity (m/s)			F Latency (ms)	
			Right	Left	Normal	Right	Left	Normal	Right	Left	Normal	Right	Left
Radial (s)	Distal forearm	Thumb base	10	20	≥18	2.4	2.2	≤2.7					
Median (s)	Wrist	Index finger	23		≥20	3.0		≤3.3					
Median (s)	Wrist	Middle finger	22		≥20	3.1		≤3.3					
Ulnar (s)	Wrist	Little finger	20		≥18	2.8		≤3.1					
Radial (m)*	Elbow	EDC	**5.8**	7.5	≥6	2.3	2.6	≤3.0					
Radial (m)*	Below spiral gr.	EDC	**5.6**	7.2					66	68	≥51		
Radial (m)*	Above spiral gr.	EDC	**2.0**	6.8					**57**	69	≥51		
Median (m)	Wrist	APB	10.0		≥6	3.2		≤3.9				28	
Median (m)	Elbow	APB	9.0						58		≥51		
Ulnar (m)	Wrist	ADM	14.0		≥8	3.0		≤3.0				26	
Ulnar (m)	Above elbow	ADM	13.0						64		≥51		

ADM = abductor digiti minimi; APB = abductor policis brevis; EDC = extensor digitorum communis; m = motor; s = sensory; spiral gr. = spiral groove.
Data in bold type are abnormal.
*See Figure C12–1 and EMG interpretation.

Case 12: Needle EMG

Muscle	Insertional Activity	Spontaneous Activity		Voluntary Motor Unit Action Potentials (MUAPs)							
				Recruitment				Configuration			
		Fibs	Fascs	Normal	Activation	Reduced	Early	Duration	Amplitude	% Polyphasia	Others
R. extensor indicis	↑	1+	0			↓↓		Normal	Normal	Normal	
Extensor digitorum com.	↑	1+	0			↓↓		Normal	Normal	Normal	
Brachioradialis	↑	1+	0			↓↓		Normal	Normal	Normal	
Triceps	Normal	0	0	X				Normal	Normal	Normal	
Anconeus	Normal	0	0	X				Normal	Normal	Normal	
Deltoid	Normal	0	0	X				Normal	Normal	Normal	
First dorsal interosseous	Normal	0	0	X				Normal	Normal	Normal	
Flexor pollicis longus	Normal	0	0	X				Normal	Normal	Normal	
Pronator teres	Normal	0	0	X				Normal	Normal	Normal	
Biceps	Normal	0	0	X				Normal	Normal	Normal	

Extensor digitorum com. = extensor digitorum communis; Fascs = fasciculations; Fibs = fibrillations; R. = right; ↑ = increased; ↓↓ = moderately reduced.

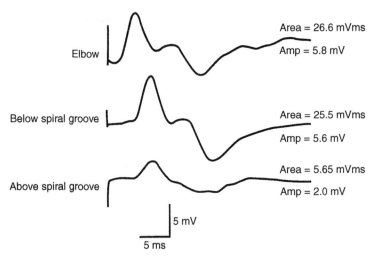

Elbow   Area = 26.6 mVms
                         Amp = 5.8 mV

Below spiral groove   Area = 25.5 mVms
                         Amp = 5.6 mV

Above spiral groove   Area = 5.65 mVms
                         Amp = 2.0 mV

5 mV

5 ms

Figure C12–1. *Right radial motor conduction studies, recording from the extensor digitorum communis. Note the significant drop in compound muscle action potential (CMAP) amplitude and area during stimulation below compared with above the spiral groove (see also Nerve Conduction table).*

axonal loss distal to the site of the lesion (wallerian degeneration).

4. There is moderate impairment of recruitment with fibrillation potentials in all radial-innervated muscles except the triceps and anconeus. Abnormal muscles include the brachioradialis, which is innervated by the radial nerve proper, and the extensor indicis proprius and extensor digitorum communis, both of which are innervated by the posterior interosseous nerve. The recruited motor unit action potentials (MUAPs) are normal in configuration, a finding consistent with a recent injury prior to the establishment of sprouting.

This case is consistent with a right radial mononeuropathy at the spiral groove, manifested mostly by segmental demyelination (partial conduction block within the spiral groove) with modest sensory and motor axonal loss. The presence of wristdrop and fingerdrop with weak brachioradialis but normal triceps and deltoid, along with superficial radial sensory deficit, makes the clinical diagnosis of radial nerve lesion in the region of the spiral groove very likely. Identifying a conduction block across the spiral groove localizes the lesion precisely to that segment of the radial nerve. In addition, the lesion could not be due to a posterior interosseous neuropathy because the radial sensory SNAP and brachioradialis muscle are abnormal; the motor branch to the brachioradialis (and the branch to the extensor carpi radialis longus) originates from the main trunk of the radial nerve before it divides into its terminal branches (posterior interosseous and radial cutaneous). In a posterior cord brachial plexus lesion, the deltoid, triceps, and anconeus muscles are abnormal. Finally, the SNAPs are normal in cervical radiculopathy (because the root lesion is proximal to the dorsal root ganglia), and muscles innervated by other nerves that share the same root should be affected.

In the case presented, the NCSs were done 5 weeks after the onset of the patient's symptoms, long after the time required for wallerian degeneration (10–11 days). Thus, the conduction block seen cannot be due to early axonal loss, and the primary pathophysiologic process here is *focal demyelinative block*. Conduction slowing also is caused by demyelination and can accompany conduction block, although they often occur independently. Sensory and motor axonal degeneration has occurred, as confirmed by low-amplitude distal radial CMAP, low-amplitude distal radial SNAP, and fibrillation potentials in radial innervated muscles. The prognosis for this patient should be good but biphasic because it is dependent on the relatively rapid remyelination process and slower reinnervation. Reinnervation in this case should be efficient because the lesion is partial and sprouting is likely to be vigorous.

DISCUSSION

Applied Anatomy

The radial nerve is the largest nerve in the upper extremity (Figure C12–2). It is a direct extension of the posterior cord of the brachial plexus, after takeoff of the axillary nerve, and contains fibers from all the contributing roots of the plexus (i.e., C5 through T1).

To attain better understanding of the anatomy and innervation of this long and serpiginous nerve, its path is best dissected into multiple segments:

• In the upper arm, while lying medial to the humerus, the radial nerve innervates all three heads of the triceps muscle (lateral, long, and medial) and the anconeus muscle; it does so through two or three separate branches, with extreme individual variability. Before entering the spiral

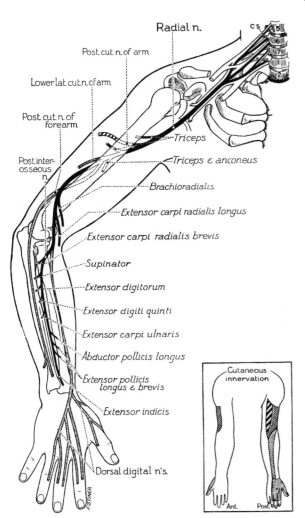

Figure C12–2. *Anatomy of the radial nerve and its branches. (From Haymaker W, Woodhall B. Peripheral nerve injuries: principles of diagnosis. Philadelphia, PA: WB Saunders, 1953, with permission.)*

groove in the midarm, it gives off the posterior cutaneous nerve of the arm (which innervates a strip of skin overlying the triceps muscle), the lower lateral cutaneous nerve of the arm (which innervates the lateral half of the arm), and the posterior cutaneous nerve of the forearm (which innervates the skin of the extensor surface of the forearm). The latter two cutaneous nerves may originate more distally, while the radial nerve is traversing the spiral groove.

- The nerve passes obliquely behind the humerus, first between the lateral and medial heads of the triceps, and then through the *spiral groove*, a shallow groove formed deep to the lateral head of the triceps muscle. To exit into the anterior compartment of the arm, the nerve pierces the lateral intermuscular septum below the deltoid insertion.

- In the anterior compartment of the arm, the radial nerve, lying lateral to the humerus, innervates the brachioradialis and the extensor carpi radialis longus. Then, the nerve passes anterior to the lateral epicondyle and travels the so-called "radial tunnel."

- The *"radial tunnel"* is not a true bony tunnel but a potential space between the humeroradial joint to the proximal edge of the supinator muscle, called the *arcade of Frohse*, which is a tendinous arch in over half of the population (Figure C12–3). The tunnel is formed by the capitulum of the humerus posteriorly, the brachialis muscle medially, and the brachioradialis and extensor carpi radialis anterolaterally. The radial nerve travels over approximately 5 cm through the tunnel, innervates the extensor carpi radialis brevis and supinator and provides sensory branches to the periosteum of the lateral epicondyle and to the humeroradial joint. The radial

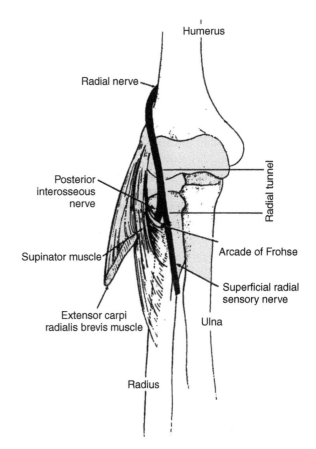

Figure C12–3. *Anatomy of the radial nerve at the elbow and proximal forearm. The radial nerve passes through the so-called "radial tunnel" and divides proximal to the edge of the supinator muscle (arcade of Frohse) into the superficial radial and posterior interosseous nerves. The posterior interosseous nerve passes under the arcade of Frohse. (Reprinted from Wilbourn AJ. Electrodiagnosis with entrapment neuropathies. AAEM plenary session I. Charleston, SC, 1992, with permission.)*

nerve divides, about 2.5 to 3 cm distal to the lateral epicondyle and slightly proximal to the edge of the supinator muscle, into its terminal branches: the superficial radial and posterior interosseous nerves.

- The posterior interosseous nerve, a terminal pure motor branch, passes under the arcade of Frohse and travels in the forearm and innervates all the remaining wrist and finger extensors through two terminal branches; a lateral branch, which innervates extensors and abductors of the thumb and the extensor of the index (the extensor pollicis longus and brevis, abductor pollicis longus, and extensor indicis); and a medial branch, which innervates the wrist extensor and all other finger long extensors (the extensor carpi ulnaris, extensor digitorum communis, and extensor digiti minimi).

- The superficial radial nerve is a terminal pure sensory nerve. It travels distally to become superficial in the midforearm. It innervates the skin of the proximal two thirds of the extensor surfaces of the thumb, index and middle fingers, and half of the ring finger, along with the corresponding dorsum of the hand (see Figure C12–2).

Clinical Features

Radial nerve lesions are usually acute and located around the spiral groove. Table C12–1 lists the common causes of radial nerve lesions in the arm. Among them, acute compression at the spiral groove, where the nerve comes in close contact with the humerus, is by far the most common. The radial nerve is compressed most often in the spiral groove after piercing the lateral intermuscular ligament, where the nerve lies unprotected by the triceps, against the humerus.

In lesions of the spiral groove, the patient usually presents with acute painless wrist drop with variable sensory loss mostly over the dorsum of the hand. On examination, there is wrist and finger drop due to weakness of all wrist and finger extensors with mild weakness of elbow flexion (along with the loss of brachioradialis reflex and belly on elbow flexion). Otherwise, elbow extension and shoulder abduction are normal. Sensory loss is limited to the territory of the radial cutaneous nerve over the dorsum of

Table C12–1. Causes of Radial Mononeuropathy in the Arm

Acute compression at the spiral groove ("Saturday night palsy," "honeymoon palsy," intraoperative, coma)

Humeral fracture

Strenuous muscular effort

Injection injury

Open trauma (gunshot or knife wound)

the hand. Occasionally, this extends to the dorsal aspect of the forearm because of involvement of the posterior cutaneous nerve of the forearm.

Radial nerve lesions, which often present with wrist- and finger-drop, should be distinguished from lesions of the posterior interosseus nerve and of the posterior cord of the brachial plexus, and from severe cervical radiculopathies (C7 and C8 radiculopathies). Table C12–2(A) lists the clinical findings inpatients presenting with prominent wrist and/or finger extensor weakness.

Electrodiagnosis

Acute radial nerve lesions at the spiral groove are similar to acute common peroneal nerve lesions at the fibular head (see Case 8). Both are frequently caused by compression of the nerve between an external object and an internal rigid structure, such as the humerus or fibula. Also, their EDX findings are similar, with signs of axonal loss, conduction block due to segmental demyelination, or both. Except for open trauma (such as a gunshot or knife wound), which often results in axon loss lesions, one cannot predict the prognosis of radial nerve lesions, without EDX studies and quantitation of the extent of demyelination and axonal loss.

In addition to the routine median and ulnar NCSs, radial sensory and motor NCSs are essential in the accurate diagnosis of radial nerve lesions. The distal radial CMAP (recording the extensor digitorum communis, EDC, or extensor indicis proprius, EIP) assesses the integrity of the motor axons terminating in these muscles. Because the EDC and EIP are C7-, C8-, and T1-innervated muscles through the posterior cord, the radial nerve, and the posterior interosseous nerve, a low-amplitude radial CMAP, recording EDC or EIP, by itself, is not necessarily indicative of a radial nerve lesion. In fact, lesions of any of these structures may result in a low-amplitude radial CMAP. The proximal radial CMAPs, on stimulation below and above the spiral groove are, however, important in detecting the presence or absence of conduction block (and occasionally focal slowing). The radial SNAP evaluates the integrity of postganglionic radial sensory axons.

The needle EMG examination is essential in axon-loss lesions that are not localizable by NCS and confirmatory in lesions associated with conduction block (due to segmental demyelination or early axonal loss). The branches of the radial nerve are fortunately placed strategically in the arm and forearm, spanning the nerve length in its entirety. This renders the radial nerve one of the most convenient nerves to study in the EMG laboratory. Thus, even when the pathologic process is axonal, it frequently is possible to localize the lesion to a short segment of the nerve. This contrasts with many other human peripheral nerves, wherein the nerve travels in long segments without giving off any sensory or motor branches developing. Examples include the median and ulnar nerves, which have no branches in the arm, and the common peroneal nerve, which has a single motor branch in the proximal thigh (to the short head of the biceps femoris).

The aims of the EDX examination in radial nerve lesions are to localize the lesion, gauge the extent of axonal loss or demyelination, and approximate the prognosis. The study also assists in planning surgical treatment, if necessary, and gauging the degree and progress of reinnervation.

The first step in the diagnosis of a radial nerve lesion is to establish that the lesion involves the main trunk of the radial nerve; this is done by excluding restricted lesions of the posterior interosseus nerve, the posterior cord of the brachial plexus, and the C7 and C8 roots (Table C12–2(B)).

Table C12–2. Differential Diagnosis of Common Causes of Wristdrop/Fingerdrop

	Radial Neuropathy at the Spiral Groove	Posterior Interosseous Neuropathy	Severe C7 and C8 Radiculopathies	Posterior Cord Brachial Plexopathy
(A) Clinical				
Common causes	Compression, humeral fracture, injection	Benign tumors, trauma, ?radial tunnel and arcade of Frohse	Disc herniation, spondylosis,	Trauma, gunshot
Wrist extension	Weak	Normal	Weak	Weak
Finger extension	Weak	Weak	Weak	Weak
Radial deviation (during wrist extension)	Absent	Present	Absent	Absent
Brachioradialis	Weak	Normal	Normal	Weak
Triceps	Normal*	Normal	Weak	Weak
Wrist flexion, forearm pronation	Normal	Normal	Weak	Normal
Deltoid	Normal	Normal	Normal	Weak
Sensory loss distribution	Radial cutaneous +/−Post. cutaneous of forearm	None	Poorly demarcated to middle, ring, and little fingers	Radial cutaneous, post. cutaneous of forearm and arm, axillary
Brachioradialis reflex	Absent or depressed	Normal	Normal	Absent or depressed
Triceps reflex	Normal*	Normal	Absent or depressed	Absent or depressed
(B) Electrodiagnosis				
Radial motor study (recording EDC)	Low in amplitude or conduction block across the spiral groove	Low in amplitude	Normal or low in amplitude	Low in amplitude
Superficial radial sensory study	Low or absent†	Normal	Normal	Low or absent
Axillary motor study (recording deltoid)	Normal	Normal	Normal	Low in amplitude
Posterior interosseous muscles‡	Abnormal	Abnormal	Abnormal	Abnormal
Brachioradialis	Abnormal	Normal	Normal	Abnormal
Other C7, C8 muscles¶	Normal	Normal	Abnormal	Normal
Triceps§	Normal*	Normal	Abnormal	Abnormal
Deltoid	Normal	Normal	Normal	Abnormal
Paraspinal muscles fibrillations	Absent	Absent	May be absent	Absent

*Triceps weakness, loss of triceps reflex and triceps (and anconeus) denervation can occur when the radial lesion is at the axilla.

†Can be normal in purely demyelinating lesions.

‡Lateral branch (extensor pollicis longus and brevis, abductor pollicis longus and extensor indicis) and medial branch (extensor carpi ulnaris, extensor digitorum communis, and extensor digiti minimi).

¶Pronator teres, flexor pollicis longus, flexor carpi radialis, in addition to the triceps and anconeus.

§And anconeus.

A radial nerve lesion at the spiral groove, studied after the potential time to complete wallerian degeneration, is characterized by the following:

1. Low-amplitude (or absent) radial SNAP. Occasionally, this study is normal when the pathology at the spiral groove is purely demyelinating.
2. Conduction block across the spiral groove (segmental demyelinating lesion) or uniformly low-amplitude radial CMAP (axon-loss lesion) or a low-amplitude distal radial CMAP with additional conduction block across the spiral groove (mixed lesion).
3. Denervation (fibrillation potentials, decreased recruitment, and large MUAPs) of all posterior interosseous-innervated muscles as well as the brachioradialis and/or extensor carpi radialis longus. As mentioned above, these two muscles originate from the main trunk of the radial nerve while in the anterior compartment of the arm, before it bifurcates into its terminal branches.
4. Normal triceps and anconeus muscles. The triceps and anconeus muscles are innervated by the radial nerve, proximal to its entrance into the spiral groove. However, both muscles are affected when the radial lesion is at the axilla (such as with crutch palsy).
5. Normal deltoid muscle. The deltoid muscle is innervated by the axillary nerve, which is another terminal branch of the posterior cord.

Another aim of the EDX examination is to prognosticate the radial nerve lesion based on the primary pathologic process. This is achieved by studying the radial CMAP amplitude and area after 10–11 days, the time needed to complete wallerian degeneration. To better assess the distal radial CMAP and SNAP, radial motor and sensory NCS should be performed on the affected and asymptomatic limbs, for comparison purposes. In axonal lesions where the radial CMAPs are uniformly low in amplitudes, the distal radial CMAP, stimulating at the elbow, and the distal radial SNAP estimates the degree of motor and sensory axonal loss, respectively. However, in demyelinating lesions in which conduction block is present, comparison between the distal and the proximal radial CMAP on the symptomatic side, stimulating above the spiral groove estimates the number of fibers that underwent segmental demyelination across the spiral groove. In mixed (axonal and demyelinating) lesions, as in this patient, one must compare the distal radial CMAP and SNAP amplitudes to their contralateral counterparts as well as contrast the distal to the proximal radial CMAPs.

Radial Tunnel Syndrome

Radial tunnel syndrome (RTS) is a term coined by Roles and Maudsley in 1972 to describe patients with lateral forearm pain and "persistent tennis elbow" who improved after surgical decompression of the posterior interosseous nerve within the radial tunnel. This syndrome continues to be debated by many physicians, while many orthopedic and hand surgeons continue to decompress the nerve within the radial tunnel.

According to its *proponents*, the patient with RTS complains of lateral forearm pain and tenderness in the region of the radial tunnel, which may radiate to the arm and/or wrist. The pain is worse with resisted extension of the middle finger with the elbow extended or resisted supination with the elbow extended. These maneuvers contract the extensor carpi radialis or the supinator muscles. On examination, there are either no findings or subtle abnormalities. Tenderness in the proximal arm that is usually maximal near the supinator is common. Apart from these findings, there is usually no other weakness, sensory loss, or reflex changes. In almost all cases of RTS, the EDX studies (NCS and needle EMG) are normal. Rarely, there are mild chronic denervation and reinnervation changes of posterior interosseous-innervated muscles on needle EMG, often with normal radial sensory and motor NCS. Perineural injection of local anesthetic and corticosteroid around the radial nerve within the tunnel as a diagnostic test for radial nerve entrapment. Advocated treatment of this syndrome is decompression of the posterior interosseous and radial nerves by severing the arcade of Frohse and any other compressive elements within the radial tunnel.

Despite its popularity among orthopedic and hand surgeons, there are many *opponents* to the existence of this syndrome. These physicians argue that (1) the symptoms of the RTS are seldom substantiated by clinical or electrophysiologic findings, (2) the tender points correlate with the "trigger points" described in regional myofascial pain syndromes, (3) the pain relief from corticosteroid injection is not a proof that the radial nerve is compressed, since patients with local musculoskeletal complaints, such as lateral epicondylitis or trigger points often get pain relief by blocks, and (4) cases of true compression of the posterior interosseous nerve are often due to mass lesions (e.g., ganglion), trauma, and, occasionally, entrapment at the arcade of Frohse and have definite neurological and EDX abnormalities that are consistent with axon-loss (Table C12–3). Many opponents believe that most patients with this alleged syndrome have actually a lateral epicondylitis ("tennis elbow") that is resistant to treatment or have a regional myofascial syndrome rather than true nerve compression.

FOLLOW-UP

The patient's wristdrop and hypesthesia began to improve within 2 weeks. Three months after the accident, he

Table C12–3. Differences Between a "True" Posterior Interosseous Neuropathy and a "Presumed" Posterior Interosseous Nerve Entrapment in Radial Tunnel Syndrome

	Posterior Interosseous Neuropathy	Radial Tunnel Syndrome
Pathophysiology	Nerve compression, usually by mass (e.g., ganglion), acute trauma, and, rarely, by the tendinous arch at the arcade of Frohse	Presumed nerve entrapment at the radial tunnel, mostly, by the tendinous arch at the arcade of Frohse
Clinical manifestations	Objective and subjective weakness of PIN muscles*; rarely painful	Pain is always present with finger extension or supination; often with tenderness on palpation over the proximal lateral forearm with distal and/or proximal radiation; rarely weakness
Electrodiagnostic findings	Denervation in PIN muscles*; radial motor CMAP may be low; radial SNAP is normal	Usually normal

*See Figure C12–2.

had minimal weakness limited to the long finger extensors (4–/5) and a small patch of hypesthesia over the dorsum of the hand.

DIAGNOSIS

Acute compressive radial mononeuropathy at the spiral groove, manifested by partial conduction block (due to segmental demyelination), with slight motor and sensory axonal loss.

ANSWERS

1. D; 2. E; 3. C.

SUGGESTED READINGS

Barnum M, Mastey RD, Weiss A-PC et al. Radial tunnel syndrome. Hand Clin 1996;12:679–689.

Brown WF, Watson BV. Quantitation of axon loss and conduction block in acute radial palsies. Muscle Nerve 1992;15:768–773.

Cornblath DR et al. Conduction block in clinical practice. Muscle Nerve 1991;14:869–871.

Cravens G, Kline DG. Posterior interosseous nerve palsies. Neurosurgery 1990;27:397–402.

Fowler CJ, Danta G, Gilliatt RW. Recovery of nerve conduction after a pneumatic tourniquet: observation on the hind-limb of the baboon. J Neurol Neurosurg Psychiatry 1972;35:638–647.

Kaplan PE. Posterior interosseous neuropathies: natural history. Arch Phys Med Rehabil 1984;65:399–400.

Roles NC, Maudsley RH. Radial tunnel syndrome. Resistant tennis elbow as a nerve entrapment. J Bone J Surg 1972;54B:499–508.

Rosenbaum R. Disputed radial tunnel syndrome. Muscle Nerve 1999;22:960–967.

Streib E. Upper arm radial nerve palsy after muscular effort: report of three cases. Neurology 1992;42:1632–1634.

Case 13

HISTORY AND PHYSICAL EXAMINATION

A 50-year-old woman had chronic pain in the right shoulder and arm for at least 10 years. She also experienced intermittent numbness of the right upper extremity. Both symptoms worsened after any sustained activity of that extremity, such as writing or cleaning. The numbness was ill-defined but involved mostly the little finger and the medial forearm. The patient noted some weakness in hand grip. Four years previously, she underwent anterior C6–C7 cervical laminectomy with no improvement. Symptoms worsened during the last year and she was referred to the electromyography (EMG) laboratory for further diagnostic studies.

On examination, there was atrophy of the right thenar eminence only. There was mild weakness of the right hand, especially of thumb abduction and the interossei. Phalen sign was negative and Tinel signs were negative at the wrist and elbow. Sensory examination revealed relative hypesthesia of the little finger and medial forearm. Deep tendon reflexes were normal. Peripheral pulses were normal. There was no Horner sign.

A cervical spine radiograph showed a rudimentary cervical rib on the right (Figure C13–1). An EMG examination was performed.

Please now review the Nerve Conduction Studies and Needle EMG tables.

QUESTIONS

1. Clinical and electrodiagnostic (EDX) findings are consistent with:
   A. Combined ulnar neuropathy and carpal tunnel syndrome.
   B. C8/T1 radiculopathy.
   C. Lower trunk brachial plexopathy.
   D. Combined C8/T1 radiculopathy and carpal tunnel syndrome.

2. Findings consistent with this disorder include all of the following *except:*
   A. Low-amplitude ulnar sensory nerve action potential (SNAP).
   B. Low-amplitude median compound muscle action potential (CMAP).
   C. Low-amplitude ulnar CMAP.
   D. Low-amplitude median SNAP.
   E. Denervation of thenar more than hypothenar muscles.

3. Which of the following is the least commonly encountered nerve conduction studies (NCS) finding associated with this disorder?
   A. Focal slowing of ulnar motor conduction velocity in the Erb point-to-axilla segment.
   B. Low-amplitude ulnar CMAP.
   C. Low-amplitude median CMAP.
   D. Low-amplitude ulnar SNAP.
   E. Low-amplitude medial antebrachial SNAP.

EDX FINDINGS AND INTERPRETATION OF DATA

The significant EDX findings in this case include the following:

1. Relatively low-amplitude right ulnar SNAP, with normal ulnar sensory distal latency and conduction velocity. Because the sensory fibers contributing to the ulnar SNAP originate from the C8 dorsal root ganglion (DRG), this finding is compatible with a postganglionic C8 lesion (including an extraspinal C8 lesion, a lower trunk or medial cord brachial plexus lesion, or an ulnar nerve lesion). This abnormality is not consistent with a preganglionic (intraspinal root) lesion.

Case 13: Nerve Conduction Studies

Nerve Stimulated	Stimulation Site	Recording Site	Amplitude (m = mV, s = µV)			Distal/Peak Latency (ms)			Conduction Velocity (m/s)			F Latency (ms)	
			Right	Left	Normal	Right	Left	Normal	Right	Left	Normal	Right	Left
Median (s)	Wrist	Thumb	20	19	≥15	3.0	3.0	≤3.6					
Median (s)	Wrist	Index finger	22	22	≥15	3.1	3.0	≤3.6					
Median (s)	Wrist	Middle finger	18	20	≥15	3.1	3.1	≤3.6					
Ulnar (s)	Wrist	Little finger	**8**	20	≥10	2.8	2.7	≤3.1	53	55	≥50		
Ulnar (s)	Wrist	Little finger	**4**	14									
Radial (s)	Forearm	Dorsum of hand	28		≥14	2.5		≤2.7					
Median (m)	Wrist	APB	**3.0**	9.5	≥6	3.5	3.2	≤4.0				**NR**	29.0
Median (m)	Elbow	APB	**3.0**						50		≥50		
Ulnar (m)	Wrist	ADM	10.0	11	≥7	2.8	2.5	≤3.2				28.4	28.0
Ulnar (m)	Elbow	ADM	8.5	9.5					59	54	≥50		
Ulnar (m)	Wrist	First DI	**7.5**	11.5	≥7	3.3	3.4	≤3.4					
Ulnar (m)	Elbow	First DI	**6.5**	11.0					54	56	≥50		
Lat ante cut (s)	Lat elbow	Forearm	20	18		2.5	2.6						
Med ante cut (s)	Med elbow	Forearm	**NR**	16		**NR**	2.0						

ADM = abductor digiti minimi; APB = abductor pollicis brevis; First DI = first dorsal interosseus; Lat ante cut = lateral antebrachial cutaneous; Lat elbow = lateral elbow; m = motor; Med ante cut = medial antebrachial cutaneous; Med elbow = medial elbow; NR = no response; s = sensory. Data in bold type are abnormal.

Case 13: Needle EMG

| Muscle | Insertional Activity | Spontaneous Activity | | Voluntary Motor Unit Action Potentials (MUAPs) | | | | | | | |
| | | | | Recruitment | | | | Configuration | | | Others |
		Fibs	Fascs	Normal	Activation	Reduced	Early	Duration	Amplitude	% Polyphasia	
R. first dorsal interosseous	↑	1+	0			↓↓		Normal	↑	Normal	
Abductor pollicis brevis	↑	1+	0			↓↓↓		↑	↑↑	Normal	
Abductor digiti minimi	Normal	0	0			↓↓		↑	Normal	Normal	
Flexor pollicis longus	Normal	0	0			↓↓		↑↑	↑	Normal	
Extensor indicis proprius	Normal	0	0	X				↑	Normal	Normal	
Pronator teres	Normal	0	0	X				Normal	Normal	Normal	
Flexor carpi ulnaris	Normal	0	0	X				↑	Normal	Normal	
Biceps	Normal	0	0	X				Normal	Normal	Normal	
Triceps	Normal	0	0	X				Normal	Normal	Normal	
Deltoid	Normal	0	0	X				Normal	Normal	Normal	
Low cervical paraspinal	Normal	0	0	–							
Midcervical paraspinal	Normal	0	0	–							

Fascs = fasciculations; Fibs = fibrillations; R. = right; ↑ = increased; ↑↑ = significantly increased; ↓↓ = moderately reduced; ↓↓↓ = severely reduced.

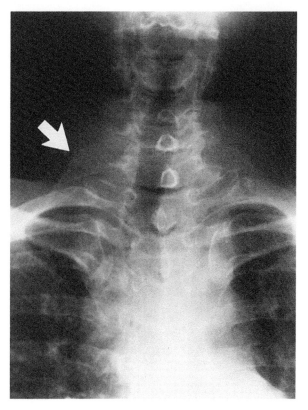

Figure C13–1. *The patient's cervical spine x-ray (anteroposterior view) revealing a rudimentary cervical rib on the right (arrow).*

2. Very low-amplitude median CMAP with normal median motor distal latency and conduction velocity, combined with normal median SNAPs amplitudes and distal latencies. This is not consistent with carpal tunnel syndrome, in which the median SNAPs are usually more affected and there is usually focal slowing at the wrist.
   - The combination of the aforementioned two findings on routine NCSs should raise the suspicion of a lower brachial plexus lesion (lower trunk or medial cord), resulting in axonal degeneration of the median motor fibers to the thenar muscles (which originate from T1 and C8 ventral roots) and of the ulnar postganglionic sensory fibers (which also originate from the C8 dorsal root ganglion). The preservation of median SNAPs is not consistent with a median nerve lesion.
3. Absent SNAP of the medial antebrachial cutaneous nerve (medial cutaneous nerve of the forearm), which branches directly from the medial cord. Its fibers originate mostly from the T1 DRGs. This abnormal NCS is a very important confirmatory evidence of lower trunk brachial plexus or extraspinal T1 lesion and excludes a selective ulnar nerve lesion.

4. Relatively low-amplitude right ulnar CMAP, recording first dorsal interosseous (when compared with the left), with normal ulnar motor distal latencies and conduction velocities. This is another supporting evidence of motor axon loss along the T1 and C8 fibers.
5. Denervation with reinnervation of muscles innervated by the T1 and C8 roots, including the median muscles (abductor pollicis brevis and flexor pollicis longus), the ulnar muscles (first dorsal interosseous, abductor digiti minimi, and flexor carpi ulnaris), and the radial muscles (extensor indicis proprius). Note that the findings are chronic (large motor unit action potentials, MUAPs) with slight ongoing denervation (fibrillation potentials), and most prominent in the abductor pollicis brevis.

In summary, these findings are pathognomonic of a lesion affecting the lower trunk of the brachial plexus. The predilection of sensory and chronic motor axonal loss to the T1 root, as supported by a most severe axon loss in the abductor pollicis brevis/thenar muscles and the medial antebrachial cutaneous SNAP, are classical findings of neurogenic thoracic outlet syndrome (TOS). In most cases of neurogenic TOS, other lower trunk/C8 structures, such as the interossei and the abductor digiti minimi/hypothenar muscles and the ulnar SNAP, are affected to a much lesser extent.

DISCUSSION

Applied Anatomy

The brachial plexus is derived from the anterior primary rami of the C5 through T1 spinal roots. As is shown in Figure C13–2, these roots intertangle at multiple sites to form structures that usually are divided into five components: roots, trunks, divisions, cords, and peripheral (terminal) nerves. Because the divisions generally are located under the clavicle, some divide the brachial plexus into two regions: *supraclavicular* (roots and trunks) and *infraclavicular* (cords and peripheral nerves). Nerve fibers from the C5 and C6 anterior primary rami combine to form the upper trunk, C8 and T1 rami combine to form the lower trunk, and the C7 ramus continues as the middle trunk. Then, each trunk divides into two divisions (anterior and posterior). All three posterior divisions unite to form the posterior cord, the upper two anterior divisions merge to form the lateral cord, and the anterior division of the lower trunk continues as the medial cord.

The terminal peripheral nerves are the main branches that extend from the brachial plexus to the upper limb. From each cord, two major nerves arise: the posterior cord gives rise to the radial and axillary nerves, the lateral cord gives rise to the musculocutaneous nerve and to the lateral

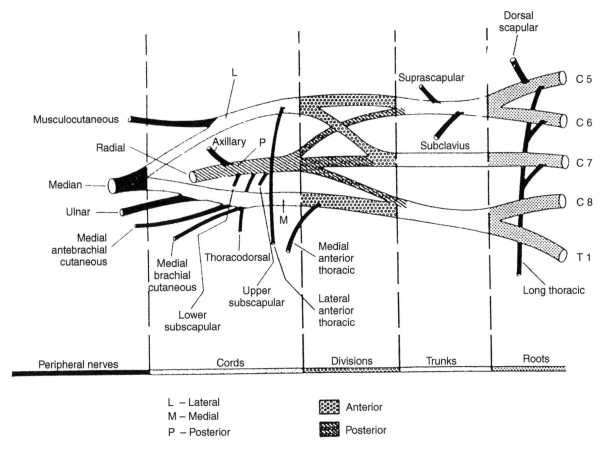

Figure C13–2. *The brachial plexus. Trunks are named upper, middle, and lower. Cords are labeled L = lateral, P = posterior, and M = medial. Roots and trunks are supraclavicular, and cords and terminal peripheral nerves are infraclavicular. (From Goodgold J. Anatomical correlates of clinical electromyography. Baltimore, MD: Williams and Wilkins, 1974, with permission.)*

half of the median nerve, and the medial cord divides into the ulnar nerve and the medial half of the median nerve.

In addition to the terminal nerves, many nerves branch directly from the main component of the brachial plexus. Except for four supraclavicular nerves, all others originate from the cords (i.e., they are infraclavicular). Except for two pure sensory nerves, all others are pure motor, and they innervate the shoulder girdle muscles. Table C13–1 lists these nerves, as they are shown in Figure C13–2, with their origin, function, destination, and segmental innervation.

Clinical Features

Thoracic outlet syndrome (TOS) is a disorder characterized by compression of the subclavian artery, subclavian vein, or brachial plexus separately or, rarely, in combination. This compression results in a vascular or neurogenic syndrome, depending on which structure is involved. Neurogenic TOS is a neurologic syndrome caused by compression

of the lower brachial plexus. Because controversy regarding this syndrome has increased during the past few decades, some have separated neurogenic TOS into *true* and *disputed* forms (see Wilbourn 1999).

1. *True or classic neurogenic TOS* (also interchangeably named cervical rib and band syndrome) is usually caused by a congenital fibrous band that originates from the tip of a rudimentary cervical rib or elongated C7 transverse process and inserts into the proximal portion of the first rib. This was described in the early twentieth century by Thornburn (1905) and Howell (1907), separately, but was better defined more than 60 years later by Gilliatt et al. (1970). In this form of neurogenic TOS, there is objective clinical and EDX evidence of peripheral nerve fiber injury: The proximal lower trunk fibers, particularly the component formed by the T1 anterior primary ramus, are angulated and stretched around the fibrous band.

Table C13–1. Motor and Sensory Nerves Arising Directly from the Brachial Plexus (Excluding the Main Terminal Nerves)

Nerve	Origin	Function	Destination
Dorsal scapular*	Anterior ramus of C5	Motor	Rhomboids (C5)
Long thoracic*	Anterior rami of C5–C6–C7	Motor	Serratus anterior (C5–C6–C7)
Suprascapular*	Upper trunk	Motor	Supraspinatus (C5–6) and infraspinatus (C5–C6)
N. to subclavius*	Upper trunk	Motor	Subclavius (C5–C6)
Lateral pectoral (lateral anterior thoracic)	Lateral cord	Motor	Pectoralis major and minor (C5 to T1)
Subscapular (upper and lower)	Posterior cord	Motor	Teres major (C5–C6) and subscapularis (C5–C6)
Thoracodorsal	Posterior cord	Motor	Latissimus dorsi (C6–C7–C8)
Medial pectoral (medial anterior thoracic)	Medial cord	Motor	Pectoralis major and minor (C5 to T1)
Medial cutaneous of arm (brachial cutaneous)	Medial cord	Sensory	Skin of medial arm (C8–T1)
Lateral cutaneous of forearm (antebrachial cutaneous)	Medial cord	Sensory	Skin of medial forearm (C8–T1)

*Are the only supraclavicular nerves.

True neurogenic TOS is a rare, unilateral disorder, which affects mainly young or middle age women. The typical patient presents with wasting and weakness of one hand. There is often several years' history of hand cramps or mild pain and paresthesias in the medial aspect of the arm, forearm and hand, both exacerbated by physical activity of the upper extremity. On examination, there is atrophy and weakness of the thenar muscles with less involvement of the hypothenar and other intrinsic hand muscles. A patchy sensory loss usually may be present along the medial arm, forearm and hand.

Most patients have a cervical rib or elongated C7 transverse process, with a translucent band extending from it to the first rib. Rarely, classical neurogenic TOS may be caused by compression by structures other than a cervical rib or band, such as a hypertrophied anterior scalenus muscle in a competitive swimmer. In most patients, cervical spine radiographs typically show a cervical rib, a rudimentary cervical rib (see Figure C13–1), or simply an elongated C7 transverse process. In these cases, surgical section of the cervical rib or band (which connects the rudimentary rib or C7 transverse process to the first rib), preferably by a supraclavicular approach, halts the progression of symptoms but does not reverse the hand atrophy or weakness, or the nerve conduction abnormalities.

True neurogenic TOS should be distinguished from carpal tunnel syndrome, ulnar neuropathy at the elbow, poststernotomy brachial plexopathy and C8 and T1 radiculopathies (Table C13–2). Occasionally, neurogenic TOS may be confused with monomelic amyotrophy and motor neuron disease.

2. *Disputed TOS*, also called nonspecific TOS, is diagnosed much more frequently and is surrounded by controversy. Pain and/or subjective sensory symptoms dominate the clinical picture, but there are no objective neurologic or convincing electrodiagnostic signs. In this situation, multiple compression sites have been advocated, resulting in many "syndromes" and recommended surgical procedures. The three common syndromes, their suggested sites of compression, and recommended surgical procedures are shown in Table C13–3 and Figure C13–3.

Electrodiagnosis

Electrodiagnostic (EDX) examination is the most useful and objective diagnostic procedure in the diagnosis of neurogenic TOS. Neurogenic TOS is the result of chronic compression and chronic axon-loss of the lower trunk of the brachial plexus, particularly fibers within the T1 anterior primary ramus. Because all ulnar sensory fibers, all ulnar motor fibers, and the C8/T1 median fibers course the lower trunk, they are among the most obviously noted abnormalities on routine NCS. Hence, the EDX findings on nerve conduction studies (NCS) and needle EMG in neurogenic TOS have a very characteristic combination of changes (Table C13–4 and Figures C13–4 and C13–5).

The *medial antebrachial cutaneous SNAP*, a sensory nerve that originates directly from the brachial plexus (medial cord) and innervates the skin of the medial forearm, is now an integral part of the EDX evaluation of patients with suspected neurogenic TOS as well as all other lower brachial plexopathies. An absent or low-amplitude

Table C13–2. Differential Diagnosis of Neurogenic Thoracic Outlet Syndrome

	Carpal Tunnel Syndrome	Cubital Tunnel Syndrome	C8 Radiculopathy	T1 Radiculopathy	Postmedian Sternotomy Brachial Plexopathy	Neurogenic Thoracic Outlet Syndrome
Lesion site	Median nerve at the wrist	Ulnar nerve at the elbow	C8 intraspinal root	T1 intraspinal root	C8 anterior primary ramus component of lower trunk	T1 anterior primary ramus component of lower trunk
Mode of symptom onset	Subacute or chronic	Subacute or chronic	Acute, subacute, or chronic	Acute, subacute, or chronic	Acute (postoperative)	Chronic
Sensory loss distribution	Lateral three digits	Medial two digits	Medial two digits and medial forearm	Medial forearm and arm	Medial two digits and medial forearm	Medial two digits and medial forearm
Muscle atrophy and/or weakness	Lateral thenars	Hypothenars, medial thenars, and interossei	Hypothenars, medial thenars, interossei, and long finger flexors	Lateral thenars	Hypothenars, medial thenars, interossei, and long finger flexors	Lateral thenars
Median SNAP	Abnormal	Normal	Normal	Normal	Normal	Normal
Ulnar SNAP	Normal	Abnormal	Normal	Normal	Abnormal	Usually abnormal
MAB SNAP	Normal	Normal	Normal	Normal	Usually abnormal	Abnormal
Median CMAP	Abnormal	Normal	Normal	Normal or abnormal	Normal or borderline	Abnormal
Ulnar CMAP	Normal	Abnormal	Normal or abnormal	Normal	Abnormal	Normal or borderline

SNAP = sensory nerve action potential; CMAP = compound muscle action potential; MAB = medial antebrachial.
Adapted from Katirji B. Thoracic outlet syndrome. In: Evans RW, ed. Saunders Manual of Neurologic Practice. Philadelphia, PA: WB Saunders, 2003, with permission.

Table C13–3. Three Disputed Syndromes Associated With Neurovascular Compression in the Thoracic Outlet Syndrome

Syndrome	Scalenus Anticus Syndrome	Costoclavicular Syndrome	Hyperabduction Syndrome
Proposed compression site	Interscalene triangle	Between first thoracic rib and clavicle	Between pectoralis minor tendon and/or between first rib and clavicle
Structures compressed	Subclavian artery or brachial plexus	Subclavian artery, subclavian vein, or brachial plexus	Subclavian/axillary artery, or brachial plexus
Suggested surgical resection of procedure	Resection of scalenus anticus muscle	Resection of first thoracic rib	Resection of first thoracic rib and pectoralis minor tendon

Adapted from Wilbourn AJ. Brachial plexus disorders. In: Dyck PPJ, Thomas PK, eds. Peripheral neuropathy, 4th ed. Philadelphia, PA: WB Saunders/Elsevier, 2005.

medial antebrachial cutaneous SNAP is a universal finding in all confirmed cases of neurogenic TOS, including the mild cases, in which thenar atrophy is subtle and an ulnar nerve lesion is also considered in the diagnosis.

Needle EMG in neurogenic TOS is confirmative and reveals decreased recruitment and large MUAPs in the T1 more than C8 innervated muscles. Hence, median-innervated thenar muscles (such as abductor pollicis brevis and opponens pollicis) are the most affected, while ulnar-innervated hand muscles (such as interossei, abductor digiti minimi, and adductor pollicis), and radial-innervated muscles (such as extensor indicis proprius) are less severely involved. Fibrillation potentials are usually rare, consistent with the chronicity of this disorder, and tend to be in the median-innervated thenar muscles (such as abductor pollicis brevis and opponens pollicis).

Though the aforementioned EDX findings are common to all patients with lower trunk brachial plexus lesions, two EDX findings are specific for neurogenic TOS and help in distinguishing this disorder from other plexopathies:

1. *Predilection of the denervation to the thenar muscles* compared to the hypothenar muscles. Clinically, this is apparent by prominent thenar atrophy with a relatively preserved hypothenar eminence (see also Table C9–1). By NCS, it is common to observe a very low-amplitude median CMAP, with a normal or borderline low-amplitude ulnar CMAP. This is explained by compression of the T1 anterior primary ramus, or predominantly the T1 component of the proximal lower trunk of the brachial plexus.

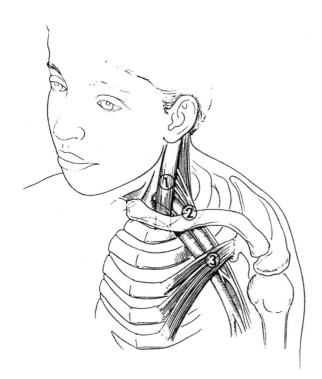

Figure C13–3. *The presumed sites of compression within the cervicoaxillary canal for the (1) scalenus anticus syndrome (interscalene triangle); (2) the costoclavicular syndrome (between the first rib and clavicle); and (3) the hyperabduction syndrome (beneath the pectoralis minor tendon). See also Table C13–3. (From Wilbourn AJ. Brachial plexus disorders. In: Dyck PPJ, Thomas PK, eds. Peripheral neuropathy, 4rd ed. Philadelphia, PA: WB Saunders/Elsevier, 2005.)*

Table C13–4. Findings on Nerve Conduction Studies That Highly Suggest True Neurogenic Thoracic Outlet Syndrome

Routine nerve conduction studies
    Low/absent ulnar sensory nerve action potential (SNAP)
    Low median compound muscle action potential (CMAP)
    Borderline/low ulnar CMAP
    Normal median SNAP
Other nerve conduction studies
    Low/absent medial antebrachial SNAP

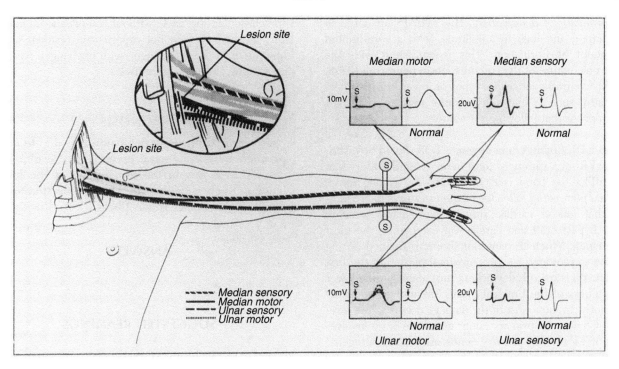

Figure C13–4. *Neurogenic thoracic outlet syndrome showing the site of compression by the cervical rib or band. (From Wilbourn AJ. Controversies regarding thoracic outlet syndrome: syllabus on controversies in entrapment neuropathies. Rochester, MN: American Association of Electrodiagnostic Medicine, 1984, with permission.)*

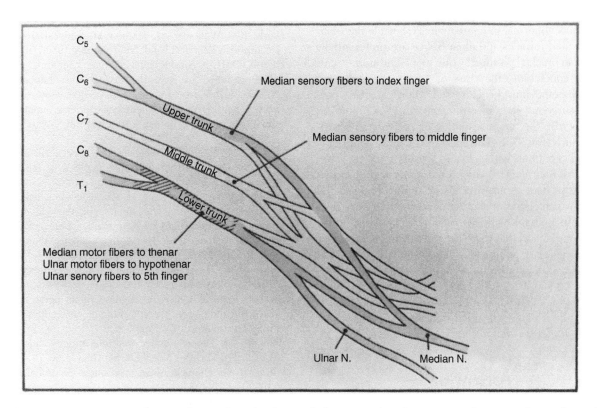

Figure C13–5. *Routine nerve conduction abnormalities (median and ulnar nerves) with neurogenic thoracic outlet syndrome (TOS). (From Wilbourn AJ. Case report #7: true neurogenic thoracic outlet syndrome. Rochester, MN: American Association of Electrodiagnostic Medicine, 1982, with permission.)*

2. *Chronicity of denervation.* The MUAPs are large in duration and high in amplitude, with a very limited amount of fibrillation. This is consistent with the chronic nature of the compression in neurogenic TOS. This contrasts with other types of lower brachial plexopathy, such as that due to tumor invasion (Pancoast tumor) or that following sternotomy.

The EDX findings in neurogenic TOS should be distinguished from a variety of focal neurogenic disorders that may afflict the hand (see Table C13–2). Among these, *brachial plexopathy following median sternotomy,* a condition that follows cardiac surgery, particularly coronary artery bypass graft and cardiac valve repair, is the most challenging. When the anterior thorax is opened during median sternotomy, the very proximal portion of the first thoracic rib is fractured which, in turn, damages the lower trunk fibers of the brachial plexus situated immediately superiorly. In fact, most of the damage occurs at the level of the C8 anterior primary ramus with little or no involvement of T1 anterior primary ramus. Although neurogenic TOS and brachial plexopathy following median sternotomy are both practically lower trunk plexopathies, these two lesions often have different predilection to fibers forming the lower trunk: T1 fibers in TOS and C8 fibers in brachial plexopathy following median sternotomy. Hence, the abductor pollicis brevis and the medial antebrachial SNAP are the most abnormal in neurogenic TOS while the ulnar C8 innervated muscles and ulnar SNAP are preferentially abnormal in brachial plexopathy due to median sternotomy.

Before concluding, the issue of "ulnar nerve slowing across Erb point" must be addressed. Many clinicians, particularly surgeons, ask electromyographers to look for slowing across the thoracic outlet in patients with suspected neurogenic TOS. This seems to be more commonly requested in patients with pain and sensory symptoms, but no objective neurologic findings on examination (disputed TOS). These data come from a few studies done in the 1970s, in which claims of slowing of conduction were documented in patients with neurogenic TOS. Specifically, the authors claimed that there is focal slowing of the ulnar nerve between Erb point and axillary stimulations, recording the abductor digiti minimi (see Urschel et al. 1971). This finding has been duplicated infrequently by electromyographers. Thus, most electromyographers, including this author, have concluded that *focal slowing across the brachial plexus is not a feature of neurogenic TOS.*

FOLLOW-UP

Following the EDX studies and radiological findings, the patient underwent resection of the cervical rib through a supraclavicular approach, without complication. One year later, she had no pain but experienced residual sensory impairment in the little finger, with unchanged weakness and atrophy of the thenar muscles.

DIAGNOSIS

Neurogenic thoracic outlet syndrome, due to compression by a congenital cervical rib, resulting in chronic axon-loss in the distribution of the lower trunk of the brachial plexus with predilection to the T1 anterior primary ramus fibers.

ANSWERS

1. C; 2. D; 3. A.

SUGGESTED READINGS

Ferrante MA, Wilbourn AJ. The utility of various sensory conduction responses in assessing brachial plexopathies. Muscle Nerve 1995;18:879–889.

Gilliatt RW et al. Wasting of the hand associated with a cervical rib or band. J Neurol Neurosurg Psychiatry 1970;33:615–624.

Gilliatt RW et al. Peripheral nerve conduction in patients with a cervical rib and band. Ann Neurol 1978;4:124–129.

Hardy RW, Wilbourn AJ, Hanson M. Surgical treatment of compressive cervical band. Neurosurgery 1980;7:10–13.

Howell CMH. A consideration of some symptoms which may be produced by seventh cervical ribs. Lancet 1907;1:1702–1707.

Katirji B, Hardy RW. Classic neurogenic thoracic outlet syndrome in a competitive swimmer: a true scalenus anticus syndrome. Muscle Nerve 1995;18:229–233.

Levin KH, Wilbourn AJ, Maggiano HJ. Cervical rib and median sternotomy-related brachial plexopathies: a reassessment. Neurology 1998;50:1407–1413.

Nishida T, Price SJ, Minieka MM. Medial antebrachial cutaneous nerve conduction in true neurogenic thoracic outlet syndrome. Electromyogr Clin Neurophysiol 1993;33:285–288.

Roos DB, Wilbourn AJ. Issues and opinions: thoracic outlet syndrome. Muscle Nerve 1999;22:126–138.

Thorburn W. The seventh cervical rib and its effects upon the brachial plexus. Med Chir Trans 1905;88:105.

Urschel HC et al. Objective diagnosis (ulnar nerve conduction velocity) and current therapy of the thoracic outlet syndrome. Ann Thorac Surg 1971;12:608–620.

Wilbourn AJ. Thoracic outlet syndrome surgery causing severe brachial plexopathy. Muscle Nerve 1988;11:66–74.

Wilbourn AJ. Thoracic outlet syndromes. Neurol Clin N Am 1999;17:477–495.

Wilbourn AJ. Brachial plexus disorders. In: Dyck PJ, Thomas PK, eds. Peripheral neuropathy, 4th ed. Philadelphia, PA: WB Saunders/Elsevier, 2005, pp. 1359–1360, 1370–1371.

Case 14

HISTORY AND PHYSICAL EXAMINATION

A 45-year-old right-handed woman had a 2-year history of numbness in both hands, worse on the right. The tingling was triggered by writing, holding a book, or driving. She frequently was awakened at night by the numbness. Shaking the hands tended to relieve the symptoms. She noticed some impairment of dexterity in the right hand. She had mild pain in the wrists. The patient was not sure whether all the fingers were equally numb. She had no weakness in the hands. There was no numbness or weakness in the legs. Similar, but less severe, symptoms had occurred 8 years before, when she was treated with ibuprofen and wrist splints, with complete resolution of symptoms. Her past medical history is relevant for congenital adrenal hyperplasia, borderline hypertension, and a history of hysterectomy and bilateral oophorectomy for fibroid tumors 2 years prior. The patient was on replacement oral dexamethasone and estrogen. She was an executive director of a local development organization.

Physical examination was relevant for positive Phalen sign bilaterally. Tinel sign could not be induced on percussion of the median nerves at the wrist. There was relative hypesthesia bilaterally in the median nerve distribution, compared with the ulnar nerve distribution. This was more pronounced in the index fingers and thumbs. There was no atrophy or weakness of the thenar muscles. There was no sensory loss in the legs. Deep tendon reflexes were normal and symmetrical. Gait and coordination were normal.

Electrodiagnostic (EDX) examination was performed.

Please now review the Nerve Conduction Studies and Needle EMG tables.

QUESTIONS

1. Among the following, the most common and specific sign of carpal tunnel syndrome (CTS) is:
   A. Positive Tinel sign.
   B. Sensory loss in the median nerve distribution.
   C. Atrophy of the thenar eminence.
   D. Weakness of thumb abduction.
   E. Positive Phalen sign.
2. Thenar atrophy is common in all of the following disorders *except:*
   A. Neurogenic thoracic outlet syndrome.
   B. Anterior interosseous syndrome.
   C. Carpal tunnel syndrome.
   D. C8/T1 radiculopathy.
3. Among the following, the EDX test most likely to reveal abnormalities in mild CTS is:
   A. Antidromic median sensory latency from wrist to index or middle finger.
   B. Comparison of median palmar to ulnar palmar mixed nerve latencies.
   C. Orthodromic median sensory latency from index or middle finger to wrist.
   D. Median motor distal latency recording the abductor pollicis brevis.
   E. Fibrillation potentials in the abductor pollicis brevis.

EDX FINDINGS AND INTERPRETATION OF DATA

Relevant EDX findings in this patient include:

1. Delayed median sensory distal latencies, with low median sensory amplitudes bilaterally.
2. Delayed median motor distal latencies bilaterally, with low right median motor amplitude and normal proximal conduction velocities.
3. Delayed median F wave latencies compared with the ulnar F wave latency.
4. Normal ulnar sensory, radial sensory, and ulnar motor conduction studies.

Case 14: Nerve Conduction Studies

Nerve Stimulated	Stimulation Site	Recording Site	Amplitude (m = mV, s = μV)			Distal/Peak Latency (ms)			Conduction Velocity (m/s)			F Latency (ms)	
			Right	Left	Normal	Right	Left	Normal	Right	Left	Normal	Right	Left
Median (s)	Wrist	Index finger	**10**	8	≥20	**4.5**	**4.6**	≤3.4					
Median (s)	Wrist	Middle finger	**10**	7	≥20	**4.8**	**4.5**	≤3.4					
Ulnar (s)	Wrist	Little finger	50		≥12	2.4		≤3.1					
Radial (s)	Distal forearm	Thumb base	35		≥18	2.0		≤2.7					
Median (m)	Wrist	APB	**4.8**	10.0	≥6	**6.8**	**6.1**	≤3.9				**33**	**30**
Median (m)	Elbow	APB	**3.7**	9.0					62	57	≥50		
Ulnar (m)	Wrist	ADM	8.5		≥7	2.5		≤3.1				26	
Ulnar (m)	Elbow	ADM	8.0						59		≥50		

ADM = abductor digiti minimi; APB = abductor pollicis brevis; m = motor; s = sensory.
Data in bold type are abnormal.

Case 14: Needle EMG

| Muscle | Insertional Activity | Spontaneous Activity | | Voluntary Motor Unit Action Potentials (MUAPs) | | | | | | | |
| | | | | Recruitment | | | | Configuration | | | |
		Fibs	Fascs	Normal	Activation	Reduced	Early	Duration	Amplitude	% Polyphasia	Others
R. abudctor pollicis brevis	Normal	0	0			↓		↑	Normal	↑	
First dorsal interosseous	Normal	0	0	X				Normal	Normal	Normal	
Flexor pollicis longus	Normal	0	0	X				Normal	Normal	Normal	
Extensor indicis proprius	Normal	0	0	X				Normal	Normal	Normal	
Pronator teres	Normal	0	0	X				Normal	Normal	Normal	
Biceps	Normal	0	0	X				Normal	Normal	Normal	
Triceps	Normal	0	0	X				Normal	Normal	Normal	
Deltoid	Normal	0	0	X				Normal	Normal	Normal	
Midcervical paraspinal	Normal	0	0	–							
Low cervical paraspinal	Normal	0	0	–							
L. abductor pollicis brevis	Normal	0	0	X				Normal	Normal	Normal	

Fascs = fasciculations; Fibs = fibrillations; L. = left; R. = right; ↓ = mildly reduced; ↑ = increased.

5. Mild reduction of recruitment and increased motor unit action potentials (MUAPs) duration in the right abductor pollicis brevis only.
6. No fibrillation potentials in the abductor pollicis brevis bilaterally.
7. Normal needle EMG of all other muscles tested particularly those innervated by the C6 and C7 roots, the median innervated muscles in the forearm, and the paraspinal muscles.

These findings are diagnostic of bilateral median mononeuropathies at or distal to the wrists and are compatible with CTS.

DISCUSSION

Applied Anatomy

The median nerve is one of the main terminal nerves of the brachial plexus, formed by contributions from the lateral and medial cords (Figure C14–1). The lateral cord component, comprised of C6–C7 fibers, provides sensory fibers to the thumb and thenar eminence (C6), index finger (C6–C7), and middle finger (C7) and motor fibers to the proximal median innervated forearm muscles. The medial cord component, comprised of C8–T1 fibers, provides sensory fibers to the lateral half of the ring finger (C8) and motor fibers to the hand and distal median innervated forearm muscles.

The median nerve descends with no branches in the arm. In the antecubital fossa, it passes between the two heads of the pronator teres and sends muscular branches to the pronator teres, flexor carpi radialis, flexor digitorum sublimis, and palmaris longus muscles. Soon after and while in the proximal forearm, the median nerve gives off the anterior interosseous nerve which is a pure motor nerve that innervates the flexor pollicis longus, medial head of the flexor digitorum profundus and the pronator quadratus muscles.

Right before entering the wrist, the median nerve gives off its first cutaneous branch, the palmar cutaneous branch, which runs subcutaneously (does not pass through the carpal tunnel) and innervates a small patch of skin over the base of the thumb and the thenar eminence (see Figure C14–1). Then, the main trunk of the median nerve, along with nine finger flexor tendons, enters the wrist through the carpal tunnel. The carpal bones form the floor and sides of the tunnel while the carpal transverse ligament, which is attached to the scaphoid, trapezoid, and hamate bones, forms its roof (Figure C14–2). The carpal tunnel cross-section is variable but is approximately 2.0 to 2.5 cm at its narrowest point in most individuals.

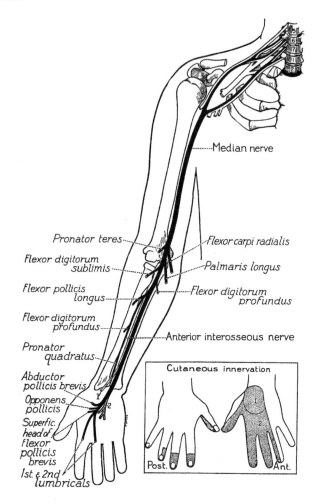

Figure C14–1. *Median nerve course and branches in the forearm and hand. 1 = the palmar cutaneous branch, and 2 = the terminal median sensory nerve. (From Haymaker W, Woodhall B. Peripheral nerve injuries. Philadelphia, PA: WB Saunders, 1953, with permission.)*

Right after exiting the tunnel, the median nerve branches into motor and sensory branches. The motor branch innervates the first and second lumbricals and gives off the recurrent motor branch, which innervates the thenar muscles (abductor pollicis brevis, opponens pollicis, and half of the flexor pollicis brevis). The sensory branch divides into terminal digital sensory branches to innervate three and one-half fingers (thumb, index, middle finger, and lateral half of the ring finger) with the corresponding palm.

Clinical Features

Carpal tunnel syndrome (CTS) is the most common entrapment neuropathy. It is slightly more common in

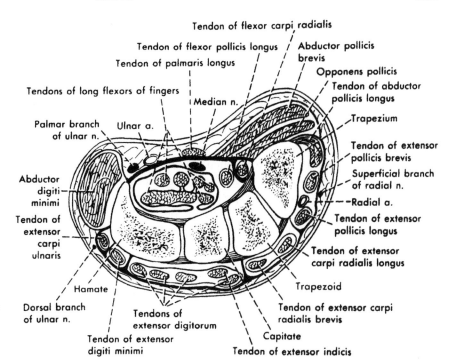

Figure C14–2. *A cross-section of the wrist revealing the carpal tunnel and its contents. (From Hollinshead WH. Anatomy for surgeons: the back and limbs, 3rd ed., vol 3. Philadelphia, PA: Harper and Row, 1982, with permission.)*

women and usually involves the dominant hand first. It is most prevalent after 50 years of age, but it may occur in younger patients, especially in association with pregnancy and certain occupations or medical conditions. Most cases of CTS are idiopathic, but many are associated with disorders that decrease the carpal tunnel space or increase the susceptibility of the nerve to pressure. Among the medical conditions with a high risk for CTS are pregnancy, diabetes mellitus, hypothyroidism, acromegaly, rheumatoid arthritis, sarcoidosis, and amyloidosis. Some patients have congenitally small carpal tunnels, while others have anomalous muscles, wrist fractures (Colles or carpal bone), or space occupying lesions (ganglia, lipoma, schwannoma). Occupational CTS, which has reached a near-epidemic level in the industrial world, is seen in patients whose jobs involve repetitive movements of the wrists and fingers. Although most cases of CTS are subacute or chronic in nature, it occasionally may be acute, such as after crush injury of the hand, fracture (Colles or carpal bone), or acute tenosynovitis.

The most common symptoms of CTS are episodic numbness and pain in the affected hand, mostly at night. A characteristic of CTS is frequent awakening at night because of hand paresthesias, hence the name, *nocturnal acroparesthesia*. Symptoms usually are relieved by shaking the affected hand. In addition, these symptoms are often exacerbated by certain activities, such as driving,

holding a book, or knitting. There is wrist and hand pain, which may radiate proximally to the forearm and, less commonly, to the arm or shoulder. Weakness of the hand and loss of dexterity are common in more advanced cases.

Phalen sign (reproduction of paresthesias in a median nerve distribution after passive flexion of the hand at the wrist) is extremely sensitive, present in 80–90% of patients with CTS with rare false positives. *Tinel sign* (paresthesias in a median nerve distribution after percussion of the median nerve at the wrist) is less common sign, present in about 50% of patients and may be false positive. On examination, there is often relative hypesthesia throughout the median nerve distribution, particularly in the fingertips and excluding the skin over the thenar eminence. Sometimes, the sensory loss is more selective to one or two fingers. Fasciculations or myokymia of the thenar muscles is not uncommon. Atrophy of the thenar muscles with weakness of thumb abduction may be evident in advanced cases. Less common associated conditions include vasomotor skin changes and Raynaud phenomenon.

The differential diagnoses of CTS include:

1. *Cervical radiculopathy*, especially a C6 or C7 radiculopathy, which commonly results in numbness of the thumb, index finger, or middle finger. Sensory symptoms or signs above the wrist, unilateral radicular pain

exacerbated by neck movements, segmental weakness in the arm and forearm, or myotatic reflex asymmetry favors a radiculopathy.

2. *Neurogenic thoracic outlet syndrome*, which frequently is associated with thenar atrophy. However, the pain and sensory manifestations in neurogenic thoracic outlet syndrome are in a C8/T1 distribution (ring and little fingers and medial aspect of the forearm).

3. *Peripheral polyneuropathy*, which may be associated with hand numbness. However, there are often sensory manifestations and motor weakness in the legs. Also, there usually is hyporeflexia or areflexia, especially at the ankles.

4. *High median mononeuropathy*, including the pronator syndrome, and compression at the ligament of Struthers in the distal arm. Both are rare syndromes and usually are associated with weakness of the long finger flexors.

5. *Cervical myelopathy*. In this condition, the numbness is not restricted to the median nerve, and there are frequently other pyramidal manifestations.

The treatment for CTS includes correcting the offending occupational factor or medical illness, wrist splinting at night, and the use of oral nonsteroidal anti-inflammatory agents or corticosteroids. Corticosteroid injection into the carpal tunnel area also is helpful to alleviate sensory symptoms and pain in patients with mild to moderate compression. Surgical decompression is indicated in patients with:

- Significant sensory loss.
- Significant thenar weakness and/or evidence of active denervation (fibrillation potentials).
- Acute median compression.
- Failure of conservative treatment.

Electrodiagnosis

Carpal tunnel syndrome (CTS) is the most common reason for referral to the EMG laboratory. Aims of the EDX studies are to confirm the diagnosis by assessing the status of the median sensory and motor fibers across the carpal tunnel, and to exclude other possible causes of the symptomatology, such as a cervical radiculopathy.

The main underlying pathophysiology in CTS early in the course is primarily paranodal demyelination. Hence, the electrophysiologic hallmark of CTS is focal slowing of conduction at the wrist, resulting in prolongation of the latencies of both motor and sensory fibers. In severe and advanced CTS, axonal loss dominates the picture.

Nerve Conduction Studies: Routine Studies

Historically, slowing of the median motor distal latency was the first described abnormality in CTS. Later, slowing of median sensory distal latencies was confirmed.

These techniques, which include orthodromic or antidromic sensory conduction studies to the digits (particularly the index and middle fingers) and motor studies to the abductor pollicis brevis, are easy to perform and are reproducible. Delayed sensory distal latencies and/or delayed motor latencies usually confirm the clinical diagnosis of CTS in one half to two thirds of patients, with a high degree of sensitivity and specificity. It is important, however, to study neighboring nerves, such as the ulnar nerve, to establish that the abnormalities are restricted to the median nerve.

The routine median sensory and motor NCSs are the most widely used techniques in the diagnosis of CTS. The median sensory studies are usually more likely to reveal abnormalities before the motor studies. The distal latencies and amplitudes of the median sensory nerve action potentials (SNAP) are often lower than those of the compound muscle action potential (CMAP). Occasionally, the SNAPs are unelicitable whenever there is axonal loss (or occasionally significant conduction block caused by segmental demyelination). In some patients with CTS, the median motor proximal conduction velocities in the forearm may be mildly slowed without implying a proximal median neuropathy. In these cases, the median CMAP is usually low in amplitude, and the proximal slowing is best explained by a conduction block or axon loss of the fastest median motor fibers at the wrist.

Nerve Conduction Studies: Comparison Studies

It is now evident that the median motor and median sensory distal latencies are not sensitive enough in the diagnosis of CTS. Relying on these measurements only will fail to detect a significant number (up to one-third) of patients with mild CTS, particularly those with symptoms precipitated by certain hand activities (e.g., drilling, typing, etc.). In addition, as the syndrome has become well known to the medical community and to the general public, it has become common practice for EMG laboratories to test patients with very early symptoms of CTS. This has resulted in the design of several NCSs with higher sensitivity and specificity than the routine median sensory and motor studies (Table C14–1). These techniques rely on one or both of the following approaches:

- Measuring the conduction time of a short segment of the median nerve across the carpal tunnel. The rationale is that the slow-conducting segment of the median nerve in CTS usually is very short. If this short segment is included in a longer nerve segment, such as the wrist-to-index segment, a mild abnormality may become "diluted" by the normal conduction in the rest of the nerve, and results in an overall conduction time (i.e., latency) that may remain within normal limits in mild and early cases of CTS.

Table C14–1. Nerve Conduction Studies in the Diagnosis of Carpal Tunnel Syndrome

Routine nerve conduction studies
  Median motor nerve conduction study
  Median sensory nerve conduction study (orthodromic or antidromic)
Internal comparison nerve conduction studies
  Comparison of median to ulnar palmar mixed latencies (orthodromic)
  Comparison of median to ulnar sensory latencies recording ring finger (antidromic)
  Comparison of median to ulnar motor latencies recording second lumbrical and second interossei, respectively
  Comparison of median to radial sensory latencies recording thumb (antidromic)
Segmental nerve conduction studies
  Inching technique (antidromic)

- Comparing the median distal latency to the distal latency of the ulnar nerve or radial nerve obtained from the same hand. With these internal comparison studies, median nerve conduction values are expressed in relative rather than absolute terms. Also, patients serve as their own controls because variables affecting nerve conduction studies, such as temperature and distance, are held constant, allowing direct comparison of distal latencies.

Table C14–2 lists and Figure C14–3 shows the most common internal comparison NCSs used in the diagnosis of CTS. Most of these procedures yield abnormal findings in symptomatic patients. However, the absence of a gold standard for the diagnosis of CTS precludes the determination of sensitivity, specificity, or predictive value for any of these tests. Applying these sensitive techniques in combination increases the diagnostic yield of EDX testing in the diagnosis of CTS to approximately 95%.

Median-Ulnar Palmar Mixed Latency Difference "Palmar Study"

Trans-palmar mixed nerve conduction studies involve the elicitation of focal slowing of the median nerve between the palm and the wrist. Although abnormal absolute values were first considered to be a satisfactory indication in the diagnosis of CTS, comparison of median to ulnar latency with palmar stimulation has proved to be more sensitive and specific. The median nerve is stimulated in the mid-palm between the second and third metacarpals, and the ulnar nerve is stimulated between the fourth and fifth metacarpals. Recording occurs at the wrist over the median and ulnar nerves 8 cm proximal to the midpalm cathode (Figure C14–3A). Extreme care must be given to measurements of nerve segments and latency analyses to prevent false-negative and false-positive results. Initial reports suggested that a median-ulnar palmar difference of

Table C14–2. Internal Comparison Nerve Conduction Studies in the Evaluation of Carpal Tunnel Syndrome (CTS)

Study	Palmar Study	Digit 4 Sensory Study	Second Lumbrical-Interossei Study	Digit 1 Sensory Study
Description	Median-ulnar mixed palmar latency comparison	Median-ulnar sensory latency comparison	Median-ulnar motor latency comparison	Median-radial sensory latency comparison
Fibers evaluated	Mixed (sensory and motor)	Sensory (antidromic)	Motor	Sensory (antidromic)
Technique	Palm stimulation of the median and ulnar nerves, recording at the wrist	Median and ulnar nerves stimulation at the wrist recording ring fingers	Median and ulnar nerves stimulation at the wrist recording 2nd lumbrical and 2nd interossei, respectively (2nd interosseous space)	Median and radial nerves stimulation at the wrist recording thumb
Distance (range)	8 cm	14 cm (11–14 cm)	9 cm (8–10 cm)	10 cm (8–10 cm)
Abnormal values	Median-ulnar peak latency difference ≥0.4 ms	Median-ulnar peak latency difference ≥0.4 ms	Median-ulnar onset latency difference ≥0.6 ms	Median-radial peak latency difference ≥0.4 ms

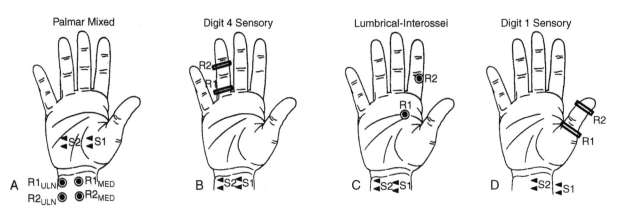

Figure C14–3. *Comparison studies in the diagnosis of carpal tunnel syndrome. S, stimulation site; R1 and R2, are active and reference recording sites, respectively. (From Katirji B, Kaminski HJ, Preston DC et al., eds. Neuromuscular disorders in clinical practice. Boston, MA: Butterworth-Heinemann, 2002.)*

greater than or equal to 0.2 ms is diagnostic of CTS; however, recent studies suggest that a difference of greater than or equal to 0.4 ms is needed for confirmation to prevent false-positive results (Figure C14–4A, A[1], and A[2]). A median-ulnar difference of 0.2 to 0.3 ms is considered borderline. It is estimated that palmar studies are abnormal in about 80% of symptomatic hands with CTS. In all published studies of CTS, palmar mixed nerve studies were far superior to the routine median sensory distal latency between the wrist and digit (index or middle finger).

Median-Ulnar Sensory Latency Difference Between the Wrist and the Ring Finger

In this study, the median and ulnar sensory distal latencies recording the ring finger are compared. When the technique is performed antidromically at a 11 to 14 cm distance (Figure C14–3B), the difference in peak latencies of greater than or equal to 0.4 ms is abnormal (Figure C14–4, B, B[1], and B[2]). This test is abnormal 80 to 90% of patients with CTS. Its only disadvantage is that the median or ulnar SNAPs may be low in amplitude and difficult to evoke, due to the variable sensory innervation of the ring finger. When done orthodromically, the response in patients with CTS has a double hump, the first peak reflecting the volume-conducted ulnar fibers, and the second peak reflecting the slowed median fibers. It is preferable, in this situation, to also record over the ulnar nerve at the wrist to confirm that the first peak represents the ulnar fibers.

Median-Ulnar Motor Latency Difference Recording the Second Lumbrical/Interossei

This motor study compares the distal motor latency of the median nerve, recording the second lumbrical muscle, to the ulnar motor latency, recording the second intersossei. The recording surface electrode is placed just lateral to the midpoint of a line over the third metacarpal bone that connects the base of the middle finger to the middle of the distal wrist crease. The reference electrode is placed over the second proximal interphalangeal joint (Figure C14–3C). The lumbrical and interosseous CMAPs are recorded when the median and ulnar nerves are stimulated at the wrist, respectively. If a standard and equal distance of 8–10 cm is used for both nerves, a median-ulnar distal latency difference of greater than or equal to 0.6 ms is consistent with CTS (Figure C14–4C, C[1] and C[2]). This technique has several advantages: (1) the motor responses are generally more easily recorded than sensory responses; (2) this study is able to localize the lesion to the wrist in over 90% of cases of severe CTS resulting in absent routine median CMAPs and SNAPs; and (3) this study can still be easily performed in patients with CTS and advanced polyneuropathy associated with absent sensory responses in the hands.

Median-Radial Sensory Latency Difference Between the Wrist and the Thumb

This technique compares the distal sensory latency of the median nerve to the latency of the radial nerve while the thumb is recorded (Figure C14–3D). This can be performed antidromically or orthodromically, but can be difficult to perform because of movement or stimulus artifacts. At an 8–10 cm distance, a difference of greater than or equal to 0.4 ms of peak latencies is considered abnormal (Figure C14–4D, D[1], and D[2]). This study is abnormal in about 80% of hands with CTS.

Other tests have been advocated but that have not proved to be superior nor specific for CTS and have no localizing value. This includes assessment for fibrillation potentials, myokymia, or chronic neurogenic changes of the thenar muscles, and delay of median minimal

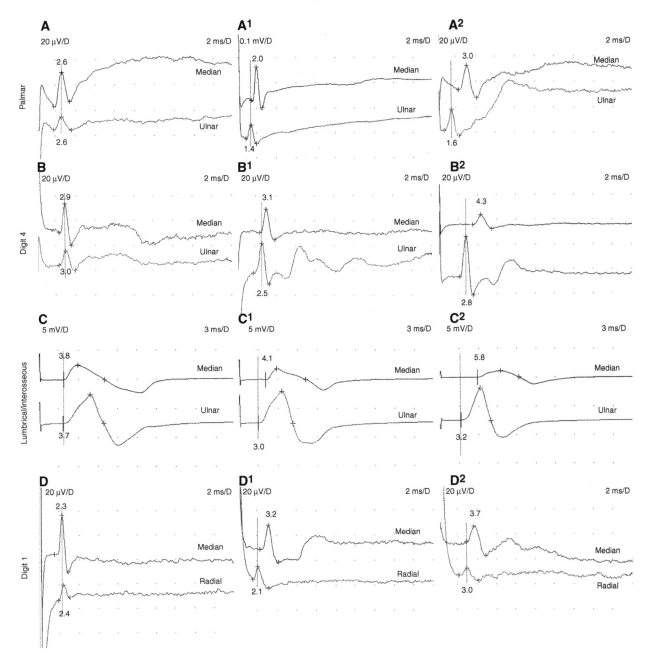

Figure C14–4. *Comparison studies in the diagnosis of carpal tunnel syndrome. The numbers shown are in ms and represent peak latencies. Palmar mixed study: (**A**) normal, (**A¹**) mildly abnormal and (**A²**) markedly abnormal. Digit 4 (median-ulnar) sensory study: (**B**) normal, (**B¹**) mildly abnormal and (**B²**) markedly abnormal. Second lumbrical/interosseous (median-ulnar) study: (**C**) normal, (**C¹**) mildly abnormal and (**C²**) markedly abnormal. Digit 1 sensory (median-radial) study: (**D**) normal, (**D¹**) mildly abnormal and (**D²**) markedly abnormal.*

F wave latencies when compared to the ulnar minimal F wave latencies.

Segmental Nerve Conduction Studies: "Inching" Studies

These studies, described by Kimura, consist of serial stimulations in 1 cm increments of the median nerve from the mid-palm to the distal forearm, recording antidromically from the index or middle finger (Figure C14–5). There usually is a latency change of 0.16 to 0.21 ms/cm between stimulation sites. In patients with CTS, there is an abrupt latency increase of greater than 0.4 to 0.5 ms across one or two adjoining segments (Figure C14–6). This most often occurs 2 to 4 cm distal to the distal wrist crease, the latter

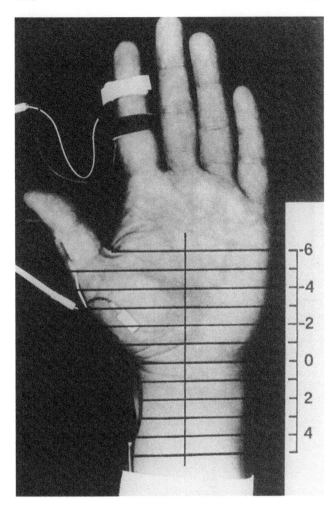

-6

-4

-2

0

2

4

Figure C14–5. *The inching technique of Kimura. Twelve sites of stimulation in 1 cm increments along the length of the median nerve. The 0 level at the distal crease of the wrist corresponds to the origin of the transverse carpal ligament. (From Kimura J. The carpal tunnel syndrome. Localization of conduction abnormalities within the distal segment of the median nerve. Brain 1979;102:619–635, with permission.)*

corresponding to the origin of the transverse carpal ligament. Although it is time consuming and subject to error (measurement error and volume conduction), the sensory study precisely localizes the lesion in more than 80% of symptomatic hands. Similar incremental study of the median nerve across the carpal tunnel, recording the abductor pollicis brevis, is also possible. However, unlike the sensory fibers, the median motor fibers are difficult to activate sequentially in 1 cm intervals because of the recurrent course of the motor branch to the thenar muscles; hence, the response is frequently contaminated by stimulus artifact because of the proximity of the recording electrode to the stimulating cathode.

Needle EMG

Needle EMG examination in patients with CTS has two objectives:

1. To evaluate the thenar muscles for evidence of axonal loss or active (ongoing) denervation. Increased spontaneous activity and fibrillation potentials is consistent with ongoing axonal loss, and is long considered a strong indication for surgical intervention. Large MUAPs and impaired recruitment suggest chronic loss of axons. Myokymic discharges are seen sometimes in the thenar muscles of patients with CTS, particularly in those with chronic axonal loss.

2. To exclude other causes of hand numbness or pain, particularly cervical radiculopathy. *It is estimated that one-quarter of patients with EDX evidence of CTS harbor a clinically significant cervical radiculopathy.* Thus, a root search, particularly of muscles innervated by the C6 and C7 roots, should be sampled in all patients with CTS. Hence, needle EMG in patients with CTS should include, in addition to the abductor pollicis brevis, at least the pronator teres, biceps, and triceps muscles.

Special Situations

Severe Carpal Tunnel Syndrome

In severe CTS, which is more common in elderly patients, absent median sensory NCS, recording all digits, and median motor NCS, recording APB, is not uncommon. This renders EDX localization of the median nerve lesion to the wrist not possible, despite classic manifestations. Traditionally, these lesions were poorly localized, by needle EMG only, at or above the wrist. In these situations, the sensory and mixed internal comparison studies are equally absent. However, the second lumbrical-interosseous motor comparison study confirms the lesion at the wrist in more than 90% of cases by revealing that the median motor response recording second lumbrical is still evokable often with marked slowing of median distal latency (Figure C14–7). The relative preservation of the motor fibers to the lumbrical muscles as compared to the thenar muscles is best explained by the fascicular distribution of the median nerve fibers within the carpal tunnel: Fibers to the lumbrical muscles, which are more centrally located, tend to be relatively spared from axonal loss late in the course of the disease while the motor fibers to the thenar muscles, as well the sensory fibers, located in the periphery of the nerve, are destroyed earlier.

Carpal Tunnel Syndrome With Peripheral Polyneuropathy

Carpal tunnel syndrome coexists not uncommonly in patients with underlying peripheral polyneuropathy, such

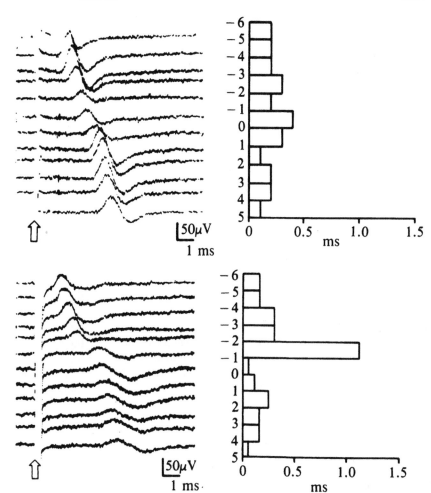

Figure C14–6. *The inching technique in a patient with carpal tunnel syndrome (CTS) (top is asymptomatic hand and bottom is symptomatic hand). The left side of the figure shows the results of 12 antidromically recorded sensory nerve action potentials (SNAPs), as shown in Figure C14–5. The right side of the figure graphs the successive time difference between traces. (From Kimura J. The carpal tunnel syndrome. Localization of conduction abnormalities within the distal segment of the median nerve. Brain 1979;102:619–635, with permission.)*

as with diabetes. In mild axonal polyneuropathies, where the SNAPs in the hands are still recorded though low in amplitudes and delayed in latencies, sensory, motor, or mixed nerve internal comparison studies are useful in showing the preferential slowing of the median fibers at the wrist due to entrapment at the carpal tunnel. In instances of severe axonal polyneuropathy, where the SNAPs are often absent in the hands, the second lumbrical-interosseous motor comparison study is the most accurate by demonstrating preferential focal slowing of median motor fibers across the carpal tunnel. In all axonal polyneuropathy cases, selective large fiber axon loss may cause slowing; hence, borderline or minimal latency differences on internal comparison studies should be cautiously interpreted.

Carpal Tunnel Syndrome With Martin-Gruber Anastomosis

Carpal tunnel syndrome occasionally occurs in a patient with Martin-Gruber anastomosis, an anomalous connection between the median and the ulnar nerves in the forearm

(see Chapter 2). When the anomalous fibers innervate the thenar muscles (usually adductor pollicis and deep head of flexor pollicis brevis), stimulation of the median nerve at the elbow activates the median nerve and the crossing ulnar fibers resulting in a large CMAP, with an initial positivity caused by volume conduction of action potential from ulnar thenar muscles to the median thenar muscles. This positive dip is not present at the wrist. Also, the median nerve conduction velocity in the forearm is spuriously fast in the presence of a CTS, since the CMAP onset represents different population of fibers at the wrist compared to the elbow (Figure C14–8). An accurate conduction velocity may be obtained by using specialized collision studies that abolish action potentials of the crossed fibers.

Carpal Tunnel Syndrome and Pregnancy

Up to 60% of pregnant women have nocturnal hand symptoms, most frequently during the third trimester of pregnancy, while the incidence of confirmed pregnancy-related CTS is about 40%. Limb edema is a significant predictor

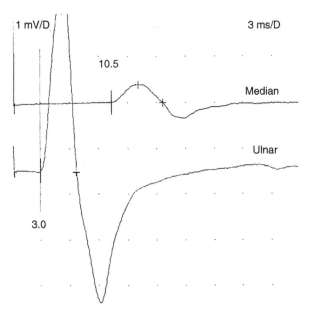

Figure C14–7. *The second lumbrical-interossei study in a patient with severe CTS resulting in absent routine median SNAPs and median CMAP recording APB. Note that the median CMAP recording second lumbrical is recorded with very long latency (and relatively low amplitude) when compared to the ulnar.*

for CTS during pregnancy. Symptoms resolve in most patients after delivery, while patients with significant weight gain, limb edema, or symptom onset during early pregnancy have lower probability for complete resolution. Treatment is usually conservative including wrist splinting,

corticosteroid injections, and oral diuretics. Most patients do not require EDX testing since symptoms usually resolve after delivery within 4–6 weeks.

When EDX studies are done during pregnancy, the pathophysiology in these patients is often median nerve demyelination resulting in focal slowing with or without conduction block across the wrist. In many of these cases, the routine NCSs reveal only slowing of distal latencies on routine or comparison studies. Some cases show low median motor or sensory amplitudes stimulating at the wrist, which may signify secondary axonal loss, conduction block, or a combination. The presence of conduction block can be confirmed by comparing motor and sensory amplitudes with stimulation at the wrist and in the palm (Figure C14–9). Palm stimulation of the median nerve recording the index or middle finger (sensory) or thenar muscles (motor) may be technically difficult because of shock artifact due to close proximity between the stimulating and recording electrodes. Due to normal (physiologic) temporal dispersion and phase cancellation of SNAP more than CMAP, median conduction block across the wrist should only be diagnosed when the drop of amplitudes exceeds 20% for median CMAPs and 40% for median SNAPs. The conduction block and slowing often resolves soon after delivery.

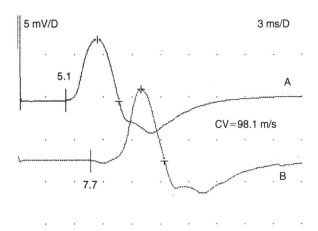

Figure C14–8. *Median motor nerve conduction study in a patient with moderately severe carpal tunnel syndrome and a Martin-Gruber anastomosis to the thenar muscle. Note the initial positive deflection stimulating the median nerve at the elbow (**B**) which is not present stimulating the nerve at the wrist (**A**). This results in a spuriously fast proximal latency (7.7 ms) and proximal conduction velocity (98.1 m/s).*

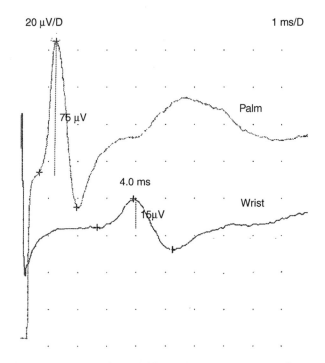

Figure C14–9. *Median antidromic sensory nerve conduction study, recording middle finger, in a pregnant woman with carpal tunnel syndrome. Note that the significant drop in SNAP amplitude across the wrist, from 75 µV at palm to 15 µV at wrist, with a significant slowing of distal latency stimulating at wrist (4.0 ms).*

FOLLOW-UP

The patient first underwent conservative treatment using splinting and nonsteroidal anti-inflammatory agents alone. Long-acting steroids were injected into the carpal tunnels, causing excellent results and reversal of symptoms. However, her paresthesias and pain recurred after 6 months. The patient then underwent bilateral carpal tunnel release with complete resolution of symptoms.

DIAGNOSIS
Bilateral carpal tunnel syndromes.

ANSWERS

1. E; 2. B; 3. B.

SUGGESTED READINGS

Al-Shekhlee A, Fernandes-Filho A, Sukul D et al. Optimal G1 placement in the lumbrical interosseous latency comparison study. Muscle Nerve 2006; 33: 289–293.

Boonyapisit K, Katirji B, Shapiro BE et al. Lumbrical and interossei recording in severe carpal tunnel syndrome. Muscle Nerve 2002;25:102–105.

Daube JR. Percutaneous palmar median nerve stimulation for carpal tunnel syndrome. Electroencephalogr Clin Neurophysiol 1977;43:139–140.

Gelberman RH, Aronson D, Weisman MH. Carpal tunnel syndrome: results of a prospective trial of steroid injection and splinting. J Bone Joint Surg 1980;52:253–255.

Giannini F et al. Electrophysiologic evaluation of local steroid injection in carpal tunnel syndrome. Arch Phys Med Rehabil 1991;72:738–742.

Eogan M, O'Brien C, Carolan D et al. Median and ulnar nerve conduction in pregnancy. Int J Gynecol Obstet 2004;87: 233–236.

Herskovitz S, Berger AR, Lipton RB. Low-dose, short-term oral prednisone in the treatment of carpal tunnel syndrome. Neurology 1995;45:1923–1925.

Hui ACF, Wong S, Leung CH et al. A randomized controlled trial of surgery vs steroid injection for carpal tunnel syndrome. Neurology 2005;64:2074–2078.

Jablecki CK et al. Literature review of the usefulness of nerve conduction studies and electromyography for the evaluation of carpal tunnel syndrome. Muscle Nerve 1993;16:1392–1414.

Jackson D, Clifford JC. Electrodiagnosis of mild carpal tunnel syndrome. Arch Phys Med Rehabil 1989;70:199–204.

Kimura J. The carpal tunnel syndrome. Localization of conduction abnormalities within the distal segment of the median nerve. Brain 1979;102:619–635.

Lesser EA, Venkatesh S, Preston DC et al. Stimulation distal to the lesion in patients with carpal tunnel syndrome. Muscle Nerve 1995;18:503–507.

Logigian EL, Busis NA, Berger AR et al. Lumbrical sparing in carpal tunnel syndrome: anatomic, physiologic, and diagnostic implications. Neurology 1987;37:1499–1505.

Loscher WN, Auer Grumbach M, Trinka E et al. Comparison of second lumbrical and interosseous latencies with standard measures of median nerve function across the carpal tunnel: a prospective study of 450 hands. J Neurol 2000;247:530–534.

McConnell JR, Bush DC. Intraneural steroid injection as a complication in the management of carpal tunnel syndrome: a report of three cases. Clin Orthop 1990;250:181–184.

Nathan PA, Meadows KD, Doyle LS. Sensory segmental latency values of the median nerve for a population of normal individuals. Arch Phys Med Rehabil 1988;69:499–501.

Padua L, Aprile I, Caliandro P et al. Symptoms and neurophysiological picture of carpal tunnel syndrome in pregnancy. Clin Neurophysiol 2001;112:1946–1951.

Padua L, Aprile I, Caliandro P et al. Carpal tunnel syndrome in pregnancy: multiperspective follow-up of untreated cases. Neurology 2002;59:1643–1646.

Pease WS, Cannell CD, Johnson EW. Median to radial latency difference test in mild carpal tunnel syndrome. Muscle Nerve 1989;12:905–909.

Phalen GS. The carpal tunnel syndrome: seventeen years' experience in diagnosis and treatment of six hundred and fifty-four hands. J Bone Joint Surg 1966;48:211–228.

Preston DC, Logigian EL. Lumbrical and interossei recording in carpal tunnel syndrome. Muscle Nerve 1992;15: 1253–1257.

Preston DC, Ross MH, Kothari MJ et al. The median-ulnar latency difference studies are comparable in mild carpal tunnel syndrome. Muscle Nerve 1994;17:1469–1471.

Redmond MD, Rivner MH. False positive electrodiagnostic tests in carpal tunnel syndrome. Muscle Nerve 1988;11: 511–518.

Report of the Quality Standards Sub-Committee of the American Academy of Neurology: practice parameter for carpal tunnel syndrome (summary statement). Neurology 1993;43:2406–2409.

Rosenbaum RB, Ochoa JL. Carpal tunnel syndrome and other disorders of the median nerve, 2nd ed. Boston, MA: Butterworth-Heinemann/Elsevier, 2002.

Schuchmann JA et al. Evaluation of local steroid injection in carpal tunnel syndrome. Arch Phys Med Rehabil 1971;52: 253–255.

Stevens JC. The electrodiagnosis of carpal tunnel syndrome. Muscle Nerve 1987;2:99–113.

Stevens JC et al. Carpal tunnel syndrome in Rochester, MN, 1961–1980. Neurology 1988;38:134–138.

Ubogu EE, Benatar M. Electrodiagnostic criteria for carpal tunnel syndrome in axonal polyneuropathy. Muscle Nerve 2006; 33: 747–752.

Uncini A, Lange DJ, Solomon M et al. Ring finger testing in carpal tunnel syndrome: a comparative study of diagnostic utility. Muscle Nerve 1989;12:735.

Wong S, Hui ACF, Tang A et al. Local vs systemic corticosteroids in the treatment of carpal tunnel syndrome. Neurology 2001;56:1565–1567.

Case 15

HISTORY AND PHYSICAL EXAMINATION

Slowly progressive weakness of right hand grip, with numbness of the right little finger developed in an 82-year-old woman over an 8- to 10-month period. She had difficulty buttoning her shirt, using her keys, and writing. At rest, she noticed that her right little finger withdrew in a semiflexed position. She had experienced chronic, deep, right elbow pain since she had a supracondylar humeral fracture 3 years earlier. Apart from a 5-year history of mild hypertension, she was in good health.

On examination, she had normal mental status and cranial nerve examination with no Horner sign. She had mild atrophy of the interossei, particularly of the first dorsal interossei. Hypothenar and thenar muscle bulk was normal. At rest, there was mild ulnar clawing, with flexion of the little and ring fingers. Manual muscle examination revealed weakness of all interossei and hypothenar muscles at Medical Research Council (MRC) 4/5. Froment sign, indicative of weak thumb adduction, was positive. Long finger flexors, thumb flexors and extensors, and wrist extensors and flexors were normal. All remaining muscle groups were normal. Sensation revealed a relatively decreased pin sensation over the right little finger, mostly close to its tip, with intact sensation in the forearm and arm. Tinel sign was negative on percussion of the ulnar nerve at the wrist and elbow. Deep tendon reflexes were normal. Gait and coordination were normal.

An electrodiagnostic (EDX) examination was performed.

Please now review the Nerve Conduction Studies and Needle EMG tables.

QUESTIONS

1. Ulnar motor nerve conductions with the elbow in extension may be:
   A. Spuriously slow.
   B. Spuriously fast.
   C. The same as expected.
2. The cubital tunnel is also referred to as all the following *except*:
   A. The humeroulnar arcade.
   B. Osborne ligament.
   C. The arcuate arcade.
   D. The ulnar groove.
3. The volume of the cubital tunnel under the humeroulnar arcade is smallest when the elbow is:
   A. Flexed at 45°.
   B. Extended.
   C. Flexed at 120°.
4. With an ulnar mononeuropathy across the elbow, which muscle is spared most often?
   A. First dorsal interosseous.
   B. Abductor digiti minimi.
   C. Adductor pollicis.
   D. Flexor carpi ulnaris

EDX FINDINGS AND INTERPRETATION OF DATA

The EDX findings in this patient include:

1. Absent ulnar sensory nerve action potential (SNAP), recording from the little finger. Although this abnormality points directly to the ulnar nerve, it has poor localizing value because it may be encountered with digital nerve lesions, most ulnar nerve lesions at or proximal to the wrist, or lower trunk/medial cord plexus lesions.
2. Low-amplitude dorsal ulnar SNAP (when compared with the contralateral SNAP). Because the dorsal ulnar cutaneous nerve arises from the ulnar nerve 6 to 8 cm

Case 15: Nerve Conduction Studies

Nerve Stimulated	Stimulation Site	Recording Site	Amplitude (m = mV, s = μV)			Distal/Peak Latency (ms)			Conduction Velocity (m/s)			F Latency (ms)	
			Right	Left	Normal	Right	Left	Normal	Right	Left	Normal	Right	Left
Ulnar (s)	Wrist	Little finger	**NR**	22	≥5	**NR**	3.1	≤3.2	**NR**	58	≥50		
Ulnar (s)	Above elbow	Little finger	**NR**	12			2.7						
Dorsal ulnar (s)	Wrist	Dorsum of hand	**8**	24	≥5	2.6		≤3.2					
Median (s)	Wrist	Index finger	25	24	≥10	3.6	3.7	≤3.8					
Median (s)	Elbow	Index finger	10	11					62	61	≥50		
Radial (s)	Forearm	Dorsum of hand	28		≥10	2.4		≤2.7					
Ulnar (m)	Wrist	ADM	**6.5**	10.0	≥7	3.2	3.0	≤3.2				**40**	27
Ulnar (m)	Below elbow	ADM	**5.0**	8.7					56	53	≥50		
Ulnar (m)	Above elbow	ADM	**2.5**	8.0					**33**	55	≥50		
Ulnar (m)	Wrist	First dors. interos.	**4.0**	10.0	≥7	4.5	4.2	≤4.6					
Ulnar (m)	Below elbow	First dors. interos.	**2.8**	8.8					56	54	≥50		
Ulnar (m)	Above elbow	First dors. interos.	**1.9**	8.2					**47**	56	≥50		
Median (m)	Wrist	APB	9.0		≥5	3.7		≤4.0				26	
Median (m)	Elbow	APB	8.0						58		≥50		

ADM = abductor digiti minimi; APB = abductor pollicis brevis; First dors. interos. = first dorsal interosseus; m = motor; NR = no response; s = sensory. Data in bold type are abnormal.

Case 15: Needle EMG

Muscle	Insertional Activity	Spontaneous Activity		Voluntary Motor Unit Action Potentials (MUAPs)							
				Recruitment				Configuration			
		Fibs	Fascs	Normal	Activation	Reduced	Early	Duration	Amplitude	% Polyphasia	Others
R. first dorsal interosseous	↑	1+	0			↓↓		↑	↑	↑	
Abductor pollicis	↑	+/–	0			↓↓		↑	↑	↑	
Abductor digit minimi	↑	Rare	0			↓↓		↑	↑	Normal	
Abductor pollicis brevis	Normal	0	0	X				Normal	Normal	Normal	
Flexor pollicis longus	Normal	0	0	X				Normal	Normal	Normal	
Extensor indicis	Normal	0	0	X				Normal	Normal	Normal	
Pronator teres	Normal	0	0	X				Normal	Normal	Normal	
Flexor carpi ulnaris	↑	0	0			↓		↑	↑	Normal	
Flexor dig. profundus	Normal	0	0	X				Normal	Normal	Normal	
Biceps	Normal	0	0	X				Normal	Normal	Normal	
Triceps	Normal	0	0	X				Normal	Normal	Normal	
Deltoid	Normal	0	0	X				Normal	Normal	Normal	
Midcervical paraspinal	Normal	0	0	–							
Low cervical paraspinal	Normal	0	0	–							

Fascs = fasciculations; Fibs = fibrillations; Flexor dig. profundus = flexor digitorum profundus; R. = right; ↑ = increased; ↓ = mildly reduced; ↓↓ = moderately reduced; ↓↓↓ = severely reduced.

above the wrist, this abnormality is extremely helpful in excluding an ulnar nerve lesion at the wrist.

3. Low-amplitude ulnar compound muscle action potential (CMAP), recording the hypothenar muscle (abductor digiti minimi [ADM]) and the first dorsal interosseous, with distal stimulation at the wrist. In the presence of a normal median CMAP, the low ulnar CMAP points to the ulnar nerve and renders a plexus lesion less likely. It also implies that the process has resulted in axonal loss.

4. Conduction block of ulnar motor fibers, recording the ADM. This is evident by comparing CMAP amplitudes and areas with below-elbow to above-elbow stimulations, recording the ADM (Figure C15–1). The former has an amplitude of 5.0 mV and the latter 2.5 mV, which amounts to a 50% amplitude decay without temporal dispersion. The block is confirmed by a decrease (33.5%) in CMAP area (from 11.7 mV ms to 7.78 mV ms). The amplitude and area decay is significant since the distance between the two stimulation sites is short (around 10 cm). Despite the conduction block to ADM, there was no conduction block across the elbow, recording the first dorsal interosseous. This is consistent with selective fascicular involvement (by a demyelinative conduction block) of the ulnar fibers directed to the hypothenar muscles.

5. Focal slowing of ulnar motor conduction velocities (CVs) across the elbow, recording the ADM. This was achieved by comparing values of below the elbow-to-wrist segment (CV = 56 m/s) with those across the elbow segment (CV = 33 m/s). Here, the difference of 23 m/s is significant and consistent with focal slowing of ulnar motor fibers across the elbow. In contrast, when recording the first dorsal interosseous, the CV difference between the same segments (56 – 47 = 9 m/s) is not significant enough to localize the lesion definitely to the elbow region (despite absolute slowing of the across the elbow segment to CV of 47 m/s). This is again compatible with preferential fascicular involvement of fibers directed to the ADM in this patient.

6. Needle EMG, revealing fibrillation potentials of mild to moderate degree in all three ulnar-innervated muscles tested in the hand (the first dorsal interosseous, the abductor digiti minimi, and the adductor pollicis). There was moderate reduction of recruited motor unit action potentials (MUAPs). All MUAPs recorded from the ulnar muscles were increased in duration and amplitude, with a significant increase in polyphasic MUAPs. The forearm muscles revealed a mildly denervated flexor carpi ulnaris (FCU) but a normal ulnar part of the flexor digitorum profundus (FDP). In contrast, all C8/T1-innervated muscles via the median (abductor pollicis brevis and flexor pollicis longus) and radial

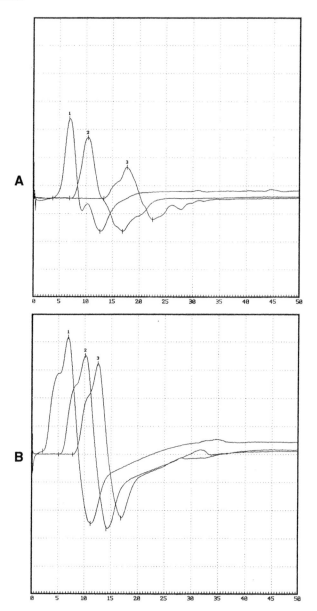

Figure C15–1. *Motor conduction studies of the right ulnar nerve, recording the abductor digiti minimi in this patient (**A**), compared with an age-matched control (**B**). The sensitivity (vertical scale) is 2 mV/division in both. Responses 1 are at the wrist, 2 below the elbow, and 3 above the elbow. Note that there is (1) partial conduction block across the elbow, evidenced by the significant decrease in amplitude (50%) and area (35%); (2) focal slowing, as easily recognized by the prominent delay in proximal latency of the third response, compared with the second (despite a shorter distance across the elbow compared with forearm), and resulting in a 33 m/s velocity across the elbow compared to a 56 m/s velocity in the forearm; and (3) slight motor fiber axonal loss, based on the low-amplitude distal compound motor action potential (Response 1A = 6.5 mV) compared with normal controls (Response 1B = 8.5 mV).*

(extensor indicis) nerves were normal, excluding a lower brachial plexopathy (lower trunk or medial cord).

In summary, this patient has a slowly progressive right ulnar mononeuropathy across the elbow, with signs of segmental demyelination (confirmed by conduction block and focal slowing) and axonal loss (evidenced by low distal/ulnar CMAPs and absent/low ulnar SNAPs); there is also ongoing denervation (fibrillation potentials) and reinnervation (demonstrated by long-duration, high-amplitude, and polyphasic MUAPs). In view of the patient's history (remote elbow fracture), this case is an example of tardy ulnar palsy.

DISCUSSION

Applied Anatomy

The ulnar nerve sensory and motor fibers are derived from the spinal nerves C8 and T1. Before arising from the plexus in the proximal axilla, the ulnar nerve fibers pass through the lower trunk and the medial cord of the brachial plexus (Figure C15–2). In the axilla and proximal arm, the ulnar nerve is closely related to the radial and median nerves and the brachial artery. Around the midarm, the ulnar nerve pierces the intermuscular septum and lies in close contact with the medial head of the triceps and humerus. The ulnar nerve develops no branches in the arm.

At the elbow level, and in contrast to most major human peripheral nerves, the ulnar nerve traverses the extensor, rather than the flexor, surface of the elbow joint. This renders the nerve more vulnerable to trauma around the elbow. At the elbow, the ulnar nerve crosses the *ulnar groove* (also called the *condylar* or *retroepicondylar groove*) behind the medial epicondyle and then passes the aponeurotic arch of the FCU to enter the *cubital tunnel* (Figure C15–3). This tunnel, also called the *humeroulnar arcade*, *Osborne ligament*, or *arcuate arcade*, is formed by the attachment of the muscle to the olecranon and medial epicondyle. Its proximal edge is variable but usually is approximately 1 cm distal to an imaginary line drawn between these two insertional points. With flexion of the elbow, the distance between the olecranon and medial epicondyle increases by approximately 1 cm, which results in tightening of the FCU aponeurosis over the nerve. In addition, the medial elbow ligament bulges, flattening the concave surface of the ulnar groove.

In the forearm, the ulnar nerve gives off its first branches. These are the motor branches to the FCU and FDP. These branches arise approximately 10 cm distal to the medial epicondyle. The ulnar nerve continues in the forearm deep to the FCU but superficial to the FDP to

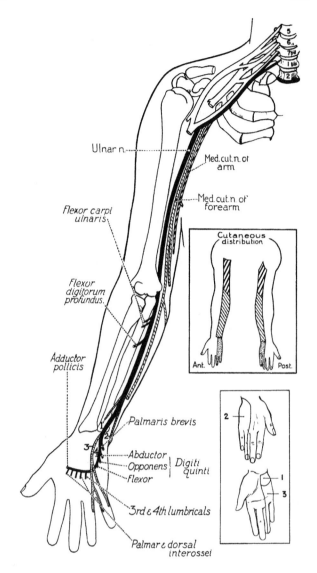

Figure C15–2. *Course of the ulnar nerve and its branches. 1. Palmar ulnar cutaneous branch; 2. dorsal ulnar cutaneous branch; 3. terminal cutaneous superficial branch; 4. terminal deep palmar motor branch. (From Haymaker W, Woodhall B. Peripheral nerve injuries. Philadelphia, PA: WB Saunders, 1953, with permission.)*

become superficial in the distal forearm, lying between the tendons of these two muscles. Two cutaneous sensory branches arise in the forearm, without passing through Guyon canal at the wrist, to innervate the skin in the hand. The first is the *palmar ulnar cutaneous branch*, which takes off at midforearm and innervates the proximal part of the ulnar border of the palm. The second is the *dorsal ulnar cutaneous branch*, which arises 6 to 8 cm proximal to the ulnar styloid, winds around the ulna, and innervates the dorsal surfaces of the little finger and half of the ring

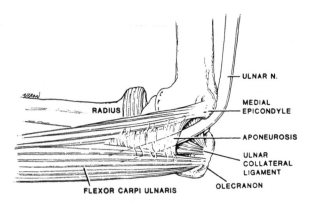

Figure C15–3. *View of the medial surface of the elbow, showing the course of the ulnar nerve through the ulnar groove and cubital tunnel. (From Kincaid JC. The electrodiagnosis of ulnar neuropathy at the elbow. Muscle Nerve 1988;11:1005–1015, with permission.)*

finger, along with the ulnar side of the dorsum of the hand (Figure C15–4).

At the wrist, the ulnar nerve enters the *distal ulnar tunnel (Guyon canal)*, where it divides into superficial (primarily sensory) and deep palmar (pure motor) branches (Figure C15–5). The superficial branch innervates the palmaris brevis muscle and the palmar aspects of digit V and half of digit IV. The deep branch innervates the hypothenar muscles, including the ADM, and travels through the palm to the dorsal and palmar interossei, the third and fourth lumbricals, the adductor pollicis, and a portion of the flexor pollicis brevis.

The flexor brevis digiti minimi (or quinti), a hypothenar muscle, has two separate attachments, at the hook of the hamate and at the pisiform bone. These musculotendinous

attachments form a fibrous arch and create the superficial boundary of the *pisohamate hiatus (PHH),* an opening through which the deep motor branch of the ulnar nerve passes. The posterior boundary of the PHH, the pisohamate ligament, extends from the pisiform bone to the hook of the hamate (Figure C15–6). The origin of the major motor branch to the ADM is proximal to this hiatus in the majority of hands.

Clinical Features

Ulnar mononeuropathy across the elbow is a common entrapment neuropathy. It is second only to carpal tunnel syndrome in the incidence of entrapment neuropathy in general. Ulnar neuropathies across the elbow are usually caused by compression, although isolated ulnar mononeuropathy resulting from nerve infarction (such as in vasculitic neuropathy) or associated with leprosy, may occur infrequently. Causes of compressive ulnar lesions across the elbow are shown in Table C15–1. Compression of the ulnar nerve in the elbow region occurs frequently at one of the two following sites: the ulnar (condylar) groove or cubital tunnel (humeroulnar (arcuate) aponeurotic arcade). In some patients with unequivocally ulnar nerve lesions around the elbow, it is difficult to identify the exact cause, even during surgery. Most surgeons presume that the lesion is within the cubital tunnel and treat it as such.

1. *Cubital tunnel syndrome.* This entrapment neuropathy accounts for many ulnar nerve lesions at the elbow, particularly in patients with no history of trauma, elbow deformity, or arthritis, and possibly congenitally tight

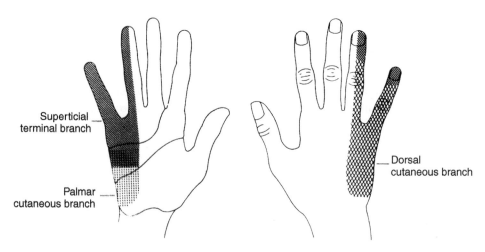

Figure C15–4. *The cutaneous distribution of the three sensory branches of the ulnar nerve. (From Stewart JD. The variable clinical manifestations of ulnar neuropathies at the elbow. J Neurol Neurosurg Psychiatry 1987;50:252–258, BMJ Publishing Group.)*

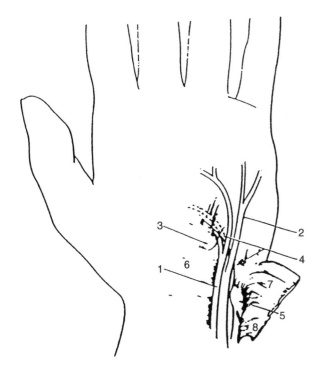

Figure C15–5. *Anatomy of the ulnar nerve within Guyon canal at the wrist. 1 = ulnar artery, 2 = superficial branch of the ulnar nerve, 3 = hamulus, 4 = fibrous arch of the hypothenar muscles (see also Figure C15–2), 5 = pisiform, 6 = transverse carpal ligament, 7 = palmaris brevis, 8 = palmar carpal ligament. (From Gross MS, Gelberman RH. The anatomy of the distal ulnar tunnel. Clin Orthop 1985;196:238–247, with permission.)*

cubital tunnels. The site of the compression in these patients is the proximal edge of the FCU aponeurosis, also called the arcuate ligament (see Figure C15–3). As outlined, the distance between the olecranon and the medial epicondyle increases during elbow flexion by

approximately 1 cm, which results in tightening of the ligament over the ulnar nerve. Also, with flexion, the medial collateral ligament bulges out into the cubital tunnel, thus further compromising the ulnar nerve.

2. *Ulnar neuropathy at the groove.* Chronic minor trauma, repetitive and persistent flexion or chronic leaning on the elbow may either exacerbate or cause ulnar neuropathy at the groove. Subluxation and reduction of the ulnar nerve from the ulnar (condylar) groove, during flexion and extension of the elbow respectively, are potential causes of repetitive ulnar nerve trauma, which results in ulnar neuropathy at the groove. It is estimated that the ulnar nerve may sublux out of the ulnar grove in approximately 16% of the population. This can be confirmed at the bedside by finding the nerve in the groove and rolling it over the medial epicondyle.

3. *Tardy ulnar palsy.* This term refers to a chronic ulnar neuropathy at the elbow, which occurs many years after a distal humeral fracture sometimes in association with a valgus deformity. This term should be restricted to this group of patients, but is unfortunately misused, particularly by surgeons, who often use it to refer to all chronic ulnar neuropathies at the elbow.

Patients with ulnar mononeuropathy at the elbow usually present with numbness and tingling of the little and ring fingers and variable degrees of hand weakness. Less commonly, patients present with weakness and wasting, with no clear sensory symptoms. Elbow pain, particularly around the medial epicondyle, is not uncommon. Weakness of hand with loss of dexterity and pinch strength are common symptoms in moderate entrapment. Patients may report that their little finger gets caught when trying to put their hand in their pocket (due to weakness of the third

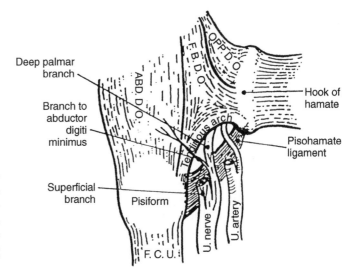

Figure C15–6. *The pisohamate hiatus (PHH) in the distal portion of Guyon canal. U. = Ulnar; F.C.U. = flexor carpi ulnaris; ABD.D.Q. = abductor digiti quinti (or minimi); F.B.D.Q. = flexor brevis digiti quinti (or minimi); Opp.D.Q. = opponens digiti quinti. (Modified from Uriburu IJF, Morchio FJ, Marin JC. Compression syndrome of the deep motor branch of the ulnar nerve [pisohamate hiatus syndrome]. J Bone Joint Surg 1976;58A:145–147, with permission.)*

Table C15–1. Causes of Compressive Ulnar Nerve Lesions Across the Elbow

Pressure
  External event (e.g., habitual elbow leaning)
  Single event (e.g., anesthesia)
  Repetitive events (e.g., occupational repetitive
    flexion/extension)
  Internal event
    Soft tissue masses
    Fibrosis following trauma
    Anomalous muscles
Bony deformities
  Acute
    Fracture/dislocation
  Chronic
    Healed fractures
    Medial epicondyle
    Lateral epicondyle
    Humeral supracondylar
    Additional elbow joint deformities
    Rheumatoid arthritis
    Valgus deformity and shallow postcondylar groove
    Supracondylar spur (ligament of Struthers)
Cubital tunnel syndrome
Chronic subluxation
Idiopathic causes

Modified from Dimitru D. Electrodiagnostic medicine. Philadelphia, PA: Hanley and Belfus, 1995.

palmar interosseous muscle). Occasionally, patients may present because of intrinsic muscle hand atrophy.

Neurologic examination may reveal a positive Tinel sign. This is produced by percussion of the ulnar nerve at the elbow; however, this sign may be positive in many healthy subjects. Sensory examination may be normal despite sensory symptoms. More often, there is a relative sensory loss in the tips of both the little and ring fingers on the palmar surface only. Unfortunately, this finding is a poor localizing sign because it is abnormal with ulnar nerve lesions (anywhere at, or proximal to, the wrist), lower brachial plexus lesions (lower trunk or medial cord), and C8 radiculopathy. However, other sensory findings are more helpful in localization. These include the following:

1. Sensory loss of the palmar and dorsal surfaces of the little and ring fingers and the ulnar side of the hand. This excludes an ulnar lesion at the wrist (i.e., at Guyon canal) because there is involvement of the territory of the dorsal ulnar cutaneous branch. This branch arises above the wrist and does not pass through Guyon canal.
2. Sensory loss of the medial half of the ring finger, which spares the lateral half. This is pathognomonic of an ulnar nerve lesion and is not seen in lower plexus or C8 root lesions.

3. Sensory loss that extends more than 2 to 3 cm above the wrist. This finding, when confirmed on objective examination, excludes an ulnar nerve lesion, because the skin of the medial forearm is innervated by the medial cutaneous nerve of the forearm, which is a branch of the medial cord of the plexus. Abnormalities in this territory suggest a lesion of the lower plexus, the C8 or T1 roots, or the medial cutaneous nerve of the forearm itself.

Inspection of the hand at rest in patients with moderate or severe ulnar mononeuropathy may reveal ulnar clawing. An *ulnar claw hand*, also called *Benediction posture* (Figure C15–7), is caused by: (1) hyperextension of the metacarpophalangeal joints of the little and ring fingers caused by weakness of the third and fourth lumbricals, thus allowing the extensor digitorum communis to exert an unopposed pull; and (2) flexion of the interphalangeal joints of the same fingers resulting from an inherent flexion muscle tone of the FDP and superficialis muscles, whose tendons are stretched over the metacarpophalangeal joints because of the above hyperextension. In ulnar lesions, this clawing is more noticeable when the FDP is spared. The *Wartenberg* sign is recognized as abduction of the little finger at rest due to weakness of the third palmar interosseous muscle.

Weakness of ulnar-innervated muscles in the hand predominates in ulnar nerve lesions across the elbow; the forearm muscles are affected less often. Weakness of the FDP to the fourth and fifth digits is assessed by flexion of the distal interphalangeal joints of these digits. Positive *Froment sign* is helpful in the clinical diagnosis of ulnar neuropathy because it shows the weakness of the adductor pollicis (ulnar muscle) and the normal flexor pollicis longus

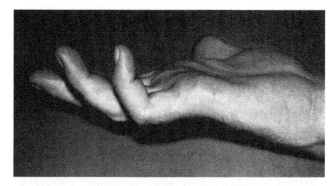

Figure C15–7. *Ulnar claw hand. Note the hyperextension of the fourth and fifth metacarpophalangeal joints with flexion of the interphalangeal joints. (From Haymaker W, Woodhall B. Peripheral nerve injuries. Philadelphia, PA: WB Saunders, 1953, with permission.)*

(median muscle), both of which are innervated by the C8/T1 roots via the lower plexus. This sign is assessed by asking the patient to grasp a piece of paper between the thumb and second digit. Because of weakness of the adductor pollicis, the patient uses the flexor pollicis longus as a substitute in an attempt to keep the paper from sliding (Figure C15–8).

Many patients with ulnar nerve lesions at the elbow have variable weakness and numbness distally. This is explained by the propensity for partial focal lesions to affect fascicles differentially within that nerve. This *fascicular phenomenon* is common in ulnar nerve lesions across the elbow and is demonstrated in Figure C15–9. Atrophy of ulnar muscles in the hand is common with long-standing lesions and is most apparent in the interossei, particularly the first dorsal interosseous (see Figure C15–8).

Treatment of ulnar neuropathy at the elbow may be conservative or surgical. Identification and reversal of the cause of repetitive compression is essential. Many patients with mild symptoms and signs who demonstrate evidence of slowing or conduction block on nerve conduction studies may be treated successfully using conservative approaches (Table C15–2). Patients with substantial weakness, particularly when progressive or associated with evidence of axonal loss or ongoing denervation, benefit from surgery. There is no clear consensus on the optimal surgical procedure. Simple decompression of the cubital tunnel may be ideal for patients with cubital tunnel syndrome, while medial epicondylectomy or submuscular transposition

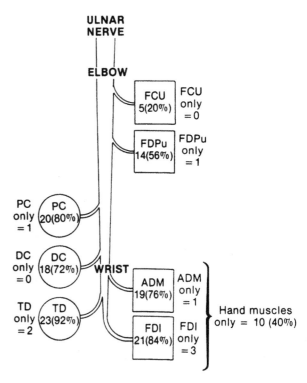

Figure C15–9. *Clinical abnormalities in the distribution of three sensory and four motor branches of the ulnar nerve in 25 patients with ulnar neuropathy at the elbow. "Only" is used to denote the number of patients in whom a single sensory area was involved, as well as to denote those patients with weakness of only one of the four muscles. ADM = abductor digiti minimi, DC = dorsal cutaneous, FCU = flexor carpi ulnaris, FDI = first dorsal interosseous, FDP = flexor digitorum profundus, PC = palmar cutaneous, TD = terminal digital branches. (From Stewart JD. The variable clinical manifestations of ulnar neuropathies at the elbow. J Neurol Neurosurg Psychiatry 1987;50:252–258, BMJ Publishing Group.)*

of the ulnar nerve are more suitable for compression at the ulnar groove. Submuscular transposition has a higher success rate but is a more complex surgery and carries a risk of nerve devascularization and ischemia.

Electrodiagnosis

Although it is the second most common site of peripheral nerve entrapment, electrodiagnostic localization of ulnar mononeuropathy at the elbow is controversial and challenging because of anatomic, technical, and pathophysiologic factors. The pathophysiologic process of ulnar nerve lesions at the elbow is extremely variable. In contrast to carpal tunnel syndrome, in which slowing across the carpal tunnel is the hallmark of the disease, ulnar mononeuropathy across the elbow may present with focal slowing, conduction block, differential slowing, axon loss, or, more

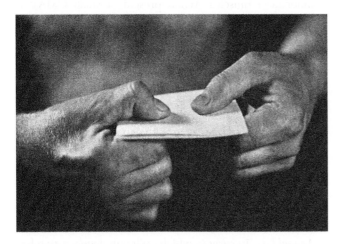

Figure C15–8. *Froment sign in an ulnar nerve lesion. The patient is asked to pull a piece of paper apart with both hands. Note that the right hand (affected hand with interosseous atrophy) flexes the thumb (by using the flexor pollicis longus) to prevent the paper from slipping out of the hand, thus substituting for the weakness of the adductor pollicis. (From Haymaker W, Woodhall B. Peripheral nerve injuries. Philadelphia, PA: WB Saunders, 1953, with permission.)*

Table C15–2. Conservative Measures in the Treatment of Mild Ulnar Neuropathy at the Elbow

In general, minimize elbow flexion

At a desk, place a pillow beneath the elbow

While sitting, the arm should not be crossed, but the elbow should be straightened and the arm rested on thigh

For extended reading, a bookstand should be used

The telephone should be held in the opposite asymptomatic hand

During sleep, a towel should be wrapped loosely around the elbow, with the elbow in no more than 30° of flexion

The aforementioned measures should be tried consistently over at least 3 months

Adapted with revision from Dellon AL, Hament W, Gittelshon A. Nonoperative management of cubital tunnel syndrome: an 8-year prospective study. Neurology 1993;43:1673–1677.

frequently, any combination of the above. Although acute lesions generally present with conduction block and/or axon loss, and chronic lesions usually present with focal slowing and/or axon loss, many ulnar lesions across the elbow do not comply with this rule.

Nerve conduction studies (NCSs) that are recommended for the evaluation of ulnar mononeuropathy across the elbow include the following.

Sensory NCS
Ulnar SNAP Recording the Little Finger

This antidromic study, or its orthodromic counterpart, is often low in amplitude or absent in ulnar nerve lesions across the elbow. Unfortunately, although this abnormality is seen with many ulnar lesions at or above the wrist, it is also encountered with lower trunk and medial cord plexus lesions because ulnar sensory fibers pass through these structures. Stimulating the ulnar nerve above the elbow while recording the little finger is helpful in the attempt to document evidence of focal slowing of sensory fibers. In practical terms, this technique is seldom helpful in localization.

Dorsal Ulnar SNAP, Recording the Dorsum of the Hand

Unfortunately, a fascicular lesion of the ulnar nerve across the elbow occasionally may spare the dorsal ulnar SNAP. Hence, an absent or low-amplitude dorsal ulnar SNAP excludes a lesion at the wrist or hand, but a normal dorsal ulnar SNAP does not exclude an ulnar lesion across the elbow. Also, there is considerable overlap between the territories of the dorsal ulnar SNAP and the radial SNAP; therefore, an absent or low-amplitude SNAP can

be occasionally misleading unless radial sensory stimulation is attempted during recording of the ulnar side of the dorsum of the hand.

Motor NCS
Ulnar Motor Conduction Studies, Recording the Hypothenar Muscles (ADM)

This is a routine motor conduction study that is performed in many laboratories. The nerve is stimulated at the wrist, below the elbow, and above the elbow. Stimulation at the axilla also is sometimes useful because it allows comparison of two segments (forearm and arm) to the across-elbow segment and also evaluate for rare ulnar nerve lesions in the arm. Erb point (supraclavicular) stimulation is also occasionally helpful in excluding a high ulnar nerve lesion (Figure C15–10). The conduction abnormalities observed across the elbow are:

- *Conduction block.* With focal segmental demyelination at the elbow, the CMAP that is elicited with above-elbow stimulation is much lower in amplitude (>20–30% decrease in amplitude and area) than the response obtained with below-elbow stimulation without CMAP dispersion. All patients with apparent conduction block of the ulnar motor fibers should undergo further investigation to rule out the presence of an anomalous connection between the median and ulnar nerves, named *Martin-Gruber anastomosis.* This occurs in approximately 20% of the population and is sometimes bilateral. It may be established easily by stimulating the median nerve while recording the ulnar-innervated muscles. When present, a small CMAP is recorded and accounts for the apparent conduction block in the forearm. Occasionally, an ulnar lesion across the elbow may occur in a patient with this anastomosis (Figure C15–11).
- *Focal slowing.* With mild (mostly paranodal) demyelination, there is slowing of conduction across the elbow. This is confirmed by comparing the conduction velocities across the elbow, such as the above-elbow-to-below elbow segment to the below-elbow-to-wrist (forearm) segment. Comparison with the contralateral side in unilateral cases also is helpful. A combination of conduction block and focal slowing is a common presentation of acute/subacute ulnar lesions across the elbow (Figure C15–12).
- *Axonal loss.* In cases in which wallerian degeneration has occurred, ulnar CMAP is low in amplitude at all points of stimulation, with no significant change in configuration, amplitude, or conduction velocity. The conduction velocities may be mildly slowed diffusely if there is significant axonal loss (due to the loss of large fibers), but no focal slowing is present. Unfortunately, motor conduction

10 mV/D   3 ms/D

20 mV/D   3 ms/D

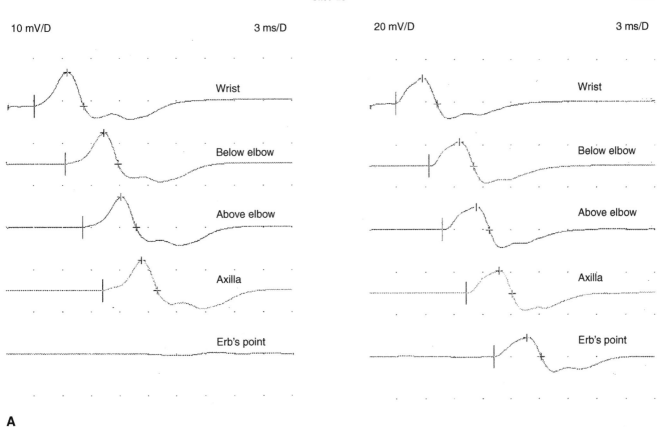

A

B

Figure C15–10. *A 35-year-old man awoke with severe left ulnar nerve palsy resulting in ulnar clawing and sensory loss in palmar and dorsal aspect of medial hand. Initial routine nerve conduction study, recording hypothenar muscles, was normal except for absent ulnar F wave. Subsequent, five point stimulation of the ulnar nerve that included axilla and Erb point stimulations revealed complete conduction block between these two points (**A**) with normal responses on the asymptomatic side (**B**). The patient reported later that he had slept in the bathtub, after drinking heavily that night, and draped his left arm over the edge of the tub to keep his head above water. He had complete recovery of function in 6 weeks.*

studies are unable to accurately localize the site of ulnar lesion in this situation.

- *Combinations of the above.* This is a common finding, particularly with chronic ulnar lesions across the elbow (Figure C15–13).

Ulnar Motor Conduction Studies Recording the First Dorsal Interosseous

This is a helpful addition to routine ulnar motor conduction studies (recording the ADM). The stimulation points are the same as those used for the routine studies, and the pathophysiologic possibilities are similar. The addition of this study increases the localizing utility of ulnar motor conduction studies by 10 to 20%, partially because of the potential fascicular and differential involvement of fibers across the elbow. For example, an ulnar lesion might

produce only axon loss to the hypothenar muscle, but it can cause a combination of axonal loss with conduction block and/or focal slowing to the fibers directed to the first dorsal interosseous. The presence of a focal conduction block or slowing to the first dorsal interosseous become diagnostically useful. Also, this study is very useful in suspected ulnar nerve lesions at the wrist or palm.

Needle EMG

Needle examination is useful in confirming an ulnar nerve lesion and in excluding a C8/T1 root lesion or a lower brachial plexopathy. It is important to establish that the C8/T1 muscles innervated by the median nerve (such as the abductor pollicis brevis or the flexor pollicis longus) and radial nerve (such as the extensor indicis proprius) are normal. In addition, in purely axonal lesions of the ulnar

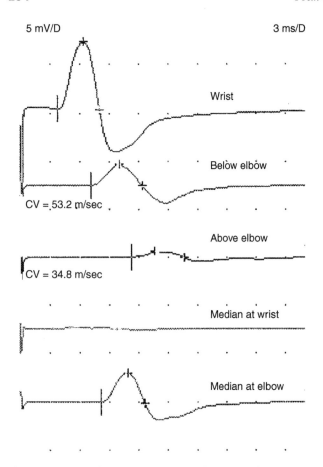

5 mV/D   3 ms/D

Wrist

Below elbow

CV = 53.2 m/sec

Above elbow

CV = 34.8 m/sec

Median at wrist

Median at elbow

Figure C15–11. *Ulnar motor nerve conduction study, recording hypothenar muscle, in a patient with Martin-Gruber anastomosis and ulnar mononeuropathy across the elbow. Note that there are two drops in amplitude and area, one in the forearm and another across the elbow. The amplitude decay in the forearm (6.8 mV at wrist and 2.5 mV below elbow) is explained by Martin-Gruber anastomosis as evidenced by a large CMAP (3.0 mV) obtained by stimulating the median nerve at the elbow, while recording the hypothenar muscles. This response is not present upon stimulating the median nerve at the wrist. The block across the elbow (2.5 mV below elbow and 1.0 mV above elbow) is also associated with focal slowing and is consistent with a concomitant ulnar mononeuropathy across the elbow.*

nerve, needle EMG is crucial in localizing the lesion to a particular segment of the nerve, which it does by establishing that muscles distal to the lesion are abnormal and muscles proximal to it are normal. Unfortunately, there are limitations to the accurate localization by needle EMG in patients with axonal ulnar neuropathies:

1. The ulnar nerve has no motor branches in the arm and only a few branches in the forearm (to the FCU and the FDP). This makes accurate localization in patients with purely axon-loss lesions (not associated with conduction block, differential slowing, or focal

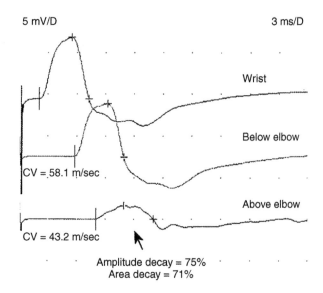

5 mV/D   3 ms/D

Wrist

Below elbow

CV = 58.1 m/sec

Above elbow

CV = 43.2 m/sec

Amplitude decay = 75%
Area decay = 71%

Figure C15–12. *Ulnar motor nerve conduction study, recording hypothenar muscle, in a patient with several months' history of ulnar mononeuropathy, revealing evidence of conduction block and focal slowing across the elbow. The distal (wrist) CMAP amplitude is normal (8.5 mV) which is consistent with no (or minimal) axon loss.*

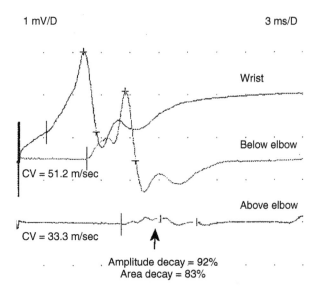

1 mV/D   3 ms/D

Wrist

Below elbow

CV = 51.2 m/sec

Above elbow

CV = 33.3 m/sec

Amplitude decay = 92%
Area decay = 83%

Figure C15–13. *Ulnar motor nerve conduction study, recording hypothenar muscle, in a patient with a year history of ulnar mononeuropathy, revealing evidence of conduction block, focal slowing, and differential slowing (dispersion) across the elbow, along with axon loss. The latter is based on very low amplitude distal (wrist) CMAP (1.8 mV).*

slowing) a difficult task. Thus, if the FCU or the FDP is denervated when the lesion is axonal (i.e., not associated with conduction block or differential or focal slowing), then the ulnar lesion could be localized only at or proximal to the elbow (i.e., at the elbow or in the arm).

2. The ulnar motor fibers directed to the hand are located anteromedially within the ulnar nerve at the elbow region. Therefore, these fibers are most closely related to the cubital tunnel and the bony ulnar groove. In contrast, the motor fibers to the forearm muscles are located far from the usual sites of compression. This explains, in part, why the forearm-innervated muscles (the FCU and the FDP) are spared with lesions around the elbow in at least half the cases. Thus, in purely axonal lesions that are associated with normal FCU and FDP muscles, the ulnar lesion is even more poorly localized at or proximal to the wrist (if the dorsal ulnar SNAP is normal), or at or proximal to the distal forearm (if the dorsal ulnar SNAP is absent/low in amplitude).

Electrodiagnostic Controversies

Ongoing controversies in the electrodiagnostic evaluation of ulnar mononeuropathy across the elbow include the following:

In Which Position Should the Elbow Be Placed During Performance of Ulnar Nerve Conduction Studies (Extension or Degree of Flexion)?

The ulnar nerve is anatomically lax and redundant in the ulnar groove when the elbow is extended. This is aimed to provide the extra nerve length needed during elbow flexion. With flexion the nerve uncoil and become more taut,

and when flexion bypass 90°, the ulnar nerve may sublux in up to 20% of individuals.

Hence, surface measurements of the ulnar nerve while the elbow is extended do not reflect the true extent of the underlying nerve. In fact, the distance measured over the skin is shorter than the true length of the nerve. Hence, the conduction velocity is spuriously slowed because the impulses travel longer distances than can be estimated on skin measurement (Figure C15–14). On the other hand, surface measurements of the ulnar nerve while the elbow is hyperflexed more than 90° may be longer than the true nerve length (due to potential nerve subluxation) resulting in artifactually fast conduction velocity.

Despite the above findings, advocates for flexion or extension techniques continue to debate this issue and whether elbow position influences the sensitivity and specificity of motor nerve conduction studies in the diagnosis of ulnar mononeuropathy across the elbow. Also, there is no consensus as to the optimal degree of elbow flexion, ranging from 45° to 135°, among advocates of flexion techniques. Surface measurement over the skin with the elbow flexed at 45° to 90° most closely correlates with the true length of the nerve. This is the angle range advocated by many electromyographers. Hyperflexion beyond 90° is, however, not recommended.

How Much Slowing of Motor Fibers Across the Elbow is Needed to Make a Diagnosis of Ulnar Mononeuropathy?

Measurement of conduction velocities is subject to error. This error is largely the result of inaccurate measurement of distance between the sites of stimulation. Because the

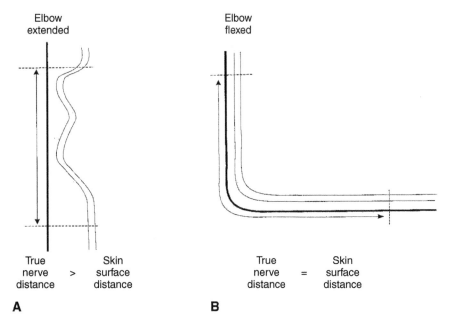

Figure C15–14. *Correlation between the true nerve distance and the skin surface distance of the ulnar nerve during extension (**A**) and flexion (**B**). The lack of correlation with the elbow in extension leads to spurious slowing of conduction velocity. (From Campbell WW. Electrophysiological approaches to the diagnosis and assessment of ulnar neuropathy: a historical and literature review. In: 2002 American Association of Electrodiagnostic Medicine plenary session, Toronto, Ontario, with permission.)*

error may involve many millimeters, using short distances between stimulation sites results in a relatively large percentage of error in the measurement of distance and, hence, in the assessment of conduction velocity. In other words, conduction velocities of longer nerve segments are more accurate and subject to less human error than velocities of shorter segments.

Based on this principle, the following is recommended:

• The distance between the below-elbow and the above-elbow stimulation sites should be kept at least at 6–10 cm.
• Comparison of motor conduction velocities of ulnar nerve segments is essential for localization, and is far more useful than are absolute values. The motor conduction velocities may be calculated using one of two methods: The short segment method compares velocities of the above-elbow-to-below-elbow segment to the below-elbow-to-wrist segment. This has more room for error in measurement. The long segment compares the above-elbow-to-wrist segment to the below-elbow-to-wrist segment. This carries the chance of false negatives by including a short area of demyelination at the elbow in a longer above-elbow-to-wrist segment.
• In general, focal slowing greater than 10 m/s across elbow compared to forearm conduction velocity is diagnostic of ulnar lesion when the study is performed with the elbow flexed between 45° and 90°. The author recommend that more stringent slowing (greater than 15 m/s) should be used when the study done while the elbow is in extension.

Are Short Segment Incremental Studies ("Inching") Required for Accurate Diagnosis?

The "inching" technique is helpful when a conduction block or slowing is seen between the above-elbow and below-elbow stimulations. It is recommended by some for precise (point) localization of the lesion in patients with suspected ulnar nerve lesions across the elbow. This may have both clinical and surgical implications, particularly in planning the optimal surgical procedure.

The stimulation site is moved progressively along the nerve across the elbow, in several equal steps (usually 1–2 cm), between the below and above elbow (over about 6–8 cm span) and CMAP amplitude, latency or morphology are recorded. This study should be done meticulously since it is subject to measurement error and volume conduction. An abrupt change in CMAP amplitude, morphology or latency (>0.5 ms) is noted (Figure C15–15). The short increment technique could also be used to point localize lesions in other segments of the ulnar nerve, such as the arm or forearm (Figure C15–16).

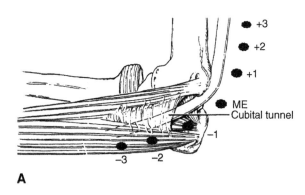

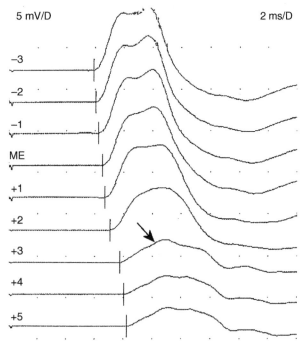

Figure C15–15. *Short incremental ("inching") motor conduction study, recording hypothenar muscles, in a patient with ulnar neuropathy across the elbow. The reference point is at the medial epicondyle (ME) and the negative numbers are successive distal stimulation points while the positive points are successive proximal stimulation sites (A). Note in (B) that there is a more prominent latency change of 0.8 ms and amplitude decay of 85% between points +2 and +3 (arrow), localizing the lesion between 2 and 3 cm above the medial epicondyle. The latency change between all other successive points ranged between 0.1 to 0.3 ms while the amplitude decay ranged between 5 and 20%.*

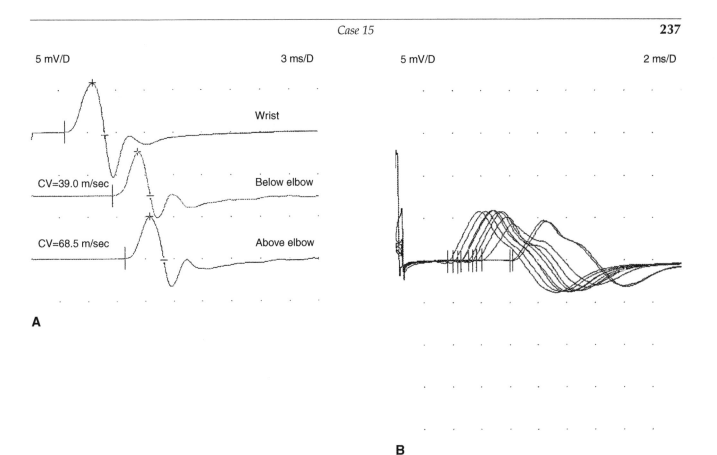

5 mV/D   3 ms/D   5 mV/D   2 ms/D

Wrist

CV=39.0 m/sec   Below elbow

CV=68.5 m/sec   Above elbow

A

B

Figure C15–16. *A 65-year-old woman presented with a year history of intermittent numbness of left little and ring fingers. All ulnar nerve conduction studies were normal except for slowing of ulnar motor fibers, recording hypothenar muscles (**A**), in the forearm segment (39 m/s) compared to across the elbow segment (68.5 m/s). Similar slowing was noted recording first dorsal interosseous muscle (not shown). Subsequent short incremental ("inching") study, recording hypothenar muscles, starting distally at the ulnar styloid and moving in 2 cm increments proximally, revealed a significant latency shift between 14 cm and 16 cm proximal to the styloid (**B**) (responses are shown superimposed). Subsequent MRI revealed a mass at the site and a schwannoma was removed successfully.*

FOLLOW-UP

The patient underwent exploration of the ulnar nerve at the elbow. Extensive fibrosis was seen around the ulnar groove. The nerve was released. The patient had some early, rapid return of function over the first 6 weeks, followed by a slower recovery phase. When seen 12 months postoperatively, she was asymptomatic and had minimal weakness and atrophy of the interossei.

DIAGNOSIS

Right ulnar mononeuropathy across the elbow, manifested by segmental demyelination and chronic axonal loss, with evidence of ongoing (active) denervation and reinnervation, after remote elbow fracture (consistent with tardy ulnar palsy).

ANSWERS

1. A; 2. D; 3. C; 4. D.

SUGGESTED READINGS

Bielawski M, Hallet M. Position of the elbow in determination of abnormal motor conduction of the ulnar nerve across the elbow. Muscle Nerve 1989;12:803–809.

Campbell WW et al. Intraoperative electroneurography: management of ulnar neuropathy at the elbow. Muscle Nerve 1988;11:75–81.

Campbell WW, Pridgeon RM, Sahni KS. Short segment incremental studies in the evaluation of ulnar neuropathy at the elbow. Muscle Nerve 1992;15:1050–1054.

Checkles NS, Russakov AD, Piero DL. Ulnar nerve conduction velocity: effect of elbow position on measurement. Arch Phys Med Rehabil 1971;53:362–365.

Dellon AL, Hament W, Gittelshon A. Nonoperative management of cubital tunnel syndrome: an 8-year prospective study. Neurology 1993;43:1673–1677.

Eisen A, Danon J. The mild cubital tunnel syndrome. Neurology 1974;24:608–613.

Jabley ME, Wallace WH, Heckler FR. Internal topography of the major nerves of the forearm and hand. J Hand Surg 1980;5:1–21.

Katirji MB, Katirji PM. Proximal ulnar mononeuropathy caused by conduction block at Erb's point. Arch Neurol 1988;45:460–461.

Kincaid JC. The electrodiagnosis of ulnar neuropathy at the elbow. Muscle Nerve 1988;11:1005–1015.

Kothari MJ, Preston DC. Comparison of the flexed and extended elbow positions in localizing ulnar neuropathy at the elbow. Muscle Nerve 1995;18:336–340.

Miller RG. The cubital tunnel syndrome: diagnosis and precise localization. Ann Neurol 1979;6:56–59.

Payan J. Electrophysiological localization of ulnar nerve lesions. J Neurol Neurosurg Psychiatry 1969;32:208–220.

Peterson AR et al. Variations in dorsomedial hand innervation. Electrodiagnostic implications. Arch Neurol 1992;49:870–873.

Stewart JD. The variable clinical manifestations of ulnar neuropathies at the elbow. J Neurol Neurosurg Psychiatry 1987;50:252–258.

Ventakesh S, Kothari MJ, Preston DC. The limitations of the dorsal ulnar cutaneous sensory response in patients with ulnar neuropathy at the elbow. Muscle Nerve 1995;18:345–347.

Case 16

HISTORY AND PHYSICAL EXAMINATION

Acute, severe right upper extremity pain developed overnight in a 22-year-old man; it peaked in 2 days, resulted in multiple visits to the emergency room, and ultimately led to admission to a community hospital on the third day. The pain was deep and maximal around the right shoulder, with radiation to the arm and forearm, and did not worsen with coughing or sneezing. Three to four days after admission, while the patient was being treated with analgesics, he noted weakness of the right upper extremity. The weakness was maximal in the shoulder and arm, and much less severe in the hand. He had slight numbness in the hand and forearm, most particularly in the right thumb. He was given a 10-day course of oral prednisone and was referred to a tertiary care center.

Two weeks before the onset of pain, the patient had an upper respiratory tract infection with cough, nasal discharge, fever, and malaise. This was treated with antibiotics for one week. There was no history of trauma. He was otherwise in excellent health.

When the patient was seen 4 weeks after the onset of symptoms, he had minimal shoulder pain. Cranial nerve examination was normal. There was no Horner sign. Findings were limited to the right upper extremity, where there was complete loss of function of the right deltoid, spinati, biceps, and brachioradialis (Medical Research Council [MRC] 0/5). The right triceps was much less involved (4/5). There was mild diffuse weakness of all finger and wrist extensors, with severe weakness of the right thumb long flexion (flexor pollicis longus) and distal interphalangeal flexion of the index and middle fingers (flexor digitorum profundus). This resulted in a positive pincer or OK sign (Figure C16–1). Deep tendon reflexes of the right upper limb were absent. Sensation revealed mild sensory loss over the thumb, and lateral arm and forearm.

An electrodiagnostic (EDX) study was performed.

Please now review the Nerve Conduction Studies and Needle EMG tables.

QUESTIONS

1. The clinical and EDX findings suggest that most of the insult involves the following two nerves:
   A. Ulnar and radial nerves.
   B. Medial cord and anterior interosseous nerve.
   C. Upper trunk and anterior interosseous nerve.
   D. Lateral cord and radial nerve.
2. The aforementioned disorder has the following characteristics *except:*
   A. It is more frequent in males.
   B. It is sometimes preceded by upper respiratory tract infection or vaccination.
   C. It is typically painful at onset.
   D. It sometimes is bilateral and rarely recurrent.
   E. It is restricted to the neural elements of the brachial plexus.
3. The routine motor nerve conduction study results in this disorder may be normal because:
   A. The illness is not associated with significant axonal loss.
   B. The lesion involves frequently the upper trunk of the brachial plexus.
   C. The process is demyelinating.
   D. All of the above.

EDX FINDINGS AND INTERPRETATION OF DATA

Abnormalities on EDX examination include:

1. Abnormal sensory nerve action potential (SNAP) amplitudes. As a rule, abnormal SNAPs point to lesions of the plexus or peripheral nerves, and are not consistent

Case 16: Nerve Conduction Studies

Nerve Stimulated	Stimulation Site	Recording Site	Amplitude (m = mV, s = µV)			Distal/Peak Latency (ms)			Conduction Velocity (m/s)			F Latency (ms)	
			Right	Left	Normal	Right	Left	Normal	Right	Left	Normal	Right	Left
Median (s)	Wrist	Thumb	6	25	≥20	3.2	2.8	≤3.3					
Median (s)	Wrist	Index finger	8	27	≥20	3.0	2.8	≤3.3					
Median (s)	Wrist	Middle finger	**19**	26	≥20	3.0	2.7	≤3.3					
Ulnar (s)	Wrist	Little finger	**16**	19	≥18	2.6	2.7	≤3.0					
Radial (s)	Wrist	Dorsum of hand	**13**	28	≥18	2.6	2.3	≤2.7					
Lat. cut. fore. (s)	Elbow	Forearm	**NR**	20	≥16	**NR**	2.5	≤2.9					
Median (m)	Wrist	APB	**6.0**	10.0	≥6.0	3.8	3.3	≤3.9				26	28
Median (m)	Elbow	APB	**6.0**	9.5					57	56	≥51		
Ulnar (m)	Wrist	ADM	9.0	12.5	≥8.0	3.0	2.9	≤3.0				27	265
Ulnar (m)	Above elbow	ADM	8.6	12.0					52	53	≥51		
Ulnar (m)	Axilla	ADM	8.0	11.7					55	57	≥51		
Ulnar (m)	Erb point	ADM	7.4	11.4					56	55	≥51		
Musculocut. (m)	Axilla	Biceps	**0.2**	5.4	≥4.0	2.9	2.6	≤3.5					
Musculocut. (m)	Erb point	Biceps	**0.1**	4.9					**45**	59	≥51		
Axillary (m)	Erb point	Deltoid	**0.2**	5.0	≥4.0	3.5	2.4	≤4.8					

ADM = abductor digiti minimi; APB = abductor pollicis brevis; Lat. cut. fore. = lateral cutaneous nerve of forearm; m = motor; Musculocut. = musculocutaneous; NR = no response; s = sensory. Data in bold type are abnormal.

Case 16: Needle EMG

| Muscle | Insertional Activity | Spontaneous Activity | | Voluntary Motor Unit Action Potentials (MUAPs) | | | | | | | |
| | | Fibs | Fasces | Recruitment | | | | Configuration | | | |
				Normal	Activation	Reduced	Early	Duration	Amplitude	% Polyphasia	Others
R. first dorsal interosseous	↑	+/−	0			↓		Normal	Normal	Normal	
Abductor pollicis brevis	↑	+/−	0			↓		Normal	Normal	Normal	
Abductor digit minimi	↑	+/−	0			↓		Normal	Normal	Normal	
Flexor pollicis longus	↑	2+	0			↓↓↓		Normal	Normal	Normal	
Pronator quadratus	↑	2+	0			↓↓↓		Normal	Normal	Normal	
Flexor digit. profundus	↑	2+	0			↓↓↓		Normal	Normal	Normal	
Extensor indicis	↑	Rare	0			↓		Normal	Normal	↑	
Extensor digit. comm.	↑	Rare	0			↓		Normal	Normal	↑	
Pronator teres	↑	1+	0			↓		Normal	Normal	Normal	
Brachioradialis	↑	3+	0	None fired							
Biceps	↑	3+	0	None fired							
Triceps	↑	+/−	0			↓		Normal	Normal	↑	
Deltoid	↑	3+	0	None fired							
Infraspinatus	↑	3+	0	None fired							
Supraspinatus	↑	3+	0	None fired							
Serratus anterior	Normal	0	0	Normal				Normal	Normal	Normal	
Rhomboidus	Normal	0	0	Normal				Normal	Normal	Normal	
Midcervical paraspinal	Normal	0	0	−							
Low cervical paraspinal	Normal	0	0	−							
L. biceps	Normal	0	0	Normal				Normal	Normal	Normal	
Deltoid	Normal	0	0	Normal				Normal	Normal	Normal	
Flexor pollicis longus	Normal	0	0	Normal				Normal	Normal	Normal	

Extensor digit. comm. = extensor digitorum communis; Fasces = fasciculations; Fibs = fibrillations; Flexor digit. profundus = flexor digitorum profundus (median part); L. = left; R. = right; ↑ = increased; ↓ = mildly reduced; ↓↓↓ = severely reduced.

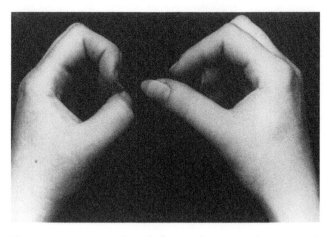

Figure 16C–1. *Normal and abnormal OK sign (pincer sign). Normal sign on the left and abnormal sign on the right, as in lesions of the anterior interosseous nerve caused by weakness of the long flexors of the thumb and index fingers. (From Mumenthaler M, Schliak H. Peripheral nerve lesions. Diagnosis and therapy. New York: Thieme Medical Publishers, 1990.)*

with root lesions (i.e., intraspinal canal lesions) because the latter interfere only with the proximal (central) axons of the dorsal root ganglia, leaving the distal (peripheral) axons intact. Although the SNAP abnormalities are diffuse, when one compares the right upper extremity to the left, the most abnormal SNAPs in order of decreasing severity are: lateral cutaneous of forearm (lateral antebrachial); median, recording the thumb and index; radial and median, recording the middle finger; and ulnar, recording the little finger. This suggests that the disorder is diffuse but has a preponderance to the upper plexus (upper trunk and lateral cord), where sensory fibers to the lateral cutaneous nerve of the forearm and median nerve are located.

2. Abnormal compound muscle action potential (CMAP) amplitudes. The CMAPs of routine motor nerve conduction studies (NCS), i.e., median and ulnar, are not as abnormal as the less commonly performed NCS, i.e., the axillary and musculocutaneous. This finding points to a pathological process that involves primarily the upper trunk of the brachial plexus or individual lesions of both the musculocutaneous and axillary nerves. The relatively lower median CMAP compared with the ulnar CMAP could be caused by a median nerve lesion or a fascicular lesion of the lower plexus (lower trunk or medial cord).

3. Needle EMG examination shows diffuse abnormalities in all muscles tested on the right, except the paraspinal, serratus anterior, and rhomboid muscles. This finding

confirms that the lesion(s) is not at the level of the roots but is located more distally into the brachial plexus or peripheral nerves. Concurrent with diffuse involvement, certain muscles are exceptionally abnormal. These include:

- Severe denervation of the flexor pollicis longus, the pronator quadratus, and the median part of the flexor digitorum profundus, consistent with severe lesion of the anterior interosseous nerve.
- Total denervation of the supraspinatus, infraspinatus, deltoid, biceps, and brachioradialis consistent with severe lesion of the upper trunk of the brachial plexus. In this situation, it is impossible to confirm or exclude additional separate lesions of the suprascapular, axillary, or musculocutaneous nerves.

The aforementioned findings point to a diffuse, likely multifocal process involving the neural elements of the upper extremity, with the most severe involvement to the upper trunk of the brachial plexus and the anterior interosseous nerve. The process is not the result of root(s) pathology (i.e., it is not due to intraspinal canal process), because of abnormal SNAPs and normal paraspinal muscles. The EDX findings are highly suggestive of neuralgic amyotrophy due to the predilection of lesions to the upper trunk and the anterior interosseous nerve.

DISCUSSION

Clinical Features

Neuralgic amyotrophy is likely an immune-mediated disorder that affects peripheral nerves of the upper limb and is not restricted to elements of the brachial plexus. Unfortunately, the disorder is known by several misleading names that result sometimes in misdiagnosis (Table C16–1). Neuralgic amyotrophy has an estimated annual incidence of 1.64 cases per 100 000 population. It most often affects adults, peaking during their twenties. Males are affected twice as often as females. It is usually unilateral, but is sometimes bilateral and asymmetrical; it is occasionally recurrent. Most cases have no specific precipitating factors, but some appear few hours to weeks of an upper respiratory tract infection, a vaccination, childbirth, or an invasive diagnostic, therapeutic or surgical procedure.

As the most popular name implies, neuralgic amyotrophy is characterized by pain and weakness of the upper limb. The pain is usually abrupt in onset with a tendency to develop at night, sometimes awakening the patient from sleep. It is a severe deep boring shoulder pain, and maximal during the first few days of illness. The pain is not exacerbated by the Valsalva maneuver (e.g., cough, sneeze)

Table C16–1. Terms Commonly Used to Describe the Syndrome of Neuralgic Amyotrophy (Listed Alphabetically)

Acute brachial plexitis
Acute brachial plexopathy
Acute brachial neuropathy
Acute brachial neuritis
Acute brachial radiculitis
Brachial plexus neuritis
Brachial plexus neuropathy
Idiopathic brachial plexopathy
Idiopathic brachial neuritis
Neuralgic amyotrophy
Parsonage-Turner syndrome
Shoulder girdle neuritis

which helps distinguishing it from a subacute cervical radiculopathy. Many patients visit the emergency department for pain control. In atypical cases, the pain is only modest and maximal over the antecubital fossa. The pain usually lasts for 7–10 days, gradually fades and becomes replaced by a dull ache.

Typically, the patient notices upper limb weakness, and sometimes wasting become apparent, during the first week as the pain starts to subside. Weakness of the shoulder girdle muscles, with or without scapular winging, is the most common since the upper plexus-innervated muscles are usually the most affected. The weakness is often restricted to multiple individual peripheral nerves and sometimes to a single nerve only (Table C16–2). Occasionally, the disorder afflicts the entire brachial plexus or exclusively the lower plexus leading to a near complete monoplegia or distal upper extremity weakness, respectively. Oddly, the main upper limb nerves, i.e., the median, ulnar, and radial nerves, are seldom exclusively affected. Occasionally, selective muscles are selectively denervated, presumably due to pathology of the motor branches. This includes the pronator teres, flexor pollicis longus and

Table C16–2. Peripheral Nerves With High Predilection to Insult During Neuralgic Amyotrophy (Listed in Order of Frequency of Occurrence)

Long thoracic nerve
Suprascapular nerve
Axillary nerve
Musculocutaneous nerve
Anterior interosseous nerve
Phrenic nerve

supraspinatus muscles (Figure C16–2). Sensory loss usually is mild but may be prominent in severe cases. Deep tendon reflexes are depressed or absent if the appropriate muscles are weakened significantly. Chest radiographs may reveal an elevated hemidiaphragm on the ipsilateral side, due to phrenic nerve palsy. Routine magnetic resonance imaging studies of the brachial plexus or upper limb usually are normal, apart from T2-weighted changes of denervated muscles. The diagnosis frequently is based on the clinical picture and is supported by EDX confirmation.

The long-term prognosis is overall good. Pain resolves within weeks. Muscle strength lags behind, but most patients recover almost completely within a few months. Some have a more protracted improvement with more prolonged pain or residual weakness and atrophy. Permanent weakness occurs when there is severe axonal loss, or when distal muscles are affected. Recurrence is rare (1–5%), usually occurring at highly irregular intervals over months to years.

There is no specific therapy for neuralgic amyotrophy. Strong analgesics are often necessary for pain control. Drugs that target neuropathic pain, such as anticonvulsants and tricyclics, are also useful. Corticosteroids often are prescribed in the acute phase, particularly in patients who have no contraindication to their use. Physical and occupational therapies are essential to maintain range of joint motion and to prevent contractures during the first months of illness.

The differential diagnosis of neuralgic amyotrophy is wide and depends upon the particular nerve(s) affected and the specific antecedent event. It includes rotator cuff tears, cervical radiculopathies, traumatic plexopathies, intraoperative nerve damage, and entrapment neuropathies. *Pack palsy* occasionally is mistaken for neuralgic amyotrophy, but the clinical circumstances and the fact that pain is not a component of its presentation help in distinguishing pack palsy from neuralgic amyotrophy. A familial disorder that is sometimes indistinguishable clinically and electrodiagnostically from the sporadic form of neuralgic amyotrophy occurs, and is inherited as an autosomal dominant trait. This disorder is often called *hereditary neuralgic amyotrophy*, or *familial brachial plexus neuropathy* and is linked to the distal long arm of chromosomes 17q25, with three mutations in the gene septin 9 identified so far. Certain features tend to help in establishing the diagnosis for these families (Table C16–3). Acute brachial plexopathy may occur after minor trauma in patients with another autosomal dominant disorder, *hereditary neuropathy with liability to pressure palsy (HNPP)*. However, the plexopathy in HNPP is typically painless and resolves more rapidly. Also, the neurological examination as well as the nerve conduction

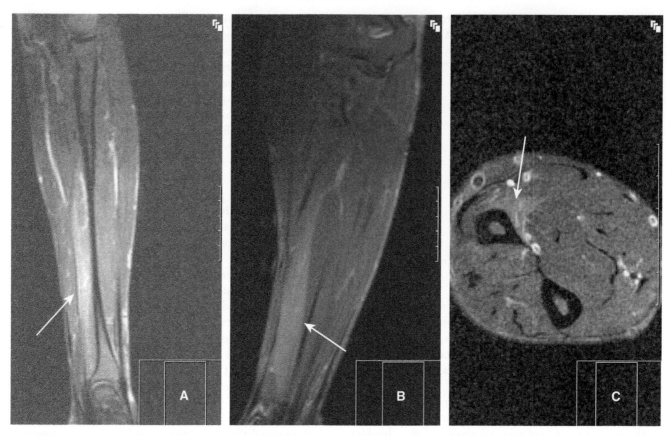

Figure 16C–2. *MRI of the forearm in a 37-year-old man who noted severe weakness of thumb flexion which was preceded by mild dull antecubital pain. Needle EMG showed prominent fibrillation potentials and no voluntary MUAPs in the flexor pollicis longus. In contrast, the median sensory and motor conduction studies, as well as needle EMG of all other muscles innervated by the median nerve, anterior interosseous nerve, and C8/T1 roots were normal. Note the high signal intensity in the flexor pollicis longus (white arrows), seen on sagittal (**A**), coronal (**B**), and axial (**C**) views of the forearm, consistent with denervation.*

studies in other limbs often reveal an underlying generalized demyelinating polyneuropathy. The diagnosis is confirmed by detecting deletion of the human peripheral myelin protein 22 (PMP22) gene, located on chromosome 17p11.2-12. Also, if done, pathologic studies of peripheral nerves reveal evidence of segmental demyelination and tomaculous or "sausage-like" formations.

Electrodiagnosis

In assessing a patient with possible neuralgic amyotrophy, the electromyographer should have a firm grasp of the anatomy of the brachial plexus and its branches (Figure C16–3), as well as the peripheral nerves of the upper extremity (Table C16–4) and the myotomal chart of all muscles of the upper limb (see Figure C11–6).

Table C16–3. Distinguishing Features of Sporadic Neuralgic Amyotrophy and Hereditary Neuralgic Amyotrophy

Feature	Sporadic Neuralgic Amyotrophy	Hereditary Neuralgic Amyotrophy
Age	Adulthood	Onset is frequently in childhood
Sex	Male predominate	Males and females equally affected
Family history	Negative	Positive (dominant trait)
Recurrence	Rare (1–5%)	Common
Lower cranial nerve involvement	Exceedingly rare	Not uncommon
Associated findings	None	Dysmorphic features (cleft palate, canthal folds, syndactyly, etc.)

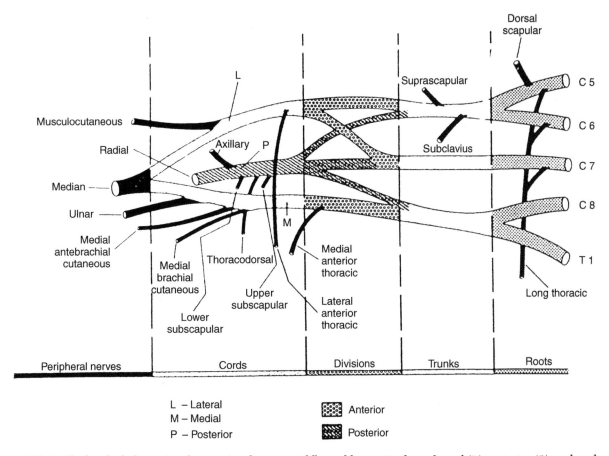

Figure 16C–3. *The brachial plexus. Trunks are named upper, middle, and lower. Cords are lateral (L), posterior (P), and median (M). Roots and trunks are supraclavicular, while cords and terminal peripheral nerves are infraclavicular. (From Goodgold J. Anatomical correlates of clinical electromyography. Baltimore, MD: Williams and Wilkins, 1974, with permission.)*

Table C16–4. Motor and Sensory Nerves Arising Directly from the Brachial Plexus (excluding the main terminal nerves)

Nerve	Origin	Function	Destination
Dorsal scapular*	Anterior ramus of C5	Motor	Rhomboids (C5)
Long thoracic*	Anterior rami of C5–C6–C7	Motor	Serratus anterior (C5–C6–C7)
Suprascapular*	Upper trunk	Motor	Supraspinatus (C5–C6) and infraspinatus
N. to subclavius*	Upper trunk	Motor	Subclavius (C5–C6)
Lateral pectoral (lateral anterior thoracic)	Lateral cord	Motor	Pectoralis major and minor (C5 to T1)
Subscapular (upper and lower)	Posterior cord	Motor	Teres major (C5–C6) and subscapularis (C5–C6)
Thoracodorsal	Posterior cord	Motor	Latissimus dorsi (C6–C7–C8)
Medial pectoral (medial anterior thoracic)	Medial cord	Motor	Pectoralis major and minor (C5 to T1)
Medial cutaneous of arm (brachial cutaneous)	Medial cord	Sensory	Skin of medial arm (C8–T1)
Lateral cutaneous of forearm (antebrachial cutaneous)	Medial cord	Sensory	Skin of medial arm (C8–T1)

*Are the only supraclavicular nerves.

Three important anatomical facts must be emphasized in localizing lesions of the brachial plexus:

1. *The median sensory fibers do not pass through the lower plexus.* The thumb SNAP is innervated by C6 through the upper trunk, the index finger by C6 and C7 through the upper and middle trunks, and the middle finger by C7 through the middle trunk. All three SNAPs traverse the lateral cord to reach the median nerve. The lateral antebrachial SNAP is similar to the median SNAP to the thumb, originating in C6 and passing through the upper trunk and lateral cord to the musculocutaneous nerve. The radial SNAP originates from the C6 and C7 roots and reaches the posterior cord via the upper and middle trunks (Figure C16–4). All these SNAPs are normal in lower brachial plexus lesions (lower trunk or medial cord) while the ulnar SNAP originating from C8, and the medial antebrachial SNAP originating from T1, are usually abnormal.

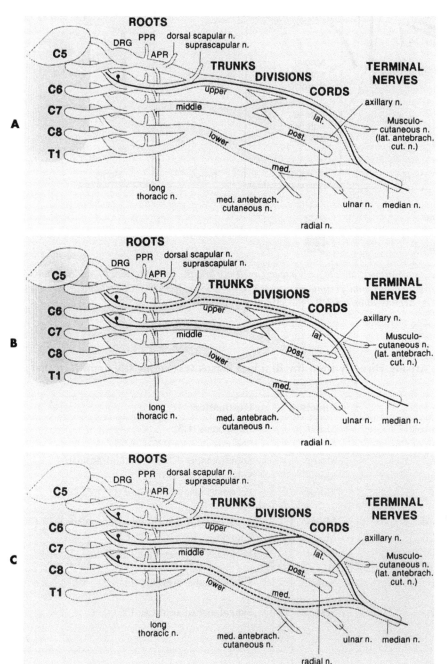

Figure C16–4. *Brachial plexus pathways for the sensory fibers assessed by median sensory nerve action potential (SNAP) (to the thumb (**A**), and index (**B**) and middle (**C**) fingers), radial SNAP (**D**), and lateral antebrachial SNAP (**E**). Solid lines represent predominant pathways and dashed lines represent possible additional pathways. (From Ferrante MA, Wilbourn AJ. The utility of various sensory nerve conduction responses in assessing brachial plexopathies. Muscle Nerve 1995;18: 879–889, with permission.)*

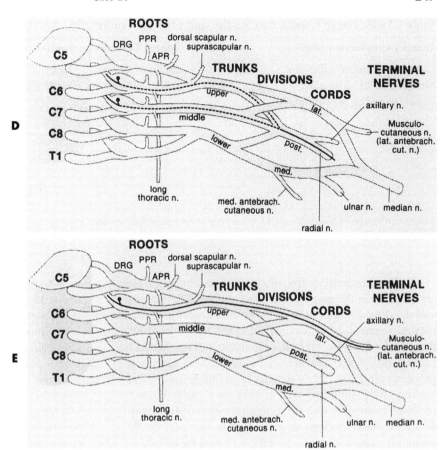

Figure C16–4, cont'd.

2. *The median motor fibers to the thenar muscles do not pass through the upper plexus.* Thus, routine median motor conduction studies are normal in upper brachial plexus lesions while their sensory counterparts are abnormal.

3. *In contrast to the median fibers to the hand, the ulnar motor fibers and ulnar sensory fibers do not separate while traversing the plexus.* They pass through the lower trunk and medial cord and continue through the ulnar nerve to their targets in the forearm and hand.

Brachial plexus lesions are divided into supraclavicular and infraclavicular plexopathies. Supraclavicular plexus lesions are further divided into the upper trunk, middle trunk, and lower trunk lesions. Infraclavicular lesions are divided into lateral cord, posterior cord and medial cord lesions. The electrodiagnosis of lesions of the brachial plexus, the largest and most complex structures of the peripheral nervous system, is more time consuming and requires performing multiple common and uncommon sensory and motor nerve conduction studies and sampling a large number of muscles with needle EMG. In lesions of the brachial plexus that are restricted to a specific trunk or cord, certain sensory and motor NCSs and muscles are likely to be abnormal based on the location of the injured fibers within the plexus (Tables C16–5 and C16–6).

In neuralgic amyotrophy, the EDX examination, particularly its needle EMG component, is very helpful in diagnosis, as well as demonstrating the severity of axon loss and showing that more muscles are involved than is clinically apparent. Routine motor nerve conduction studies (i.e., median, ulnar, and radial) often are normal because they do not assess the upper plexus, which is usually involved maximally, and these three nerves are rarely affected selectively. However, *routine sensory conduction studies (median, ulnar, and radial SNAPs) are abnormally low in amplitude in at least one-third of cases*, mostly because of upper plexus lesions. In particular, the median sensory response (recording the index or middle finger) may be abnormal as a result of upper or middle trunk axonal loss. Specialized nerve conduction studies often are required to show abnormalities of the upper plexus. In particular, the lateral antebrachial SNAP and, less commonly the median SNAP recording the thumb and index, are abnormal. Similarly, the axillary and musculocutaneous motor NCSs reveal low CMAP amplitudes.

Table C16–5. Nerve Conduction Studies and Muscles Commonly Affected in *Upper Brachial Plexus Lesions*

Sensory Conduction Studies	Motor Conduction Studies	Needle EMG
Lateral antebrachial cutaneous	Axillary (recording deltoid)	Pronator teres
Median (recording thumb)	Musculocutaneous (recording biceps)	Brachioradialis
Radial (recording base of thumb)		Biceps
		Triceps
		Deltoid
		Infraspinatus
		Supraspinatus
		Serratus anterior
		Rhomboids

Adapted with revisions from Wilbourn AJ. Assessment of the brachial plexus and the phrenic nerve. In: Johnson EW, Pease W, eds. Practical electromyography, 3rd ed. Baltimore, MD: Williams and Wilkins, 1997.

Needle examination frequently is more impressively abnormal than the nerve conduction studies. Fibrillations and decreased recruitment of motor unit action potential (MUAP) consistent with denervation are more extensive than is evident by clinical examination. The MUAPs become polyphasic and increased in duration as sprouting proceeds after one to two months from illness onset. The findings frequently are patchy, and they often do not conform to specific root or peripheral nerve distribution. At times, EMG findings in patients with shoulder girdle weakness suggest that the disorder is caused by lesions of multiple individual peripheral nerves (mononeuropathies) rather than of the upper plexus.

Certain EDX findings, when present, are highly suggestive of neuralgic amyotrophy. These include:

1. Selective denervation of multiple peripheral nerves around the shoulder girdle (the long thoracic, spinal accessory, suprascapular, axillary, and musculocutaneous). In fact, in many cases of neuralgic amyotrophy, the EDX examination often can prove that the lesion is more likely to be that of multiple mononeuropathies than a brachial plexopathy. For example, when denervation is noted in the biceps and deltoid but not in the brachioradialis or pronator teres, the findings are consistent with combined axillary and musculocutaneous mononeuropathies rather than an upper trunk plexopathy.

2. Partial proximal median mononeuropathy affecting the anterior interosseous-innervated muscles more severely, without abnormalities in median SNAPs, CMAP, or thenar muscles.

3. Severe and selective denervation of one or more muscles innervated by a specific nerve without (or with minimal) involvement of neighboring muscles innervated by the same nerve, presumably due to pathology of the motor branches. Examples include:
   - Denervation of the pronator teres muscle without involvement of other median-innervated or C6- or C7-innervated muscles. This unusual finding is almost pathognomonic of neuralgic amyotrophy.
   - Denervation of the triceps with minimal or no denervation of the more distally placed radial muscles (such as the brachioradialis, the extensor carpi radialis, and the extensor digitorum communis), or C6- or C7-innervated muscles (such as the pronator teres).

Table C16–6. Nerve Conduction Studies and Muscles Commonly Affected in *Lower Brachial Plexus Lesions*

Sensory Conduction Studies	Motor Conduction Studies	Needle EMG
Ulnar recording little finger	Ulnar recording hypothenar	All hand intrinsics*
Dorsal ulnar cutaneous	Ulnar recording 1st dorsal interosseous	Flexor pollicis longus
Medial antebrachial cutaneous	Median recording thenar	Flexor carpi ulnaris
Medial brachial cutaneous	Radial recording extensor digitorum communis	Extensor indicis
		Flexor digitorum profundus
		Extensor digitorum communis

*These include the abductor pollicis brevis, the first dorsal interosseous (and all other interossei), the adductor pollicis, and the abductor digiti minimi.
Adapted with revisions from Wilbourn AJ. Assessment of the brachial plexus and the phrenic nerve. In: Johnson EW, Pease W, eds. Practical electromyography, 3rd ed. Baltimore, MD: Williams and Wilkins, 1997.

- Denervation of the supraspinatus muscle with minimal or no involvement of the infraspinatus.
4. Absent lateral antebrachial cutaneous SNAP, with or without sensory loss along the lateral aspect of the forearm, even when there is neither clinical nor needle EMG evidence of involvement of the main trunk of the musculocutaneous nerve (i.e., normal biceps and brachialis muscles).

FOLLOW-UP

The patient's pain resolved completely in a few weeks. However, weakness was prominent and necessitated a temporary period of disability from occupation. In the ensuing 6 months, he had gradual return of function in most affected muscles, particularly the biceps, brachioradialis, spinati, and finger flexors. However, his deltoid continued to be affected severely.

Repeat EMG examination at 6 months showed significant reinnervation in all muscles, including the biceps, brachioradialis, spinati, and finger flexors. Fibrillation potentials disappeared in these muscles. However, the axillary CMAP amplitude remained very low, and the deltoid muscle continued to demonstrate fibrillations and no voluntary MUAPs. These findings point out that, in addition to an upper plexus lesion (which resulted from severe denervation of the biceps, brachioradialis, spinati, and possibly deltoid), there likely was a severe lesion of the axillary nerve proper, which explains the lack of reinnervation of the deltoid in the presence of good recovery of the other muscles innervated by the upper trunk.

Further follow-up disclosed a protracted improvement of the deltoid; at 18 months, the neurologic examination was normal except for moderate weakness of the deltoid at 4/5 and upper extremity areflexia. The patient returned to work 18 months after the initial insult.

DIAGNOSIS

Severe neuralgic amyotrophy, resulting in diffuse denervation but predominant involvement of the upper trunk of the brachial plexus, anterior interosseous nerve, and axillary nerve.

ANSWERS

1. C; 2. E; 3. D.

SUGGESTED READINGS

Airaksinen EM et al. Hereditary recurrent brachial plexus neuropathy with dysmorphic features. Acta Neurol Scand 1985;71:309–316.

Beghi E et al. Brachial plexus neuropathy in the population of Rochester, Minnesota, 1970–1981. Ann Neurol 1985;18:320–323.

England JD, Sumner AJ. Neuralgic amyotrophy: an increasingly diverse entity. Muscle Nerve 1987;10:60–68.

Flagman PD, Kelly JJ. Brachial plexus neuropathy. An electrophysiologic evaluation. Arch Neurol 1980;37:160–164.

Katirji B. Subacute lower brachial plexopathy: another form of neuralgic amyotrophy. Muscle Nerve 2000;23:1642.

Malamut RI et al. Postsurgical idiopathic brachial neuritis. Muscle Nerve 1994;17:320–324.

Parsonage MJ, Turner AJW. Neuralgic amyotrophy: the shoulder-girdle syndrome. Lancet 1948;1:973–978.

Spillane JD. Localized neuritis of the shoulder girdle. Lancet 1943;2:532–535.

Tsairis P, Dyck PJ, Mulder DW. Natural history of brachial plexus neuropathy; report of 99 cases. Arch Neurol 1972;27:109–117.

Vanneste JA, Bronner IM, Laman DM et al. Distal neuralgic amyotrophy. J Neurol 1999;246:399–402.

Weikers NJ, Mattson RH. Acute paralytic brachial neuritis: a clinical and electrodiagnostic study. Neurology 1969;19:1153–1158.

Wilbourn AJ. Assessment of the brachial plexus and the phrenic nerve. In: Johnson EW, Pease W, eds. Practical electromyography, 3rd ed. Baltimore, MD: Williams and Wilkins, 1997.

Part III
Generalized Disorders

Case 17

HISTORY AND PHYSICAL EXAMINATION

A 21-year-old woman developed intermittent binocular diplopia, primarily with distant vision. Within a few weeks, the symptoms worsened and she noted droopy eyelids, first on the right, then on the left. She had increasing fatigue and weakness, primarily after activity, and had fallen a few times. On system review, she admitted to fatigue and weakness while chewing but denied swallowing and speech difficulties. All symptoms improved after rest. The patient was otherwise in excellent health.

On examination, the patient was alert, oriented, and in no distress. She had mild bilateral ptosis, which worsened with sustained upgaze. Extraocular muscles showed bilateral lateral rectus muscle weakness with nystagmoid movements on lateral gaze. Pupils and fundi were normal. There was mild bilateral peripheral facial weakness and weakness of eye closure. Speech, tongue, and palate were normal. The patient had moderate weakness in the limb muscles particularly in the legs and worse proximally. Her outstretched arms became fatigued in 1 to 2 minutes and could not be sustained. Deep tendon reflexes were +2/4 throughout. Sensation and coordination were normal. Gait was slow and waddling. Romberg test was negative. Tensilon (Edrophonium) test was equivocal, with possible improvement of ptosis only.

An electrodiagnostic (EDX) examination was performed.

Please now review the Nerve Conduction Studies and Needle EMG tables.

QUESTIONS

1. Decremental response on slow repetitive stimulation is commonly seen in all of the following *except:*
   A. Botulism.
   B. Amyotrophic lateral sclerosis.
   C. Myasthenia gravis.
   D. Corticosteroid myopathy.
   E. Lambert-Eaton myasthenic syndrome (LEMS).
2. In patients with suspected ocular myasthenia, which test is most sensitive in establishing the diagnosis?
   A. Serum acetylcholine receptor antibody.
   B. Single-fiber jitter study of the frontalis muscle.
   C. Slow repetitive stimulation of the facial nerve.
   D. Slow repetitive stimulation of the spinal accessory nerve.
   E. Single-fiber jitter study of the extensor digitorum communis.
3. Factors that increase the sensitivity of electrodiagnosis in myasthenia gravis include all of the following *except:*
   A. Slow repetitive stimulation, recording weakened muscles.
   B. Slow repetitive stimulation before and after exercise.
   C. Rapid repetitive stimulation, recording a proximal muscle.
   D. Single-fiber EMG jitter study.
   E. Slow repetitive stimulation on warm limbs.

EDX FINDINGS AND INTERPRETATION OF DATA

Pertinent EDX findings include the following:

1. Normal sensory and motor nerve conduction studies (NCSs). In particular, the amplitudes of the compound muscle action potentials (CMAPs), of all motor nerves tested, are normal.
2. Slow repetitive stimulation (at a rate of 2 Hz) of the median and spinal accessory nerves reveals reproducible CMAP decrement at rest and after exercise (Figures C17–1 and C17–2). Also, the median nerve decrement corrects after exercise (postexercise facilitation. Compare Figure C17–1A, train 1 to train 2).

Case 17: Nerve Conduction Studies

Nerve Stimulated	Stimulation Site	Recording Site	Amplitude (m = mV, s = µV)			Distal/Peak Latency (ms)			Conduction Velocity (m/s)			F Latency (ms)	
			Right	Left	Normal	Right	Left	Normal	Right	Left	Normal	Right	Left
Sural (s)	Calf	Ankle		18	≥6		4.0	≤4.4		47	≥40		
Tibial (m)	Ankle	AH		10.0	≥8		5.4	≤5.8			≥40		47.5
Tibial (m)	Knee	AH		8.5						49			
Median (s)	Wrist	Index finger		35	≥20		3.0	≤3.3			≥50		
Median (s)	Elbow	Index finger		25						60			
Ulnar (s)	Wrist	Little finger		30	≥18		2.8	≤3.0					
Median (m)*	Wrist	APB		11.5	≥6		3.4	≤3.9			≥50		25.5
Median (m)*	Elbow	APB		11.0						62			
Ulnar (m)	Wrist	ADM		10.5	≥8		2.8	≤3.0			≥50		26.2
Ulnar (m)	Above elbow	ADM		9.5						60			
Spin access (m)*	Anterior neck	Trapezius		3.5	≥3		3.0	≤4.0					

ADM = abductor digiti minimi; AH = abductor hallucis; APB = abductor pollicis brevis; EDB = extensor digitorum brevis; m = motor; s = sensory; Spin access = spinal accessory.
*Decrement on slow, repetitive stimulation (see Figures C17–1 and C17–2).

Case 17: Needle EMG

Muscle	Insertional Activity	Spontaneous Activity		Voluntary Motor Unit Action Potentials (MUAPs)								
				Recruitment				Configuration				
		Fibs	Fascs	Normal	Activation	Reduced	Early	Duration	Amplitude	% Polyphasia	Others	
L. tibialis anterior	Normal	0	0	X				Normal	Normal	Normal		
Medial gastrocnemius	Normal	0	0	X				Normal	Normal	Normal		
Vastus lateralis	Normal	0	0	X				Normal	Normal	Normal		
Gluteus medius	Normal	0	0	X				Normal	Normal	Normal		
L. brachioradialis	Normal	0	0	X				Normal	Normal	Normal		
Biceps	Normal	0	0	X				Normal	Normal	Normal		
Triceps	Normal	0	0	X				Normal	Normal	Normal		
Deltoid	Normal	0	0	X				Normal	Normal*	Normal		

Fascs = fasciculations; Fibs = fibrillations; L. = left.
*Significant moment-to-moment variation of motor unit potentials amplitudes and configurations (see Figure C17–6).

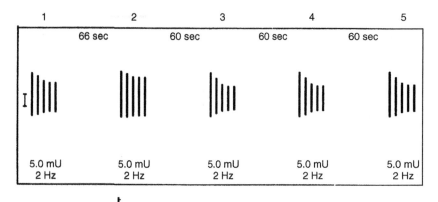

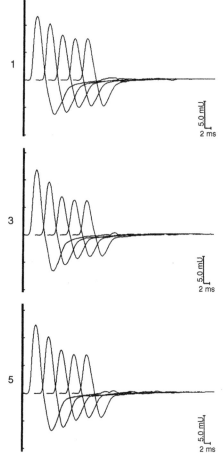

A

Figure C17–1. *Slow repetitive stimulation (2 Hz) of the median nerve, recording the abductor pollicis brevis, at rest and for 3 minutes after 1 minute of exercise in this patient with MG (**A**) and in an age-matched control (**B**). Train 1 was at rest, and Trains 2 through 5 were done every minute following 1 minute of exercise. The upper tracing of each panel shows all five stimulations, and the lower tracings represent Train 1, Train 3, and Train 5. Note the significant decrement of the compound muscle action potential (CMAP) at rest (35%) and after exercise in this patient, but not in the control. Note also the postexercise facilitation in the patient (Train 2, **A**). There was no significant postexercise exhaustion (compare Trains 1 and 3, 4, and 5 in **A**).*

3. No increment of the CMAP amplitude after brief (10 seconds) exercise (not shown).
4. Normal needle EMG, except for motor unit action potential (MUAP) instability (moment-to-moment variation of MUAP amplitude) in the deltoid muscle.

These findings are diagnostic of a neuromuscular junction defect of the postsynaptic type and are consistent with myasthenia gravis. Normal CMAP amplitude at rest and the absence of CMAP increment after brief exercise exclude a presynaptic defect, as is seen with LEMS or botulism. The absence of denervation on needle EMG excludes a lower motor neuron disease (as seen with amyotrophic lateral sclerosis), which may be associated with a decremental response on slow repetitive stimulation.

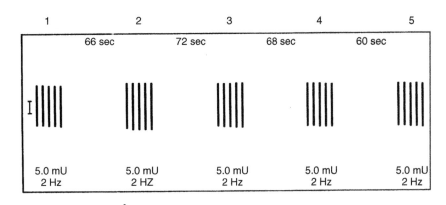

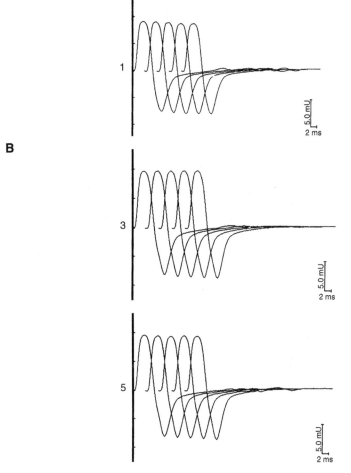

B

Figure C17–1, cont'd.

DISCUSSION

Anatomy and Physiology

Neuromuscular Junction

The neuromuscular junction (NMJ) is the site where the motor neuron makes contact with the skeletal muscle fiber's membrane (sarcolemma). It is near the center of the muscle fiber where there is a cup-shaped depression of the sarcolemma, called the endplate. The NMJ is a chemical synapse that is essential for transmitting action potentials from the terminal nerve branches to muscle fibers. This synapse utilizes acetylcholine (ACH) as a transmitter that binds to specific receptors in the junctional membrane, resulting local depolarizations that spread and trigger all-or-none muscle action potential. The NMJ is divided into a presynaptic terminal, a synaptic cleft, and a postsynaptic region (Figure C17–3).

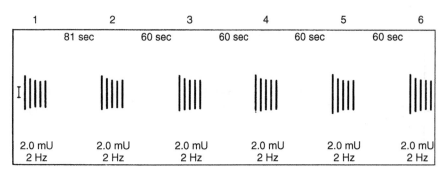

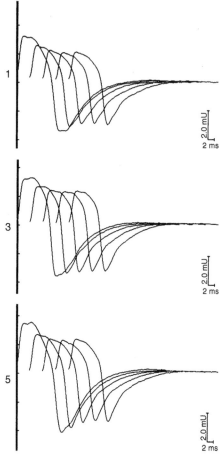

Figure C17–2. *Slow repetitive stimulation (2 Hz) of the spinal accessory nerve, recording the trapezius, at rest and for 4 minutes after 1 minute of exercise in this patient. Train 1 is at rest, and Trains 2 through 6 are done every minute following 1 minute of exercise. The upper tracing of each panel shows all six stimulations, and the lower tracings represent Train 1, Train 3, and Train 5. Note the significant decrement of the compound muscle action potential at rest (33%) and after exercise, with no significant postexercise facilitation or exhaustion.*

1. The *presynaptic terminal* is composed mainly of an unmyelinated nerve terminal covered by a Schwann cell and is loaded with synaptic vesicles. Each synaptic vesicle is 50 nm diameter in structure and contains approximately 5000 to 10 000 molecules of ACH, called the *quanta*. The synaptic vesicles cluster around the terminal's active zones, the site for their eventual release facing the muscle fiber. Acetylcholine is packaged into vesicles to protect the molecules from hydrolysis (by the presynaptic acetylcholinesterase) and to maximize the required amount of transmitter release. The ACH supply is saved in immediately available stores, which are ready for release near the active zone region. Much larger ACH depots are stored more proximally in the axon and may be mobilized to replenish the immediately available stores whenever depleted. ACH is synthesized as follows:

Acetyl-coenzyme A + choline

$$\xrightarrow{\text{Choline acetyltransferase}} \text{acetylcholine} + \text{coenzyme A}$$

2. The *synaptic cleft* is a small space (~60 nm) between the synaptic terminal and the sarcolemma. It is lined by

A   B

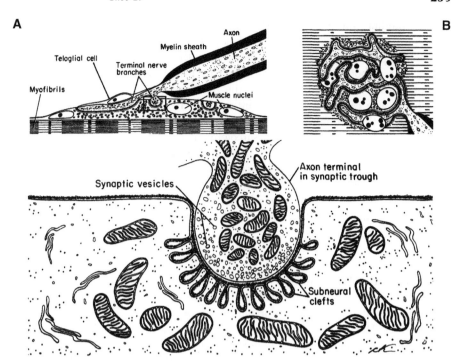

Figure C17–3. *Neuromuscular junction. (A) A longitudinal section through the endplate. (B) Overhead view of (A). (C) Enlarged view of the junction, showing the presynaptic region, the synaptic cleft, and the postsynaptic membrane and junctional clefts. (From Fawcett DW. Bloom and Fawcett: a textbook of histology. Philadelphia, PA: WB Saunders, 1986, with permission.)*

a basement membrane and is abundant in acetylcholinesterase, which breaks down ACH into choline and acetate. A large amount of acetylcholinesterase is present in neuromuscular junction, enough to quickly hydrolyze the ACH released into the synaptic cleft.

3. The *postsynaptic membrane* is the main constituent of the postsynaptic region and faces the active zone of the presynaptic terminal. The postsynaptic membrane forms highly convoluted invaginations, the junctional folds, where nicotinic ACH receptors are embedded at the top of the folds, with a density of 10 000–15 000 per μm^2, a thousand-fold more than in the rest of the sarcolemma. The *nicotinic ACH receptor* is a glycoprotein composed of five subunits ($\alpha 2\beta\delta\in$), i.e., two α subunits, one β subunit, one $\in$ subunit, and one δ subunit. The $\in$ subunit replaces the γ subunit, which is present during development. They are arranged like barrel staves around a central iron pore (Figure C17–4).

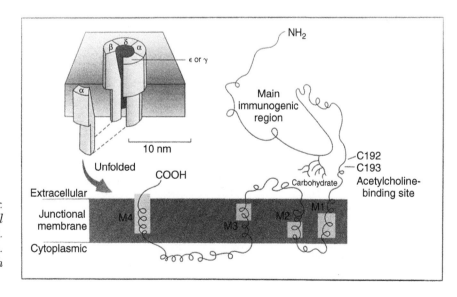

Figure C17–4. *The acetylcholine receptor. Each subunit winds through the junctional membrane four times (M1 through M4). (From Drachman DB. Myasthenia gravis. N Engl J Med 1994;330:1797–1810, with permission.)*

The binding site of the ACH molecule is located around amino acids 192 and 193 of both α subunits. The receptor channel opens transiently when the binding sites of both α subunits are locked by two ACH molecules. The opened channel of the ACH receptor behaves as a cation channel with little selectivity. The half-life of the nicotinic ACH receptor is approximately 8.5 days. A recently identified sarcolemmal protein, *muscle specific tyrosine kinase (MuSK)*, is expressed exclusively at the NMJ and is closely associated to the ACH receptor. Its exact role in adult muscle is still unknown. In the developing muscle, MuSK is essential for aggregating the ACH receptors and is activated by nerve-derived agrin.

Neuromuscular Transmission

Neuromuscular transmission involves the transmission of action potential from the motor neuron's axon to the muscle fiber. The delay between the depolarization of the presynaptic terminal and the generation of endplate potential at the postsynaptic membrane is short (0.3–1 ms), and is mostly due to the exocytotic release of ACH from the presynaptic terminal. Neuromuscular transmission may be divided into three processes: (1) presynaptic terminal depolarization and ACH release; (2) ACH binding and ion channel opening; and (3) postsynaptic membrane depolarization and muscle action potential generation.

- *Presynaptic terminal depolarization and ACH release.* With the arrival of the action potential to the nerve terminal, voltage gated calcium channels (VGCCs) open allowing calcium to enter the presynaptic terminal. With the increase in cytosolic calcium concentration, several complex interactions, that involves several proteins and receptors, lead to the ensuing docking and fusion of synaptic vesicles with the presynaptic membrane in the active zone and release of ACH release into the synaptic cleft.

- *Acetylcholine binding and ion channel opening.* The released ACH molecules diffuses through the cleft and bind with the ACH receptors on the postsynaptic junctional folds. For a single receptor channel to open and allow the rapid passage of cations, two ACH molecules must bind to the α subunits of the receptor. The channels remain open for about 1 ms after ACH binding and then they close and ACH dissociates from the receptors.

- *Postsynaptic membrane depolarization and muscle action potential generation.* The passage of cations through the open cation channels following their electrochemical gradients (Na^+ ions flow inward, and K^+ ions flow outward) leads to a local depolarization in the endplate region. This endplate potential (EPP) is a slow potential with a large amplitude that ranges from 50 to 70 mV. It spreads electrotonically to the depths of the synaptic folds triggering the opening of Na^+ voltage-gated channels and the development of a muscle action potential that propagates along the muscle fiber. After closure of the nicotinic receptor, ACH is released and subsequently is hydrolyzed by acetylcholinesterase into choline and acetate. Choline is taken back by the presynaptic terminal and ACH is resynthesized (Figure C17–5).

Clinical Features

Myasthenia gravis (MG) is the best understood and most thoroughly studied of all human organ-specific

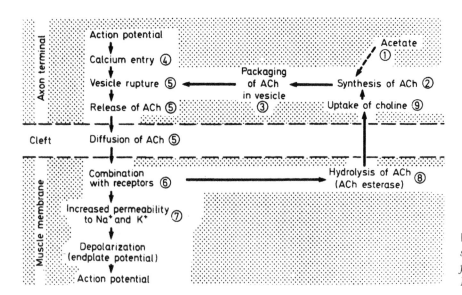

Figure C17–5. *Neuromuscular transmission. (From McComas AJ. Neuromuscular function and disorders. Boston, MA: Butterworth, 1977, with permission.)*

autoimmune diseases. It is characterized by a reduction of skeletal muscle postsynaptic ACH receptors resulting in a decrease in the EPP necessary for action potential generation. In the majority of patients, MG is *caused by an antibody-mediated attack on the postsynaptic nicotinic ACH receptors* in the neuromuscular junction. In a small number of patients, other antigenic targets, such as the muscle specific tyrosine kinase (MuSK), may exist. Myoid cells and other stem cells within the thymus gland, which is hyperplastic in at least two-thirds of patients with MG, may serve as autoantigens by expressing on their surface the ACH receptor or one of its protein components.

The prevalence of MG is between 50 and 125 cases per million population. There is strong evidence that its prevalence is increasing, which may be in part attributed to better case recognition and aging of the population. As with many other autoimmune disorders, the disease afflicts mostly women, affected nearly twice as often as men. The annual incidence of MG ranges between 1.1 and 6 per million. MG incidence has two distinct peaks: the first occurs in the second and third decades and affects mostly women; and the second peak strikes mostly men during the sixth and seventh decades.

The hallmarks of MG are muscle weakness and fatigability. The symptoms are intermittent and are usually worse with activity and improve after rest. Generally, patients are much better in the morning than in the evening. Ocular symptoms (diplopia and/or ptosis) are extremely common and are the presenting signs in more than one half of patients. Most importantly, almost all patients at some point during the course of their illness develop ocular manifestations. Also, the disorder continues to be restricted to the extraocular muscles in 15% of patients, hence the designation *ocular myasthenia*. Additionally, only 3–10% of patients with ocular myasthenia generalize if no other symptoms appear after three years from initial presentation. Bulbar muscle weakness is the initial presenting manifestation in about 20% of patients and is seen in over 30% of patients during the course of their disease. Bulbar weakness is a major contributor to disability throughout the course of the disease. It manifests as dysarthria, nasal speech, dysphagia, chewing difficulties, or nasal regurgitation. Occasionally, the jaw muscle weakness may be severe leading to a "jaw drop" and patients often hold their jaw closed, a highly pathognomonic manifestation of MG. Limb weakness, mostly of proximal muscles, is seen as the initial symptom in 20% of patients. At times, the generalized weakness is severe and involves the respiratory muscles, resulting in respiratory failure that requires mechanical ventilation, a situation often referred to as *myasthenic crisis*. Because of variable clinical severity, MG is usually classified into five main categories (Table C17–1).

Table C17–1. Myasthenia Gravis Foundation of America Clinical Classification

Class I	Any ocular muscle weakness
	May have weakness of eye closure
	All other muscle strength is normal
Class II	Mild weakness affecting other than ocular muscles
	May also have ocular muscle weakness of any severity
IIa	Predominantly affecting limb, axial muscles or both
	May also have lesser involvement of oropharyngeal muscles
IIb	Predominantly affecting oropharyngeal, respiratory muscles, or both
	May also have lesser involvement of limb, axial muscles, or both
Class III	Moderate weakness affecting other than ocular muscles
	May also have ocular muscle weakness of any severity
IIIa	Predominantly affecting limb, axial muscles or both
	May also have lesser involvement of oropharyngeal muscles
IIIb	Predominantly affecting oropharyngeal, respiratory muscles, or both
	May also have lesser involvement of limb, axial muscles, or both
Class IV	Severe weakness affecting other than ocular muscles
	May also have ocular muscle weakness of any severity
IVa	Predominantly affecting limb, axial muscles or both
	May also have lesser involvement of oropharyngeal muscles
IVb	Predominantly affecting oropharyngeal, respiratory muscles, or both
	May also have lesser involvement of limb, axial muscles, or both
Class V	Defined by intubation, with or without mechanical ventilation, except when employed during routine postoperative management. The use of a feeding tube without intubation places the patient in class IVb

The findings on neurologic examination parallel the symptoms, often revealing ptosis, weakness of extraocular muscles, flaccid dysarthria, or neck extensor or proximal muscle weakness. Although many muscles are fatigable, *the most objective finding is fatigable eyelids*, i.e., ptosis developing within 1–2 minutes of sustained upgaze. Deep tendon reflexes are preserved. Sensation is normal.

The *diagnosis* of MG may be made on clinical grounds, especially when reproducible fatigability of eyelids or extraocular muscles is confirmed. However, laboratory

Table C17–2. Confirmatory Diagnostic Tests in Myasthenia Gravis

Edrophonium (Tensilon) test
Serum antibody assay
   Acetylcholine receptor antibody
   Muscle specific kinase (MuSK) antibody
   Antistriatal muscle antibody
Repetitive nerve stimulation
Single-fiber electromyography

testing is frequently needed, and recommended, for confirmation (Table C17–2):

1. *Tensilon test.* Edrophonium (Tensilon) is a short-acting anticholinesterase inhibitor that transiently improves muscle strength in myasthenic patients. By inhibiting ACH degradation, it allows the ACH that is released into the junction to interact repeatedly with the decreased number of nicotinic ACH receptors. When given intravenously, its effect is quick (20–30 seconds) but transient, lasting around 5 minutes. Before the test, baseline muscle weakness should be established, preferably of muscles that can be tested objectively, such as eyelids or extraocular muscles. Difficulties in interpretation of the test are common when attempting to evaluate improvement in limb strength or bulbar function. A 1 to 2 mg test dose is given intravenously; if no improvement occurs within 45 seconds, the rest of the10 mg dose is administered. For results to be considered positive, the weakness should correct or improve unequivocally. False-positive and false-negative results are rare. Side effects usually are minor and include abdominal cramps, bradycardia, and hypotension. The patient's pulse and blood pressure should be monitored during the test, and atropine should be readily available to counteract significant bradycardia.

2. *Acetylcholine receptor antibodies.* Approximately 85 to 90% of patients with generalized MG have elevated serum ACH receptor antibody, while the test is positive in only about 50 to 65% of patients with ocular myasthenia. A positive serum ACH receptor binding antibody is the most sensitive test and is highly specific for MG. ACH receptor modulating antibody test increases the diagnostic yield slightly. ACH receptor antibodies may be found in all subtypes of immunoglobulin G (IgG) and are heterogenous. They can be directed against many different epitopes of one or more of the five peptide chains of the ACH receptor. The majority of these antibodies bind at sequences of the α chains, particularly in the main immunogenic region (see Figure C17–4). There is no correlation between total ACH receptor binding, as measured in routine radioimmunoassay, and the severity of the disease. However, there is some correlation between antibody titer and clinical status in individual patients in response to various treatment modalities.

3. *Muscle specific tyrosine kinase (MuSK) antibody.* It has been long known that seronegative MG is also an autoimmune disease and likely mediated by antibodies directed at epitopes of other constituents of the motor endplate. Antibodies to MuSK antibody, a NMJ sarcolemmal protein, are present in about 40 to 70% of patients with generalized seronegative MG. These antibodies probably interfere with maintenance of normal ACH receptor density at the NMJ, since they were shown, *in vivo*, to interfere with ACH receptor clustering. Patients with MuSK positive antibodies are difficult to distinguish from other myathenics. However, they often may show a preponderance to bulbar, facial, and shoulder muscles and may not be responsive to cholinesterase inhibitors.

4. *Striated muscle antibodies.* These autoantibodies may be positive but only assist in suggesting the diagnosis of MG. Antistriated muscle antibodies are, however, useful markers for thymoma, particularly in patients between the ages of 20 and 50 years, since false positive and negative tests are common in children and older adults.

5. *Repetitive nerve stimulation and single-fiber EMG.* These are discussed separately in the electrodiagnosis section.

The *differential diagnosis* of *generalized MG* includes Lambert-Eaton myasthenic syndrome (LEMS), botulism, congenital myasthenic syndromes, and chronic fatigue syndrome. LEMS presents with generalized weakness, areflexia, and autonomic symptoms, but it is not uncommon to confuse its EDX findings with those of MG (Table C17–3). Botulism is subacute and has usually prominent autonomic manifestations, including dilated pupils and ileus. Congenital myasthenic syndromes are extremely rare disorders and usually begin in childhood. The fatigue associated with chronic fatigue syndrome may mimic generalized MG, except for normal ocular and bulbar strength and normal serologic and EDX studies. *Ocular myasthenia* should be distinguished from Graves disease (thyroid orbitopathy), progressive external ophthalmoplegia, Kearns-Sayre syndrome, oculopharyngeal muscular dystrophy, congenital myasthenic syndromes, and orbital apex or cavernous sinus mass compressing cranial nerves. In Graves disease, there is proptosis, conjunctival edema, and muscle enlargement (on imaging of the orbit); the forced duction test is positive. Progressive external ophthalmoplegia and Kearns-Sayre syndrome

Table C17–3. Differential Diagnosis Between Generalized Myasthenia Gravis and Lambert-Eaton Myasthenic Syndrome

	Myasthenia Gravis	Lambert-Eaton Myasthenic Syndrome
Ocular involvement	Common and prominent	Uncommon and subtle
Bulbar involvement	Common and prominent	Uncommon and subtle
Myotatic reflexes	Normal	Absent or depressed
Sensory symptoms	None	Paresthesias are common
Autonomic involvement	None	Dry mouth, impotence and gastroparesis
Tensilon test	Frequently positive	May be positive
Serum antibodies directed against	Postsynaptic Ach receptors or MuSK	Presynaptic voltage-gated calcium channels
Baseline CMAPs	Normal	Low in amplitude
Postexercise CMAPs	No change	Significant facilitation
Slow repetitive stimulation	Decrement	Decrement
Rapid repetitive stimulation	No change or decrement	Increment
Single-fiber EMG	Increased jitter with blocking	Increased jitter with blocking
Rapid-rate stimulation jitter	Does not change or worsens jitter	Improves jitter

CMAPs = compound muscle action potentials; EMG = electromyography, Ach = acetylcholine, MuSK = muscle-specific kinase.

have usually symmetrical and slowly progressive ophthalmoplegia and ptosis. In Kearns-Sayre syndrome, there is associated multisystem involvement including pigmentary retinopathy, cerebellar ataxia, and cardiac conduction defects. Oculopharyngeal muscular dystrophy is a late onset autosomal dominant disease with slowly progressive dysphagia and ophthalmoplegia. In compressive mass lesions, the extraocular weakness usually follows one or more oculomotor nerve distribution and the pupils are frequently involved. Imaging studies, such as magnetic resonance imaging (MRI), might be required to rule out such a mass lesion within the orbit or cavernous sinus.

Once the diagnosis of MG is confirmed, certain commonly associated disorders must be considered and excluded. *Thymoma* occurs in approximately 10% of all patients with MG. This is age specific and is most common in adult patients between the ages of 20 and 60 years. Elevated antistriated muscle antibodies, which occur in certain myasthenics, are useful markers for thymoma,

particularly in patients between the ages of 20 and 50 years, while false positive and negative tests are common in the young (<20 years) and older (>60 years) MG patients. Thus, a computed tomography (CT) scan or an MRI of the chest should be performed on all patients with MG. Because *hyperthyroidism* occurs in 3 to 8% of patients with MG, all patients should have thyroid function tests at the time of diagnosis. Other autoimmune disorders, such as systemic lupus erythematosus and rheumatoid arthritis, may coexist with myasthenia; screening for these should be performed by obtaining at least antinuclear antibodies and rheumatoid factor.

Therapy for MG has improved dramatically over the past 30 years, and the current mortality from this disorder is near zero. Treatment consists of one or more of several modalities, often used separately or in combination (Table C17–4). Treatment choices are usually individualized to the patient depending on severity of illness, age, life style and career, associated complicating disorders, and the risk and benefit of various therapies.

Table C17–4. Therapeutic Modalities in Myasthenia Gravis

Therapy	Mechanism of Action
Cholinesterase inhibitors (e.g., pyridostigmine)	Enhances neuromuscular transmission
Corticosteroids, azathioprine, cyclosporine, mycophenolate mofetil, cyclophosphamide, etc.	Immunosuppression
Plasmapheresis	Removes antibodies from circulation
Intravenous immunoglobulins	Unknown (?downregulates antibody production)
Thymectomy	Unknown (?eliminates a source of antigenic stimulation [thymic myoid cells] and/or removes a reservoir of B lymphocytes)

Electrodiagnosis

Electrodiagnostic (EDX) abnormalities encountered in MG are related to the blockade of the NMJ at the post-synaptic membrane. Although the changes are observed most often with repetitive stimulation of motor nerves or single-fiber EMG, other less specific changes may be encountered on routine EMG examination.

Nerve Conduction Studies

Sensory conduction studies are normal in MG. Similarly, routine motor conduction studies are usually normal. However, on rare occasions, the CMAP amplitudes are borderline or slightly decreased. This occurs in patients with prominent weakness, such as that associated with a myasthenic crisis, and is explained by prominent neuro-muscular blockade beyond the safety factor (see repetitive nerve stimulation). In these situations, many muscle fibers do not reach threshold with a single stimulus, as is used with routine motor conduction studies, resulting in a small summated CMAP. It should be noted again that this is an extremely rare finding in MG. In fact, a presynaptic disorder, such as LEMS and botulism, should always be considered and excluded when the CMAP amplitudes are low or borderline. A presynaptic disorder is confirmed by looking for a significant (>50–100%) increment of CMAP amplitude after brief exercise and/or rapid, repetitive stimulation (*see* repetitive stimulation). *Compound muscle action potential increment after brief exercise and/or rapid, repetitive nerve stimulation is not a feature of MG.*

Needle EMG Examination

Needle EMG results usually are normal in MG. Three changes may, however, be seen. These include:

1. *Unstable MUAPs (moment-to-moment variation of MUAPs).* In healthy subjects, individual MUAPs are morphologically stable between successive discharges with no variation in amplitude and configuration, since all muscle fibers of the motor unit fire with every discharge. The morphology of a repetitively firing MUAP may fluctuate in patients with MG, if individual muscle fibers intermittently block within the unit (Figure C17–6). Technically, MUAP variation is best achieved during recording of a single MUAP by minimal voluntary activation. Care should be taken to record from no more than a single MUAP because MUAP overlap can lead to an erroneous assumption of MUAP instability. This finding is, however, not specific because it is observed in other neuromuscular junction disorders as well as in neurogenic disorders associated with active reinnervation such as motor neuron disease, subacute radiculopathy, or polyneuropathy. During reinnervation, the newly formed endplates are imma-ture and demonstrate poor efficacy of neuromuscular transmission.

2. *Short-duration, low-amplitude, and polyphasic MUAPs.* These MUAPs, which are observed primarily in proximal muscles, are similar to the MUAPs seen in primary myopathies. They are caused, in MG, by physiologic blocking and slowing of neuromuscular transmission at many muscle fibers during voluntary activation. This leads to exclusion of many muscle fiber action potentials (MFAPs) from the MUAP (hence the short duration and low amplitude) and to a delay in neuromuscular transmission of other fibers (hence the polyphasia).

3. *Fibrillation potentials.* These potentials are extremely rare in MG. Their presence should raise the question of another diagnosis, or an associated diagnosis.

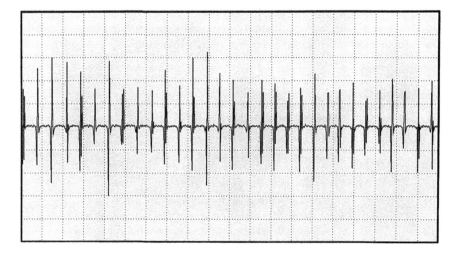

Figure C17–6. *Moment-to-moment variation (i.e., instability) of a single motor unit action potential recorded from the deltoid muscle in a patient with generalized myasthenia gravis (sensitivity = 0.2 mV/division, sweep speed = 100 ms/division).*

When observed, they are inconspicuous and present mostly in proximal muscles. Their exact mechanism in MG is not known, but they are believed to be the result of persistent transmission block, which causes "effective" denervation of some muscle fibers.

Repetitive Nerve Stimulation (RNS)

Basic Concepts

To comprehend the effects of repetitive stimulation of motor nerves in both healthy individuals and those with myasthenic conditions, one must review important facts regarding the transmission of action potential through the presynaptic terminal and the postsynaptic membrane. These physiologic facts dictate the type and frequency of repetitive nerve stimulation (RNS) and the type of single fiber EMG study utilized in the accurate diagnosis of NMJ disorders.

- *Quantum.* A quantum is the amount of ACH packaged in a single vesicle, which contains approximately 5000 to 10 000 ACH molecules. Each quantum (vesicle) released results in a 1 mV change in postsynaptic membrane potential. This occurs spontaneously during rest and forms the basis of miniature endplate potential (MEPP).

- *Acetylcholine release and stores.* The number of quanta released after a nerve action potential depends on the number of quanta in *the immediately available (primary) store* and the probability of release, i.e., m = p × n, where m = the number of quanta released during each stimulation, p = the probability of release (effectively proportional to the concentration of calcium and typically about 0.2, or 20%), and n = the number of quanta in the immediately available store. In normal conditions, a single nerve action potential triggers the release of 50–300 vesicles (quanta) with an average of about 60 vesicles (quanta). In addition to the immediately available store of ACH, located beneath the presynaptic nerve terminal membrane, *a secondary (or mobilization) store* starts to replenish the immediately available store after 1–2 seconds of repetitive nerve action potentials. A large *tertiary (or reserve) store* is also available in the axon and cell body.

- *Calcium influx into presynaptic terminal.* After depolarization of the presynaptic terminal, VGCCs open, leading to calcium (Ca^{2+}) influx. Through a calcium-dependent intracellular cascade, vesicles are docked into the active zones, where they open into the synaptic cleft and release their ACH content. When this process is completed, Ca^{2+} then diffuses slowly out of the presynaptic terminal in 100 to 200 ms. The different rates at which motor nerves are repetitively stimulated in the EMG laboratory is extrapolated from the Ca^{2+} diffusion rate (see below).

- *Endplate potential (EPP).* EPP is the potential generated at the postsynaptic membrane after a nerve action potential and neuromuscular transmission. In humans, its amplitude is equivalent to approximately 60 quanta (60 vesicles), which are released from the presynaptic terminal. This results in approximately a 60 mV change in membrane potential amplitude.

- *Safety factor.* In normal conditions, the number of quanta (vesicles) released at the junction after the arrival of the nerve action potential at the presynaptic terminal (approximately 60 vesicles) far exceeds the change in postsynaptic membrane potential that is required to reach the *threshold* needed to generate a postsynaptic muscle action potential (7 to 20 mV). The safety factor results in an EPP that always reaches threshold, results in an all-or-none muscle fiber action potential (MFAP), and prevents neuromuscular transmission failure despite repetitive action potentials. In addition to quantal release, several other factors contribute to the safety factor and EPP, including ACH receptor conduction properties, ACH receptor density, and acetylcholinesterase activity.

- *Compound muscle action potential (CMAP).* CMAP is the summation of all propagated MFAPs within a muscle. The value is obtained after supramaximal stimulation of the motor nerve during recording through a surface electrode that is placed over the belly of a muscle.

Electrophysiology

When repetitive stimulation is applied to a normal motor nerve, the amount of ACH released during the first several stimulations exceeds what is released during ensuing stimulations. Despite this decrease, the amount of ACH released continues to exceed the ACH required to reach action potential threshold because of the safety factor. The decline in ACH release also levels off to a constant amount because of mobilization of large amount of ACH from depot stores into the active zone. This allows indefinite release of ACH during prolonged stimulation at physiologic rates.

The rate at which motor nerves are stimulated dictates whether calcium plays a role in enhancing the release of ACH. Because Ca^{2+} diffuses out of the presynaptic terminal within 100 to 200 ms, a slow rate of stimulation (slower than every 200 ms) implies that the subsequent stimulus arrives long after calcium has dispersed. Thus, an interstimulus interval of greater than 200 ms, or a stimulation rate of less than 5 Hz, is considered a slow rate of repetitive stimulation. At this slow rate, the role of Ca^{2+} in ACH release is not enhanced. In contrast, with rapid repetitive stimulation (i.e., at an interstimulus interval of less than 200 ms, or a stimulation rate greater than 5–10 Hz),

Ca^{2+} influx is enhanced greatly, which results in larger releases of ACH and a larger EPP.

In normal conditions (Figures C17–7 and C17-8), both rates of stimulation generate MFAPs in all muscle fibers since the EPPs remain above threshold because of the safety factor. Thus, at both stimulation rates, all muscle fibers generate MFAPs, and the CMAP (summated MFAPs) does not change (i.e., no decrement or increment).

However, the *postsynaptic disorders*, such as MG, are characterized by the following (Tables C17–3 and C17–5):

- The CMAP is normal since a single stimulus usually leads to normal EPPs and MFAPs in all fibers due the presence of safety factor and despite ACH receptor blockade.
- Slow RNS (2–5 Hz) results in the decline of many muscle fiber EPPs which often fail to reach thresholds. This leads to a progressive loss of MFAPs and a decremental CMAP (see Figure C17–7).
- Rapid RNS (10–50 Hz) results in no change of CMAP since the depleted stores are compensated by the Ca^{2+} influx. In severe myasthenics, rapid RNS may result is CMAP decrement since the increased ACH release cannot compensate for the marked postsynaptic neuromuscular block (see Figure C17–8).

In contrast, the *presynaptic disorders*, such as Lambert-Eaton myasthenic syndrome, are characterized by the following (See Tables C17–3 and C17–5):

- The CMAP is low in amplitude since many muscle fibers do not reach threshold after a single stimulus due to the inadequate release of quanta (vesicles).
- Slow RNS (2–5 Hz) results in CMAP decrement since the decline in ACH release with subsequent stimuli results in lower amplitude EPPs and further loss of MFAPs (see Figure C17–7).
- Rapid RNS (10–50 Hz) results in CMAP increment due to the accumulation of Ca^{2+} in the presynaptic vesicles. This, in turn, significantly enhances ACH release, and results in many EPPs reaching the threshold required for the generation of MFAPs (see Figure C17–8).

Technical Considerations

Repetitive nerve stimulation often follows routine motor NCS. Electromyographers and nerve conduction technologists should master the various motor NCS and RNS techniques to avoid false positive and false negative results. There are certain prerequisites that are essential for performing reliable RNS and for increasing the sensitivity and specificity of the test in the diagnosis of RNS.

1. Limb temperature should be kept warm since neuromuscular transmission is enhanced in a cool limb which may mask a CMAP decrement. Warming the extremity studied is important because cooling improves neuromuscular transmission and can result in a false negative RNS. Hand skin temperature should be maintained

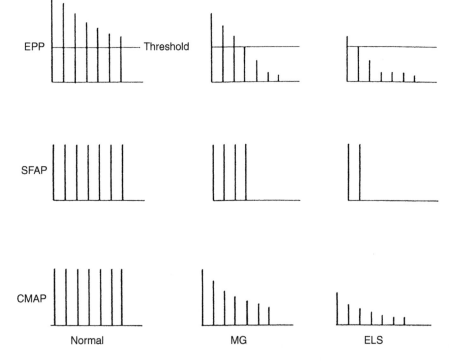

Figure C17–7. *Slow repetitive stimulation effect on endplate potential (EPP), single-fiber action potential (SFAP, also referred to as muscle fiber action potential [MFAP]), and compound muscle action potential (CMAP) in normal health, myasthenia gravis (MG), and Lambert-Eaton myasthenic syndrome (ELS). (Adapted from Oh S. Clinical electromyography, neuromuscular transmission studies. Baltimore, MD: Williams and Wilkins, 1988, with permission.)*

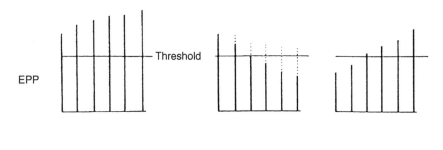

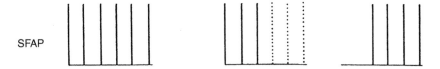

Figure C17–8. *Rapid repetitive stimulation effect on endplate potential (EPP), single-fiber action potential (SFAP, also referred to as muscle fiber action potential [MFAP]), and compound muscle action potential (CMAP) in normal health, myasthenia gravis (MG), and Lambert-Eaton myasthenic syndrome (ELS). (Adapted from Oh S. Clinical electromyography, neuromuscular transmission studies. Baltimore, MD: Williams and Wilkins, 1988, with permission.)*

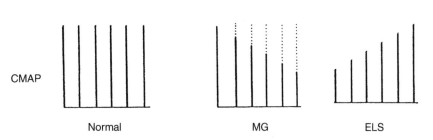

greater than 32°C, and foot skin temperature greater than 30°C.

2. Patients on cholinesterase inhibitors (such as pyridostigmine) should be asked to withhold their medication for 12–24 hours before RNS, if medically not contraindicated.

3. The limb tested should be immobilized as best as possible. Particular attention should be given to the stimulation and recording sites. Movement at either site may result in CMAP amplitude decay or increment, potentially leading to a false diagnosis of an NMJ disorder.

4. Though a supramaximal stimulation (i.e., 10–20% above the intensity level needed for a maximal response) is needed to obtain a CMAP, unnecessary high intensity or long duration stimuli should be avoided to prevent movement artifact and excessive pain.

5. The choice of nerve to be stimulated and muscle to be recorded from depends on the patient's clinical manifestations. The aim is to record from clinically weakened muscles, if these muscles are accessible. Easily tested and well-tolerated nerves for RNS are the median and ulnar nerves, recording abductor pollicis brevis and abductor digiti minimi respectively, since they are accompanied by minimal movement artifact and the upper limb is easily immobilized. However, since distal muscles are frequently spared in MG, recording from a proximal muscle is often necessary. Slow RNS of the spinal accessory nerve, recording the upper trapezius muscle, is the most common study of a proximal nerve. It is relatively well tolerated, less painful, and subject to less movement artifact when compared to RNS of other

Table C17–5. Compound Muscle Action Potential and Repetitive Abnormalities Characteristic of Common Neuromuscular Junction Disorders

NMJ Defect	Disorder	CMAP	Slow RNS	Fast RNS
Postsynaptic	Myasthenia gravis	Normal	Decrement	Normal or decrement
Presynaptic	Lambert-Eaton myasthenic syndrome	Low	Decrement	Increment

CMAP = compound muscle action potential; NMJ = neuromuscular junction; RNS = repetitive nerve stimulation.

proximal nerves such as the musculocutaneous or axillary nerves, recording the biceps or deltoid muscles, respectively. Finally, facial RNS, recording orbicularis oris, is indicated in patients with suspected ocular MG, particularly when RNS recording proximal muscles are normal or equivocal. However, the facial CMAP is low in amplitude and often plagued by large stimulation artifacts. This renders measurement of decrement difficult and subject to error.

6. In addition to RNS at rest, it is very useful to perform slow RNS after exercise to try to achieve *postexercise exhaustion*, a finding that is often seen in patients with MG. This phenomenon is analogous to the clinical exhaustion that is observed in these patients after exercise. Postexercise RNSs are particularly useful in patients with suspected MG who show only equivocal CMAP decrement at rest (10%). Voluntary exercise is preferable to tetanic stimulation (30–50 Hz) since the latter is extremely painful. After performing slow RNS at rest, the patient is asked to activate the recorded muscle for 1 minute. Then, slow RNS is repeated every 30 to 60 seconds for 4 to 6 minutes looking for postexercise exhaustion, i.e., worsening of decrement compared to baseline decrement at rest. The postexercise study may also result in a phenomenon, known as *postexercise facilitation*. This manifests as improvement or reversal of CMAP decrement, during the first minute of stimulation after exercise (see Figure C17–1A, and compare train 1 to train 2).

Measurements

In MG, slow RNS results in a CMAP decrement. The greatest decrement in amplitude occurs between the first and second responses, while the maximal amplitude decrement is often between the first and or third fourth responses. By the fifth response, the decrement levels off (see Figures C17–1A and C17–2). For these reasons, a train of four or five stimuli at 2 Hz usually is satisfactory and is best tolerable. The decrement is calculated as follows:

$$\% \text{ decrement} = \frac{\text{Amplitude (1st response)} - \text{Amplitude (3rd/4th response)}}{\text{Amplitude (1st response)}} \times 100$$

CMAP decrement of greater than 10% is considered positive and eliminates the potential for a false-positive result. Technical artifacts, such as movement of stimulating or recording electrodes, can lead to CMAP changes that may be mistakenly interpreted as a decrement. These can be minimized by immobilizing the tested limb and securing the stimulating and recording electrodes.

Single-Fiber EMG
Basic Concepts

Single-fiber EMG (SFEMG) is the selective recording from a single or a small number of muscle fibers innervated by a single motor unit. SFEMG recording requires a special expertise and understanding of the micro-environment of motor unit physiology and may be applied to many neuromuscular disorders. However, SFEMG jitter study is most useful in the diagnosis of MG and other NMJ disorders.

Neuromuscular jitter is defined as the random variability of the time interval between two potentials of two muscle fibers of the same motor unit. In healthy subjects, there is a slight variability in the amount of ACH released at the synaptic junction from one moment to another. Although a nerve action potential results in a muscle action potential at all times, the rise in EPP is variable, which results in a small variation in the interpotential interval of the pair of muscle fibers.

Technical Considerations

Recording of neuromuscular jitter requires specific requisites that are essential for the completion and accurate interpretation of data. These include the following:

1. A *concentric single-fiber needle electrode* with a small recording surface (25 mm) is inserted into a muscle. The small recording surface of this electrode restricts the number of recordable MFAPs to an effective area of 300 μm^3, as compared with a concentric needle electrode that records from approximately 1 cm^3.

2. A *500 Hz low-frequency filter* effectively eliminates signals from distant fibers that are more than 500 μm from the electrode. Filter settings should be set at 500 Hz for the high pass filter, and 10–20 kHz for the low pass filter.

3. An *amplitude threshold trigger and a delay line* in the EMG equipment to be capable of isolating individual muscle fiber potentials by triggering them onto a screen with a delay line capability.

4. Computerized equipment assists in calculating the SFEMG jitter.

5. Selected single MFAPs should have an ideal rise time of 300 μs and a preferable peak-to-peak amplitude of 200 μV or more.

6. Patients on cholinesterase inhibitors (such as pyridostigmine) should be asked to withhold their medication for 12–24 hours before single fiber jitter studies, if medically not contraindicated. Also, interpretation of results should be cautiously done in patients who received botulinum toxin injections 6 months prior to study,

since botulinum toxin may interfere with NMJ in muscles that are distant from the site of injection.

Voluntary Single-Fiber EMG

Voluntary (recruitment) SFEMG is the most commonly used method for activating motor units: the patient activates and maintains the firing rate of the motor unit. This technique is not possible if the patient cannot cooperate (e.g., child, dementia, coma, or severe weakness), and is difficult if the patient is unable to maintain a constant firing rate (e.g., tremor, dystonia, or spasticity). With minimal voluntary activation, the needle is positioned until at least two muscle potentials (a pair) from a single motor unit are recognized. When a muscle fiber pair is identified, one fiber triggers the oscilloscope (triggering potential), and the second precedes or follows the first (slave potential). Normal values for jitter (mean and individual values) are available from a multicenter international collaborative effort (Table C17–6). Jitter values differ between muscles, and tend to increase with age, particularly over the age of 50 years.

The muscle(s) tested should be customized according to the patient's symptoms. Frequently tested muscles in patients with suspected MG are the extensor digitorum communis, the orbicularis oculi, and the frontalis. The latter two are particularly helpful in the diagnosis of ocular myasthenia. They are ideal because most patients can control and sustain their voluntary activity to the minimum required for the test. *The diagnostic yield of jitter study is increased by the examination of affected muscle(s) performed by an experienced electromyographer on a fully cooperative patient.*

With voluntary activation, 50 to 100 consecutive discharges of a single pair are recorded. After the interpotential intervals (IPIs) of the pairs are measured, a mean consecutive difference (MCD or jitter) is calculated as follows:

$$\text{MCD} = \frac{(\text{IPI1} - \text{IPI2}) + (\text{IPI2} - \text{IPI3}) + n + (\text{IPI}N - 1 - \text{IPI}N)}{N - 1}$$

where MCD is mean consecutive difference, IPI is interpotential interval, and N is the number of discharges (intervals) recorded. In practice, an MCD should be calculated from at least 50 interpotential intervals. Analysis of 10 to 20 pairs frequently is needed for a mean MCD to be reported. Although the jitter can be measured using a mean and a standard deviation, it is measured more reliably by the MCD because of the potential change in the mean IPI over time. *Jitter is best expressed as the mean MCD of approximately 10 to 20 muscle fiber pairs* (Figure C17–9).

Neuromuscular blocking is defined as the failure of transmission of one of the potentials. Blocking represents the most extreme abnormality of the jitter. Blocking is calculated as the percentage of discharges of a motor unit in which a single-fiber potential does not fire. For example, during 100 discharges of the pair, if a single potential is missing 30 times,

Table C17–6. Reference Values* for Jitter Measurements During Voluntary Muscle Activation (μs)

Muscle	10 Years	20 Years	30 Years	40 Years	50 Years	60 Years	70 Years	80 Years	90 Years
Frontalis	33.6/49.7	33.9/50.1	34.4/51.3	35.5/53.5	37.3/57.5	40.0/63.9	43.8/74.1		
Orbicularis oculi	39.8/54.6	39.8/54.7	40.0/54.7	40.4/54.8	40.9/55.0	41.8/55.3	43.0/55.8		
Orbicularis oris	34.7/52.5	34.7/52.7	34.9/53.2	35.3/54.1	36.0/55.7	37.0/58.2	38.3/61.8	40.2/67.0	42.5/74.2
Tongue	32.8/48.6	33.0/49.0	33.6/50.2	34.8/52.5	36.8/56.3	39.8/62.0	44.0/70.0		
Sternocleidomastoid	29.1/45.4	29.3/45.8	29.8/46.8	30.8/48.8	32.5/52.4	34.9/58.2	38.4/62.3		
Deltoid	32.9/44.4	32.9/44.5	32.9/44.5	32.9/44.6	33.0/44.8	33.0/45.1	33.1/45.6	33.2/46.1	33.3/46.9
Biceps	29.5/45.2	29.6/45.2	29.6/45.4	29.8/45.7	30.1/46.2	30.5/46.9	31.0/48.0		
Extensor digitorum communis	34.9/50.0	34.9/50.1	35.1/50.5	35.4/51.3	35.9/52.5	36.6/54.4	37.7/57.2	39.1/61.1	40.9/66.5
Abductor digiti minimi	44.4/63.5	44.7/64.0	45.2/65.5	46.4/68.6	48.2/73.9	51.0/82.7	54.8/96.6		
Quadriceps	35.9/47.9	36.0/48.0	36.5/48.2	37.5/48.5	39.0/49.1	41.3/50.0	44.6/51.2		
Tibialis anterior	49.4/80.0	49.3/79.8	49.2/79.3	48.9/78.3	48.5/76.8	47.9/74.5	47.0/71.4	45.8/67.5	44.3/62.9

*Values were derived from a multicenter international collaborative study: 95% confidence limits for mean jitter/95% confidence limits for upper limit of jitter values of individual fiber pairs.

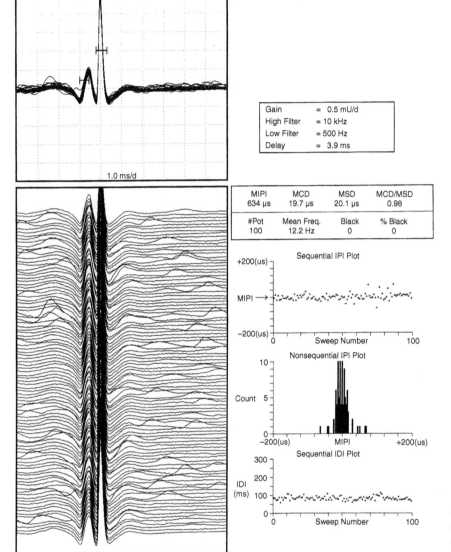

Gain	= 0.5 mU/d
High Filter	= 10 kHz
Low Filter	= 500 Hz
Delay	= 3.9 ms

MIPI	MCD	MSD	MCD/MSD
634 μs	19.7 μs	20.1 μs	0.98

#Pot	Mean Freq.	Black	% Black
100	12.2 Hz	0	0

Figure C17–9. *Normal jitter analysis of a muscle fiber pair, recording the extensor digitorum communis, from a 40-year-old woman with fatigue.*

the blocking occurs at a rate of 30%. In general, blocking occurs when jitter values are significantly abnormal.

In patients with MG, abnormal jitter values are common and frequently are accompanied by blocking (Figure C17–10). This reflects the failure of one of the muscle fiber pairs to transmit an action potential because of the failure of the EPP to reach threshold. The results of SFEMG jitter study are expressed by: (1) the mean jitter of all potential pairs, (2) the percentage of pairs with blocking, and (3) the percentage of pairs with normal jitter.

Jitter analysis is highly sensitive, but it is not specific. It is frequently abnormal in MG and other neuromuscular junction disorders; however, it also may be abnormal in a variety of neuromuscular disorders, including neuropathy,

myopathy, and anterior horn cell disorder. Thus, a diagnosis of MG obtained by jitter analysis must be considered in the context of the patient's clinical manifestations, nerve conduction studies, and needle EMG findings.

Stimulation Single-Fiber EMG

Stimulation (axonal-stimulated) SFEMG records the jitter between a stimulus artifact and a single potential that is generated by stimulation of a motor unit near the end-plate zone. It has the advantage of requiring no patient participation; thus, it may be performed on children, as well as uncooperative or comatose patients. It is performed by inserting another monopolar needle electrode near the intramuscular nerve twigs, and stimulating at a low current

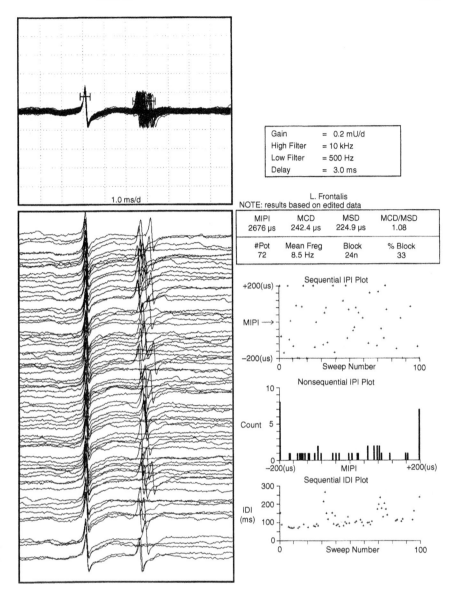

Gain	= 0.2 mU/d
High Filter	= 10 kHz
Low Filter	= 500 Hz
Delay	= 3.0 ms

L. Frontalis
NOTE: results based on edited data

MIPI	MCD	MSD	MCD/MSD
2676 µs	242.4 µs	224.9 µs	1.08

#Pot	Mean Freq	Block	% Block
72	8.5 Hz	24n	33

Figure C17–10. *Abnormal jitter analysis of a muscle fiber pair, recording the frontalis muscle, from a 70-year-old man with mild ptosis. Note the intermittent blocking of the slave (second) potential (33%).*

and constant rate. The electromyographer has to manipulate two electrodes, a stimulating and recording electrode, until one or more potentials are recorded. The IPI is calculated between the stimulus artifact and a single potential generated by stimulating a motor unit near the endplate zone. Since jitter (MCD) values are calculated on the basis of one endplate, the normal values are lower than those obtained by voluntary activation. To calculate the normal stimulation jitter value, the reference data for voluntary activation are multiplied by 0.80.

In addition to its relative ease in performing, the rate of stimulation can be adjusted from a slow rate (2–5 Hz) to a rapid rate (20–50 Hz). This is helpful in the differentiation of presynaptic and postsynaptic disorders because neuromuscular transmission, jitter and blocking improve significantly with a rapid rate stimulation in LEMS, but it does not change or it worsens in MG (Figure C17–11).

Diagnostic Sensitivity of Electrodiagnostic Tests

In general, the diagnostic utility of the EDX studies correlates well with the severity of MG. The tests are more often abnormal in patients with significant generalized weakness while they may be normal in those with mild ocular disease. The exact sensitivity of the various EDX tests is not known, since there is no gold standard for diagnosis and many seropositive patients are not subjected to these time consuming tests. Using the clinical examination and a positive Tensilon test as a gold standard for the diagnosis of MG, the diagnostic sensitivity of various diagnostic tests is shown in Figure C17–12. Most importantly,

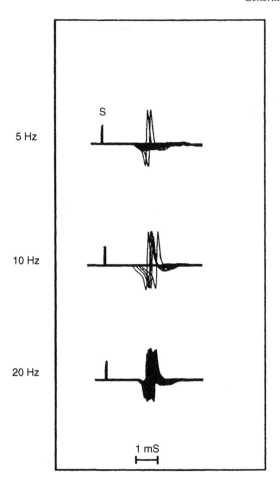

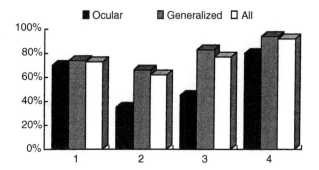

Figure C17–12. *The diagnostic sensitivity of the laboratory tests in myasthenia gravis. 1 = acetylcholine receptor antibody; 2 = slow RNS, recording distal muscle; 3 = slow RNS, recording proximal muscle; 4 = single-fiber electromyography of the forearm muscle (extensor digitorum communis). (Adapted from Oh SJ et al. Diagnostic sensitivity of the laboratory tests in myasthenia gravis. Muscle Nerve 1992;15:720–724, with permission.)*

Figure C17–13 highlights the proposed EDX work-up for such a patient.

FOLLOW-UP

Acetylcholine receptor antibodies, anti-MuSK antibodies, antistriated muscle antibody, thyroid function tests, antithyroid antibodies, antinuclear antibodies (ANAs), and rheumatoid factor were all negative. A CT scan of the chest did not show an enlarged thymus.

The diagnosis of MG was established based on the clinical findings and the decremental response to slow repetitive stimulation. The patient was started on treatment with pyridostigmine (Mestinon) 60 mg qid, with significant improvement of weakness and chewing. However, because of persistent ocular symptoms and fatigability, she underwent an extended transsternal thymectomy. Pathologic examination revealed thymus hyperplasia (germinal center formation). Two months later, she felt much stronger and demonstrated no ocular symptoms. She slowly tapered her pyridostigmine and discontinued it 18 months postoperatively. Three years after thymectomy, she still was in complete remission.

Figure C17–11. *The effect of stimulation rate on the jitter and blocking in an endplate in the extensor digitorum communis of a patient with Lambert-Eaton myasthenic syndrome. Single-fiber electromyographic recordings were made during stimulation of an intramuscular nerve twig. Each trace represents the superimposition of ten consecutive responses. Eighty percent of responses are blocked at 5 Hz, compared with 50% at 10 Hz and none at 20 Hz. S = stimulus artifact. (From Saunders DB. Lambert-Eaton myasthenic syndrome: clinical diagnosis, immune-mediated mechanisms and update on therapies. Ann Neurol 1995;37(S1): S63–S73, with permission.)*

it is extremely rare for patients with MG to have an entirely negative work-up that includes repetitive nerve stimulation recording both distal and proximal muscles, single-fiber jitter analysis of an affected muscle, and ACH receptor antibody.

Suggested Electrodiagnostic Work-Up
When a patient is suspected to have MG, routine nerve conduction studies should be performed initially. If the CMAP amplitudes are low, a presynaptic defect should be suspected and excluded, but a postsynaptic defect is surmised if the CMAP amplitudes are normal.

DIAGNOSIS
Generalized seronegative myasthenia gravis.

ANSWERS

1. D; 2. B; 3. C.

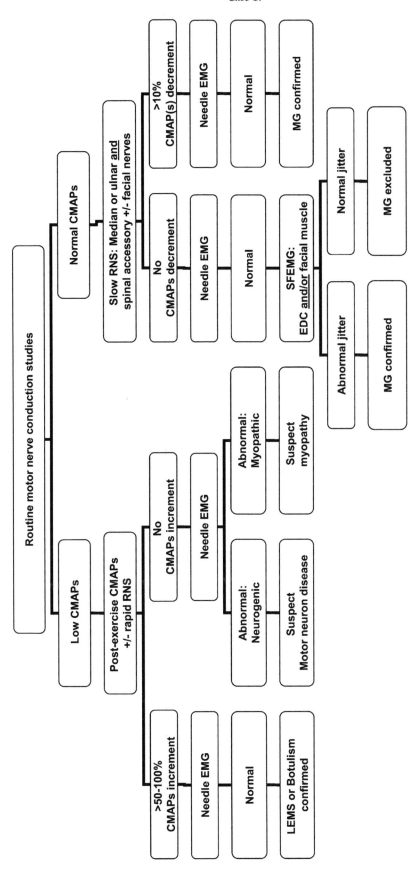

Figure C17–13. *Suggested electrodiagnostic strategy for patients with suspected myasthenia gravis in particular, or a neuromuscular junction defect in general. All patients will have normal sensory nerve conduction studies. (CMAP = compound muscle action potential, RNS = repetitive nerve stimulation, LEMS = Lambert-Eaton myasthenic syndrome, MG = myasthenia gravis, SFEMG = single fiber EMG, EDC = extensor digitorum communis.)*

SUGGESTED READINGS

Barberi S, Weiss GM, Daube JR. Fibrillation potentials in myasthenia gravis. Muscle Nerve 1982;5:S50.

Boonyapisit K, Kaminski HJ, Ruff RL. The molecular basis of neuromuscular transmission disorders. Am J Med 1999;6: 97–113.

Daroff RB. The office Tensilon test for ocular myasthenia gravis. Arch Neurol 1986;43:843–844.

Drachman DB. Myasthenia gravis. N Engl J Med 1994;330: 1797–1810.

Gilchrist JM. Ad hoc committee of the AAEM special interest group on SFEMG. Single fiber EMG reference values: a collaborative effort. Muscle Nerve 1992;15:151–161.

Gilchrist JM. Single fiber EMG. In: Katirji B, Kaminski HJ, Preston DC, Ruff RL, Shapiro EB, eds. Neuromuscular disorders in clinical practice. Boston, MA: Butterworth-Heinemann, 2002, pp. 141–150.

Howard JH, Sanders DB, Massey JM. The electrodiagnosis of myasthenia gravis and the Lambert-Eaton syndrome. Neurol Clin 1994;12:305–330.

Kaminski HJ, ed. Myasthenia gravis and related disorders. Totowa, NJ: Humana Press, 2003.

Katirji B, Kaminski HJ. An electrodiagnostic approach to the patient with neuromuscular junction disorder. Neuro Clin 2002;20:557–586.

Kelly JJ et al. The laboratory diagnosis of mild myasthenia gravis. Ann Neurol 1982;12:238–242.

Kupersmith MJ, Moster M, Bhuiyan S et al. Beneficial effects of corticosteroids on ocular myasthenia gravis. Arch Neurol 1996;53:802–804.

Lanska DJ. Diagnosis of thymoma in myasthenic using anti-striated muscle antibodies. Neurology 1991;41:520–524.

Lewis RA, Selwa JF, Lisak RP. Myasthenia gravis: immunological mechanisms and immunotherapy. Ann Neurol 1995;37(S1): S51–S62.

Oh SJ. Electromyography: neuromuscular transmission studies. Baltimore, MD: Williams & Wilkins, 1988.

Oh SJ et al. Electrophysiological and clinical correlation in myasthenia gravis. Ann Neurol 1982;12:348–354.

Oh SH et al. Diagnostic sensitivity of the laboratory tests in myasthenia gravis. Muscle Nerve 1992;15:720–724.

Stalberg E, Trontelj JV. Single fiber electromyography, 2nd ed. Philadelphia, PA: Lippincott-Raven Press, 1994.

Tindall RSA et al. Preliminary results of a double-blind, randomized, placebo-controlled trial of cyclosporine in myasthenia gravis. N Engl J Med 1987;316:719–724.

Zinman L, Ng E, Bril V. IV immunoglobulin in patients with myasthenia gravis: A randomized controlled study. Neurology 2007; 68:837–841.

Case 18

HISTORY AND PHYSICAL EXAMINATION

A 76-year-old woman had been in excellent health until 1 year before presentation when she noticed a gradual development of numbness and pain in both legs. This feeling ascended slowly and began to involve the hands. Progressive imbalance followed, and she first required a cane and later a walker for ambulation. She had leg weakness, with difficulty getting up the steps and rising from a sitting position. She denied any bowel or bladder symptoms. Past medical history was negative.

Her neurological examination was relevant for areflexia, marked loss of position and vibration sense at the toes and ankles, and symmetrical weakness of hand grips (Medical Research Council [MRC] 4+/5) and hip flexors (4/5), with more pronounced weakness in the distal leg muscles (4–/5). Gait was wide-based and ataxic, with a positive Romberg test.

Electrodiagnostic (EDX) study was performed.

Please now review the Nerve Conduction Studies and Needle EMG tables.

QUESTIONS

1. The clinical and EDX findings in this case are consistent with:
   A. Acute axonal polyneuropathy.
   B. Chronic inherited demyelinating polyneuropathy.
   C. Acute acquired demyelinating polyneuropathy.
   D. Chronic acquired demyelinating polyneuropathy.
   E. Multifocal motor neuropathy with conduction block.
2. The etiologic differential diagnosis might include all the following *except:*
   A. Charcot-Marie-Tooth disease type 2 (hereditary motor sensory neuropathy (HMSN) type II).
   B. Neuropathy associated with osteosclerotic myeloma.
   C. Neuropathy associated with monoclonal gammopathy of unknown significance (MGUS).
   D. Chronic inflammatory demyelinating polyradiculoneuropathy (CIDP).
   E. Neuropathy associated with early human immunodeficiency virus (HIV) infection.
3. Peripheral neuropathy is commonly associated with all of the following *except:*
   A. Amyloidosis.
   B. Immunoglobulin M (IgM) MGUS.
   C. IgE MGUS.
   D. Multiple myeloma.
   E. IgG MGUS.

EDX FINDINGS AND INTERPRETATION OF DATA

The abnormal EDX findings in this case include:

1. Absent upper and lower limb sensory nerve action potentials (SNAPs).
2. Multiple partial conduction blocks bilaterally in the forearms. In comparing of responses obtained by distal versus proximal stimulation, the left median compound muscle action potential (CMAP) declined in amplitude from 2.5 mV distally to 1.2 mV proximally (52% amplitude loss), without increase in duration and with an obvious change in waveform morphology (Figure C18–1A). The left ulnar CMAP decreased in amplitude from 3.8 mV distally to 1.0 mV proximally below the elbow (74% amplitude loss), with slight increase in duration (Figure C18–1B). Also, the right ulnar CMAP amplitude dropped from 4.2 mV to 1.0 mV (76% amplitude loss). The CMAP amplitude decay of these nerves was also confirmed by greater than 50% concomitant drop in CMAP areas. The amplitude change of the right median nerve (from 3.3 mV distally to 2.7 mV proximally) was borderline (18%) and probably not significant.

Case 18: Nerve Conduction Studies

Nerve Stimulated	Stimulation Site	Recording Site	Amplitude (m = mV, s = µV)			Distal/Peak Latency (ms)			Conduction Velocity (m/s)			F Latency (ms)	
			Right	Left	Normal	Right	Left	Normal	Right	Left	Normal	Right	Left
Sural (s)	Calf	Ankle	NR		≥3.0	NR		≤4.6	NR				
Peroneal (m)	Ankle	EDB	0.66	2.5*	≥2.5	11.2	7.2*	≤6.0				NR	
Peroneal (m)	Knee	EDB	0.38	1.2*					12		≥40		
Tibial (m)	Ankle	AH	0.70	3.8*	≥4.0	10.0	6.4*	≤6.0				NR	
Tibial (m)	Knee	AH	0.44	1.0*					12		≥40		
H reflex	Knee	Soleus	NR			NR							
M response	Knee	Soleus	1.0			6.7							
Median (s)	Wrist	Index finger	NR		≥10	NR		≤3.8					
Median (s)	Elbow	Index finger	NR			NR			NR		≥50		
Ulnar (s)	Wrist	Little finger	NR		≥5	NR		≤3.2					
Radial (s)	Distal forearm	Thumb base	NR		≥10	NR		≤2.8					
Median (m)*	Wrist	APB	3.3	2.5*	≥5	7.4	7.2*	≤4.0	21	23*	≥50	57.6	57.6
Median (m)*	Elbow	APB	2.7	1.2*									
Ulnar (m)*	Wrist	ADM	4.2	3.8*	≥7	4.8	6.4*	≤3.1				57.6	58
Ulnar (m)*	Below elbow	ADM	1.0	1.0*					19	18*	≥50		
Ulnar (m)*	Above elbow	ADM	0.8	1.0*					18	20*	≥50		

ADM = abductor digiti minimi; APB = abductor pollicis brevis; EDB = extensor digitorum brevis; m = motor; NR = no response; s = sensory.
Data in bold type are abnormal.
*See Figure C18–1.

Case 18: Needle EMG

Case 18: Needle EMG

Muscle	Insertional Activity	Spontaneous Activity		Recruitment				Voluntary Motor Unit Action Potentials (MUAPs) Configuration			
		Fibs	Fascs	Normal	Activation	Reduced	Early	Duration	Amplitude	% Polyphasia	Others
R. tibialis anterior	↑	Few	0			↓↓		↑	Normal	Normal	
Medial gastrocnemius	↑	Few	0			↓↓		↑	Normal	Normal	
Tibialis posterior	↑	Few	0			↓		Normal	Normal	Normal	
Abductor hallucis	↑	0	0			↓↓		↑	Normal	Normal	
Vastus lateralis	Normal	0	0			↓		Normal	Normal	Normal	
Gluteus medius	Normal	0	0	X				Normal	Normal	Normal	
Middle lumbar paraspinal	0	0	–								
R. first dorsal interosseous	Normal	0	0			↓		Normal	Normal	Normal	
Brachioradialis	Normal	0	0	X				Normal	Normal	Normal	

Fascs = fasciculations; Fibs = fibrillations; R. = right; ↑ = increased; ↓ = mildly reduced; ↓↓ = moderately reduced.

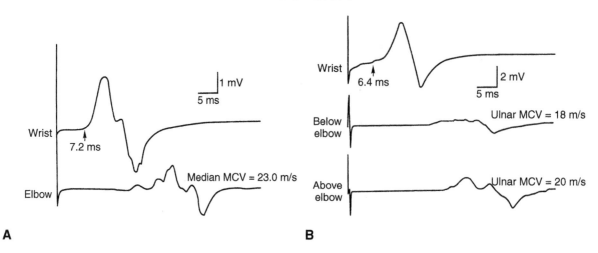

Figure C18–1. *Motor nerve conduction studies of the left median nerve, recording abductor pollicis brevis (**A**) and the left ulnar nerve, recording abductor digiti minimi (**B**). Note the conduction blocks and dispersion between distal and proximal stimulations and the marked slowing of velocities and distal latencies. (See also the Nerve Conduction Studies table.)*

3. There is significant slowing of conduction velocities (18 to 23 m/s), distal latencies, and F wave latencies in the arms, despite relatively spared distal amplitudes.

4. Abnormalities in the leg are severe. Although there is marked slowing of both conduction velocities and distal latencies, the distal CMAP amplitudes are extremely low representing only few motor units; thus one cannot use these data with confidence to foresee primary pathology (demyelination versus axonal loss). The upper extremities, which are less affected in this patient, are much more useful for such a prediction.

5. Inconspicuous fibrillation potentials and large motor unit action potentials (MUAPs), more pronounced distally, are evidence that axonal loss has occurred and is minimal and chronic.

The clinical and EDX findings are consistent with *chronic, progressive, acquired, demyelinating sensorimotor polyneuropathy* because of the following:

- The clinical history is one of slow and steady progression without exacerbations.
- The presence of both relatively few fibrillation potentials and few chronic neurogenic MUAP changes.
- The diagnosis of sensorimotor polyneuropathy is based on the clinical manifestations (weakness and sensory loss) and is supported by diffusely abnormal sensory and motor studies.
- The disorder is demyelinating because there are multiple conduction blocks and significant slowing of conduction velocities and distal latencies in the upper limbs, despite relatively preserved distal CMAP amplitudes.
- This patient's polyneuropathy is acquired because of the presence of multifocal conduction blocks in peripheral

nerve segments that are not susceptible to common entrapments.

This EDX study is not compatible with multifocal motor neuropathy with conduction block because of abnormal (unevokable) SNAPs. The polyneuropathy is obviously not acute (such as with Guillain-Barré syndrome) based on the history of slow progression (longer than 3 months) and the MUAP changes which are consistent with chronic reinnervation. The conduction slowing in the inherited demyelinating polyneuropathy, such as in Charcot-Marie-Tooth disease (CMT) type I (HMSN I), is uniform and there are no conduction blocks. Finally, the nerve conduction studies are not consistent with Charcot-Marie-Tooth disease type 2 (also called HMSN type II), because this latter disorder is a manifestation of a primary axonal polyneuropathy.

DISCUSSION

Clinical Features

Peripheral Polyneuropathies

Peripheral polyneuropathy is a common presenting illness in neurologic practice with multiple, sometimes overwhelming, list of potential etiologies. *Pattern recognition* is a useful diagnostic approach but applies to a minority of patients who usually have advanced disease and often requires vast clinical experience such as by a seasoned neurologist. For an example, an asymmetrical polyneuropathy with predilection to cool skin areas (nipples, buttocks, and fingers) and skin ulcerations is highly suggestive of leprous neuropathy. Also, a distal sensory polyneuropathy with brisk reflexes, mild cognitive impairment, and a red tongue suggests combined system degeneration due to vitamin B12 deficiency. Another approach to the etiologic diagnosis of peripheral polyneuropathy is to order all available tests, including costly serology evaluations, on every patient with a polyneuropathy. Unfortunately, this *irrational "shotgun" approach* is quite common and often utilized by internists and some neurologists. It sometimes results in an incorrect diagnosis secondary to incidental abnormalities such as an elevated glucose on glucose tolerance test or anti-neuronal antiboby on serological testing.

A recommended and more *rational approach* may be initiated on every patient presenting with a peripheral polyneuropathy. This could be achieved by performing a thorough history and physical examination followed by EDX studies (see Figure C26–1, Case 26), and often results in limited and cost effective investigations (Table C18–1). Despite extensive investigations in specialized centers that includes EDX testing, antibody panels and genetic testing, up to 20% of patients with peripheral polyneuropathies will not have their exact causation identified. Of those with

Table C18–1. Essential Facts Important in the Classification and Etiologic Diagnosis of Peripheral Polyneuropathy

Temporal Profile of the Polyneuropathy
Is the polyneuropathy subacute or chronic?
If chronic, is the disorder progressive, relapsing and remitting, or stepwise?

   Subacute – consider Guillain-Barré syndrome, porphyria, diphtheria, critical illness, and drugs/toxins

   Chronic relapsing and remitting – consider CIDP and drugs/toxins

   Chromic progressive – consider CIDP, metabolic disturbance*, nutritional deficiency, and toxins

Anatomic Pattern of the Polyneuropathy
Is the polyneuropathy distal, proximal or both?
Are there any foot or spine deformities (pes cavus or kyphoscoliosis)?
Is the polyneuropathy symmetric or asymmetric?
If asymmetric, do the findings follow specific peripheral nerve distribution?

   Distal – consider metabolic disturbance*, vitamin deficiency, toxins, drugs, critical illness, hereditary

   Distal and proximal – consider Guillain-Barré syndrome, CIDP, porphyria

   Asymmetric – consider vasculitis, CIDP, HNPP

   Involvement of specific peripheral nerves – consider multifocal motor neuropathy, Lewis-Sumner syndrome, HNPP, vasculitis, leprosy

   Pes cavus or kyphoscoliosis – consider CMT, HNPP

Type(s) of Nerve Fiber Involvement
Is the polyneuropathy sensory, motor or mixed?
If sensory, is it small fiber, large fiber or both?
Are the autonomic fibers involved?

   Large fiber sensory – consider Sjögren syndrome, anti-Hu paraneoplastic disease, vitamin E deficiency, and vitamin B6 intoxication

   Small fiber sensory – consider diabetes, amyloidosis, HIV, metabolic disturbance*, toxins, drugs, or amyloidosis

   Autonomic – consider Guillian-Barré syndrome, metabolic disturbance*, amyloidosis, HIV infection

Family History of Polyneuropathy
Is there a family history of polyneuropathy?
Is there a family history of foot deformities (pes cavus) or the spine (kyphoscoliosis)?

   Autosomal dominant – consider CMT1, CMT2, CMT3, HNPP

   X-linked – consider CMTX

   Autosomal recessive – consider CMT3, CMT4

Medical Illness and Exposure to Drugs or Toxins
Is the exposure time locked to the onset of symptoms?
Did eliminating the exposure stopped progression of polyneuropathy?

   Medical illness – consider diabetes mellitus, chronic renal insufficiency, hypothyroidism, HIV infection, connective tissue disease, myeloproliferative disorders (+/– paraproteinemia), celiac disease, and paraneoplastic disease

   Drugs – consider vincristine, paclitaxil, cisplatin, amiodarone, hydralazine, isoniazid, metronidazole, nitrofurantoin, disulfiram, thalidomide, gold, and pyridoxine (toxicity)

   Toxins – consider ethyl alcohol, arsenic, thallium, acrylamide, nitric oxide, ethylene oxide, n-hexane, perhexiline, and methyl n-butyl ketone

Continued

Table C18–1. —cont'd

Primary Pathology (axonal or demyelinating)
Is the polyneuropathy primarily axonal or demyelinating?
If demyelinating, is it segmental (multifocal) or uniform?
    Axonal – consider metabolic disturbance,* toxins, drugs, critical illness, CMT2, CMT4
    Demyelinating and segmental (multifocal) – consider Guillain-Barré syndrome, CIDP, CIDP with paraproteinemia, HNPP
    Demyelinating and uniform – consider CMT1, CMT3, CMTX, CMT4

CIDP = chronic inflammatory demyelinating polyradiculoneuropathy, HNPP = hereditary neuropathy with liability to pressure palsy, CMT = Chercot-Marie-Tooth disease, HIV = human immunodeficiency virus.
*Include diabetes mellitus, uremia, thyroid disorders.

idiopathic etiology, it is estimated that a familial neuropathy accounts for about 40% if a meticulous family history is taken and relatives are carefully examined.

Chronic Demyelinating Polyneuropathies

In most peripheral polyneuropathies, it is often possible to define the predominant pathophysiologic mechanism, based on electrophysiologic and pathologic features, as being either primarily axonal or demyelinating. In demyelinating polyneuropathy, it is also useful to distinguish between neuropathies with segmental (multifocal) versus uniform slowing, based on electrophysiologic studies (see electrodiagnosis). Multifocal or segmental demyelinating polyneuropathies are almost always acquired, while uniform demyelinating polyneuropathies are typically hereditary.

The causes of chronic axonal neuropathies are abundant, while chronic demyelinating polyneuropathies have a fairly restrictive differential diagnosis (Table C18–2). Many acquired demyelinating polyneuropathies are immune in nature and respond to immunosupression or immunomodulation, while most axonal polyneuropathies are metabolic or toxic in nature. Since the differential diagnosis of chronic acquired demyelinating polyneuropathies is quite limited, the diagnostic work-up for patients with such entities is much less laborious and is quite different from that of patients with axonal neuropathies (Table C18–3).

Chronic Inflammatory Demyelinating Polyradiculoneuropathy

Chronic inflammatory demyelinating polyradiculoneuropathy (CIDP) is the prototype of all chronic acquired demyelinating polyneuropathies. It is an autoimmune disorder of the peripheral nervous system that affects individuals at any age and may be relapsing and remitting or slowly progressive usually over several months. Proximal and distal symmetrical weakness is the most common manifestation. Many patients have also numbness and paresthesias, usually of the feet and hands. Generalized areflexia is very common while some patients have only hyporeflexia or distal areflexia.

Table C18–2. Common Causes of Chronic Demyelinating Peripheral Polyneuropathy

Acquired (nonuniform multifocal slowing)
1. CIDP
2. CIDP associated with HIV infection (early phase)
3. Multifocal motor neuropathy with conduction block (with or without associated anti-GM$_1$ antibody)
4. Chronic demyelinating polyneuropathy occurring with anti-MAG antibody
5. Chronic demyelinating polyneuropathy associated with monoclonal gammopathy
    MGUS (IgG, IgM, or IgA)
    Osteosclerotic myeloma (POEMS syndrome)
    Multiple myeloma
    Waldenstrom macroglobulinemia
    Castleman disease
    Amyloidosis
6. CIDP associated with central nervous system demyelinating disease

Hereditary (uniform slowing)
1. HMSN I and III (CMT1 and 3)
2. HNPP*
3. Congenital hypomyelinating neuropathy
4. Leukodystrophies
    Adrenomyeloneurpathy
    Metochormatic
    Krabbes
    Cockayne
5. Cerebrotendinous xanthomatosis
6. Refsum disease
7. Tangiers disease

CIDP = chronic inflammatory demyelinating polyradiculoneuropathy; HIV = human immunodeficiency virus; GM$_1$ = ganglioside M$_1$; MAG = myelin-associated glycoprotein; MGUS = monoclonal gammopathy of unknown significance; Ig = immunoglobulin; POEMS syndrome = polyneuropathy, organomegaly, endocrinopathy, monoclonal protein, and skin changes; HMSN = hereditary motor and sensory neuropathy; CMT = Charcot-Marie-Tooth disease; HNPP = hereditary neuropathy with liability to pressure palsy.
*May have multifocal slowing also, usually across common entrapment sites.

Table C18–3. Recommended Work-Up of Chronic Acquired Demyelinating Peripheral Polyneuropathy

CBC, serum calcium, BUN, creatinine

CSF examination

HIV antibody (especially if high risk, or if CSF pleocytosis >50 cells)

Serum protein electrophoresis *and* immunofixation*

Urine immunofixation (preferably on a 24-hour collection)

Serum anti-MAG antibody (especially if predominantly sensory)

Serum anti-GM$_1$ antibody (if pure motor with multifocal blocks)

Skeletal bone survey

Bone marrow aspirate (particularly with bone lesion(s), a paraprotein of more than 1 to 2 g/dL, or rising paraprotein value)

BUN = blood urea nitrogen; CBC = complete blood count; CSF = cerebrospinal fluid; GM$_1$ = ganglioside M$_1$; HIV = human immunodeficiency virus; MAG = myelin-associated glycoprotein.

*Serum immunofixation is often necessary because routine serum protein electrophoresis may miss patients with a small amount of circulating paraprotein (M-protein).

Patients with CIDP must be distinguished from patients with the more prevalent acquired axonal peripheral polyneuropathies. CIDP should also be separated from hereditary polyneuropathies, particularly those with demyelinating features such as CMT1, CMTX, and CMT3. CIDP should also be distinguished from other polyradiculopathies, such as meningeal carcinomatosus, Lyme disease, or sarcoidosis. When predominantly motor, CIDP may mimic neuromuscular junction disorders (such as the Lambert-Eaton myasthenic syndrome), motor neuron disorders, and myopathies.

Chronic inflammatory demyelinating polyradiculoneuropathy (CIDP) is a diagnosis of pattern recognition, based on clinical manifestations, EDX, cerebrospinal fluid examination, laboratory tests appropriate to the specific clinical situation, and, occasionally, results from nerve biopsy. The American Academy of Neurology defined criteria for the diagnosis of CIDP (Table C18–4). Four features are set as the basis of diagnosis: clinical, electrodiagnostic, pathologic, and cerebrospinal fluid studies. These are further divided into mandatory, supportive, and, where appropriate, exclusion. Mandatory features are those required for diagnosis and should be present in all definite cases. Supportive features are helpful in clinical diagnosis but by themselves do not make a diagnosis. Exclusion features strongly suggest alternative diagnoses.

Peripheral Polyneuropathy and Monoclonal Gammopathy of Undetermined Significance

The prevalence of monoclonal gammopathy of undetermined significance (MGUS) increases with age. It is present in 1% of patients older than 50 years of age and in 3% of patients older than 70 years of age. This entity must be distinguished from the more malignant myeloproliferative disorders, such as multiple myeloma, by obtaining complete blood count (CBC), calcium, blood urea nitrogen (BUN)/creatinine, a skeletal survey, and, at times, a bone marrow aspirate. Table C18–5 lists both the criteria needed to confirm the diagnosis of MGUS and its common

Table C18–4. American Academy of Neurology Criteria for Diagnosis of Chronic Inflammatory Demyelinating Polyneuropathy

I. *Clinical*
   A. *Mandatory*
   1. Progressive or relapsing motor and sensory, rarely, only motor or sensory, dysfunction of more than one limb of a peripheral nerve nature, developing over at least 2 months
   2. Hypo- or areflexia. This usually involves all four limbs
   B. *Supportive*
   Large-fiber sensory loss predominates over small-fiber sensory loss
   C. *Exclusion*
   1. Mutilation of hands or feet, retinitis pigmentosa, ichthyosis, appropriate history of drug or toxic exposure known to cause a similar peripheral neuropathy, or family history of an inherited peripheral neuropathy
   2. Sensory level
   3. Unequivocal sphincter disturbance

II. *Electrodiagnostic Studies*
   A. *Mandatory*
   Nerve conduction studies including studies of proximal nerve segments in which the predominant process is demyelination
   Must have *three of four*:
   1. Reduction in conduction velocity (CV) in two or more motor nerves:
      a. <80% of lower limit of normal (LLN) if amplitude >80% of LLN
      b. <70% of LLN if amplitude <80% of LLN

Continued

Table C18–4. —cont'd

II. Electrodiagnostic Studies—cont'd

 2. Partial conduction block* or abnormal temporal dispersion[†] in one or more motor nerves: either peroneal nerve between ankle and below fibular head, median nerve between wrist and elbow or ulnar nerve between wrist and below elbow

 3. Prolonged distal latencies in two or more nerves:

 a. >125% of upper limit of normal (ULN) if amplitude >80% of LLN

 b. >150% of ULN if amplitude <80% of LLN

 4. Absent F waves or prolonged minimum F-wave latencies (10 to 15 trials) in two or more motor nerves:

 a. >120% of ULN if amplitude >80% of LLN

 b. >150% of ULN if amplitude <80% of LLN

 B. *Supportive*

 1. Reduction in sensory CV <80% of LLN

 2. Absent H reflexes

III. CSF Studies

 A. *Mandatory*

 1. Cell count <10/mm^3 if HIV-seronegative or <50/mm^3 if HIV-seropositive

 2. Negative VDRL

 B. *Supportive*

 Elevated protein

IV. Pathologic Features

 A. *Mandatory*

 Nerve biopsy showing unequivocal evidence of demyelination and remyelination[‡]

 B. *Supportive*

 1. Subperineurial or endoneurial edema

 2. Mononuclear cell infiltration

 3. "Onion-bulb" formation

 4. Prominent variation in the degree of demyelination between fascicles

 C. *Exclusion*

 Vasculitis, neurofilamentous swollen axons, amyloid deposits, or intracytoplasmic inclusions in Schwann cells or macrophages indicating adrenoleukodystrophy, metachromatic leukodystrophy, globoid cell leukodystrophy, or other evidence of specific pathology

---

*Criteria suggestive of partial conduction block: >20% drop in area or amplitude with <15% change in duration between proximal and distal sites.

[†]Criteria for abnormal temporal dispersion and possible conduction block: >20% drop in area or amplitude between proximal and distal sites with >15% change in duration between proximal and distal sites and. These criteria are only suggestive of partial conduction block as they are derived from studies of normal individuals. Additional studies, such as stimulation across short segments or recording of individual motor unit potentials, are required for confirmation.

[‡]Demyelination by either electron microscopy (>5 fibers) or teased fiber studies (>12% of 50 teased fibers, minimum of four internodes each, demonstrating demyelination/remyelination).

Diagnostic categories. *Definite:* Clinical A and C, Electrodiagnostic A, CSF A, and Pathology A and C. *Probable:* Clinical A and C, Electrodiagnostic A, and CSF A. *Possible:* Clinical A and C and Electrodiagnostic A.

---

characteristics. Although MGUS is relatively benign and is commonly asymptomatic, follow-up reveals that malignant myeloproliferative disorders will develop in up to one-third of these patients within 20 years. A good indication for this malignant transformation is a rising M-protein (paraprotein) value, especially one greater than 3 g/dL. Thus, a regular follow-up of the paraprotein value is warranted in all patients with MGUS.

Up to 10% of patients with peripheral polyneuropathy have a monoclonal protein; this is significantly higher than the prevalence in the general population (1–3%). The paraprotein is commonly of the IgG or IgM class and less often of the IgA class. Almost half of patients with IgM-associated neuropathy have elevated serum antibody titers to myelin-associated glycoprotein (anti-MAG). However, patients with elevated anti-MAG antibody do not all have a detectable IgM paraprotein on immunofixation.

The polyneuropathies associated with paraproteinemia (e.g., MGUS, myeloma) are heterogeneous; they can be axonal or demyelinating, sensory or sensorimotor. Their characteristics correlate poorly with the class of abnormal paraprotein. Certain important points need to be emphasized:

1. When it is demyelinating in nature, MGUS-associated polyneuropathy is indistinguishable from CIDP, both clinically and electrophysiologically, except by the presence of the serum paraprotein.

Table C18–5. Monoclonal Gammopathy of Unknown Significance (MGUS)

Criteria for Diagnosis	Characteristics
1. Paraprotein (M-protein) value less than 3 g/dL	Common monoclonal type: IgM or IgG
2. No lytic bony lesions	Common light chain: kappa
3. Plasma cell in bone marrow less than 5%	Urine monoclonal protein: rare
4. No anemia, hypercalcemia, or renal failure	

2. Immunoglobulin M-associated neuropathy is predominantly sensory and ataxic, and often is demyelinating.
3. Anti-MAG-associated polyneuropathy, similar to IgM-associated neuropathy, is frequently predominantly sensory, ataxic, and demyelinating.
4. A subgroup of patients with myeloma, those with osteosclerotic myeloma, commonly present with a chronic demyelinating polyneuropathy. Typically, there is a single or multiple sclerotic bone lesion that harbors monoclonal plasma cells. This disorder also is termed POEMS (*p*olyneuropathy, *o*rganomegaly, *e*ndocrinopathy, *m*onoclonal protein, and *s*kin changes) because of other frequently associated features (hepatosplenomegaly, gynecomastia, atrophic testicles, hyperpigmentation, hypertrichosis, and clubbing).

There is continuous debate regarding the various acquired demyelinating polyneuropathies, namely CIDP, MGUS neuropathy, anti-MAG-associated neuropathy, and multifocal motor neuropathy with conduction block. Our current knowledge of the exact etiology and pathogenesis of these immune disorders is lacking. Figure C18–2 reveals a schematic representation of the significant overlap between all these disorders. Apart from the presence of a monoclonal protein, the clinical and EDX features of CIDP – with or without MGUS – are quite similar. However, as is shown in Table C18–6, there are certain features in the presentation and clinical course that tend to help differentiate between these disorders.

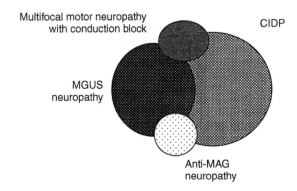

Figure C18–2. *Spectrum of acquired demyelinating polyneuropathies.*

The treatment of patients with MGUS-associated polyneuropathy depends on its clinical presentation. Patients with sensory symptoms only, particularly the elderly, may be treated symptomatically with drugs that alter neuropathic pain. Plasma exchange is effective, particularly in neuropathies with IgG and IgA type MGUS, but should be reserved for patients with significant motor weakness or ataxia. Intravenous gamma globulin is useful particularly in patients with a CIDP-MGUS presentation. Prednisone, rituximab, azathioprine, chlorambucil, and cyclophosphamide have resulted in benefit.

Electrodiagnosis

In a patient with suspected peripheral polyneuropathy, the EDX study:

1. Provides an unequivocal diagnosis of peripheral polyneuropathy.
2. Defines the anatomic distribution of a neuropathy, as a single mononeuropathy, multiple mononeuropathies, or a generalized peripheral polyneuropathy.
3. Excludes mimickers of polyneuropathies such as bilateral L5 and S1/S2 radiculopathies, bilateral tarsal tunnel syndromes and, occasionally, bilateral carpal tunnel syndromes, or distal myopathies.
4. Establishes the type of fiber(s) affected (sensory, motor, or both).
5. Estimates the chronicity and activity of the process.
6. Most importantly, identifies its primary pathologic process (demyelination or axonal loss).

Thus, at the completion of an EDX test, the clinician should be able to better characterize the polyneuropathy and classify its pathophysiology. This helps establish a relatively short differential diagnosis and work-up aimed at identifying the cause of the neuropathy and planning its management (see Table C18–1).

Analyzing conduction times (velocities and latencies), as well as CMAP amplitude, area and duration, is an essential exercise in the EMG laboratory for establishing the primary pathologic process of a polyneuropathy. In most situations, the polyneuropathy falls in one of the following categories based on one of two primary nerve dysfunctions: the

Table C18–6. Distinctive Features for Differentiating Between Chronic Inflammatory Demyelinating Polyradiculoneuropathy (CIDP) Without and With MGUS

Feature	CIDP Without MGUS	CIDP With MGUS
Age	Relatively younger	Relatively older
Course	Progressive or relapsing	Frequently progressive
Neuropathy	Predominantly motor	Predominantly sensory with ataxia
Clinical deterioration	More rapid	Slow indolent
Functional impairment	Moderate to severe	Mild
Spontaneous improvement	Common	Rare
Response to therapy	Good	Less responsive

axon or its supporting myelin. Occasionally, such as in very mild polyneuropathies or in severe situations associated with absent responses, it may be difficult to establish the primary pathology based on EDX studies.

- *Primary axonal polyneuropathies (axonopathies)* affect the axon primarily and produce a length-dependent dying-back degeneration of axons. The major change on NCS is a decrease of the CMAP and SNAP amplitudes, more marked in the lower extremities. In contrast, conduction times (velocities, distal latencies, and F wave minimal latencies) are normal. Sometimes, there is a slight slowing of distal latencies, conduction velocities

and F wave minimal latencies when the polyneuropathy is advanced (Figure C18–3). This is explained by the fact that the loss of axons is distributed in a random fashion, which results in survival of some fast-conducting fibers (Figure C18–4B). Figure C18–5 reveals the theoretical distribution of conduction velocity in motor nerves of healthy patients and patients with axonal neuropathy. Unless there is selective loss of largely myelinated, fast-conducting fibers, the axonal loss is indiscriminate, resulting in survival of some fast-conducting fibers and leading to normal velocities. It is only when axonal loss is severe, surpassing 75 to 80% of the total population of

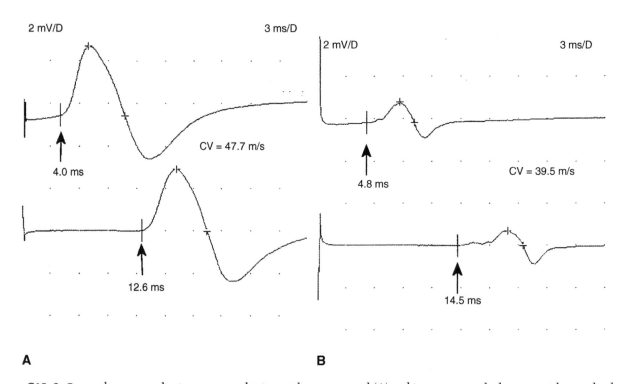

Figure C18–3. *Peroneal motor conduction nerve conduction studies in a control (**A**) and in an age-matched patient with axonal polyneuropathy due to chronic alcoholism (**B**). Note the significant decrease in CMAP amplitudes in (**B**) compared to (**A**), while there is only slight slowing of distal latencies and conduction velocities.*

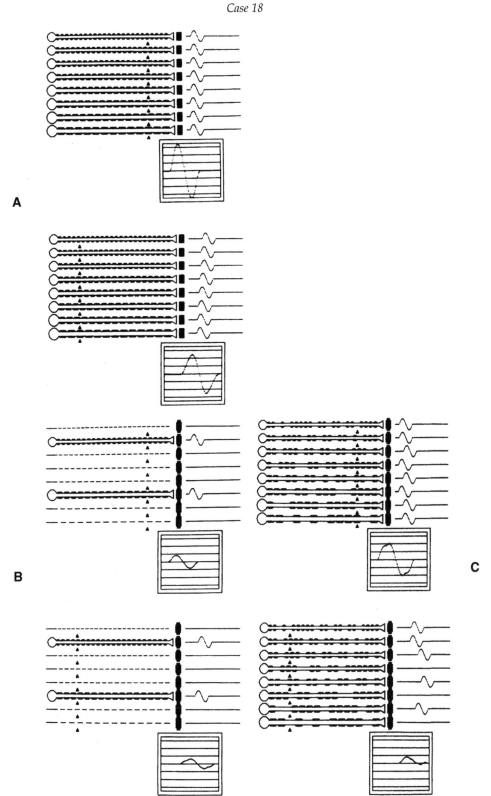

Figure C18–4. *Computerized model of peripheral motor nerve in normal nerve (**A**), axonal degeneration (**B**), and segmental demyelination (**C**). (Adapted from Albers JW. Inflammatory demyelinating polyradiculoneuropathy. In: Brown WF, Bolton CF, eds. Clinical electromyography. Boston, MA: Butterworth-Heinemann, 1989.)*

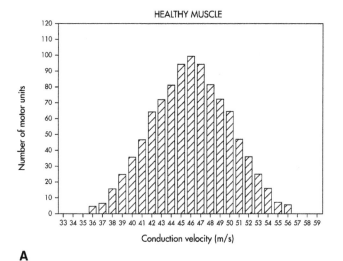

A

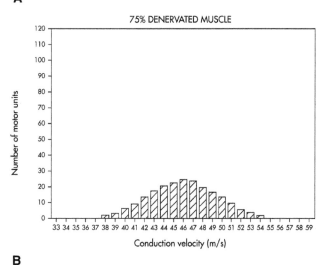

B

Figure C18–5. *Computer simulation of the effect on the distribution of conduction velocities of a loss of 75% of the motor units. (**A**) Normal. (**B**) Abnormal. (From Osselton JW et al., eds. Clinical neurophysiology, EMG, nerve conduction and evoked potentials. Oxford: Butterworth-Heinemann, 1995.)*

axons, that slight slowing of velocities occurs. In these situations, conduction velocities should be no less than 70% of the lower limit of normal.

- *Primary demyelinating polyneuropathies (myelinopathies)* are, however, characterized by significant slowing of conduction times (velocities, distal latencies, and F wave latencies) because the pathologic process results in myelin disruption (segmental and paranodal demyelination) which impedes saltatory conduction. Commonly, the CMAP amplitudes are relatively preserved distally, although conduction blocks and dispersion are common, mainly in the acquired forms (such as CIDP). With distal stimulation, the CMAP is mildly reduced in amplitude because of

temporal dispersion and phase cancellation. The distal latency is slowed (>130% of upper limit of normal) because of demyelination. With more proximal stimulation, the CMAP is much lower in amplitude, which results from temporal dispersion and conduction block along some fibers. The proximal conduction velocities are markedly slow (<70% of lower limit of normal) because of increased probability for the action potentials to pass through demyelinated nerve segments (Figure C18–4C). If untreated, CIDP is often progressive and debiltating with secondary axonal loss (Figure C18–6).

Multiple *criteria* have been set for the diagnosis of CIDP and are aimed at distinguishing the primary demyelinating polyneuropathy from the primary axonal polyneuropathy. Criteria proposed by Cornblath and Asbury were adopted by consensus to apply to patients with suspected CIDP (see Report from an Ad Hoc subcommittee, 1991). Table C18–7 reveals common nerve conduction criteria used to identify the acquired demyelinating polyneuropathies.

Conduction block is defined as the loss of CMAP amplitude and area with proximal stimulation. The diagnosis of conduction block on nerve conduction studies requires a special detailed analysis of several CMAP parameters, including amplitude, duration, and area. In general, physiologic temporal dispersion, due to interphase cancellation, is length-dependent (i.e., more prominent in longer than shorter nerves, and in tall versus short subjects). This results in some loss in amplitude and area between distal and proximal stimulations in normal subjects, and even greater loss in long nerves and tall subjects.

Based on this, when the diagnosis of conduction block is being considered and criteria are being established in EMG laboratories, special thought should be given to the following:

- Criteria for conduction block should not be universal but should be individualized to the specific nerve and the specific segment of the nerve being studied.
- During analysis, special attention should be paid to the duration of the CMAP while a drop in amplitude is being evaluated. The diagnosis of conduction block can be difficult to confirm if significant (pathologic) temporal dispersion is present. This usually results in significant (>15%) prolongation of CMAP negative peak duration. Measurement of the negative peak area, which requires the use of computerized equipment, is extremely useful in these situations. Many criteria have been advocated for the diagnosis of conduction block, some based on normal controls and others on patients with demyelinating neuropathy. Table C18–8 reveals a practical approach for the diagnosis of conduction block and Figure C18–7 shows a practical algorithm in the diagnosis of conduction block, temporal dispersion or both.

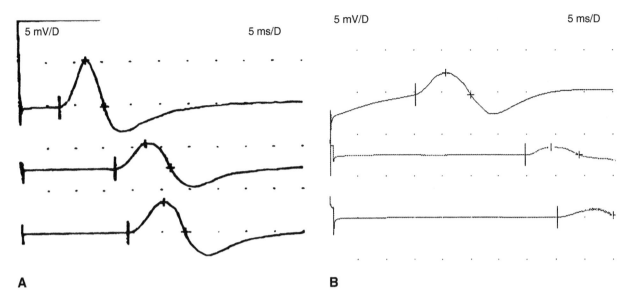

5 mV/D   5 ms/D   5 mV/D   5 ms/D

A   **B**

Figure C18–6. *A 75-year-old man developed an indolent distal sensory loss and mild ataxia beginning in the summer of 2003. He was diagnosed with CIDP in November 2003 but was not treated. He continued to worsen steadily and, in December 2004, became wheelchair bound with complete areflexia, severe sensory loss, and severe proximal weakness. His EDX studies showed significant worsening. The ulnar motor conduction study in November 2003 (**A**) compared to December 2004 (**B**). Note the worsened latencies and amplitudes and evidence of conduction block in December 2004.*

Table C18–7. Electrophysiologic Criteria for Acquired Demyelinating Polyneuropathy

Criteria	Albers and Kelly	Asbury and Cornblath
Required	***≥3 Criteria***	***≥3 Criteria***
1. Conduction block/w temporal dispersion	? number of nerve*	in ≥ 1 nerve†
2. Slowing of MCV	in ≥ 2 nerves <90% LLN if CMAP >50% LLN <80% LLN if CMAP <50% LLN	in ≥ 2 nerves <80% LLN if CMAP >80% LLN <70% LLN if CMAP <80% LLN
3. Slowing of MDL	in ≥2 nerves >115% ULN if CMAP >LLN >125% ULN if CMAP <LLN	in ≥ 2 nerves >125% ULN if CMAP >80% LLN > 150% ULN if CMAP <80% LLN
4. F wave latency	in ≥ 1 nerve >125% ULN	in ≥ 2 nerves Absent, or latency >120% ULN if CMAP >80% LLN >150% ULN if CMAP <80% LLN

*Conduction block = >30% drop in CMAP amplitude between distal and proximal stimulations.
†Conduction block = >20% drop in CMAP area or amplitude between distal and proximal stimulations with <15% increase in CMAP duration; temporal dispersion = >20% drop in CMAP area or amplitude between distal and proximal stimulations with >15% increase in CMAP duration.
MCV = motor conduction velocity; MDL = motor distal latency; ULN = upper limit of normal; LLN = lower limit of normal; CMAP = compound muscle action potential.
Adapted from Brown WF. Acute and chronic inflammatory demyelinating neuropathies. In: Brown WF, Bolton CF, eds. Clinical electromyography. Boston, MA: Butterworth-Heinemann, 1993, pp. 533–559; Albers JW, Kelly JJ. Acquired inflammatory demyelinating polyneuropathies: clinical and electrophysiologic features. Muscle Nerve 1989;12:435–451; Cornblath DR. Electrodiagnostic abnormalities in Guillain-Barré syndrome. Ann Neurol 1990;27(suppl):S17–S20.

Table C18–8. Electrodiagnostic Criteria of Conduction Block

Definite in any nerve*
  1. ≥50% drop in CMAP amplitude with ≤15% prolongation of CMAP duration
  2. ≥50% drop in CMAP area
  3. ≥30% drop in area or amplitude over a short nerve segment (e.g., radial across the spiral groove, ulnar across the elbow, peroneal across the fibular head)

Possible in median, ulnar, and peroneal nerves only
  1. 20–50% drop in CMAP amplitude with ≤15% prolongation of CMAP duration
  2. 20–50% drop in CMAP area

All Amplitudes, areas and durations reflect negative-peak areas, amplitudes and durations.
*Caution should be taken in evaluating the tibial nerve, where stimulation at the knee can be submaximal, resulting in 50% or at times >50% drop in amplitude, especially in overweight patients.

Patients with axonal polyneuropathy are sometimes erroneously diagnosed as demyelinating polyneuropathies and lead to wrong therapies that are potentially harmful. For example, a patient with alcoholic polyneuropathy misdiagnosed as CIDP may be treated with steroids, IVIG, or plasma exchange, all with potential adverse effects. The reasons for these misdiagnoses include the following:

1. Nerve conduction studies are sometimes conducted on cool limbs which results in slowing of distal latencies, conduction velocities, and F wave latencies, and sometimes results in shifting these conduction times in patient with axonal polyneuropathies into the demyelinating range.
2. There is a general overemphasis on slowing of nerve conduction velocities with no regards to the distal CMAPs. Very low amplitude CMAPs often reflect the status of only few surviving nerve fibers, which may be medium or small in size and hence with slow velocities.
3. Cases of axonal polyneuropathy associated with slowing at common entrapment sites (e.g., ulnar across elbow, median at wrist), overstimulation of motor nerves at

distal sites (resulting in apparent conduction blocks due to volume conduction), or normal anatomical variants (e.g., Martin-Gruber anastomosis) may be erroneously diagnosed as a demyelinating polyneuropathy.

FOLLOW-UP

The patient had no risk factors for HIV infection, and her serum HIV antibody was negative. Serum immunoelectrophoresis showed a monoclonal IgM kappa band measuring 1 g/L. The paraprotein was consistent with MGUS; her complete blood count was normal without anemia. Serum calcium, BUN, and creatinine values were normal, as were results of the skeletal bone survey. Bone marrow aspirate showed 2% plasma cells. Serum anti-MAG antibody was negative. A sural nerve biopsy showed marked loss of myelin, with preservation of axon cylinders and proliferation of Schwann cells.

The patient was treated with weekly courses of plasma exchange, along with oral corticosteroids. She showed significant improvement in strength, pain level, and gait over the next 3 months. This was confirmed by repeat

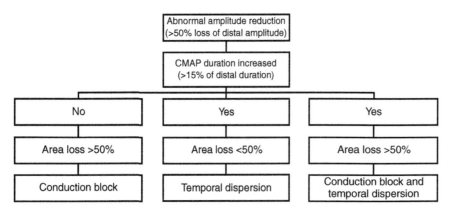

Figure C18–7. *Algorithmic evaluation of a CMAP drop (decay) between distal and proximal stimulation, defining conduction block, temporal dispersion, or both.*

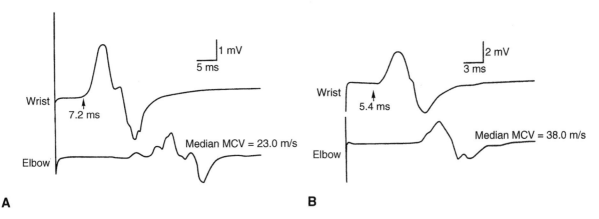

Figure C18–8. *Left median motor conduction studies at baseline (A) and 6 months following treatment (B). Note the amplitude and sweep speed scale change. There is resolution of conduction block and significant improvement of distal latency and conduction velocity in the forearm (between the wrist and elbow stimulations).*

conduction studies, 6 months after treatment, which showed marked improvement, with resolution of most conduction blocks and improvement of both distal latencies and conduction velocities (Figure C18–8). Because of osteopenic vertebral fractures, steroids were discontinued, and the patient was maintained on bimonthly plasma exchange and azathioprine. Because of loss of appropriate venous access, she was then shifted to monthly intravenous immunoglobulin infusions (2 g/kg infused in 2 days). The patient strength was satisfactory on this regimen and a follow-up after 4 years showed no change in the paraprotein value

DIAGNOSIS

Chronic demyelinating polyneuropathy, associated with monoclonal gammopathy of undetermined significance (MGUS) of the IgM-kappa type.

ANSWERS

1. D; 2. A; 3. C.

SUGGESTED READINGS

Ad hoc subcommittee of the American Academy of Neurology AIDS task force. Criteria for diagnosis of chronic inflammatory demyelinating polyneuropathy (CIDP). Neurology 1991;41:617–618.

Albers JW, Kelly JJ. Acquired inflammatory demyelinating polyneuropathies: clinical and electrophysiologic features. Muscle Nerve 1989;12:435–451.

Braun PE, Frail DE, Latov N. Myelin-associated glycoprotein is the antigen for monoclonal IgM polyneuropathy. J Neurochem 1982;39:1261–1265.

Bromberg MB, Feldman EV, Albers JW. Chronic inflammatory demyelinating polyradiculoneuropathy: comparison of patients with and without an associated monoclonal gammopathy. Neurology 1992;42:1157–1163.

Cook D et al. High dose intravenous immunoglobulin in the treatment of demyelinating neuropathy associated with monoclonal gammopathy. Neurology 1990;40:212–214.

Cornblath DR. Electrodiagnostic abnormalities in Guillain-Barré syndrome. Ann Neurol 1990;27(suppl):S17–S20.

Cornblath DR et al. Conduction block in clinical practice. Muscle Nerve 1991;14:869–871.

Dyck PJ et al. Plasma exchange in polyneuropathy associated with monoclonal gammopathy of undetermined significance. N Engl J Med 1991;325:1482–1486.

Eurelings M et al. Malignant transformation in polyneuropathy associated with monoclonal gammopathy. Neurology 2005; 64:2079–2084.

Gorson KC, Allan G, Ropper AH. Chronic inflammatory demyelinating polyneuropathy: clinical features and response to treatment in 67 consecutive patients with and without a monoclonal gammopathy. Neurology 1997;48:321–328.

Katirji B. Chronic relapsing axonal neuropathy responsive to intravenous immunoglobulins. Neurology 1997;48:1690–1694.

Kelly JJ Jr. The electrodiagnostic findings in polyneuropathies associated with monoclonal gammopathies. Muscle Nerve 1990;13:1113–1117.

Kelly JJ Jr et al. Prevalence of monoclonal proteins in peripheral neuropathy. Neurology 1981;31:1480–1483.

Kelly JJ Jr et al. Polyneuropathies associated with IgM monoclonal gammopathies. Arch Neurol 1988;45:1355–1359.

Kyle RA. "Benign" monoclonal gammopathy: a misnomer? JAMA 1984;251:1849–1854.

Kyle RA, Dyck PJ. Neuropathy associated with monoclonal gammopathies. In: Dyck PJ, Thomas PK, eds. Peripheral neuropathy, 3rd ed. Philadelphia, PA: WB Saunders, 1993.

Latov N et al. Plasma-cell dyscrasia and peripheral neuropathy with a monoclonal antibody to peripheral-nerve myelin. N Engl J Med 1980;303:618–621.

Lewis RA, Sumner AJ. The electrodiagnostic distinctions between chronic familial and acquired demyelinative neuropathy. Neurology 1982;32:592–596.

Notermans NC et al. Polyneuropathy associated with monoclonal gammopathy of undetermined significance: a prospective study of the prognostic value of clinical and laboratory abnormalities. Brain 1994;117:1385–1393.

Notermans NC et al. Intermittent cyclophosphamide and prednisone treatment of polyneuropathy associated with monoclonal gammopathy of undetermined significance. Neurology 1996;47:1227–1233.

Report from an ad hoc subcommittee of the American Academy of Neurology AIDS Task Force. Research criteria for the diagnosis of chronic inflammatory demyelinating polyneuropathy (CIDP). Neurology 1991;41:617–618.

Rhee RK, England DR, Sumner AJ. Computer simulation of conduction block: effects produced by actual block versus interphase cancellation. Ann Neurol 1990;28:146–159.

Simmons Z et al. Presentation and initial clinical course in patients with chronic inflammatory demyelinating polyradiculoneuropathy: comparison of patients without and with monoclonal gammopathy. Neurology 1993;43:2202–2209.

Simmons Z et al. Long term follow-up of patients with chronic inflammatory demyelinating polyradiculoneuropathy, without and with monoclonal gammopathy. Brain 1995;118: 339–368.

Case 19

HISTORY AND PHYSICAL EXAMINATION

Progressive weakness developed over 7 months in the left hand of a 53-year-old right-handed woman. Initially, she noted that she had difficulty picking up small objects, buttoning shirts, or pulling snaps. This worsened and she recently has been unable to use her left hand to assist during meals. The weakness had not affected her left upper arm and her right upper extremity was normal. She denied any limb or neck pain, numbness, or cramps. She denied any bulbar, ocular, cognitive, or sphincteric symptoms.

Her medical history was relevant for diabetes mellitus since 45 years of age, hypertension, and cigarette smoking. She takes insulin injections and furosemide. There is no family history of neuromuscular disorder.

On examination, she had normal mental status and cranial nerves. There was no facial weakness, neck weakness, or tongue atrophy or fasciculations. She had slight atrophy of all intrinsic muscles of the left hand only. No fasciculations were observed. Tone was normal. There was moderate weakness that was restricted to the left upper extremity muscles. Manual muscle examination, using Medical Research Council (MRC) grading (1 to 5), showed the following:

- Hand grip 4–/5
- Interossei 4–/5
- Long finger flexors 4/5
- Long finger extensors 4/5
- Wrist extensors 4+/5
- Wrist flexors 4+/5
- Elbow flexion 5–/5
- Elbow extension 5–/5
- Shoulder abduction 5–/5

Deep tendon reflexes were pathologically brisk in both upper extremities, but knee jerks were normal and ankle jerks were absent. Jaw jerk was brisk. She had a right Babinski sign and bilateral Hoffmann signs.

Sensory examination was normal to all modalities. Results of gait and cerebellar examinations were normal.

The patient was evaluated by a neurologist who found normal x-rays of the cervical spine. Magnetic resonance imaging of the cervical spine revealed mild disk bulging at C3–C4 and C5–C6. An electrodiagnostic (EDX) study of the left upper extremity, done 3 months after onset of symptoms, revealed fibrillations and large motor units in left C7-, C8-, T1-innervated muscles, with normal sensory and motor nerve conduction studies. Because of progressive left hand weakness, the patient was referred for a repeat EDX examination 7 months after the onset of symptoms.

Please now review the Nerve Conduction Studies and Needle EMG tables.

QUESTIONS

1. The aforementioned EDX findings can be seen with all of the following *except:*
   A. Widespread polyradiculopathy.
   B. Diffuse anterior horn cell disease.
   C. Axonal motor neuropathy.
   D. Diabetic distal polyneuropathy.
2. Diffusely low-amplitude compound muscle action potentials (CMAPs) may be caused by all of the following *except:*
   A. Cool limbs.
   B. Amyotrophic lateral sclerosis (ALS).
   C. Duchenne muscular dystrophy.
   D. Lambert-Eaton myasthenic syndrome.
   E. Widespread polyradiculopathy.
3. In a patient with diffuse degenerative spine disease, the presence of fibrillations in the upper and lower limbs, as well as the tongue and masseter muscles, is diagnostic of ALS:
   A. True.
   B. False.

Case 19: Nerve Conduction Studies

Nerve Stimulated	Stimulation Site	Recording Site	Amplitude (m = mV, s = μV)			Distal/Peak Latency (ms)			Conduction Velocity (m/s)			F Latency (ms)	
			Right	Left	Normal	Right	Left	Normal	Right	Left	Normal	Right	Left
Sural (s)	Calf	Ankle		5	≥3		3.7	≤4.6					
Peroneal (m)	Ankle	EDB		**1.5**	≥2.5		4.4	≤6.0		48	≥40		55.8
Peroneal (m)	Knee	EDB		**1.0**									
Tibial (m)	Ankle	AH		7.0	≥4		4.7	≤6.0		45	≥40		57.9
Tibial (m)	Knee	AH		4.5									
H reflex	Knee	Soleus	**NR**	**NR**		**NR**	5.8						
M response	Knee	Soleus	15	12		6.6							
Median (s)	Wrist	Index finger	25	30	≥10	2.8	2.9	≤3.6					
Median (s)	Elbow	Index finger		15						57	≥50		
Ulnar (s)	Wrist	Little finger	12	15	≥8	2.7	2.6	≤3.1					
Radial (s)	Wrist	Dorsum of hand		25	≥10		2.4	≤2.7					
Median (m)	Wrist	APB	**3.0**	**NR**	≥5	3.7	**NR**	≤4.0	49	**NR**	≥50	31.0	**NR**
Median (m)	Elbow	APB	**2.2**	**NR**									
Ulnar (m)	Wrist	ADM	7.0	**3.0**	≥7	3.3	3.3	≤3.1	49	49	≥50	33.4	34.7
Ulnar (m)	Elbow	ADM	5.5	**2.8**									

ADM = abductor digiti minimi; AH = abductor hallucis; APB = abductor pollicis brevis; EDB = extensor digitorum brevis; m = motor; NR = no response; s = sensory. Data in bold type are abnormal.

Case 19: Needle EMG

| Muscle | Insertional Activity | Spontaneous Activity | | Voluntary Motor Unit Action Potentials (MUAPs) | | | | | | | |
| | | Fibs | Fascs | Recruitment | | | | Configuration | | | |
				Normal	Activation	Reduced	Early	Duration	Amplitude	% Polyphasia	Others
L. first dorsal interosseous	↑	2+	0	−		↓↓↓		↑	Normal	↑	1 MUP
Abductor digiti minimi	↑	2+	0			↓↓↓		↑	Normal	Normal	
Abductor pollicis brevis	↑	2+	0	No voluntary MUAPs							
Flexor pollicis longus	↑	2+	0			↓↓↓		↑	↑	Normal	
Extensor indicis proprius	↑	2+	0			↓↓		↑	Normal	Normal	
Pronator teres	↑	3+	0			↓↓		Normal	↑	Normal	
Biceps	↑	2+	0			↓↓		Normal	Normal	↑	
Triceps	↑	2+	0			↓↓		Normal	↑	Normal	
Deltoid	↑	1+	0			↓↓↓		Normal	Normal	↑	
Low cervical paraspinal	↑	+/−	0	−							
Midcervical paraspinal	↑	+/−	0	−							
R. first dorsal interosseous	↑	+/−	0			↓↓		↑	Normal	Normal	
Abductor pollicis brevis	↑	1+	0			↓↓↓		↑	Normal	Normal	1 MUP
Flexor pollicis brevis	↑	+/−	0			↓↓		↑	Normal	Normal	
Pronator teres	↑	1+	+/−	X				Normal	Normal	Normal	
Biceps	↑	+/−	1+	X				Normal	Normal	Normal	
Triceps	Normal	0	1+			↓		Normal	↑	Normal	
R. deltoid	↑	+/−	0			↓		Normal	Normal	↑	
Midcervical paraspinal	Normal	0	0	−							

Continued

Case 19: Needle EMG—cont'd

Muscle	Insertional Activity	Spontaneous Activity Fibs	Fascs	Recruitment Normal	Activation	Reduced	Early	Configuration Duration	Amplitude	% Polyphasia	Others
Low cervical paraspinal	Normal	0	0	–							
L. tibialis anterior	↑	1+	0	X				Normal	Normal	Normal	
Medial gastrocnemius	↑	1+	+/–	X				Normal	Normal	Normal	
Flexor digitorum longus	↑	1+	0			→		Normal	Normal	Normal	
Extensor digitorum brevis	↑	1+	0			↓↓		↑	Normal	Normal	
Vastus lateralis	↑	+/–	0	X				Normal	Normal	Normal	
Gluteus medius	Normal	0	0			→		Normal	Normal	Normal	
Midlumbar paraspinal	Normal	0	0	–							
Low lumbar paraspinal	↑	0	0	–							
R. tibialis anterior	↑	+/–	0	X				Normal	Normal	Normal	
Medial gastrocnemius	Normal	0	0	X				Normal	Normal	Normal	
Flexor digitorum longus	↑	+/–	0			→		↑	Normal	Normal	
Vastus lateralis	↑	+/–	+/–			→		↑	Normal	Normal	
Midlumbar paraspinal	Normal	0	0	–							

Fascs = fasciculations; Fibs = fibrillations; L. = left; MUP = motor unit potential; R. = right; ↑ = increased; ↓ = mildly reduced; ↓↓ = moderately reduced; ↓↓↓ = severely reduced.

4. A patient with weakness in the right hand has fibrillation potentials in the right C5 through T1 roots, with normal left upper limb, lower limbs, thoracic paraspinal and bulbar muscles. These findings rule out ALS:
   A. True.
   B. False.

EDX FINDINGS AND INTERPRETATION OF DATA

Pertinent EDX findings in this patient include:

1. Normal sensory nerve action potentials (SNAPs) throughout, including all sensory amplitudes, distal latencies, and conduction velocities.
2. Low-amplitude (or absent) median and ulnar CMAPs, recording the thenar and hypothenar muscles, bilaterally and asymmetrically (worse on the left), with borderline distal latencies, conduction velocities, and F-wave latencies, and no conduction blocks.

These two findings are suggestive of a cervical intraspinal canal lesion, affecting the lower C8/T1 roots or cord segments bilaterally, worse on the left, and producing axonal loss. The slight slowing of motor distal latencies and conduction velocities, and F wave latencies, with values not lower than 70 to 80% of the normal limit, is compatible with an axonal loss lesion, and reflects relative loss of the large, fast-conducting motor fibers. Normal ulnar SNAPs, which derive their fibers from C8 roots, are evidence in support of a preganglionic lesion (i.e., a lesion of the lower cervical roots or cord).

3. Low left peroneal CMAP, recording the extensor digitorum brevis (EDB), with normal latency and conduction velocity.

This, when added to the aforementioned findings, might suggest a diffuse intraspinal canal disease, which extends to the lumbosacral roots or cord. However, it should be remembered that selective atrophy of the extensor digitorum brevis is a common finding, of no definite clinical significance; thus, a low-amplitude CMAP, recording EDB, does not automatically indicate a pathologic process at the L5 root, S1 root, or peroneal nerve.

4. On needle examination, it is clear that the disorder is much more diffuse than can be determined either clinically or by nerve conduction studies. Fibrillation potentials, reduced recruitment, and reinnervated long-duration polyphasic motor unit action potentials (MUAPs) are detected diffusely. Fasciculation potentials are not prominent, seen primarily in asymptomatic limbs. Axonal loss is widespread, affecting muscles of multiple roots and multiple nerve distribution in multiple extremities. The needle EMG findings also mirror the weakness and CMAP abnormalities; they are worst in the left upper extremity, and they are early and subtle in the other three limbs.

In summary, using strict EDX definitions, the findings are pathognomonic of a diffuse pathologic process that involves all ventral roots or spinal cord segments and produces axonal loss, worse in the left cervical myotomes, with evidence of prominent active (ongoing) denervation. These findings may result from an active polyradiculopathy (such as carcinomatous meningitis), a diffuse myelopathy, or rapidly progressive motor neuron disease (such as amyotrophic lateral sclerosis). Obviously, this EDX study is most compatible with ALS in this patient due to the associated upper motor neuron findings, as well as the lack of pain or any other sensory manifestations. The extensive denervation seen in this patient is not consistent with diabetic distal sensorimotor polyneuropathy, because of the predominant loss of motor units in the upper extremities, the marked asymmetry, and the preservation of all the SNAPs. Finally, cool extremities result in high (not low) CMAP and SNAP amplitudes with slow latencies.

DISCUSSION

Pathology and Etiology

Amyotrophic lateral sclerosis (ALS), a term first coined by Charcot in 1875, is the prototypical disease among disorders of the motor neuron. It is a relentlessly progressive and fatal neurodegenerative disorder caused by loss of both upper motor neurons (UMN) and lower motor neurons (LMN). ALS is usually sporadic while 5 to 10% of cases are familial, usually following an autosomal dominant inheritance pattern.

The pathology of sporadic ALS is represented by the selective loss of motor neurons in the spinal cord and brain stem, and cortical motor neurons (Betz cells). Classic findings on spinal cord sections include the loss of anterior horns, with degeneration of the pyramidal tracts (crossed and uncrossed) and dramatic preservation of the dorsal columns and spinocerebellar tracts. Although all motor neurons ultimately degenerate, there is relative sparing of the oculomotor nuclei in the brain stem and Onuff nucleus in the lumbosacral cord. Microscopically, there is, in addition to the loss of anterior horn motor neurons, frequent accumulation of neurofilaments in surviving neurons and dilatation of axons ("spheroids"). The pathologic findings in familial ALS are identical to those in the sporadic form, except that Lewy-like bodies frequently are identified in surviving motor neurons.

Amyotrophic lateral sclerosis is a fatal disorder of unknown etiology. It is likely that there are initiating and propagating factors that lead to motor neuron cell death. Currently, there are five major hypotheses about the development of ALS, although many theories are interrelated:

1. *The excitatory amino acid hypothesis.* This theory suggests that glutamate excitotoxicity could contribute to neuronal cell loss. It implies that excessive synaptic glutamate, caused in part by its insufficient clearance due to the loss of glutamate transport (likely astroglial-specific), is followed by increased cytosolic calcium, which activates motor neuron cell death.

2. *The oxidative stress hypothesis.* This theory suggests that increased free radicals lead to neuronal death. It is supported by the discovery that a subset of patients with familial ALS have a mutation in SOD1, the gene that encodes copper-zinc superoxide dismutase (Cu, Zn SOD). This cytoplasmic enzyme, present in all neurons and glia, "dismutes" superoxide into molecular oxygen and hydrogen peroxide, which is catalyzed further into water. How mutation of human Cu, Zn SOD might cause degeneration of motor neurons is unclear. Hypotheses include (1) the generation of hydroxyl radical (HO) from hydrogen peroxide, (2) the release of free copper, which could promote free radical damage to the membranes, or (3) the formation of a nitronium-like intermediate with peroxynitrite, resulting in the nitration of tyrosine residues in critical proteins.

3. *The neurofilament poisoning hypothesis.* This theory proposes that neurofilament gene mutation results in disorganization and/or decreased transport of neurofilaments, leading to accumulation of axonal neurofilaments, neuronal dysfunction, and degeneration.

4. *The immune hypothesis.* Certain antibodies directed against the motor neuron population may be found in ALS patients and animal models. Antiganglioside antibodies, especially anti-GM1, are occasionally detected in ALS sera usually in medium titers. These antibodies are present in high titer in acute motor axonal neuropathy (AMAN), and multifocal motor neuropathy with conduction block. Antibodies to – and L-type calcium channels, present in the sera of some patients with ALS, results in increased calcium entry into the cell, leading to degeneration. The lack of response to various immunomodulatory treatments, including intravenous immunoglobulin, cyclophosphamide, and corticosteroids, is perhaps the most telling that there is no convincing evidence of conventional autoimmunity in ALS.

5. *The viral hypothesis.* HIV and HTLV1 infections may cause ALS-like syndromes, but neither viruses have been shown to cause ALS. However, the possibility of an unconventional infection, such as prions, cannot be excluded.

Clinical Features

Amyotrophic lateral sclerosis, also known as motor neuron disease, Lou Gehrig disease, or maladie de Charcot, occurs in a fairly uniform distribution worldwide with no true differences in geographical incidence, except for small clusters in Guam, the Kii peninsula of Japan, and West New Guinea. The worldwide incidence of ALS is 0.6 to 2.6 per 100 000 population, and its lifetime risk is 1 in 1000. Since 5 to 10% of ALS cases are dominantly inherited, the risk to siblings of a patient with ALS is approximately 2.5 to 5%. The disorder affects both sexes, with a slight preponderance to males. The mean age of onset is 55 years, with a wide range from 17 to 77 years. The illness is fatal within 5 years in 80% of patients; however, some survive as long as 20 years. Patients with initial weakness in the bulbar muscles and older patients have a poorer prognosis for survival. Most patients with ALS die of respiratory failure and fewer than 10% of ALS patients in the United States choose long-term mechanical ventilation to sustain their lives.

More than two-thirds of patients with ALS present with weakness, atrophy, or both. The weakness involves one arm, one leg, or asymmetrically both legs in almost half of patients, while generalized weakness, bilateral upper extremities, or unilateral hemiparesis are less common. Bulbar manifestations are present at onset in a quarter of patients. Fasciculations, cramps, shortness of breath, head drop, or weight loss are rare initial presentations. UMN findings include weakness, spasticity, hyperreflexia, and Babinski and Hoffman signs. LMN findings are usually more pronounced and include weakness, muscle atrophy, fasciculations, and hyporeflexia. Bulbar manifestations in ALS typically include dysarthria, dysphagia, sialorrhea, aspiration, and pseudobulbar affect (inappropriate, spontaneous, forced laughing, crying, or yawning).

A typical patient with ALS is a man in his fifties in whom asymmetrical weakness and atrophy of the muscles develop in one limb, usually those in one hand or one foot. The weakness progresses over time to adjacent myotomes in the same limb and thence to the contralateral limb or the other limb on the same side. The weakness ultimately generalizes to involve all limb, bulbar and respiratory muscles. At its advanced stage, there is usually generalized diffuse muscular atrophy and weakness, fasciculations, spasticity with hyperreflexia, and possibly dysphagia and dysarthria. In typical ALS, there is sparing of sphincteric function, eye movement, sensory function, and cognitive capability.

The *diagnosis* of ALS is based on the presence of a progressive disorder with the characteristic combination of upper and lower motor neuron involvement. Many criteria have been proposed but most are inadequate, particularly those pertaining to early diagnosis and the definition of upper motor neuron involvement. Among them, the revised El Escorial diagnostic criteria currently are the most widely accepted for the diagnosis of ALS (Table C19–1).

Although lower motor neuron dysfunction dominates the clinical picture in many patients, there usually is evidence of upper motor neuron involvement as well. Extreme cases of "pure" lower motor neuron or "pure" upper motor neuron involvement exist, but they are less common than classic ALS. Because of this variability and the preponderance to lower or upper motor neurons, ALS variants commonly are separated from the classic form (Table C19–2).

Table C19–1. Revised El-Escorial Criteria for the Diagnosis of Amyotrophic Lateral Sclerosis

Features Present
Evidence of lower motor neuron degeneration by clinical, electrophysiological or pathological examination

Evidence of upper motor neuron degeneration by clinical examination

Progressive spread of signs within a region, or to other regions as determined by history or examination

Four Topographical Anatomic Regions
Bulbar (brainstem)

Three spinal cord regions

Cervical

Thoracic

Lumbosacral

Levels of Diagnostic Certainty
Definite ALS

UMN as well as LMN signs, in the bulbar region and at least two spinal regions

or

UMN and LMN signs in three spinal regions

Probable ALS

UMN and LMN signs in at least two regions with some UMN signs necessarily rostral to the LMN signs

Probable ALS-laboratory supported

Clinical signs of UMN and LMN dysfunction in only one region

or

UMN signs alone in one region

and

LMN signs defined by electrophysiologic criteria in at least two regions

Possible ALS

Clinical signs of UMN and LMN dysfunction are found together in only one region

or

UMN signs are found in two or more regions

or

LMN signs are found rostral to UMN signs

LMN = lower motor neuron; UMN = upper motor neuron.

Although ALS often can be readily diagnosed clinically, especially when both upper and lower motor neuron features are present, a definitive diagnosis sometimes may be difficult to attain, particularly during the early stages of the disease. Table C19–3 lists common disorders that may mimic ALS, thus posing difficulties in the diagnostic process.

There is no cure for ALS. Treatment options for ALS have been disappointing, although major strides have been made during the past few years. Effort is ongoing to identify drugs with potential effects on the progression of ALS. The various classes of therapy that currently are used or are being investigated in slowing the progression of disease include antiexcitotoxins, nerve growth factors, and neuroprotective agents. Since glutamate excess is neurotoxic, then drugs that decrease synaptic glutamate might be beneficial. These drugs could decrease glutamate release, block postsynaptic receptors (N-methyl-D-aspartate [NMDA] and non-NMDA), decrease glutamate synthesis, or increase glutamate transport. Drugs in this group include riluzole (Rilutek®), which is the only drug that has been approved to treat ALS in the United States. It decreases glutamate release but also blocks voltage-activated sodium channels. Nerve growth factors regulate the survival of developing and mature motor neurons, ameliorate neuron loss in animal models of motor neuron degeneration, and are important in muscle innervation and sprouting. Subcutaneous ciliary neurotrophic factor (CNTF) and brain-derived neurotrophic factor (BDNF), and intraventricular glial cell line-derived neurotrophic factor (GDNF) have failed to show benefit or had poorly tolerated adverse effects. Insulin-like growth factor-1 (IGF-1) is the most promising in the treatment of ALS, with some evidence that IGF-1 has a positive effect in slowing the progress of human ALS. Neuroprotective agents such vitamin E, deprenyl, and coenzyme Q10 have not yet shown a positive effect.

Electrodiagnosis

Nerve Conduction Studies

Although the major changes in ALS are seen on needle EMG, nerve conduction studies (NCS) should be done in all patients with suspected ALS to exclude other possible causes of weakness. Sensory NCSs are normal, although a subtle decrease in SNAP amplitudes has been reported in a few studies. Motor NCSs may show abnormalities that vary with the stage of disease. Normal study results are not uncommon early in the disease course. Later, low-amplitude CMAPs are frequently revealed; these may be regional (i.e., the result of motor conduction studies performed on weakened limb(s) because of anterior horn cell loss). In more advanced stages of the disease, diffusely low CMAP amplitudes with normal SNAP amplitudes, so called *"low motor-normal sensory pattern,"* is characteristic.

Table C19–2. Amyotrophic Lateral Sclerosis (ALS) and Its Variants

Disorder	Frequency (%)	Characteristics
Sporadic ALS	*90–95*	
Classic ALS	82	LMN and UMN dysfunctions
LMN-dominant ALS		LMN dysfunctions with subtle UMN signs
UMN-dominant ALS		UMN dysfunctions with subtle or needle EMG signs of LMN dysfunctions
Progressive bulbar palsy	9	Bulbar with or without pseudobulbar dysfunctions
Progressive muscular atrophy	7	Pure LMN dysfunctions
Primary lateral sclerosis	2	Pure UMN dysfunctions
Familial ALS	*5–10*	
Autosomal dominant ALS		
SOD 1-linked	20 (2% of ALS)	Linked to chromosome 21q22, associated with >50 mutations in gene for Cu, Zn SOD (Ala^4 to valine)
Non-SOD 1-linked		Not linked to chromosome 21q22
Autosomal recessive ALS		Some are linked to chromosome 2q33

ALa^4 = alanine^4; Cu, Zn SOD = copper-zinc superoxide dismutase; LMN = lower motor neuron; SOD1 = superoxide dismustase; UMN = upper motor neuron.

This NCS pattern is not specific for the diagnosis and may be seen in spinal muscular atrophies, diffuse myelopathies or polyradiculopathies, axonal motor polyneuropathies, presynaptic neuromuscular junction disorders, and severe myopathies (see Figure C17–13). In contrast to CMAP amplitudes, motor conduction velocities, distal latencies, and F wave latencies are usually normal in ALS until significant degrees of axon loss have occurred, when mild slowing may be detected due to the loss of large and fast conducting axons. This slowing is proportional to the reduction in CMAP amplitude, and the conduction velocity does not decrease to less than 70 to 80% of the lower limit of normal. Motor conduction block, or significant CMAP temporal dispersion, should raise the suspicion of another disorder that may, at times, mimic motor neuron disease: multifocal motor neuropathy with conduction block.

Table C19–3. Differential Diagnosis of Amyotrophic Lateral Sclerosis

Cervical spondylotic myelopathy (cervical myelopathy with cervical polyradiculopathy)

Cervical and lumbar spondylosis (cervical and lumbosacral polyradiculopathy)

Multifocal motor neuropathy with conduction block

Chronic polymyositis (when lower motor neuron involvement only)

Inclusion-body myositis (when lower motor neuron involvement only)

Myasthenia gravis (when bulbar)

Needle EMG

Needle EMG is the most powerful tool in confirming the diagnosis of ALS. Needle EMG findings in motor neuron disease in general and in ALS in particular are dependent on the extent of lower motor neuron degeneration. Changes seen on needle EMG consist of abnormal spontaneous activity and loss of motor neurons; this loss is characterized by impaired MUAP recruitment and altered MUAP configuration that is consistent with reinnervation.

Fasciculation potentials are sporadic or quasi-rhythmic, spontaneous (involuntary) contractions of a group of muscle fibers that are innervated by a single motor unit. They can be of any shape and size, depending on the motor units from which they arise (Figure C19–1). They reflect irritability of the motor unit and usually originate from the distal nerve terminals, with spread by axon reflex to other parts of the unit. They frequently are visible on inspection. During needle EMG, fasciculation potentials are characterized by a random firing pattern. Fasciculations are particularly prominent in patients with ALS and have been closely linked to the disease since its first description by Charcot. Using simultaneous multichannel EMG recordings from different sites and muscles, it has been estimated that more than 90% of patients with ALS have fasciculations.

Although fasciculation potentials are extremely common in ALS, they also occur in other lower motor neuron disorders (radiculopathies and peripheral polyneuropathies), with the use of anticholinesterase medication, in hyperthyroidism and hypocalcemia, and in healthy muscles (particularly the calves). Thus, fasciculation

0.1 mV/D   20 ms/D

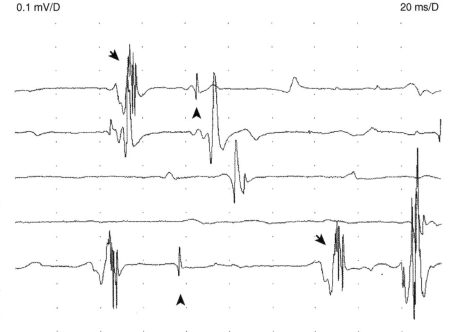

Figure C19–1. *Fasciculation potentials recorded, in raster mode, from the vastus lateralis in a patient with motor neuron disease. Note that the sweep speed is set at 20 ms/division. Note that the morphology of the potentials is of motor units but with extreme variability in configuration among the individual discharges and their irregular firing pattern. Individual fasciculation potential may recur irregularly (arrows and arrowheads).*

potentials are nonspecific and may be benign, unless they are accompanied by fibrillation potentials or by MUAP changes.

Because they can occur in healthy individuals, an attempt has been made to distinguish "benign" from "malignant" fasciculations. On average, malignant fasciculations have a slower rate of discharge and higher amplitudes compared with the benign ones. However, these differences are not sufficient to provide a reliable method of distinguishing between them. The best way to differentiate is to look for accompanying changes on needle EMG, such as fibrillation potentials, impaired recruitment, and MUAP configuration abnormalities.

Fibrillation potentials are spontaneous action potentials of denervated muscle fibers that usually fire regularly. They can take one of two forms: a brief spike or a long-duration positive wave. They are seen most commonly in processes associated with axonal or neuronal loss, although they may occur in necrotizing myopathies. In ALS, the identification of fibrillation potentials is extremely important because they confirm the occurrence of axonal loss and support the suspicion that the accompanied fasciculation potentials are pathologic. Because fibrillation potentials are abolished by sprouting, which usually is an active process early in the disease course, these potentials can be of limited number and of scattered distribution during the first stages of ALS. In general, fibrillation potentials are more prominent in rapidly progressive than in slowly progressive motor neuron disease.

Reduced MUAP recruitment is caused by degeneration and loss of motor neurons in ALS, with the result that only a few can be activated voluntarily. The activated motor units fire more rapidly as anterior horn cells are lost (Figure C19–2). This EDX finding always is abnormal but, when isolated, does not mean automatically that axonal loss has occurred because it may happen if there is demyelination anywhere along the motor axon that results in the block of conduction transmission. In ALS patients, slow recruitment frequency (poor activation) of MUAPs in limbs where UMN loss predominates may also be evident but is a less frequent finding.

Reinnervated MUAPs dominate as collateral sprouting increases the number of muscle fibers per motor unit resulting in increased duration and amplitude MUAPs (Figure C19–2). Also, because of conduction slowing along the newly formed collateral sprouts, muscle fiber action potentials become asynchronous. This results in increased polyphasic MUAPs (more than four phases). Thus, a mixture of MUAPs often is seen on needle EMG, dependent on the stage of illness. Normal MUAPs are intermixed with polyphasic MUAPs, with or without satellite potentials (Figure C19–3), and with long-duration, high-amplitude MUAPs (Figure C19–4). Moment-to-moment MUAP amplitude variation, representing motor unit instability, may also be appreciated.

In *summary*, the findings on needle EMG are variable and depend on the stage of illness. At any one point in a patient's illness, sampling many muscles in four limbs and

0.2 mV/D

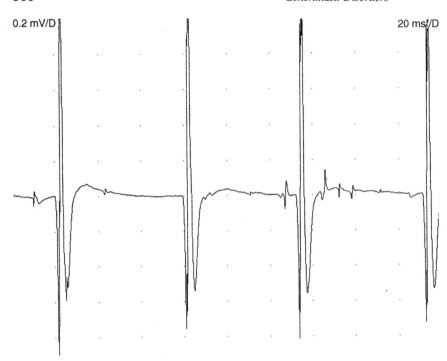

20 ms/D

Figure C19–2. *Reduced recruitment with maximal effort from the biceps muscle of a 55-year-old man with ALS revealing a single unit, with long duration and high amplitude, firing rapidly at a rate of 20 Hz. Note that the sweep speed is set at 20 ms/division.*

the head often reveals a mixture of the following findings (listed in worsening severity):

1. Normal muscles.
2. Muscles with fasciculation potentials only.
3. Muscles with fasciculations, a slight reduction in MUAP recruitment, and polyphasia of MUAPs.
4. Muscles with profuse fibrillation potentials, rare fasciculations, and marked impairment of recruitment, with long-duration, high-amplitude MUAPs.
5. Muscles with severe atrophy, few fibrillations, and no or very few voluntary MUAPs.

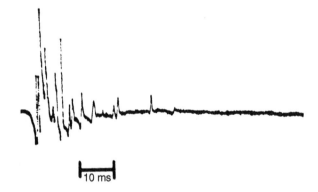

10 ms

Figure C19–3. *Polyphasic motor unit potential (MUAP) with satellite (linked) potentials, also called complex MUAP. (From Daube J. AAEM minimonograph 11: needle electromyography in clinical electromyography. Muscle Nerve 1991;14:685–700, with permission.)*

Other Electrodiagnostic Tests

Other EDX tests sometimes used in the assessment of ALS including repetitive nerve stimulation, single fiber EMG and motor unit number estimate. Repetitive stimulation of motor nerves at a slow rate may result in a modest decrement of the CMAP in many patients with ALS, usually by less than 20 to 25%. This decrement is more likely to occur during recording of a denervated muscle, particularly in patients with rapidly progressive ALS. Single-fiber EMG reveals a marked increase in fiber density (2–10 times), which is consistent with collateral sprouting. Jitter analysis is abnormal in 90% of patients with ALS. Both increased fiber density and abnormal jitter are seen more commonly in muscles with denervation than in healthy muscles. Finally, motor unit number estimation (MUNE), is a promising technique with potentials in studies of the natural history and prognosis of ALS, and of the response to experimental treatment. MUNE is a technique that measures the approximate number of LMNs innervating a single muscle or a small group of muscles. At least four methods for this have been described; In general, MUNE count is determined through division of the supramaximal CMAP amplitude or area by the mean surface-recorded motor unit potential amplitude or area. At this time, there is no role for MUNE in the routine diagnosis of ALS.

Electrodiagnostic Criteria

Amyotrophic lateral sclerosis is a clinical disorder in which the EDX study plays a major role in supporting the diagnosis

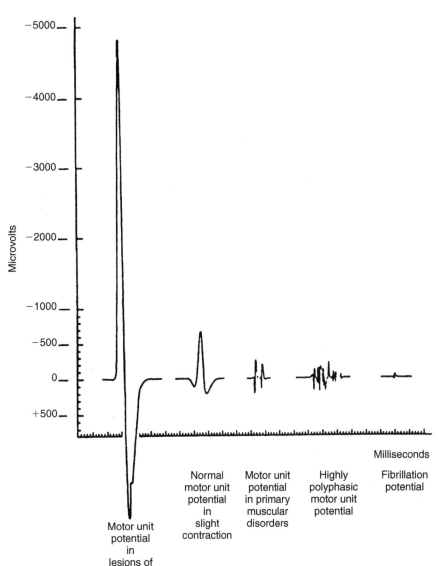

Figure C19–4. *Relative average durations and amplitudes of some motor unit potentials (MUAPs) seen in myopathic and neurogenic disorders. (From Daube J. AAEM minimonograph 11: needle electromyography in clinical electromyography. Muscle Nerve 1991;14:685–700, with permission.)*

and in excluding entities that can mimic ALS. Electrophysiologic confirmation of ALS requires evidence of a widespread LMN degeneration, and hence the needle EMG examination should be performed on three or more regions of the neuraxis and should assess all the major segments in the limbs examined. When the bulbar region is assessed, changes must be observed in at least one muscle (including tongue, jaw muscles, and facial muscles). Needle EMG of the tongue is difficult due to failure to achieve adequate relaxation which results in inability to appreciate fibrillation or fasciculation potentials. Also, the tongue MUAPs normally are small and may appear similar to fibrillation potentials. The thoracic

segment can only be assessed by needle EMG of the thoracic paraspinal muscles at or below the T6 level, and occasionally the abdominal muscles. Evaluation of higher thoracic segments may be misleading as denervation changes derived from lower cervical segments may manifest as far caudally as the T6 level.

The criteria proposed by Lambert in 1969 had been the most widely accepted for the diagnosis of ALS. These criteria require fibrillation with fasciculation potentials in three limbs, with the head counting as a "limb." El Escorial criteria have adopted these standards with some revisions. Table C19–4 provides a summary of definitive EDX criteria for ALS.

Table C19–4. Electrodiagnostic Criteria for the Diagnosis of Amyotrophic Lateral Sclerosis (ALS)

1. Active denervation (fibrillation potentials), with or without fasciculation potentials, in at least two muscles, of different root innervation and different peripheral or cranial nerve innervation, in two or more regions*
2. Evidence of reinnervation of motor unit action potentials (MUAPs), with decreased recruitment
3. Normal sensory nerve action potentials (SNAPs)
4. Normal motor conduction studies or low compound muscle action potential (CMAP) amplitudes, with normal or borderline conduction velocities, and distal and F wave latencies†

*Regions are defined as follows: brain stem (bulbar), cervical (upper limbs), thoracic (back and abdomen), and lumbosacral (lower limbs). Involvement in a region is without regard to right or left side, but location is indicative of the level of neuraxis involved.
†Motor conduction velocities may be slowed but should not be lower than 70 to 80% of lower limits of normal values, in nerves with very low CMAP amplitudes (less than 50% of the lower limits of normal or less than 30% of normal mean).

The aforementioned criteria are fulfilled at the time of diagnosis in approximately two-thirds of patients with ALS. However, a significant proportion of patients with a clinical diagnosis of ALS fail to show these findings on EDX testing, particularly on initial studies. This is caused by the following *limitations*:

- Insufficient distribution of fibrillation potentials and loss of MUAPs. Some patients have evidence of diffuse anterior horn cell loss on their first EDX examination, but testing results in other patients may not fulfill these strict criteria. These limitations are related to the fact that the EDX may fail to reveal dissemination of anterior horn cell loss of all segments of the neuraxis, such as in patients experiencing LMN degeneration in its earlier stages that is restricted to one extremity or one region (cervical, lumbosacral, or bulbar only). Hence, it is not uncommon for patients with ALS to have earlier EDX examinations, sometimes performed by experienced electromyographers, that revealed findings of cauda equina syndrome, lumbosacral radiculopathy, or cervical radiculopathy. Unfortunately, this often may lead to unnecessary spinal operations, especially in elderly patients in whom spine imaging often is abnormal. The EDX examination may also lead to inconclusive findings when the UMN findings are predominant and there is little or a restricted degree of LMN degeneration or when the disorder is associated with a concomitant disorder such as a peripheral polyneuropathy.
- Abnormal SNAP amplitudes. Although sensory function and SNAPs usually are normal in ALS patients, subtle abnormalities in the SNAPs may be detected in some patients. These are supported by morphologic abnormalities in sensory nerves, which are sometimes demonstrated in ALS. In addition, abnormal SNAP amplitudes are more common proportionately in elderly patients (>70 years) because normal controls are not available for these populations in most EDX laboratories. These patients often lack SNAPs in the lower extremities, a finding that can be misinterpreted as a sign of peripheral polyneuropathy. Thus, one must avoid "over-interpretation" of SNAP amplitudes in elderly patients.

Thus, clinicians must understand the drawbacks of EDX study and use this test as an adjunct to clinical examination. Sequential EDX examinations are sometimes necessary to confirm progression and worsening of denervation in the affected limb(s), and even more importantly, to document evidence of dissemination of denervation. In practical terms, it frequently is more important for the electromyographer to test extensively an asymptomatic or mildly symptomatic limb than a limb with severe atrophy and weakness because the documentation of denervational changes in all limbs is essential to show dissemination of disease and to solidify the diagnosis.

Although the role of EDX study in ALS is complementary to the clinical suspicion, there are many *advantages* associated with use of the EDX examination that:

- Detect evidence of LMN degeneration in limbs before any clinical weakness or atrophy is evident.
- Identify evidence of LMN degeneration in prominently spastic limbs in which atrophy and weakness are difficult to assess. In UMN-dominated ALS, needle EMG signs of denervation occur on average of 6 months prior to clinical appearance of LMN signs.
- Exclude other disorders of motor nerves, such as multifocal motor neuropathy with conduction block.
- Distinguish motor neuron disease from other neuromuscular disorders such as inclusion body myositis.

FOLLOW-UP

The patient's weakness progressed and spread to other extremities. Initially, her left upper extremity became weak. Six months later, she developed early dysphagia and dysarthria. Her follow-up examination revealed tongue fasciculations and asymmetrical weakness of the upper extremities, worse on the right. The deep tendon reflexes became less active. Vital capacity declined to 1.31 liters (45% of predicted value) and she became dyspneic at rest. Arterial blood gases on room air showed pH = 7.44, carbon dioxide partial pressure (PCO_2) = 85, partial pressure of oxygen (PO_2) = 85, bicarbonate radical (HCO_3) = 30.7. The patient refused tracheostomy and the use of assisted ventilation. She died of respiratory failure 28 months after the onset of symptoms.

DIAGNOSIS

Classic amyotrophic lateral sclerosis.

ANSWERS

1. D; 2. A; 3. A; 4. B.

SUGGESTED READINGS

Behina M, Kelly J. Role of electromyography in amyotrophic lateral sclerosis. Muscle Nerve 1991;14:1236–1241.

Bensimon G et al. A controlled trial of riluzole in amyotrophic lateral sclerosis. N Engl J Med 1994;330:585–591.

Bernstein LP, Antel JP. Motor neuron disease: decremental responses to repetitive stimulation. Neurology 1981;31: 204–205.

Bradley WG et al. Morphometric and biochemical studies of peripheral nerves in amyotrophic lateral sclerosis. Ann Neurol 1983;14:267–277.

Brooks BR, Miller RG, Swash M et al. El Escorial revisited: revised criteria for the diagnosis of amyotrophic lateral sclerosis. Amyotroph Lateral Scler Other Motor Neuron Disord 2000;1:293–299.

Brown RH. Superoxide dismutase and familial amyotrophic lateral sclerosis: new insights into mechanisms and treatments. Ann Neurol 1996;39:145–146.

Brown RH, Swash M, Pasinelli P, eds. Amyotrophic lateral sclerosis. 2nd edn. Informa Healthcare, 2006.

Chancellor AM, Warlow CP. Adult onset motor neuron disease: worldwide mortality, incidence and distribution since 1950. J Neurol Neurosurg Psych 1992;55: 1106–1115.

Drachman DB, Kuncl RW. Amyotrophic lateral sclerosis: an unconventional autoimmune disease? Ann Neurol 1989;26: 269–274.

Gooch CL, Harati Y. Motor unit number estimation, ALS and clinical trials. Amyotroph Lateral Scler Other Motor Neuron Disord 2000;1:71–82.

Gurney ME et al. Benefit of vitamin E, Riluzole, and Gabapentin in a transgenic model of familial amyotrophic lateral sclerosis. Ann Neurol 1996;39:147–157.

Hjorth RJ, Walsh JC, Willison RG. The distribution and frequency of spontaneous fasciculations in motor neuron disease. J Neurol Sci 1973;18:469–474.

Killian JM et al. Decremental motor responses to repetitive nerve stimulation in ALS. Muscle Nerve 1994;17:747–754.

Kuncl RW, Cornblath DR, Griffin JW. Assessment of thoracic parapsinal muscles in the diagnosis of ALS. Muscle Nerve 1988;11:484–492.

Lacomblez L et al. Dose-ranging study of riluzole in amyotrophic lateral sclerosis. Lancet 1996;347:1425–1431.

Lambert EH. Electromyography in amyotrophic lateral sclerosis. In: Kurland LT, Norris FH, eds. Motor neuron diseases. New York: Grune and Stratton, 1969.

Lambert EH, Mulder DW. Electromyographic studies in amyotrophic lateral sclerosis. Mayo Clin Proc 1957;32:441–446.

Miller RG, Rosenberg JA, Gelinas DF et al. Practice parameter: rhe care of the patient with amyotrophic lateral sclerosis (an evidence based review). Neurology 1999;52:1311–1323.

Mitsumoto H, Chad D, Pioro EP, eds. Amyotrophic lateral sclerosis. Philadelphia, PA: FA Davis, 1998.

Moss AH et al. Home ventilation for amyotrophic lateral sclerosis. Neurology 1993;43:438–443.

Quality Standards Subcommittee of the American Academy of Neurology. Practice advisory on the treatment of amyotrophic lateral sclerosis with riluzole: report of the Quality Standards Subcommittee of the American Academy of Neurology. Neurology 1997;49:657–659.

Rosenfeld J, Swash M. What's in a name? Lumping or splitting ALS, PLS, PMA and the other motor neuron diseases. Neurology 2006;66:6214–625.

Roth G. The origin of fasciculation potentials. Ann Neurol 1982;12:542–547.

Rothstein JD. Excitotoxic mechanisms in amyotrophic lateral sclerosis. In: Seratrice G, Munsat T, eds. Pathogenesis and therapy of amyotrophic lateral sclerosis, advances in neurology, vol. 68. Philadelphia, PA: Lippincott-Raven, 1995.

Rothstein JD, Martin LJ, Kuncl RK. Decreased glutamate transport by the brain and spinal cord in amyotrophic lateral sclerosis. N Engl J Med 1992;326:1464–1468.

Shefner JM, Tyler HR, Krarup C. Abnormalities in the sensory action potential in patients with amyotrophic lateral sclerosis. Muscle Nerve 1991;14:1242–1246.

Siddique T et al. Linkage of a gene causing familial amyotrophic lateral sclerosis to chromosome 21 and evidence of genetic-locus heterogeneity. N Engl J Med 1991;324:1381–1384.

Smith RG et al. Serum antibodies to L-type calcium channels in patients with amyotrophic lateral sclerosis. N Engl J Med 1992;327:1721–1728.

Sorenson EJ, Stalker AP, Kurland LT et al. Amyotrophic lateral sclerosis in Olmsted County, Minnesota, 1925 to 1998. Neurology 2002;59:280–282.

Urban PP, Vogt T, Hopf HC. Corticobulbar tract involvement in amyotrophic lateral sclerosis: a transcranial magnetic stimulation study. Brain 1998;121:1099–1108.

Case 20

HISTORY AND PHYSICAL EXAMINATION

A 32-year-old white woman developed progressive weakness in the legs over 2 months. She noticed gradually increasing difficulty climbing stairs and standing from a sitting position. She began using a walker for assistance 4 days before admission to the hospital. She reported muscle pain in both legs but denied any ocular, bulbar, or sphincteric symptoms. There was no history of skin rash or arthralgia. Three weeks earlier, she was found to have "abnormal liver function tests" and received a diagnosis of possible "toxic hepatitis." She was taking no medications and denied any history of alcohol or drug abuse.

On examination, she was in no apparent distress. There was no skin rash. She had normal cranial nerves. She had significant difficulty getting up from a chair and needed assistance when walking. There was generalized mild muscle tenderness. Manual muscle examination revealed significant symmetrical proximal more than distal muscle weakness, worse in the legs. Deep tendon reflexes were normal. Sensation was normal. Using the Medical Research Council (MRC) grading system, her muscle strength was rated as follows:

	Right	Left
Deltoid	4/5	4/5
Triceps	4/5	4/5
Biceps	4/5	4/5
Hand grip	4+/5	4+/5
Iliopsoas	4–/5	4–/5
Quadriceps	4–/5	4–/5
Hamstrings	4–/5	4–/5
Ankle dorsiflexion	4+/5	4+/5
Plantar dorsiflexion	4+/5	4+/5

Abnormal laboratory values were: creatine kinase (CK) 14 857 units/liter (U/L) (normal, <140 U/L), aldolase 589.1 U/L (normal, 3.5–17.5 U/L), lactate dehydrogenase (LDH) 1475 U/L (normal, 60–210 U/L), serum alanine aminotransferase (ALT) 478 U/L (normal, 8–54 U/L), and serum aspartate aminotransferase (AST) 566 U/L (normal, 10–50 U/L). Normal laboratory studies included the following: Westergren erythrocyte sedimentation rate (ESR; 10 mm/h), serum gamma-glutamyl transferase (GGT) level, antinuclear antibody (ANA), rheumatoid factor, thyroxine (T_4), thyroid-stimulating hormone (TSH), complete blood count (CBC), bilirubin, alkaline phosphatase, electrolytes, and serum protein electrophoresis. Negative results included the following: human immunodeficiency virus (HIV) antibody, urine myoglobin, serum lyme titers, toxoplasma immunoglobulin M (IgM) and Venereal Disease Research Laboratory (VDRL).

An electrodiagnostic (EDX) examination was performed.

Please now review the Nerve Conduction Studies and Needle EMG tables.

QUESTIONS

1. In this disorder fibrillation potentials are most common in:
   A. Paraspinal muscles.
   B. Proximal muscles of the lower extremities.
   C. Proximal muscles of the upper extremities.
   D. Distal muscles.
   E. Anterior neck muscles.
2. Motor unit action potentials (MUAPs) seen in the chronic form of this disorder are:
   A. Short in duration and low in amplitude.
   B. Long in duration and complex.
   C. Normal.
   D. All of the above.

Case 20: Nerve Conduction Studies

Nerve Stimulated	Stimulation Site	Recording Site	Amplitude (m = mV, s = µV)			Distal/Peak Latency (ms)			Conduction Velocity (m/s)			F Latency (ms)	
			Right	Left	Normal	Right	Left	Normal	Right	Left	Normal	Right	Left
Sural (s)	Calf	Ankle		20	≥5		4.0	≤4.5		42	≥40		
Peroneal (m)	Ankle	EDB		3.8	≥3		5.0	≤5.0			≥40		
Peroneal (m)	Knee	EDB		3.5						44			48
Median (s)	Wrist	Index finger		30	≥20		2.6	≤3.4					
Median (m)	Wrist	APB		7.8	≥6		3.2	≤3.9			≥50		
Median (m)	Elbow	APB		7.3						56			27

APB = abductor pollicis brevis; EDB = extensor digitorum brevis; m = motor; s = sensory.

Case 20: Needle EMG

Muscle	Insertional Activity	Spontaneous Activity Fibs	Spontaneous Activity Fascs	Recruitment Normal	Recruitment Activation	Recruitment Reduced	Recruitment Early	Configuration Duration	Configuration Amplitude	Configuration % Polyphasia	Others
L. tibialis anterior	↑	3+	0	X				↓	↓	↑	
Medial gastrocnemius	↑	1+	0	X				Normal	Normal	↑	
Vastus lateralis	↑	2+	0				X	↓	Normal	↑	
Vastus intermedius	↑	2+	0				X	↓	↓	↑↑	
Midlumbar paraspinal	↑	2+	0	–							
Lower lumbar paraspinal	↑	2+	0	–							
L. brachioradialis	↑	2+	0	X				↓	↓	↑	
Biceps	↑	2+	0				X	↓↓	↓↓	↑↑	
Triceps	↑	2+	0	X				↓	↓	↑	
Deltoid	↑	2+	0				X	↓	↓	↑↑	

Fascs = fasciculations; Fibs = fibrillations; L. = left; ↑ = increased; ↓ = slightly reduced; ↑↑ = significantly increased; ↓↓ = significantly reduced.

3. Increasing weakness developed in a 45-year-old woman with polymyositis who was taking corticosteroids. Which of the following findings suggests steroid myopathy rather than relapsing polymyositis?
   A. Rising CK.
   B. Fibrillation potentials.
   C. Short-duration, low-amplitude MUAPs.
   D. Complex repetitive discharges.
   E. Normal insertional activity.

EDX FINDINGS AND INTERPRETATION OF DATA

Pertinent EDX findings in this case include the following:

1. Normal sensory and motor nerve conduction studies (amplitudes, distal latencies, and conduction velocities), including F-wave latencies.
2. Fibrillation potentials in all muscles tested in the lower and upper extremities, including the paraspinal muscles.
3. Prominent MUAP changes in many muscles tested, mostly resulting in short-duration, low-amplitude, and polyphasic MUAPs.
4. Early MUAP recruitment in proximal muscles.

These findings are consistent with a diffuse myopathy associated with fibrillation potentials, compatible with a necrotizing myopathy, such as an inflammatory myopathy (e.g., polymyositis).

DISCUSSION

Classification and Pathology

The inflammatory myopathies are a heterogeneous group of disorders that share a common pathologic feature: inflammatory cells in muscles. They comprise three major categories of muscle disease, polymyositis (PM), dermatomyositis (DM), and inclusion body myositis (IBM), conditions that are clinically, histologically, and pathogenetically distinct. Inflammatory myopathies are often classified into two major types (Table C20–1), a primary and secondary (associated with systemic or other identifiable disorders).

Polymyositis and dermatomyositis are organ-specific autoimmune disorders in which the skeletal muscles and skin (in DM only) are the primary target(s). In IBM, there is evidence that the disorder is primarily degenerative while the immune mechanisms are secondary.

Pathologically, the inflammatory myopathies are characterized by mononuclear cell inflammation, segmental

Table C20–1. General Classification of Inflammatory Myopathies

Primary
Dermatomyositis
  Adult
  Juvenile
  Amyopathic
Polymyositis
Inclusion body myositis

Secondary
With connective tissue diseases (overlap syndromes), e.g., scleroderma, systemic lupus erythematosus
With cancer (paraneoplastic), e.g., breast, ovary, lung, and gastrointestinal malignancies
Giant cell and granulomatous disorders, e.g., sarcoidosis
Infection, e.g., trichinosis, cysticercosis

Others
Eosinophilic syndromes, e.g., diffuse fascitis of Schulman
Local nodular myositis

muscle fiber necrosis, and muscle fiber regeneration. The pathologic findings in PM and DM have both common and diverse features. Both also are different from the findings in inclusion body myositis. Table C20–2 shows the major differences among these three primary inflammatory myopathies.

Clinical Features

Polymyositis and dermatomyositis affect patients of all ages, with a predilection to women. In the United States, these disorders are twice as common among blacks than whites (incidence rate of 0.77 versus 0.32 per 100 000, respectively). Most patients present with muscle weakness that develops subacutely over weeks to months, and affects predominantly the proximal pelvic and shoulder girdle muscles, including the neck flexors. Dysphagia and myalgia/muscle tenderness are common, each occurring in one-third of patients. Extramuscular manifestations are not uncommon. They include involvement of the lungs (interstitial lung disease) and the heart (cardiomegaly, congestive heart failure, and conduction defects), and manifestations of diffuse necrotizing vasculitis (especially in juvenile DM).

In DM only, there is an associated skin rash that can be the presenting symptom. Two classic rashes are characteristic. The first is a "heliotrope rash," an erythematous, violaceous (hence the name) rash over the malar and periorbital areas that may extend to involve other sun-exposed areas, such as the dorsum of the hands, knees, elbows, or forehead. The second rash is Gottron papules, an erythematous papular rash over the knuckles of the fingers. Subcutaneous calcinosis complicates up to half of children with

Table C20–2. Pathologic and Treatment Response Differences Between Polymyositis, Dermatomyositis, and Inclusion Body Myositis

	Polymyositis	**Dermatomyositis**	**Inclusion Body Myositis**
Fiber necrosis	Single	Single or group	Single
Perifascicular atrophy	No	Yes	No
Capillaries	Normal	Reduced	Normal
Inflammation	Endomysial CD8 cells	Perimysial/vascular B, CD4 cells	Endomysial CD8 cells
Complement activation	No	Capillaries	No
Rimmed vacuoles	No	No	Yes
15–18 nm tubular filaments	No	No	Yes
Response to corticosteroids	Good	Good	Poor
Response to IVIG	Fair	Good	Poor

IVIG = intravenous immunoglobulin.

juvenile DM and may be present in chronic DM. These lesions are most often seen in the buttocks, thighs, knuckles, and elbows (Figure C20–1). They may be painful, ulcerate through the skin, or get infected.

In contrast to PM and DM, IBM affects patients over the age of 50, has a male predominance, and is more common in the white than black population. The onset is insidious and it progresses slowly, evolving over years. It is the most common inflammatory myopathy in patients over the age of 50. Clinically, IBM has a unique muscle involvement that easily distinguishes it from the other inflammatory myopathies. There is usually asymmetrical involvement of the finger flexors and wrist flexors in the upper extremities,

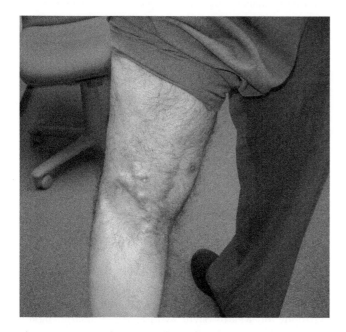

Figure C20–1. *Calcinosis in the popliteal fossa of a patient with a long history of dermatomyositis.*

and the knee extensors and ankle dorsiflexors in the lower extremities (Figure C20–2). Dysphagia is common and afflicts up to 60% of patients as the disease progresses.

Up to a quarter of patients with DM/PM have an associated connective tissue disease. The "overlap syndrome" links PM and DM with other connective tissue disease such as scleroderma, systemic lupus erythematosus, Sjögren syndrome, rheumatoid arthritis, and mixed connective tissue disease.

Laboratory features include an elevated serum CK in 90% of patients (at least 5 to 10 times normal values). LDH, ALT, and AST may be elevated, which can lead to the erroneous diagnosis of liver disease. In these situations, the ALT/AST ratio is useful. In hepatocellular disease, the ratio is greater than 1 while in myopathies, the ratio should be reversed (i.e., ALT/AST < 1). Also, measuring serum GGT activity is helpful in excluding concomitant hepatic disease, since this enzyme highly specific for hepatocellular disease and has a low level or is absent in muscle. Serum aldolase may also be elevated, but the utility of this enzyme in the diagnosis and follow-up of myopathies is of limited value for two reasons. First, aldolase is less sensitive or specific than CK since it is present in lower amounts in skeletal muscle. Second, serum aldolase is elevated in primary muscle as well as liver disease. ESR is normal or mildly elevated. Autoantibodies, such as ANA, SSA, or SSB, are positive in overlap syndromes. Anti-Jo-1 antibody is the most prevalent in DM/PM, occurring in 20% of patients and in 50 to 75% of patients with associated interstitial lung disease.

The incidence of malignancy in patients with DM and PM older than 40 years of age is higher than that expected for the general population, suggesting that DM and PM may be paraneoplastic. The increased risk in patients older than 40 years of age is 6-fold for DM and 2-fold for PM compared with that of the general population. The neoplasms are variable, but most are reported as carcinoma of the breast, ovary, and lung and gastrointestinal tract.

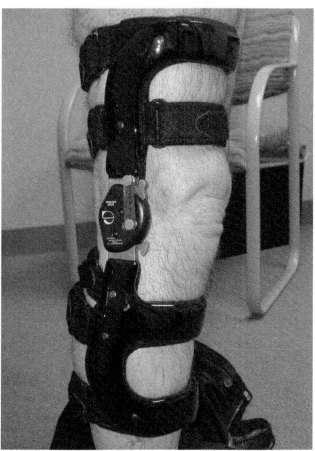

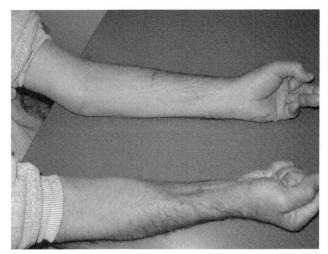

A   **B**

Figure C20–2. *Bilateral asymmetrical hand weakness and atrophy (**A**) with severe bilateral asymmetrical quadriceps weakness, necessitating an assisted knee brace (**B**), in a 67-year-old man with inclusion body myositis.*

The diagnoses of DM and PM are confirmed based on the combination of clinical, laboratory, electrophysiologic, and pathologic findings. In 1975, Bohan and Peter proposed a classification that has been used since, with some revisions, in confirming the diagnoses of PM and DM. Based on these criteria, the confidence limits in the diagnosis of PM or DM range from definite to probable to possible (Table C20–3). The differential diagnoses of PM include IBM, polymyalgia rheumatica, metabolic myopathies (such as acid maltase deficiency), and limb girdle muscular dystrophy. In dermatomyositis, the presence of typical skin rash combined with muscle weakness often is diagnostic.

Nearly all patients with DM and PM respond favorably to corticosteroids. The initial recommended dose of prednisone is 1.0 to 1.5 mg/kg/day. One must treat with adequate prednisone as long as there is evidence of active disease. This should be titrated based on objective serial clinical evaluations and CK determinations. The effectiveness of intravenous immunoglobulin is proven in DM, but it is also effective in PM. Other immunosuppressive agents such as azathioprine, methotrexate, and cyclophosphamide also are effective. The prognosis is favorable for children and with early diagnosis and treatment. A significant number of patients require a small dose of prednisone for maintenance.

In contrast to PM/DM, IBM is a treatment-resistant myositis. No immunosuppresive or immunomodulating agent has been shown to alter the natural course of disease.

Electrodiagnosis

Electrodiagnostic Findings of Myopathies in General

Sensory nerve conduction studies (NCS) in myopathy are normal, except in certain myopathies in which an associated peripheral polyneuropathy may occur (such as myotonic dystrophy or Kearns-Sayre syndrome). Similarly, motor NCSs usually are normal; however, motor studies may reveal low-amplitude compound muscle action potentials (CMAPs)

Table C20–3. Criteria and Confidence Limits in the Diagnosis of Polymyositis and Dermatomyositis

Criteria

1. Clinical	Predominantly proximal (limb girdle and neck flexor muscles), usually symmetrical, muscle weakness progressing over weeks or months, with or without myalgia, dysphagia or respiratory muscle involvement
2. Laboratory	Elevation of serum levels of skeletal muscle enzymes, particularly CK (MM isoenzyme), and sometimes aldolase, ALT, and LDH
3. Electromyography	Multifocal needle EMG changes of myopathy (short, small, polyphasic motor unit potentials), fibrillations and, sometimes, complex repetitive discharges*
4. Muscle biopsy	Necrosis affecting all types of muscle fibers, phagocytosis, muscle fiber regeneration, and lymphocytic infiltration in the absence of cytoplasmic inclusion bodies†
5. Dermatological	Lilac (heliotrope) discoloration of the eyelids and/or Grotton signs (scaly, erythematous dermatitis over the dorsum of the hands, particularly over the metacarpophalangeal and proximal interphalangeal joints which may extend to knees, elbows, medial malleoli, neck, face and upper trunk)

Confidence Limits

Diagnosis	Polymyositis	Dermatomyositis
Definite	4 criteria without rash	3 or 4 criteria plus rash
Probable	3 criteria without rash	2 criteria plus rash
Possible	2 criteria without rash	1 criteria plus rash

*See electrodiagnosis discussion for details.
†See Table C20–2 for differences between PM, DM, and inclusion body myositis.

when recording severely affected muscles. Examples include median and ulnar motor NCSs in adults with myotonic dystrophy, advanced Duchenne muscular dystrophy or critical illness myopathy. Proximal motor NCSs, such as musculocutaneous and femoral studies, may be low in amplitudes if performed on children with Duchenne muscular dystrophy. F waves and H reflexes are universally normal except when there is an associated polyneuropathy.

Repetitive nerve stimulations (RNS) generally are normal in myopathy, with certain exceptions. In non-dystrophic myotonic disorders, rapid RNS (usually at 20 Hz) may result in a decrementing response, particularly after prolonged stimulation. Also, during a paralytic attack of hyperkalemic periodic paralysis, rapid RNS may result in an increment of the low-amplitude baseline CMAP.

Electrodiagnostic findings in myopathies generally are limited to those attained with needle EMG. This has led few electromyographers to perform only needle EMG, without NCSs, on patients with suspected myopathy. However, this is not recommended because other neuromuscular disorders, such as neuromuscular junction disorders and early anterior horn cell disorders, may result in MUAP changes similar to those seen in myopathy.

The changes seen on needle EMG in myopathy include one or more of the following.

1. *Abnormal insertional and spontaneous activities.*
   - *Fibrillation potentials.* These are commonly seen in neurogenic disorders (hence, the designation "denervation potentials"), but they also frequently accompany certain necrotizing myopathies, namely the inflammatory myopathies and the progressive muscular dystrophies. Morphologically, fibrillation potentials seen in myopathies do not differ from the ones observed in neurogenic disorders, except that fibrillation potentials associated with myopathies tend to fire at slower rates. The pathogenesis of these potentials in myopathy is discussed in a forthcoming section.
   - *Myotonic discharges.* These potentials are induced by needle insertion and usually are "waxing and waning" in character because of variability in frequency and amplitude (Figure C20–3). They are associated with a distinctive sound that can be compared with the sound of a diving airplane ("dive-bomber"). These discharges, generated by single muscle fibers, can be accompanied by clinical myotonia (percussion myotonia,

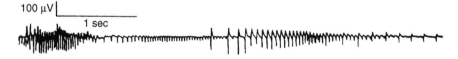

100 µV
1 sec

Figure C20–3. *Myotonic discharge. Note the change in both amplitude and frequency of the discharge. This discharge is recorded at a compressed screen (sweep speed = 200 ms). (From Sethi RK, Thompson LL. The electromyographer's handbook, 2nd ed. Boston, MA: Little, Brown, 1989, with permission.)*

grip myotonia, or lid myotonia). Myotonic discharges are specific for ce311rtain myopathies, including myotonic dystrophy, non-dystrophic myotonias (such as myotonia congenita), and acid maltase deficiency (see Table 2–4, p. 33).

- *Complex repetitive discharges (CRDs)*. CRD is a composite waveform that contains several distinct spikes and often fires at a constant and fast rate of 30 to 50 Hz. These discharges are recognized as polyphasic and complex potentials; hence the former name "bizarre repetitive potentials" (Figure C20–4). CRD remains uniform from one discharge to another, a feature that helps distinguishing it from myokymic discharge. CRDs are spontaneous discharges of muscle fibers

50 µV/D   50 ms/D

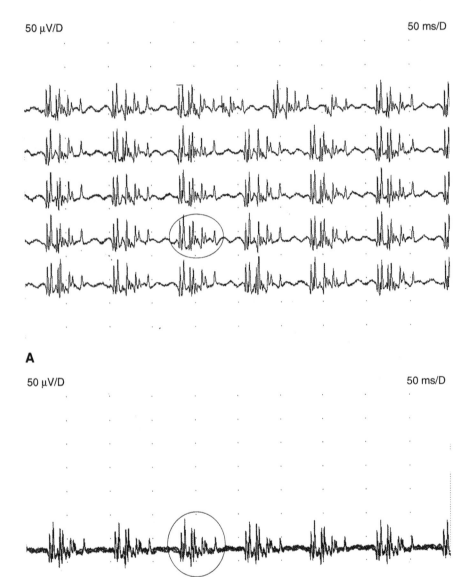

A

50 µV/D   50 ms/D

B

Figure C20–4. *Complex repetitive discharge. Note that the complex (circled) is stable and remains exactly the same between discharges with a constant firing rate. (**A**) The discharge is shown as a triggered rastered form. (**B**) The five rasters are superimposed. Note that the complex superimposes perfectly reflecting its uniform configuration.*

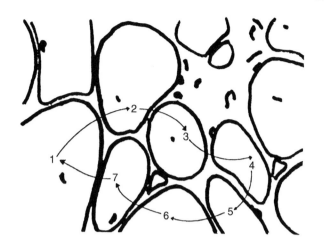

Figure C20–5. *Pathophysiology of a complex repetitive discharge (CRD): an ephaptic transmission from muscle fiber to muscle fiber that creates a circus movement without an intervening synapse. (Courtesy of Dr. David Preston.)*

during which a single muscle fiber spontaneously depolarizes, which is followed by ephaptic spread to adjacent denervated fibers. Often, a circus movement is created, which leads to a recurrent discharge (Figure C20–5). The chain reaction eventually blocks resulting in abrupt cessation. These recurrent discharges give a distinctive machine-like sound over the loudspeaker during needle EMG. Complex repetitive discharges are most often seen in myopathies and neuropathic disorders such as radiculopathies. They accompany most commonly chronic conditions but may be observed in subacute disorders.

2. *Changes in MUAP morphology.*

Although MUAP changes were suspected to exist in myopathy, Kugelberg (1949) is credited for a major contribution to our current understanding of the characteristic MUAP changes that occur in myopathy. These MUAP changes reflect the disintegration of motor unit structure in myopathy caused by muscle fiber loss, the variation in muscle fiber diameter, and an increased amount of connective tissue, along with the presence of regenerated and reinnervated muscle fibers. In general, MUAPs in myopathy are short in duration, low in amplitude and polyphasics (Figure C20–6). These units are very small compared with both normal MUAPs and sprouted ("neurogenic") MUAPs (Figure C20–7). Typical MUAP changes seen in myopathy include:

- *Short-duration MUAPs.* In myopathy, there is a shift toward a shorter mean MUAP duration (Figure C20–8). This is probably caused by the loss of muscle fibers within the motor unit. Short-duration MUAPs are the most consistent MUAP change associated with myopathy.
- *Polyphasic MUAPs.* In myopathy, MUAPs with more than four phases are increased in number, resulting in an increased percentage of polyphasic potentials, beyond the 10 to 20% seen in healthy individuals. This is probably caused by variability in muscle fiber conduction velocities and desynchronization of muscle action potentials within the territory of the motor unit.

0.2 mV/D   20 ms/D

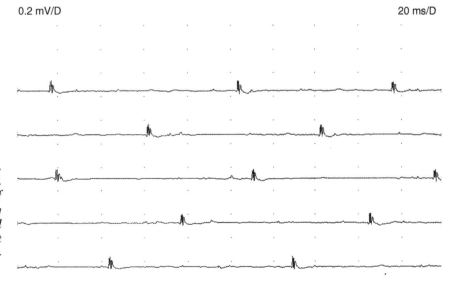

Figure C20–6. *Typical short-duration, low-amplitude, and polyphasic MUAP, recorded in a raster form, from the deltoid of a 55-year-old patient with a 3-month history of proximal weakness, elevated CK, and elevated anti-Jo1 antibody. Subsequent work-up revealed polymyositis with interstitial lung disease.*

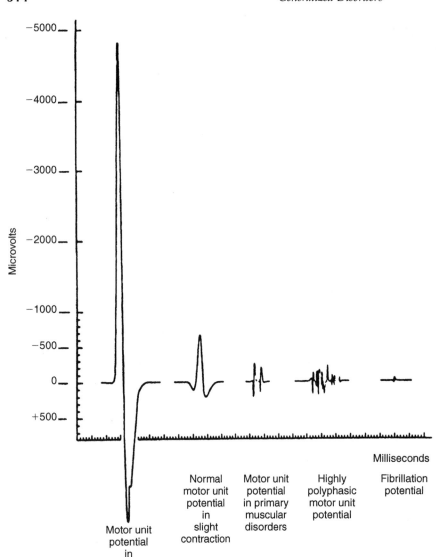

Microvolts

Motor unit
potential
in
lesions of
anterior horn
cells

Normal
motor unit
potential
in
slight
contraction

Motor unit
potential
in primary
muscular
disorders

Highly
polyphasic
motor unit
potential

Fibrillation
potential

Milliseconds

Figure C20–7. *Relative average durations and amplitudes of some motor unit action potentials (MUAPs) seen in myopathic and neurogenic disorders. (From Daube J. AAEM minimonograph 11: needle electromyography in clinical electromyography. Muscle Nerve 1991;14:685–700, with permission.)*

- *MUAPs with satellite (linked) potentials.* Sometimes, an MUAP may be divided into two or more time-locked sections that are separated by baseline. The MUAP portion with the greatest duration or amplitude is considered the main body of the MUAP, while the remaining portions are called "linked" or "satellite" potentials (Figures C20–8 and C20–9). These MUAPs are easily seen with trigger/delay techniques. Including the satellite potentials may yield very long duration values that may be misleading. Therefore, these satellite potentials should be excluded from duration analysis.
- *Low-amplitude MUAPs.* This is the least reliable and most debated MUAP change in myopathy. Low-amplitude

MUAPs are caused by the loss of muscle fiber and collagen tissue replacement, which results in increasing the distance between many muscle fibers and the recording electrode.

The alterations in MUAP configuration that occur in myopathy are not absolute. Instead, the MUAP changes form a continuum that ranges from normal to grossly abnormal MUAPs, with many MUAPs falling at points on the continuum between these two. Hence, identifying a myopathic process by needle EMG is one of the most difficult tasks for electromyographers. Evaluation of a patient with suspected myopathy requires meticulous analysis of the morphology of many MUAPs, within different areas of

0.2 mV/D   20 ms/D

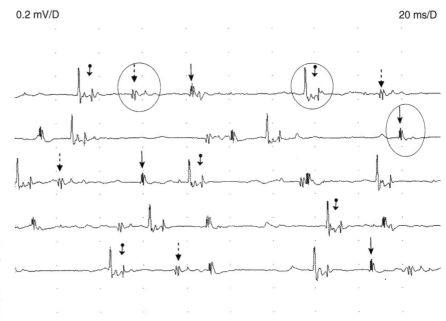

Figure C20–8. *Several MUAPs recorded from the biceps muscle, recorded in a raster form, of the same patient as Figure C20–5. Note the short-duration, low-amplitude, and polyphasic MUAPs (solid arrow and dashed-line arrow) and the MUAP with satellite (linked) potentials (bulleted arrow).*

the muscle, in many muscles and in multiple extremities including the paraspinal muscles. Automated analysis of MUAPs, using computer-assisted EDX equipment that incorporates triggered and delayed sweeps, has allowed better determination of MUAP changes, especially those associated with myopathy (Figure C20–10).

3. *Changes in MUAP recruitment.*

The EDX assessment of recruitment is the most subjective parameter studied in the EMG laboratory, and attainment of accurate results is highly dependent on experience. Interpretation of recruitment is a particularly difficult task in myopathy. Interference pattern computer-assisted analysis,

0.2 mV/D   20 ms/D

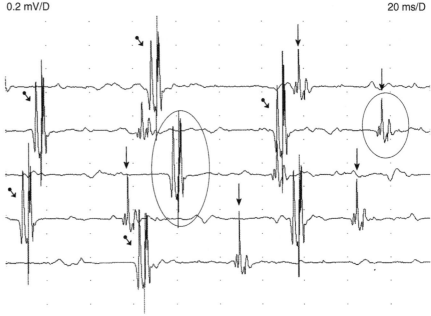

Figure C20–9. *MUAP recording from the quadriceps of a 61-year-old woman with a 3-year history of partially responsive chronic polymyositis. Note the two complex MUAPs that are polyphasic and with satellite potentials (arrow and bulleted arrow) leading to an initial misdiagnosis of motor neuron disease. These complex MUAPs with satellite potentials may yield long-duration values that may be misleading. Therefore, satellite potentials should be excluded from duration analysis and only the MUAP portion with the greatest duration or amplitude (main body of the MUAP) should be measured.*

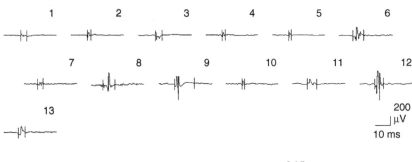

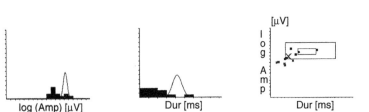

Figure C20–10. *Quantitative MUAP analysis (Multi-MUP system, Medtronic) from the deltoid muscle of a 65-year-old man with polymyositis. Thirteen MUAP were collected for analysis. Note the shift to the left of both amplitude and duration depicting short-duration and low-amplitude MUAPs compared to normal (bell-shaped curves).*

which typically judges the "turns and amplitudes," has gained some popularity but has not been used extensively in routine EDX studies.

The recruitment of MUAPs in various myopathies may take one of these forms:

- *Normal recruitment.* This is common in mild to moderate myopathies.
- *Early recruitment.* There is increased recruitment of MUAPs in relation to effort, which results from the inability of an individual MUAP to generate any significant force (because of the loss of muscle fibers). This phenomenon sometimes is referred to as an "increase in the interference pattern." An early recruitment pattern is the most common recruitment abnormality seen in myopathy.
- *Reduced recruitment with a rapid firing rate.* This recruitment, which imitates neurogenic recruitment, is the least common in myopathy. It occurs in advanced myopathy when loss of muscle fibers is severe, resulting in the functional loss of many motor units.

In summary, the EDX evaluation in patients with suspected myopathy is challenging to electromyographers because the findings may be subtle and patchy. Meticulous care in analyzing MUAP configuration and recruitment and a rather extensive sampling of muscles in both upper and lower extremities are needed in most cases.

Despite its complexity, there are many *advantages* to the use of EDX studies in the diagnosis of myopathy:

1. The EDX study excludes other neuromuscular disorders (neuromuscular junction, peripheral nerve, anterior horn cell), which sometimes mimic a myopathy.
2. The EDX study permits widespread muscle sampling and may detect abnormalities that are regional (such as in facioscapulohumeral muscular dystrophy or IBM) or patchy (such as in polymyositis). This is in contrast to

muscle biopsy, which is usually limited to analysis of one or two muscle specimens.
3. The EDX study may identify specific features of myopathy and helps in attaining a final diagnosis (see forthcoming section). These include myotonia (as seen with myotonic dystrophy) and fibrillation potentials (as seen in the inflammatory myopathies).
4. When abnormal, The EDX study is often able to identify muscle(s) that are significantly affected by the pathological process, thereby guiding the clinician to a suitable site for biopsy (usually from the contralateral side).
5. The EDX study may be used to follow the progress of certain myopathies, such as an inflammatory myopathy during treatment or in cases of relapse.

The EDX examination, however, has two relevant *limitations* in the diagnosis of myopathy:

1. In general, the diagnostic sensitivity of EDX in myopathy is not high. This is because needle EMG is dependent on the muscle action potential and is not related to the contractile function of muscle. In general, needle EMG more readily detects myopathies in which muscle necrosis has occurred and tends to miss myopathies in which the integrity of both muscle fibers and their action potentials is spared. Thus, needle EMG findings in myopathy are diverse. At one end of the spectrum, if myonecrosis is prominent, such as in muscular dystrophy or inflammatory myopathy, the MUAPs are small and the EMG is abnormal and sensitive. At the other extreme, the needle EMG may be normal (or the changes too subtle to detect) in certain myopathies, such as the metabolic and endocrine myopathies, because the integrity of most muscle fibers and their action potentials is maintained. Thus, *a normal needle EMG never excludes a myopathy.*

2. The EDX findings in myopathy are not always specific enough to provide a specific diagnosis. In other words, the needle EMG changes in many myopathies are similar, which may prevent the electromyographer from making a specific diagnosis of the myopathic process. Hence, the EDX examination is certainly not the final step in the work-up in many of these patients. Except in certain situations, as in a patient with a classic rash of dermatomyositis or in assessment of a sibling of a patient with documented myotonic dystrophy, a muscle biopsy or genetic testing is necessary to identify the exact cause of myopathy.

Certain needle EMG features may accompany the MUAP changes and are helpful in the differential diagnosis of myopathies. Two features are instrumental in the accurate diagnosis of myopathy: fibrillation potentials and myotonic discharges. Based on these electrical potentials and the MUAP changes associated with myopathy, the EDX findings in myopathy may be easily divided into six general categories (Table C20–4):

- Myopathies commonly presenting with normal EMG.
- Myopathies commonly presenting with MUAP changes and fibrillation potentials.
- Myopathies commonly presenting with MUAP changes only.
- Myopathies commonly presenting with fibrillation potentials only.
- Myopathies commonly presenting with MUAP changes and myotonic discharges.
- Myopathies commonly presenting with myotonic discharges only.

Electrodiagnostic Findings in Polymyositis/Dermatomyositis

Although the clinical manifestations of PM and DM are diffuse, the EDX findings, similar to their pathologic counterparts, are frequently patchy. Thus, a meticulous needle EMG often is required to identify these abnormalities. This should include sampling of the proximal and distal muscles, the upper and lower extremity muscles, and the paraspinal muscles.

Needle EMG findings during the active phases of PM/DM consist of the following.

1. *Increased insertional activity with fibrillation potentials.* These potentials, when associated with PM and DM, have certain features:
   - They are patchy in distribution and are not present in every muscle sampled. Thus, extensive needle EMG often is required, particularly in early or mild cases, to allow identification of these potentials.

- They are detected in nearly all patients with PM or DM, as long as an extensive search is performed. In more than two-thirds of patients with PM/DM, fibrillation potentials are present in all or at least half of the sampled muscles. In the minority of patients, these potentials are limited to only a few muscles.
- They have a predilection to the paraspinal muscles in the cervical, thoracic, and lumbar regions, presumably because of the propensity of the disease to affect proximal and truncal muscles. In fact, fibrillation potentials are found in the paraspinal muscles in 90 to 100% of patients during the active phase of disease.
- When serial studies are performed, there is a rough correlation between the number of fibrillation potentials and the severity or level of activity of the disease (i.e., the degree of ongoing myonecrosis).
- Fibrillation potentials decrease after successful treatment. Along with the decline in serum CK, the disappearance of fibrillation potentials is among the earliest signs of a favorable response to treatment.
- Fibrillation potentials recur as PM or DM relapses. Thus, in patients treated with corticosteroids who develop increasing weakness, the presence of fibrillation potentials is generally consistent with recurring disease and not with "steroid myopathy," which is not accompanied by these potentials. In these situations, comparative studies are important.

The exact cause of fibrillation potentials in the necrotizing and inflammatory myopathies is not well understood. Because fibrillation potentials are spontaneous action potentials that are generated by denervated muscle fibers, two possible explanations for their occurrence have been proposed:

- *Segmental myonecrosis* leading to effective denervation of the distant segments of muscle fibers as they become separated physically from the neuromuscular junction. The denervated segment of the muscle fiber generates the fibrillation potentials. This phenomenon may also initiate collateral sprouting to these segments, which may lead to fiber type-grouping (as seen histologically), increased fiber density (as measured by single-fiber EMG), and long-duration and complex MUAPs (as seen on conventional needle EMG).
- *Damage to the terminal intramuscular motor axons*, presumably by the inflammatory or necrotizing process, which results in denervation of some muscle fibers. Here again, collateral sprouting accounts for reinnervation (fiber type-grouping, increased fiber density, and long-duration, complex MUAPs).

2. *Small MUAPs.* In subacute PM or DM, the MUAPs frequently are short in duration, low in amplitude, and polyphasic in configuration, and they are frequently intermixed with normal MUAPs. However, in chronic

Table C20–4. Patterns of Needle EMG Findings in Myopathies

Normal	Myopathic MUAPs With Fibrillation Potentials	Myopathic MUAPs only	Fibrillation Potentials Only	Myopathic MUAPs and Myotonia	Myotonia Only
Metabolic myopathies	*Inflammatory myopathies*	*Muscular dystrophies*	*Inflammatory myopathies**	*Myotonic dystrophies (DM)*	*Myotonia congenita*
McArdle disease	Polymyositis	FSH	Polymyositis	DM1	Thomsen disease
Tarui disease	Dermatomyositis	Limb girdle	Dermatomyositis	DM2	Becker disease
Brancher deficiency	Inclusion body myositis	Oculopharyngeal Congenital	Sarcoid myopathy		*Other myotonic disorders*
Debrancher deficiency	Sarcoid myopathy		HIV-associated myopathy	*Muscle channelopathies*	Atypical painful myotonia
CPT deficiency	HIV-associated myopathy	*Congenital myopathies*		Paramyotonia congenita	Myotonia fluctuans
Carnitine deficiency		Central core	*Others*	Hyperkalemic periodic paralysis[†]	
Adenylate deaminase deficiency	*Muscular dystrophies*	Nemaline rod	Chloroquine		
	Duchenne			*Others*	
	Becker	*Endocrine myopathies*		Acid maltase deficiency	
Mitochondrial myopathies	Distal	Steroid (severe)		Myotubular myopathy	
Kearns-Sayre syndrome	*Others*	Hypothyroid Hyperthyroid		Colchicine	
MELAS	Critical illness myopathy	Hyperparathyroid			
MERRF	Myotubular myopathy	*Toxic myopathies*			
	Parasitic infections (trichinosis)	Alcohol			
Endocrine myopathies		Emetine			
Steroid (mild)		Statins			
Hypothyroid					
Hyperthyroid		*Acute rhabdomyolysis*			
Hyperparathyroid					
Cushing					
Others					
Fiber type disproportion					
Acute rhabdomyolysis					
Periodic paralysis[†]					

*Early or mild.
[†]Between attacks.
CPT = carnitine palmitoyltransferase deficiency; FSH = facioscapulohumeral; HIV = human immunodeficiency virus; McArdle disease = myophosphorylase deficiency; MELAS = mitochondrial encephalomyopathy, lactic acidosis, and stroke-like episodes; MERRF = myoclonic epilepsy and ragged-red fibers; Tarui disease = phosphofructokinase deficiency.
Adapted with revisions from Katirji B, Kaminski HJ, Preston DC et al., eds. Neuromuscular disorders in clinical practice. Boston, MA: Butterworth-Heinemann, 2002.

cases of PM/DM (as well as in other chronic myopathies, such as IBM), it is common to find long-duration, complex MUAPs with many components and satellites (Figure C20–11). These potentials result from collateral sprouting or from significant variation of muscle fiber conduction velocities within the motor unit caused by segmental degeneration and regeneration.

The EDX findings in polymyositis and dermatomyositis follow a cyclic pattern. Fibrillation potentials appear first at relapse and disappear early during remission, but abnormal MUAPs become evident later in relapse and last longer before resolution (Figure C20–12). This changing pattern must be recognized after treatment, when serial studies are performed on patients with PM/DM. For example, when fibrillations are not detected in a patient

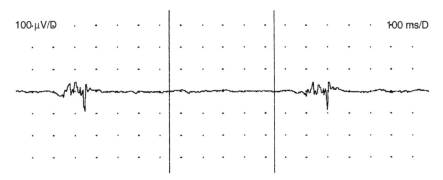

A

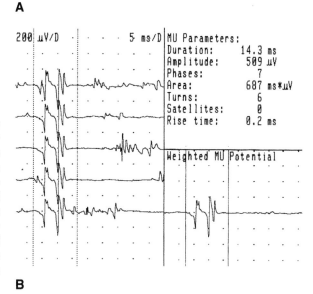

Figure C20–11. *MUAPs recording from the quadriceps of a 74-year-old man with 3-year history of inclusion body myositis. Although the MUAP in (**A**) is very low in an amplitude, it is polyphasic and complex, resulting in an increase in absolute duration to 25 ms. The increased duration of this unit may suggest a neurogenic disorder. (**B**) This MUAP has also a slightly prolonged duration (14.3 ms). It has a well-defined satellite, which precedes the main body of the MUAP. The satellite potential should not be counted in the measurement of the duration.*

B

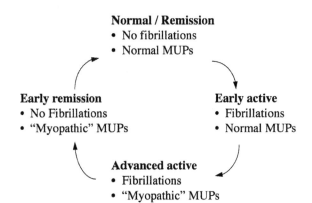

Figure C20–12. *Needle electromyography changes seen during the various phases of polymyositis and dermatomyositis. (Adapted, with revisions, from Wilbourn AJ. Electrodiagnostic examination with myopathies. J Clin Neurophysiol 1993;10: 132–148, with permission.)*

with PM/DM who is experiencing worsening weakness while taking corticosteroids, the diagnosis of iatrogenic "steroid myopathy" becomes more likely because the latter is not associated with fibrillation potentials.

FOLLOW-UP

A muscle biopsy was obtained from the quadriceps muscle. The findings were diagnostic of inflammatory myopathy, particularly PM (Figure C20–13). No rimmed vacuoles were seen. The patient was started on prednisone 80 mg/day. She showed a dramatic improvement in strength, accompanied by a decline in CK. Prednisone was tapered slowly with no evidence of recurrence. One year later, she displayed normal strength and CK while taking prednisone 10 mg every other day.

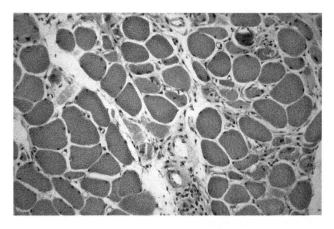

Figure C20–13. *Quadriceps muscle biopsy of a patient, revealing myofiber degeneration and regeneration, variability in muscle fiber size, and endomysial and perivascular inflammatory infiltration by lymphocytes (hematoxylin and eosin).*

DIAGNOSIS

Idiopathic polymyositis.

ANSWERS

1. A; 2. D; 3. E.

SUGGESTED READINGS

Bohan A, Peter JB. Polymyositis and dermatomyositis. N Engl J Med 1975;292:344–347, 403–407.

Buchthal F. Electromyography in the evaluation of muscle diseases. Neurol Clin 1985;3(3):573–598.

Chad D. Inflammatory myopathies. In: Katirji B, Kaminski HJ, Preston DC, Ruff RL, Shapiro EB, eds. Neuromuscular disorders in clinical practice. Boston, MA: Butterworth-Heinemann, 2002, pp. 1169–1180.

Dalakas MC. Polymyositis, dermatomyositis, and inclusion body myositis. N Engl J Med 1991;325:1487–1498.

Dalakas MC. Inflammatory, immune, and viral aspects of inclusion-body myositis. Neurology 2006;66(2 Suppl 1):S33–38.

Dalakas MC, Hohlfeld R. Polymyositis and dermatomyositis. Lancet 2003;362(9388):971–982.

Dalakas MC et al. A controlled trial of high-dose intravenous immune globulin infusions as treatment for dermatomyositis. N Engl J Med 1993;329:1993–1998.

Daube JR. Application of quantitative methods in neuromuscular disorders. In: Halliday AM, Butler SR, Paul R, eds. A textbook of clinical neurophysiology. New York: John Wiley, 1987.

Fellows LK, Foster BJ, Chalk CH. Clinical significance of complex repetitive discharges. A case-control study. Muscle Nerve 2003;28:504–507.

Katirji B, Al-Jaberi M. Creatine kinase revisited. J Clin Neuromusc Dis 2001;2:158–163.

Kugelberg E. Electromyogram in muscular disorders. J Neurol Neurosurg Psychiatry 1947;10:122–133.

Lacomis D. Electrodiagnostic approach to the patient with suspected myopathy. Neurol Clin N Am 2002;20:587–603.

Lambert EH, Sayre GP, Eaton LM. Electrical activity in muscle in polymyositis. Trans Am Neurol Assoc 1954;79:64–69.

Mastaglia FL, Ojeda VJ. Inflammatory myopathies: parts 1 and 2. Ann Neurol 1985;7:215–227, 317–323.

Mitz M et al. Electromyographic and histologic paraspinal abnormalities in polymyositis/dermatomyositis. Arch Phys Med Rehabil 1981;62:118–121.

Sandstedt PER, Henriksson KG, Larsson LE. Quantitative electromyography in polymyositis and dermatomyositis. Acta Neurol Scand 1982;65:110–121.

Sigurgeirsson B et al. Risk of cancer in patients with dermatomyositis or polymyositis. N Engl J Med 1992;326:363–367.

Streib E. Differential diagnosis of myotonic disorders. Muscle Nerve 1987;10:603–615.

Streib E, Daube JR. Electromyography of paraspinal muscles. Neurology 1975;25:386.

Streib EW, Wilbourn AJ, Mitsumoto H. Spontaneous electrical muscle fiber activity in polymyositis and dermatomyositis. Muscle Nerve 1979;2:14–18.

Trojaborg W. Quantitative electromyography in polymyositis: a reappraisal. Muscle Nerve 1990;13:964–971.

van der Meulen MFG, Bronner IM, Hoogendijk JE et al. Polymyositis. An overdiagnosed entity. Neurology 2003;61:316–321.

Wilbourn AJ. Electrodiagnostic examination with myopathies, J Clin Neurophysiol 1993;10:132–148.

Case 21

HISTORY AND PHYSICAL EXAMINATION

A 51-year-old, white, previously healthy woman noted a gradual onset of progressive fatigue and general weakness. At first this was attributed to depression, and she was treated in a psychiatric hospital with haloperidol without effect. Within 3 months, her weakness had worsened so that she was unable to walk more than a few steps and could not manage stairs. Weakness was variable, and was much less of a problem in the morning. When the patient was first seen by a neurologist, a diagnosis of myasthenia gravis was made. She was placed on pyridostigmine (Mestinon®), which resulted in some improvement. At that time, a computed tomography (CT) scan of the chest, obtained to look for thymoma, was reported as normal. On questioning, the patient complained of difficulty swallowing, related to dry mouth, intermittent horizontal double vision and drooping of eyelids, and "burning" of the arms and legs. She denied sphincteric symptoms, loss of weight, loss of appetite, or shortness of breath.

Medical history was relevant for long-standing hypertension and hiatal hernia. She underwent an aortic bypass graft for intermittent claudication, cholecystectomy for gallstones, and hysterectomy for fibroid tumor. She had a long history of heavy cigarette use, at least 70 pack-years. She was on pyridostigmine (Mestinon®), captopril (Capoten®), and ranitidine (Zantac®).

Neurologic examination revealed normal mental status. The patient was not in distress and she used a wheelchair. She had mild bilateral ptosis, which was fatiguable on sustained upgaze. Fundi, pupils, extraocular movements, visual fields, and visual acuity were all normal. There was no facial weakness or asymmetry. The tongue was normal. Muscle bulk and tone were normal. She had proximal weakness, worse in the legs (Medical Research Council [MRC] 4/5 in legs and 4+/5 in arms). Deep tendon reflexes were diffusely hypoactive (trace to 1/4). Neither strength nor reflexes were accentuated by brief exercise. Sensation and cerebellar examination were normal. Gait was slow and waddling. Romberg test was negative.

Electrodiagnostic (EDX) studies were performed 24 hours after discontinuation of pyridostigmine (Mestinon®).

Please now review the Nerve Conduction Studies and Needle EMG tables.

QUESTIONS

1. The abnormalities seen on routine nerve conduction studies in this case are *least often* observed in:
   A. Amyotrophic lateral sclerosis.
   B. Myopathy.
   C. Lambert-Eaton myasthenic syndrome.
   D. Postpoliomyelitis syndrome.

2. Characteristics of this disorder include all of the following *except:*
   A. It results from impaired release of acetylcholine from the presynaptic terminal.
   B. It is caused by blockage of the voltage-gated calcium channel (VGCC) in the presynaptic terminal.
   C. It usually manifests with generalized weakness and minimal extraocular muscle weakness.
   D. It frequently is associated with thymoma.

3. Both myasthenia gravis and Lambert-Eaton myasthenic syndrome (LEMS) result in:
   A. Low-amplitude compound muscle action potentials (CMAPs).
   B. Significant facilitation of CMAPs after brief exercise.
   C. Decrement of CMAPs with slow repetitive stimulation.
   D. Significant increment of CMAPs with rapid repetitive stimulation.

Case 21: Nerve Conduction Studies

Nerve Stimulated	Stimulation Site	Recording Site	Amplitude (m = mV, s = µV)			Distal/Peak Latency (ms)			Conduction Velocity (m/s)			F Latency (ms)	
			Right	Left	Normal	Right	Left	Normal	Right	Left	Normal	Right	Left
Median (s)	Wrist	Index		30	≥15		3.2	≤3.6		57	≥50		
Median (s)	Elbow			22									
Ulnar (s)	Wrist	Little finger		18	≥10		2.8	≤3.1					
Radial (s)	Forearm	Thumb base		45	≥14		2.5	≤2.7					
Median (m)*	Wrist	APB		**2.8†**	≥6		3.9	≤4.0					
Median (m)*	Elbow	APB		**2.0**						56	≥50		29.0
Ulnar (m)*	Wrist	ADM		**1.8†**	≥7		3.0	≤3.1					
Ulnar (m)*	Wrist	ADM		**1.5**						58	≥50		28.8
Sural (s)	Calf	Ankle		9	≥4		3.9	≤4.6					
Peroneal (m)	Wrist	EDB		**1.0†**	≥2.5		3.6	≤6.0					
Peroneal (m)	Elbow	EDB		**1.0**						49	≥40		51.0
Tibial (m)	Wrist	AH		**4.2†**	≥6		5.4	≤6.0		44	≥40		53.0
Tibial (m)	Wrist	AH		**3.8**									

ADM = abductor digiti minimi; AH = abductor hallucis; APB = abductor pollicis brevis; EDB = extensor digitorum brevis; m = motor; s = sensory.

Data in bold type are abnormal.

*See Figure C21–1.

†Significant postexercise potentiation ranging from 260 to 300%; see EDX interpretation for details.

Case 21: Needle EMG

Muscle	Insertional Activity	Spontaneous Activity		Voluntary Motor Unit Action Potentials (MUAPs)							
		Fibs	Fasces	Recruitment				Configuration			
				Normal	Activation	Reduced	Early	Duration	Amplitude	% Polyphasia	Others
L. tibialis anterior	Normal	0	0	X				Normal	Normal	Normal	
Medial gastrocnemius	Normal	0	0	X				Normal	Normal	Normal	
Vastus lateralis	Normal	0	0	X				Normal	Normal	Normal	
Vastus intermedius	Normal	0	0	X				Normal	Normal	Normal	
L. first dorsal interosseous	Normal	0	0	X				Normal	Normal	Normal	
Brachioradialis	Normal	0	0	X				Normal	Normal	Normal	
Biceps	Normal	0	0	X				Normal	Normal	Normal	
Triceps	Normal	0	0	X				Normal	Normal	Normal	
Deltoid	Normal	0	0	X				Normal	Normal	Normal	

Fasces = fasciculations; Fibs = fibrillations; L. = left.

EDX FINDINGS AND INTERPRETATION OF DATA

Relevant EDX findings in this case include:

1. Low CMAP amplitudes with normal distal latencies and conduction velocities throughout the upper and lower limbs.
2. Normal sensory nerve action potentials (SNAPs) throughout.
3. Normal needle EMG.
4. Prominent postexercise potentiation of all motor amplitudes (i.e., CMAPs) after a single stimulus following brief exercise (10 seconds). This facilitation was universal (i.e., it occurred when applied to all motor nerves studied) and ranged from 260 to 300%. These postexercise potentiation values are as follows:

Nerve	Preexercise CMAP (mV)	Postexercise CMAP (mV)	Facilitation (%)
Median*	2.8	7.3	260
Ulnar*	1.8	5.3	294
Peroneal	1.0	3.0	300
Tibial	4.2	11.0	260

*See Figure C21–1.

5. Prominent CMAP increment after rapid repetitive stimulation (30 and 50 Hz) of the left median nerve at 250% (Figure C21–2).
6. A decrement of the CMAP after slow repetitive stimulation of the left median nerve at 35%.
7. Normal needle EMG.

These findings are consistent with presynaptic neuromuscular junction blockade, such as that seen in LEMS. Classic electrophysiologic findings include low CMAP amplitudes, significant facilitation after brief exercise, and prominent increment after rapid repetitive stimulation.

DISCUSSION

Pathophysiology

Lambert-Eaton myasthenic syndrome (LEMS) is a rare autoimmune disorder of the neuromuscular junction, caused by autoantibodies against the presynaptic P/Q type voltage-gated calcium channels (VGCC). The block of VGCCs results in a decrease in calcium influx during depolarization of the presynaptic membrane, and interferes with the calcium-dependent release of acetylcholine (ACH) from its stores in vesicles into the synaptic cleft. Passive transfer of IgG of patients with LEMS to animals produces the same physiologic and morphologic changes as those seen in humans.

Lambert-Eaton myasthenic syndrome is paraneoplastic, associated with small-cell lung cancer (SCLC) in approximately 50% of patients. A significant predictor for developing SCLC in patients with LEMS is smoking at the time of diagnosis. SCLC is commonly detected soon after the onset of LEMS symptoms, but this latency rarely extends beyond five years. Cultured SCLC cells exhibit VGCC activity, suggesting that SCLC cells expresses VGCCs and initiate the autoimmune process. Serum IgG antibodies against P/Q type VGCCs are present in 90% of patients with LEMS with SCLC, and in 3% of patients with SCLC with no neurological symptoms. Other malignancies associated with LEMS are relatively rare, and most have been intrathoracic such lymphoma, thymoma, and carcinoid tumors. The remaining LEMS patients do not have cancer, are usually younger women, and have other autoimmune disorders such as systemic lupus erythematosus, pernicious anemia, and juvenile-onset diabetes mellitus.

Clinical Features

Lambert-Eaton myasthenic syndrome, also referred to as the *myasthenic syndrome*, affects primarily adults older than 40 years of age, with a slight predilection to men. Patients present with proximal muscle weakness (especially of the lower extremities) and minimal ocular and bulbar

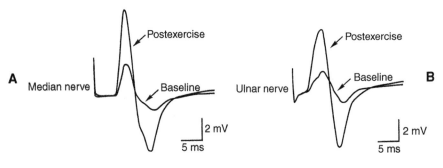

Figure C21–1. *Baseline compound motor action potentials (CMAPs) with superimposed postexercise CMAPs of the left median nerve, recording the abductor pollicis brevis (**A**), and the left ulnar nerve, recording the abductor digiti minimi (**B**). Note the prominent facilitation following 10 seconds of exercise (260% for median and 294% for ulnar).*

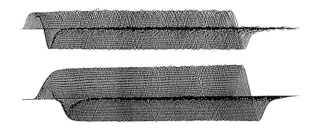

Figure C21–2. *Rapid, repetitive stimulation (50 Hz) of the median nerve at the wrist, recording the abductor pollicis brevis in a normal control* (top), *and in this patient* (bottom). *Note the significant facilitation of compound motor action potential (CMAP) (250%) in the patient but not the control.*

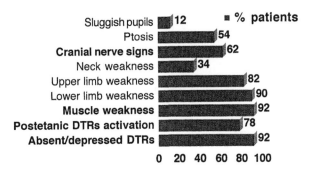

Figure C21–4. *Lambert-Eaton myasthenic syndrome. Signs during the course of illness in 50 cases. (Adapted from O'Neil JH, Murray NMF, Newsom-Davis J. The Lambert-Eaton myasthenic syndrome: a review of 50 cases. Brain 1988;11:577–596.)*

weakness, and are susceptible to fatigue. Deep tendon reflexes are characteristically absent or reduced. Autonomic complaints (especially dry mouth) and transient paresthesias may also occur. A helpful and distinctive clinical finding is muscle facilitation: after a brief period (~10 seconds) of intensive exercise of a muscle, muscle power is much transiently stronger and the deep tendon reflex to that muscle is enhanced. Unfortunately, this sign cannot always be confirmed during bedside evaluation. Figures C21–3 and C21–4 show the common signs and symptoms of LEMS patients, based on series of 50 patients.

The disorder may be mistaken for myasthenia gravis or myopathy. However, the *diagnosis* of LEMS is highly dependent on the electrophysiologic characteristics of the neuromuscular junction defect. Also, anti-P/Q-type VGCC antibodies are detected in the serum of 90% of patients with LEMS who have SCLC and in less than 50% of patients with LEMS without cancer. Elevated titers are detected in more than 10% of patients with SCLC and

paraneoplastic cerebellar degeneration with no LEMS manifestations. Low titers may also be present in patients with other autoimmune diseases, such as systemic lupus erythematosus and rheumatoid arthritis. *All patients with LEMS should be screened for cancer, particularly lung cancer, by CT scan or magnetic resonance imaging (MRI) of the chest.*

Treatment of LEMS is difficult. Treatment of the primary cancer is essential but seldom results in improvement of the neurologic symptoms. Figure C21–5 outlines a practical algorithmic treatment plan of weakness for patients with LEMS. Measures to combat weakness include:

1. Drugs, such as pyridostigmine (a choline esterase inhibitor), guanidine, or 3-4 aminopyridine. *3-4 Aminopyridine* blocks voltage-sensitive potassium channels, thereby increasing evoked transmitter release by prolonging the action potential duration and increasing calcium influx at the nerve terminal. Potential side effects include paresthesias and seizures. It is available commercially in Europe but limited to research studies in the United States. *Guanidine* also enhances the release of ACH from presynaptic terminal, but its serious adverse effects, including hepatotoxicity and bone marrow suppression, are limiting factors.
2. Plasmapheresis and intravenous immunoglobulins produce short-term clinical improvement and repeated treatments are needed to maintain improvement of muscle power.
3. Immunosuppressive drugs, particularly oral corticosteroids, azathioprine, or cyclosporine, may be helpful.

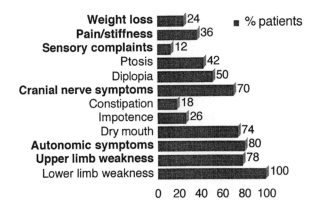

Figure C21–3. *Lambert-Eaton myasthenic syndrome. Symptoms during the course of illness in 50 cases. (Adapted from O'Neil JH, Murray NMF, Newsom-Davis J. The Lambert-Eaton myasthenic syndrome: a review of 50 cases. Brain 1988:11:577–596.)*

Electrodiagnosis

Nerve Conduction Studies

Nerve conduction studies (NCSs) in LEMS reveal normal sensory responses. However, motor NCSs disclose low or

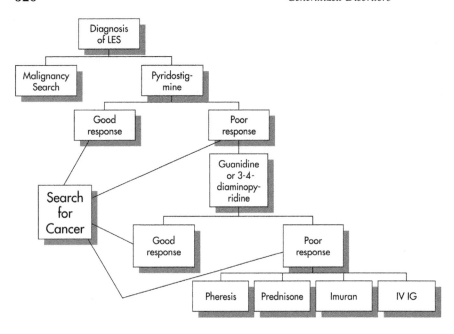

Figure C21–5. *Suggested treatment plan in patients with Lambert-Eaton myasthenic syndrome (LES = Lambert-Eaton myasthenic syndrome; IV IG = intravenous immunoglobulin).*

borderline-low CMAP amplitude in all motor nerves (discussed in a later section). These are usually associated with normal distal latencies, conduction velocities, and F wave latencies.

In general, *low-amplitude CMAPs with normal SNAPs* are infrequent findings in the EMG laboratory, especially when the findings are diffuse (i.e., every motor NCS has low CMAP, and every sensory NCS reveals normal SNAP). Figure C21–6 outlines the common site of pathology in patients manifesting low-amplitude CMAP responses in all or most motor nerves. These disorders are distinguished by a detailed needle EMG and repetitive nerve stimulation. Table C21–1 lists the common causes of such findings, as seen in the EMG laboratory.

Repetitive Nerve Stimulation

Abnormal repetitive nerve stimulations (RNSs) are the hallmark of neuromuscular junction defects. Since calcium diffuses out of the presynaptic terminal within 100 to 200 ms after a single-action potential, repetitive nerve stimulations are separated into slow and rapid stimulations, based on the stimulus rate (number of stimuli per second = hertz) applied to motor nerves. Slow RNS is performed at a rate slower than the time required for calcium diffusion (an interstimulus interval of >200 ms, i.e., slower than 5 stimuli/second, usually 2–3 Hz), and rapid stimulation occurs at a rate faster than this diffusion (an interstimulus interval of <100 ms, i.e., faster than 10 stimuli/second, usually 20–50 Hz) (for more details, refer to Case 17).

RNS in Healthy Individuals

Slow or fast rates of motor nerve stimulation do not abolish any endplate potential (EPP); all remain above threshold because of the presence of a "safety factor" (many more quanta (vesicles) are released with a single stimulus than are needed to generate an EPP). Thus, the CMAP (= summated muscle fiber action potentials, MFAPs) does

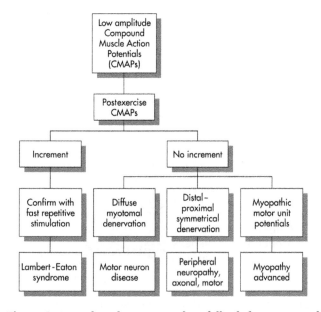

Figure C21–6. *Algorithmic approach to diffusely low compound motor action potential (CMAP) amplitudes (with normal sensory nerve action potential [SNAPs]).*

Table C21–1. Causes of Diffuse Low-Amplitude CMAPs (Compound Muscle Action Potentials) and Normal SNAPs (Sensory Nerve Action Potentials)

Anterior horn cell disease (e.g., amyotrophic lateral sclerosis and poliomyelitis)

Diffuse polyradiculopathies (e.g., concomitant cervical and lumbar spondylosis)

Pure motor axonopathy (e.g., acute motor axonal neuropathy (AMAN) and hereditary motor neuropathy)

Neuromuscular junction defect (e.g., Lambert-Eaton myasthenic syndrome and botulism)

Myopathy (severe; e.g., critical illness myopathy and advanced muscular dystrophy)

not change (no decrement). After rapid RNS or following brief exercise, there usually is a slight physiologic increment of the CMAP, which does not exceed 25% of the baseline CMAP. This *physiologic post-tetanic facilitation* is believed to be caused by increased synchrony of MFAPs after tetanic stimulation (Figures C21–7 and C21–8).

RNS in Patients With Lambert-Eaton Myasthenic Syndrome

1. *CMAP is low in amplitude.* Many muscle fibers do not reach threshold after a single stimulus because

of the inadequate release of quanta (vesicles). Thus, many muscle fibers will not generate an MFAP which results in a low-amplitude baseline CMAP at rest.

2. *Slow RNS* (<5/second, i.e., an interstimulus interval of >200 ms, usually 2–3 Hz) *results in decrement of the CMAP.* Acetylcholine (ACH) release is reduced because of depletion of the immediately available ACH stores. At this slow rate, the role of calcium (Ca^{2+}) in ACH release is not enhanced because Ca^{2+} diffuses out of the terminal in 100 to 200 ms. Thus, subsequent stimuli result in further loss of many EPPs and MFAPs (see Figure C21–7).

3. *Rapid RNS* (>5–10/second, i.e., an interstimulus interval of <100 ms, usually 20–50 Hz, or following brief exercise CMAP) greatly enhances Ca^{2+} influx, which results in larger releases of quanta and larger EPPs. This results in many muscle fibers reaching the threshold required for the generation of EPPs. Thus, more MFAPs are summated; hence the *increment of the CMAP* (see Figure C21–8). The post-tetanic facilitation should exceed 50%, and preferably 100%, to be diagnostic. This marked postexercise facilitation of the CMAP is the electrical correlate of the clinical facilitation of muscle strength and reflexes sometimes seen after brief exercise.

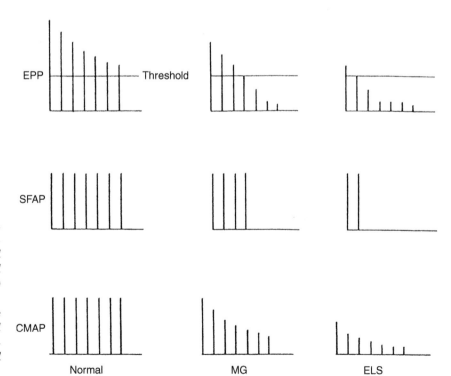

Figure C21–7. *Slow, repetitive stimulation effect on endplate potential (EPP), single-fiber action potential (SFAP), also referred to as muscle action potential (MAP), and compound muscle action potential (CMAP) in normal nerve, myasthenia gravis (MG), and Lambert-Eaton myasthenic syndrome (LEMS or ELS). (Adapted from Oh S. Clinical electromyography, neuromuscular transmission studies. Baltimore, MD: Williams and Wilkins, 1988, with permission.)*

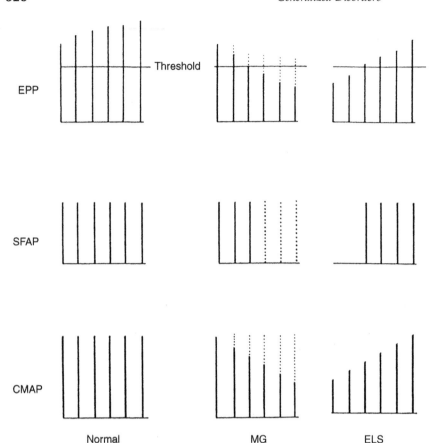

Figure C21–8. *Rapid, repetitive stimulation effect on endplate potential (EPP), single-fiber action potential (SFAP, also referred as muscle action potential [MAP]), and compound muscle action potential (CMAP) in normal nerve, myasthenia gravis (MG), and Lambert-Eaton myasthenic syndrome (LEMS or ELS). (Adapted from Oh S. Clinical electromyography, neuromuscular transmission studies. Baltimore, MD: Williams and Wilkins, 1988, with permission.)*

RNS in Patients With Myasthenia Gravis (MG)

1. *CMAP is normal.* A single stimulus usually leads to normal EPPs and MAPs in all fibers, which results in normal CMAP. This occurs despite the loss of ACH receptors and is due to the effect of the safety factor (many more quanta (vesicles) are released with a single stimulus than are needed to generate an EPP).
2. *Slow RNS* (<5/second, i.e., an interstimulus interval of >200 ms, usually 2–5 Hz) results in the progressive loss of many muscle fiber EPPs, owing to their failure to reach threshold. This results in loss of MFAPs and in a *decremental CMAP* (summated MAPs) (see Figure C21–7).
3. *With rapid repetitive stimulation* (>5–10/second, i.e., an interstimulus interval of <100 ms, usually 20–50 Hz or following brief exercise CMAP), the depleted stores are compensated by the Ca^{2+} influx, resulting in *no change of CMAP*. In severe myasthenics, there is a decrement in CMAP because the increased ACH release cannot compensate for the marked postsynaptic neuromuscular block (see Figure C21–8).

Single-Fiber EMG

Single-fiber jitter analysis is abnormal with frequent blocking in LEMS, as well as in myasthenia gravis. It is difficult to distinguish MG from LEMS using recruited (voluntary) single-fiber EMG because both disorders lead to a prolonged jitter, with or without blocking (for details, refer to Case 17). However, with stimulation jitter techniques, one can differentiate LEMS from myasthenia. Using a rapid rate of stimulation (>10 Hz), block or jitter or both improve significantly in LEMS owing to enhancement of ACH release by the influx of Ca^{2+} into the presynaptic terminal (Figure C21–9). However, at this rate of stimulation, the jitter does not change or worsen in myasthenia gravis.

Needle EMG

Needle EMG in LEMS usually is normal; rarely, short-duration, low-amplitude motor unit action potentials (MUAPs) are recorded, when severe neuromuscular blockade exists.

Conclusion

The EDX findings in LEMS include low-amplitude CMAP, increment of CMAP after brief exercise, and increment of CMAP after rapid RNS. Table C21–2 summarizes the EDX findings in LEMS and myasthenia gravis.

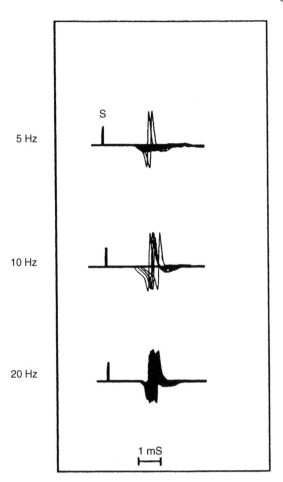

Figure C21–9. *The effect of stimulation rate on jitter and blocking in an endplate in the extensor digitorum communis in a patient with Lambert-Eaton myasthenic syndrome (LEMS). Single-fiber EMG recordings were made during stimulation of an intramuscular nerve twig. Each trace represents the superimposition of ten consecutive responses. Eighty percent of responses are blocked at 5 Hz, compared to 50% at 10 Hz and none at 20 Hz. S = stimulus artifact. (From Saunders DB. Lambert-Eaton myasthenic syndrome: clinical diagnosis, immune-mediated mechanisms and update on therapies. Ann Neurol 1995;37(S1): S63–S73, with permission.)*

The diagnosis of LEMS must be considered and excluded in all patients whose nerve conduction studies show low or borderline-low baseline CMAP amplitudes at rest, with normal sensory responses. Low or borderline-low CMAP amplitudes at rest should be followed by a repeat distal nerve stimulation after 10 seconds of exercise to exclude the possibility of LEMS. Assessing CMAP after brief exercise in patients with suspected LEMS is as accurate as results obtained after rapid RNS. It has the advantage of being much less painful and thus can be done on many motor nerves. It is recommended that postexercise CMAP is performed on several motor nerves, as a screening, in patients with suspected LEMS. If postexercise facilitation is present, then one motor nerve (such as a median or ulnar nerve) is stimulated with a rapid train (20–50 Hz) to verify the diagnosis.

Patients with LEMS are often misdiagnosed as MG. This occurs when slow RNSs (2–3 Hz) are only performed and result in CMAP decrements that are frequent and common finding in MG and LEMS. Most of these patients have low amplitude or borderline CMAPs on NCSs that are overlooked. Repeating distal nerve stimulation after 10 seconds of exercise on all nerves with low amplitude or borderline CMAPs, which is often done prior to slow RNS, should exclude or confirm the diagnosis of LEMS. If postexercise facilitation is present, a rapid RNS would be then done for confirmation. Table C21–3 lists the common differentiating clinical and electrophysiologic features of LEMS and MG.

FOLLOW-UP

A review of the CT scan performed earlier revealed a small mass in the azygoesophageal recess. A barium swallow confirmed the presence of an extrinsic indentation of the lower esophagus. After an unrevealing bronchoscopy, a right thoracotomy was performed. The mass was consistent with SCLC, with 9 of 27 positive lymph nodes. An extensive search for distant metastases was negative. The patient underwent radiation therapy and a 6-month course of chemotherapy. Her muscle weakness did not respond despite 3 months of plasmapheresis (twice per week) and

Table C21–2. Electrodiagnostic Findings in Lambert-Eaton Myasthenic Syndrome and Myasthenia Gravis

NMJ Defect (Disorder)	Baseline CMAP	Postexercise CMAP	Slow RNS	Fast RNS
Postsynaptic (MG)	Normal	Normal	Decrement	Normal or decrement
Presynaptic (LEMS)	Low	Increment	Decrement	Increment

CMAP = compound muscle action potential; LEMS = Lambert-Eaton myasthenic syndrome; MG = myasthenia gravis; NMJ = neuromuscular junction; RNS = repetitive nerve stimulation.

Table C21–3. Differential Diagnosis Between Generalized Myasthenia Gravis and Lambert-Eaton Myasthenic Syndrome

	Myasthenia Gravis	Lambert-Eaton Myasthenic Syndrome
Ocular involvement	Common and prominent	Uncommon and subtle
Bulbar involvement	Common and prominent	Uncommon and subtle
Deep tendon reflexes	Normal	Absent or depressed
Sensory symptoms	None	Paresthesias are common
Autonomic involvement	None	Dry mouth, impotence and gastroparesis
Tensilon test	Frequently positive	May be positive
Serum antibodies directed against	Postsynaptic Ach receptors or MuSK	Presynaptic voltage-gated calcium channels
Baseline CMAPs	Normal	Low in amplitude
Postexercise CMAPs	No change	Significant facilitation (>50–100%)*
Slow repetitive stimulation	Decrement	Decrement
Rapid repetitive stimulation	No change or decrement	Increment[†]
Single-fiber EMG	Increased jitter with blocking	Increased jitter with blocking
Rapid-rate stimulation jitter	Does not change or worsens jitter	Improves jitter[‡]

Ach = acetylcholine; CMAPs = compound muscle action potentials; EMG = electromyography; MuSK = muscle-specific kinase.
*See Figure C21–1.
[†]See Figure C21–2 (bottom tracing).
[‡]See Figure C21–9.

pyridostigmine, 120 mg every 3 hours. After the completion of chemotherapy, she was placed on guanidine, and the dose was increased to 500 mg qid, with no effect. Prednisone, 80 mg daily, was added, also with no beneficial result.

Eight months later, diarrhea developed increasingly. Pyridostigmine (Mestinon) was stopped, but the diarrhea became so severe that the patient required intravenous hyperalimentation. There was no clinical or radiologic evidence of SCLC recurrence. Then acute tubular necrosis developed, and the patient declined treatment with dialysis. She died 14 months after the onset of neurologic symptoms, 10 months after being diagnosed with LEMS and SCLC.

DIAGNOSIS

Lambert-Eaton myasthenic syndrome, associated with small-cell lung carcinoma.

ANSWERS

1. B; 2. D; 3. C.

SUGGESTED READINGS

Chalk CH et al. Response of the Lambert-Eaton myasthenic syndrome to treatment of associated small-cell lung carcinoma. Neurology 1990;40(10):1552–1556.

Eaton LM, Lambert EH. Electromyography and electric stimulation of nerves in diseases of motor unit: observations on myasthenic syndrome associated with malignant tumors. JAMA 1957;163:1117–1124.

Hughes R, Katirji MB. The Eaton-Lambert (myasthenic) syndrome in association with systemic lupus erythematosus. Arch Neurol 1986;43:1186–1187.

Jablecki C. Lambert-Eaton myasthenic syndrome. Muscle Nerve 1984;7:250–257.

Katirji B. Lambert-Eaton myasthenic syndrome: a harbinger to transitional cell carcinoma of the urinary bladder. J Clin Neuromusc Dis 2000;1:134–136.

Lambert EH, Eaton LM, Rooke ED. Defect of neuromuscular conduction associated with malignant neoplasms. Am J Physiol 1956;187:612–613.

Lennon VA et al. Calcium-channel antibodies in the Lambert-Eaton syndrome and other paraneoplastic syndromes. N Engl J Med 1995;332:1467–1474.

Leys K et al. Calcium channel autoantibodies in the Lambert-Eaton myasthenic syndrome. Ann Neurol 1991;29(3):307–314.

Maddison P, Newsom-Davis J. The Lambert-Eaton myasthenic syndrome. In: Katirji B, Kaminski HJ, Preston DC, Ruff RL, Shapiro EB, eds. Neuromuscular disorders in clinical practice. Boston, MA: Butterworth-Heinemann, 2002, pp. 931–941.

Maddison P, Newsom-Davis J, Mills KR. Distribution of electrophysiological abnormality in Lambert-Eaton myasthenic syndrome. J Neurol Neurosurg Psychiatry 1998;65:213–217.

Maddison P, Newsom-Davis J, Mills KR et al. Favourable prognosis in Lambert-Eaton myasthenic syndrome and small-cell lung carcinoma. Lancet 1999;353:117–118.

McEvoy KM et al. 3,4-Diaminopyridine in the treatment of Lambert-Eaton syndrome. N Engl J Med 1989;321:1567–1571.

O'Neil JH, Murray NMF, Newsom-Davis J. The Lambert-Eaton myasthenic syndrome: a review of 50 cases. Brain 1988;111:577–596.

Saunders DB. Lambert-Eaton myasthenic syndrome: clinical diagnosis, immune-mediated mechanisms and update on therapies. Ann Neurol 1995;37(S1):S63–S73.

Tim RW, Saunders DB. Repetitive nerve stimulation studies in Lambert-Eaton myasthenic syndrome. Muscle Nerve 1994;17:995–1001.

Ueno S, Hara Y. Lambert-Eaton myasthenic syndrome without anti-calcium channel antibody: adverse effect of calcium antagonist, diltiazem. J Neurol Neurosurg Psychiatry 1992;55(5):409–410.

Case 22

HISTORY AND PHYSICAL EXAMINATION

A 60-year-old woman presented with a 5- to 10-year history of leg weakness and a sense of unsteadiness of insidious onset. Recently, she had become aware of mild impairment of sensation over the tips of the fingers and toes. She had mild low back pain with no radicular pain. For many years before this, she had aching discomfort in both feet, which worsened with activity and weight bearing.

Her medical history was benign, except for hypertension and chronic anxiety disorder. Her medications included alprazolam (Xanax®) and diltiazem (Cardizem®). Family history was relevant for a 30-year-old son with hammer toes, high-arched feet, and "thin legs" since childhood. She had a daughter and a maternal cousin with high-arched feet. Parents were deceased, with no definite history of neuromuscular disease.

The general examination was relevant for bilateral pes cavus deformities without hammer toes. There were no skin trophic changes. On neurologic examination, the fundi were normal without retinal pigmentary changes. Cranial nerves were normal. There was atrophy of all intrinsic muscles of both hands. Distal legs were thin with inverted-champagne bottle appearance. She could not wiggle her toes. Manual muscle examination revealed bilateral symmetrical weakness, worse distally. Toe flexors and extensors were 0/5 (Medical Research Council [MRC]), ankle dorsiflexors and plantar flexors were 4–/5, and hand intrinsics 4+/5. Deep tendon reflexes were +1 in the upper extremities but absent in the legs. Sensation revealed decreased position and vibration sense at the toes, and to a lesser extent at the ankles. Pin and touch sensation was relatively decreased in all four extremities, symmetrically worse distally with a stocking-and-glove distribution. Gait was steppage due to foot weakness. She could not walk on heels or toes. Romberg test was negative.

An electrodiagnostic (EDX) examination was performed.

Please now review the Nerve Conduction Studies and Needle EMG tables.

QUESTIONS

1. The EDX findings observed in this patient are common to all of the following disorders *except:*
   A. Refsum disease.
   B. Charcot-Marie-Tooth disease type I.
   C. Metachromatic leukodystrophy.
   D. Diabetic polyneuropathy.
   E. Adrenomyeloneuropathy.

2. Characteristics of hereditary demyelinating motor and sensory neuropathies include all of the following *except:*
   A. Conduction blocks.
   B. Symmetrical slowing of latencies and velocities.
   C. Uniform slowing of velocities in different segments of the same nerve.
   D. Onion bulb formation on histological evaluation of nerve.

3. Characteristics of Charcot-Marie-Tooth disease type 1 (CMT1) include all of the following *except:*
   A. Has a common subtype that is associated with tandem duplication on chromosome 17.
   B. Commonly is associated with pes cavus and hammer toes.
   C. Has wide phenotypic variability.
   D. Has abnormal sensory nerve action potentials (SNAPs).
   E. Has low-amplitude compound muscle action potentials (CMAPs), with slight slowing of distal latencies and conduction velocities.

Case 22: Nerve Conduction Studies

Nerve Stimulated	Stimulation Site	Recording Site	Amplitude (m = mV, s = µV)			Distal/Peak Latency (ms)			Conduction Velocity (m/s)			F Latency (ms)	
			Right	Left	Normal	Right	Left	Normal	Right	Left	Normal	Right	Left
Sural (s)	Calf	Ankle	NR	NR	≥3	NR	NR	≤4.6					
Peroneal (m)	Ankle	EDB	NR	NR	≥2.5	NR	NR	≤6.0	NR	NR	≥40	NR	NR
Peroneal (m)	Knee	EDB	NR	NR									
Tibial (m)	Ankle	AH	NR	NR	≥4	NR	NR	≤6.0	NR	NR	≥40	NR	NR
Tibial (m)	Knee	AH	NR	NR									
Median (s)	Wrist	Index finger	NR	NR	≥10	NR	NR	≤3.8					
Ulnar (s)	Wrist	Little finger	NR	NR	≥5	NR	NR	≤3.2					
Radial (s)	Distal forearm	Dorsum of hand	NR	NR	≥10	NR	NR	≤2.8					
Median (m)*	Wrist	APB	**4.2***	**3.4**	≥5	**10.9**	**11.3**	≤4.0				**53.1**	**49.5**
Median (m)*	Elbow	APB	**3.8**	**2.9**					**24**	**22**	≥50		
Ulnar (m)*	Wrist	ADM	**3.9***	**3.7**	≥7	**6.9**	**7.1**	≤3.1				**51.5**	**53.8**
Ulnar (m)*	Above elbow	ADM	**3.1**	**2.7**					**21**	**23**	≥50		

ADM = abductor digiti minimi; AH = abductor hallucis; APB = abductor pollicis brevis; EDB = extensor digitorum brevis; m = motor; NR = no response; s = sensory.
Data in bold type are abnormal.
*See Figure C22–1B.

Case 22: Needle EMG

Muscle	Insertional Activity	Spontaneous Activity		Voluntary Motor Unit Action Potentials (MUAPs)							
				Recruitment				Configuration			
		Fibs	Fascs	Normal	Activation	Reduced	Early	Duration	Amplitude	% Polyphasia	Others
L. tibialis anterior	↑	1+	0			↓↓		↑	↑	Normal	
Medial gastrocnemius	↑	1+	0			↓↓		↑	↑	Normal	
Flexor digitorum longus	↑	1+	0			↓↓		↑	↑	Normal	
Abductor hallucis	↓	Rare	0	No voluntary motor unit potentials (MUAPs)							
Extensor digitorum brevis	↓	Rare	0	No voluntary motor unit potentials (MUAPs)							
Vastus lateralis	Normal	0	0	X				Normal	Normal	Normal	
R. tibialis anterior	↑	1+	0			↓↓		↑	↑	Normal	
Abductor hallucis	↓	Rare	0	No voluntary motor unit potentials (MUAPs)							
L. first dorsal interosseous	↑	+/−	0			↓		↑	↑	Normal	
Pronator teres	Normal	0	0	X				↑	Normal	Normal	
Deltoid	Normal	0	0	X				Normal	Normal	Normal	
R. first dorsal interosseous	↑	0	0			↓		↑	↑	Normal	

Fascs = fasciculations; Fibs = fibrillations; L. = left; R. = right; ↑ = increased; ↓ = mildly reduced; ↓↓ = moderately reduced.

EDX FINDINGS AND INTERPRETATION OF DATA

Relevant EDX findings in this case include:

1. Absent SNAPs throughout the upper and lower extremities.
2. Absent CMAPs and F waves in both lower extremities.
3. Marked slowing of motor distal latencies, conduction velocities, and F wave latencies in the upper extremities, along with moderate reduction of distal CMAP amplitudes (Figure C22–1). Distal latencies are 200 to 300% of the upper limit of normal values, conduction velocities are 45 to 50% of the lower limit of normal, and F wave latencies are 154 to 168% of the upper limit of normal values.
4. Motor slowing is uniform (affecting all motor nerve segments equally) and symmetrical (affecting motor nerves equally in both upper extremities). Also, there is no evidence of conduction block or significant temporal dispersion (see Figure C22–1).
5. Needle EMG reveals neurogenic changes that are mostly distal and symmetrical, but highly chronic, based on very large motor unit action potentials (MUAPs).

These findings are compatible with a chronic, demyelinating, sensorimotor peripheral polyneuropathy. Uniform and symmetrical slowing of motor conduction studies and the absence of conduction blocks are more consistent with an inherited, rather than an acquired, demyelinating polyneuropathy.

Based on the clinical manifestations, family history, and EDX findings, this case is consistent with an inherited demyelinating, sensorimotor peripheral polyneuropathy, as is seen with autosomal dominant hereditary motor sensory neuropathy (HMSN) type I (Charcot-Marie-Tooth disease type I).

DISCUSSION

Classification

Hereditary neuropathies are a heterogeneous group of peripheral nerve disorders (Figure C22–2). Some have a known metabolic basis and potential therapies (Table C22–1). The hereditary neuropathies that are not based on known specific metabolic defect are classified into three clinical groups: (1) hereditary motor and sensory neuropathies (HMSNs); (2) hereditary sensory and autonomic neuropathies (HSANs); and (3) hereditary motor neuropathies (HMNs).

The *hereditary motor and sensory neuropathies (HMSNs)* were classified by Dyck and Lambert into three predominant types (1) HMSN I, a demyelinating type; (2) HMSN II, a neuronal (axonal) type; and (3) HMSN III (Dejerine-Sottas disease), a severe demyelinating neuropathy of infancy and early childhood. HMSN I and II are

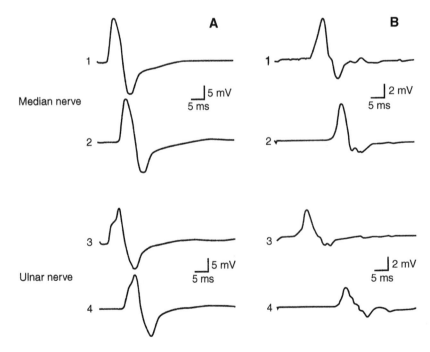

Figure C22–1. *Right median and ulnar motor conduction studies in an age-matched normal control (**A**) compared with patient (**B**). Note the significant slowing of distal and proximal latencies and the slight reduction of compound muscle action potential (CMAP) amplitudes in the patient. There is minimal temporal dispersion and no conduction block.*

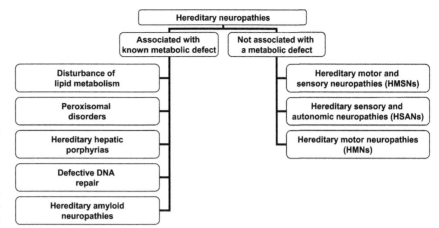

Figure C22–2. *Classification of hereditary neuropathies. (Adapted, with revisions, from Thomas PK. Classification and electrodiagnosis of hereditary neuropathies. In: Brown WF, Bolton CF, eds. Clinical electromyography, 2nd ed. Boston, MA: Butterworth-Heinemann, 1993, pp. 391–425.)*

Table C22–1. Classification of Hereditary Neuropathies Associated With Specific Metabolic Defects

Disturbance of Lipid Metabolism	Peroxisomal Disorders	Hereditary Hepatic Porphyrias	Defective DNA Repair	Familial Amyloid Neuropathies
Metachromatic leukodystrophy (sulfatide lipidosis, arylsulfatase deficiency)	Adrenoleukodystrophy	Acute intermittent porphyria	Ataxia telangiectasia	Transthyretin (TTR) amyloidosis (familial amyloid polyneuropathy I and II, Portuguese–Swedish–Japanese type and Indiana/Swiss or Maryland/German types)
Krabbe disease (Globoid cell leukodystrophy, galactosylceramide lipidosis)	Adrenomyeloneuropathy Hyperoxaluria type 1 (glycolic aciduria) Infantile Refsum disease	Variegate porphyria Hereditary coproporphyria	Xeroderma pigmentosa Cockayne syndrome	
Refsum disease (phytanic acid storage disease)		Delta aminolevulinic acid (ALA) dehydratase deficiency		Apoporotein A1 amylodosis (familial amyloid polyneuropathy III, Iowa type)
Tangier disease (high-density lipoprotein deficiency)				Gelsolin amyloidosis (familial amyloid polyneuropathy IV, Finnish/Danish type)
Bassen-Kornzweig disease (abetalipoproteinemia)				
Fabry disease (galactosidase A deficiency)				
Cerebrotendinous xanthomatosis (cholestanolosis)				
Niemann-Pick disease (acute neuropathic type, Crocker type A)				

characterized by skeletal deformities (pes cavus, hammer toes, scoliosis), insidious onset of distal lower more than upper extremities weakness, atrophy and sensory loss, and reduced or absent deep tendon reflexes. Based on clinical examination, these disorders are difficult to distinguish from each other because of similar phenotypes. With the recent influence of chromosomal linkage and gene identification, the term Charcot-Marie-Tooth disease (CMT) reemerged which created some confusion in the nomenclature and classifications of these disorders.

Charcot-Marie-Tooth disease (CMT) is subdivided into six major types with some but not perfect correlation to the HMSN classification (Table C22–2). CMT1 and CMT2 are interchangeable with HMSN I and HMSN II. The name

Dejerine-Sottas syndrome (DSS, Dejerine-Sottas disease) is preserved and is the same condition as HMSN III. The term CMT3 is not commonly used since the genes involved with DSS are the same as CMT1. CMT4 is a new designation for a group of autosomal recessive CMT and should not be confused with HMSN IV which is Refsum disease. CMTX is an X-linked disorder and hereditary neuropathy with liability to pressure palsy (HNPP) is a distinct disorder characterized by recurrent mononeuropathies.

The *hereditary sensory and autonomic neuropathies (HSANs)* are very rare and familial neuropathies with selective involvement of the primary sensory, with or without the autonomic, fibers. They should be distinguished from inherited disorders that affect large primary afferent

Table C22–2. Charcot-Marie-Tooth Disease (CMT, Hereditary Motor and Sensory Neuropathy, HMSN) Subtypes, Its Variants and Their Genetic Causes

Disorder	Locus/Gene	Protein
Charcot-Marie-Tooth Disease Type 1 (CMT1, HMSN I, Autosomal-Dominant, Demyelinating)		
CMT1A	17p11.2-12 /PMP22*	Peripheral myelin protein 22
CMT1B	1q22-23 / MPZ	Myelin protein zero
CMT1C	16p13.1-12.3 / LITAF	SIMPLE
CMT1D	10q21.1-22.1 / EGR2	Early growth response protein 2
Charcot-Marie-Tooth Disease Type 2 (CMT2, HMSN II, Autosomal-Dominant, Axonal)		
CMT2A	1p35-36/KFI1B	Kinesin-like protein Mitousin 2
CMT2B	3q13-22/RAB7	Ras-related protein
CMT2C	12q23-24/?	? (unknown)
CMT2D	7p15/GARS	Glycy-tRNA synthetase
CMT2E	8P21/NEFL	Neurofilament triplet L protein
CMT2F	7q11-21/HSP27	Small heat shock protein
CMT2	1q22/MPZ	Myelin protein zero
Dejerine-Sottas Syndrome (DSS, HMSN III, CMT3, Autosomal-Dominant or Recessive, Demyelinating)		
DSS A	17p/PMP22	Peripheral myelin protein 22
DSS B	1q/MPZ	Myelin protein zero
DSS C	10q/EGR2	Early growth response protein 2
DSS D	8q23	Unknown
Charcot-Marie-Tooth Disease Type 4 (CMT4, Autosomal-Recessive, Axonal or Demyelinating)		
CMT4A	8q13-21/GDAP1	Ganglioside-induced differentiation-associated protein-1
CMT4B1	11q22/MTMR2	Myotubularin-related protein-2
CMT4B2	11p15/MTMR13	Myotubularin-related protein-13
CMT4C	5q23-33/KIAA1985	–
CMT4D	8q24.3/NDRG1	N-myc downstream-regulated gene-1
CMT4E	10q21.1-22.1/EGR2	Early growth response protein 2
CMT4F	19q13.1-13.2/PRX	Periaxin gene
X-linked Charcot-Marie-Tooth Disease (CMTX, Axonal or Demyelinating)		
CMTX (X-linked)	Xq13-q21/CX32(GJB1)	Connexin 32 (gap junction protein-β-1)
Hereditary Neuropathy with Liability to Pressure Palsy (HNPP, Demyelinating)		
HNPP (autosomal dominant)	17p11.22/PMP22[†]	Peripheral myelin protein 22

*Duplication (98%) and point mutation (2%).
[†]Deletion (80%) and point mutation (20%).

Table C22–3. Hereditary Sensory and Autonomic Neuropathy (HSAN)

Disorder	Locus/Gene	Protein
HSAN I (hereditary sensory radicular neuropathy)	9q22.1-q22.3/SPTLC1	Serine-palitoyltransferase-1
HSAN II (congenital sensory neuropathy)	12p13-33	
HSAN III (familial dysautonomia, Riley-Day syndrome)	9q31-33/IKBKAP	Inhibitor of kappaB-kinase complex associated polypeptide
HSAN IV (congenital sensory neuropathy with anhidrosis)	1q21-22/TRKA	
HSAN V	1q21-22/NTRK1	

neurons (spinocerebellar degeneration). They are currently subdivided into five types, based on mode of inheritance, natural history, electrophysiologic characteristics and histopatologic findings (Table C22–3).

The *hereditary motor neuropathies (HMNs)* are loosely subdivided into proximal and distal (Table C22–4). The proximal HMNs are better known as spinal muscular atrophies (SMAs). These are among the most common autosomal recessive disorders in childhood affecting 1/10 000 live births with carrier frequency of 1/50. Spinal muscular atrophy is caused by a deficiency of the ubiquitous survival motor neuron (SMN) protein, which is encoded by the SMN genes, SMN1 and SMN2, on chromosome 5q. The distal HMNs are a genetically and clinically heterogeneous group of disorders that are also known as spinal CMT because of their overlap with CMT. They are characterized by distal weakness with or without foot deformities, but without sensory or autonomic involvement. Sensory nerve action potentials are normal while the motor NCSs reveal low-amplitude CMAPs with normal or borderline velocities, consistent with motor axonopathy. The inheritance of HMNs is either dominant or recessive. Only few have been mapped to a chromosome or have a defined gene mutation.

Table C22–4. Hereditary Motor Neuropathy (HMN)

Proximal HMN (Spinal Muscular Atrophy, SMA, Autosomal-Recessive, Mutations of the Survival Motor Neuron 1 (SMN 1) Gene on Chromosome 5q13)

SMA I	Werdnig-Hoffmann disease. Onset before the age of 6 months, inability to sit or walk, and fatal before the age of 2 years
SMA II	Intermediate, arrested Werdnig-Hoffmann disease. Onset between 6 and 18 months of age, able to sit but not walk and survive beyond the age of 4 years
SMA III	Kugelberg-Welander disease
SMA IIIa	Onset between the age of 2 to 3 years, survive into adulthood and able to walk independently usually until age 20–40 years
SMA IIIb	Onset after the age of 3 years and able to walk independently till age 30–50 years
SMA IV	Adult SMA. Variable age of onset, but rarely before the age of 20 years and usually after the age of 30 years

Bulbospinal (Kennedy Disease, X-Linked CAG Repeat Expansion of the Androgen Receptor Gene on Chromosome Xq13.1)
Distal HMN (Spinal Form of Charcot-Marie-Tooth Disease)

HMN I	Juvenile onset, autosomal dominant
HMN II	Adult onset, autosomal dominant (12q24)
HMN III	Mild juvenile, autosomal recessive (11q13)
HMN IV	Severe juvenile, autosomal recessive
HMN V	Upper limb predominance, autosomal dominant (7p)
HMN VI	Severe infantile with respiratory distress, autosomal recessive
HMN VII	Vocal cord paralysis, autosomal dominant (9p21.1-p12)

Scapuloperoneal

Type I	Autosomal dominant
Type II	Autosomal recessive

Bulbar

Type I	Autosomal recessive (Vialetto-Van Laere syndrome)
Type II	Autosomal recessive (Fazio-Londe disease)

Clinical Features and Genetics

Electrodiagnostic studies have proven to be the most important distinguishing test. CMT1, is also known as HMSN I or the demyelinating form of CMT, is a predominantly demyelinating polyneuropathy that is characterized by prominent uniform slowing of motor conduction velocities, with relative preservation of CMAP amplitudes. CMT2, also known as HMSN II or the neuronal form of CMT, is a predominantly axonal polyneuropathy that can be distinguished by normal or near-normal motor distal latencies and conduction velocities and decreased CMAP amplitudes. CMTX is an X-linked disorder characterized by intermediate slowing of conduction velocities, placing this disorder in the midst between CMT1 and CMT2.

Charcot-Marie-Tooth Disease 1 (CMT1, HMSN I)

Hereditary motor and sensory neuropathy I (HMSN I, CMT1) is the prototype of all inherited neuropathies. It is an autosomal-dominant disorder with complete penetrance and with a marked interfamily and intrafamily clinical phenotypic variability. The age of symptom onset varies from birth through the forties. Many adult patients can trace, in retrospect, their symptoms before the age of 20. These childhood or adolescence manifestations may include incoordination, frequent ankle or foot trauma, or poor athletic ability. The disorder is a slowly progressive, distal, symmetrical, motor more than sensory, peripheral polyneuropathy. The most common presenting symptoms are related to muscle weakness, muscle atrophy, or foot deformity (pes cavus, hammer toes, pes equinovarus, or pes planus). Many patients undergo surgical correction of foot deformity before correct diagnosis. Sometimes, the diagnosis is made during EDX studies for other, unrelated symptoms, or it may occur as part of an evaluation of family members. There is poor correlation in CMT1 between the clinical findings and conduction velocities.

Common findings on examination include distal muscle weakness, atrophy, distal areflexia, pes cavus, and hammer toes (Figure C22–3). The atrophy is predominant in the foot but may extend into the distal legs, resulting in an "inverted champagne bottle" appearance to the leg, and into the hands, resulting in "claw hands." Although most patients do not complain of positive sensory symptoms, there is distal loss of all sensory modalities. Pain, other than that related to foot deformity and callus formation, is rare. Scoliosis is present in a minority of patients. Enlarged and palpable peripheral nerves may be identified in some patients with HMSN I. Late in the disease, steppage gait and claw hands are common. Although the disorder is frequently disabling, the life expectancy of patients with the disease is normal.

Molecular and genetic studies have further subdivided CMT1 into four subtypes, with no definitive phenotypic characteristics that could accurately distinguish among them. These are named 1A, 1B, 1C, and 1D (see Table C22–2). *CMT1A is the most common inherited neuropathy*. Most patients have a tandem duplication of a 1.5 Mb region, which contains the peripheral myelin protein-22 (PMP22) gene, on chromosome 17p11.2p12. Duplication of PMP22 gene leads to overexpression (increased dosage) of the

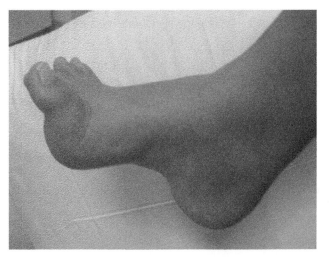

A

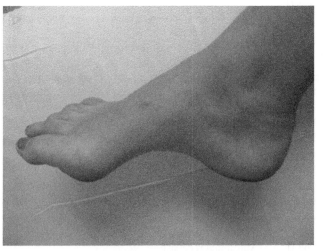

B

Figure C22–3. *Classic foot deformity (pes cavus and hammer toes) of a 25-year-old woman with CMT1A (**A**). Her 35-year-old sister, who was asymptomatic, had milder foot deformities and marked slowing of conduction velocities (**B**).*

peripheral myelin protein. Occasional patients have point mutations of the PMP22 gene complex. CMT1B is associated with mutations of the myelin protein zero (MPZ) gene located on chromosome 1q22-23. The exact function of PMP22 and MPZ is not well understood, but both proteins are integral parts that likely play a major role in myelin compaction. CMT1C and CMT1D have been mapped to chromosome 16p and 10q with gene loci, named LITAF and EGR2, respectively.

Charcot-Marie-Tooth Disease 2 (CMT2, HMSN II)

Hereditary motor and sensory neuropathy II (HMSN II, CMT2) is a heterogeneous group of inherited neuropathies that are due to primary axonal degeneration. They are not distinguishable from CMT1 except by having preserved conduction velocities (>38 m/s) and absence of onion bulb formation on nerve biopsy. In contrast to CMT1, CMT2 phenotypes do not have palpable or enlarged nerves, but tend to have a later age of onset, diffuse areflexia and less involvement of hand muscles. CMT2 is divided into several subtypes based on gene locus and product (see Table C22–2).

Dejerine-Sottas Syndrome (DSS, HMSN III)

Hereditary motor and sensory neuropathy III (HMSN III, CMT3, Dejerine-Sottas syndrome or hypertrophic neuropathy of infancy or congenital hypomyelinating neuropathy) is a rare and severe autosomal-recessive demyelinative neuropathy that presents at birth or during early infancy with hypotonia, weakness, and delayed motor milestones. It is characterized by severe demyelination and profound slowing of motor conduction velocities, with hypertrophic nerves and prominent onion bulb formations.

Charcot-Marie-Tooth Disease 4 (CMT4)

Autosomal-recessive forms of hereditary neuropathies are rare, usually present in small ethnic groups, and named collectively CMT4 (see Table C22–2). These disorders may present in infancy and childhood with delayed motor milestones, severe neuropathies, and areflexia. Some patients become wheelchair bound by adulthood.

Charcot-Marie-Tooth Disease X (CMTX)

CMTX is the second most common type of CMT, after CMT1A. It is an X-linked disorder with no male-to-male inheritance. Males have more severe phenotypes while female carriers are usually asymptomatic or minimally affected. Characteristics of CMTX include an earlier age of onset, faster rate of progression, and modest slowing of conduction velocities.

Mutations in the gap junction protein-β-1 gene, also previously known as connexin 32 (CX32), on chromosome Xq13-q21 is the cause of most cases of CMTX. Unlike PMP22 and MPZ, which are present in compact myelin, CX32 is located at uncompacted folds of Schwann cell cytoplasm around the nodes of Ranvier and at Schmidt-Lanterman incisures. This suggests a role for CX32 in providing a pathway for the transfer of ions and nutrients around and across the myelin sheath.

Hereditary Neuropathy With Liability to Pressure Palsy (HNPP)

Hereditary neuropathy with liability to pressure palsy (HNPP), also known as *tomaculous neuropathy*, is an autosomal-dominant disorder that often presents with recurrent, painless, focal mononeuropathies, often at common compression or entrapment sites. These lesions develop after minor compression or trauma or with no identifiable precipitating factor, and recover spontaneously over days to weeks. The onset of the first episode is usually during adolescence, though the diagnosis is often delayed till adulthood. Recurrent peroneal palsy at the fibular neck, ulnar neuropathy across the elbow and painless brachial plexopathy are common presentations. In severe cases, there is an underlying slowly progressive demyelinating polyneuropathy, with pes cavus, hammer toes, and distal weakness, areflexia and sensory loss that is difficult to distinguish from CMT1.

The majority of patients with HNPP have a 1.5 Mb deletion of the PMP22 gene on chromosome 17p11. The same gene that, when duplicated, results in CMT1A. The deletion in HNPP results in underexpression of the gene. In the remainder of HNPP patients, a point mutation is present that results in frame-shift or insertion of stop codon.

Electrodiagnosis

Electrodiagnostic (EDX) examination provides important information for the clinician suspecting a diffuse peripheral polyneuropathy or hereditary neuropathy.

1. Motor and sensory nerve conduction studies (NCSs) are very helpful in determining the fibers affected, i.e., motor, sensory, or both. In all HMSN (CMT) subtypes, the sensory nerve action potentials (SNAPs) are diminished in amplitudes or absent, while the compound muscle action potentials (CMAPs) and motor conduction velocities are more variably reduced depend on the different HMSN subtype. This distinguishes them from the distal types of HMNs, which share with CMT many of their clinical features (foot deformity and distal weakness/atrophy), but lack clinical and EDX involvement of sensory fibers. In the distal HMNs, the CMAPs are reduced while the SNAPs are normal. In HSANs, the SNAPs are either reduced/absent or normal

dependent on involvement or sparing of large sensory fibers, while the CMAPs and motor conduction velocities are usually normal.

2. Motor and sensory NCSs are key in determining the principal pathologic process (demyelination versus axonal degeneration). This differentiation is an important step in the final diagnosis of hereditary neuropathies since it helps in guiding the decision of which genetic test to order.

In dying-back axonal peripheral polyneuropathy, the amplitudes of the CMAPs are diminished with stimulation at any site along the nerve without conduction blocks or significant temporal dispersion; however, the conduction velocities are normal or only slightly reduced (values usually are more than 80% of the lower limits of normal). By contrast, slowing of conduction velocities is pronounced in demyelinating polyneuropathy; values usually are less than 60% of the lower limits of normal, and there is relative preservation of CMAP amplitudes. When evoked, the sensory distal latencies and conduction velocities parallel the motor latencies and velocities. Conduction velocity values of the sural sensory nerve are less than 60% of the lower limits of normal in HMSN I, and are either normal or greater than 80% of the lower limits of normal in HMSN II.

3. The EDX features may also help in distinguishing chronic familial from chronic acquired demyelinating neuropathy (Table C22–5). This is particularly useful when the neuropathy is protracted and the familial history is indeterminate.

- In familial neuropathy, such as HMSN type I, the slowing is uniform, affecting all segments of the nerve equally and symmetrically. However, in acquired neuropathy, such as chronic inflammatory demyelinating polyneuropathy (CIDP), the slowing of distal latencies and conduction velocities is multifocal and asymmetrical due to random demyelination.

- The slowing in hereditary neuropathy is symmetrical, with minimal variability between adjacent nerves in the same limb or in contralateral limbs. For example, slowing of conduction velocities of the ulnar and median nerves is comparable in both upper extremities in

patients with HMSN type I. This contrasts with acquired demyelinating neuropathy in which deviation of conduction velocities between adjacent nerves or contralateral nerves of 5 to 10 m/s is common.

- In the acquired forms of demyelinating polyneuropathy such in CIDP, findings compatible with conduction block and significant temporal dispersion (e.g., prolongation of CMAP duration with proximal stimulation of 50–100% compared with the CMAP duration with distal stimulation) are common. However, in hereditary neuropathy, there is no associated conduction block, and temporal dispersion is minimal (10–20%).

In summary, hereditary demyelinating neuropathy are characterized by diffuse, uniform, and symmetrical slowing, without conduction block or temporal dispersion. Common causes of hereditary demyelinating peripheral neuropathy with uniform slowing are shown in Table C22–6.

4. The distinction between the major subtypes of HMSN (CMT) may be guided on the basis of motor conduction velocities, since the clinical features of these disorders are similar enough that it often is difficult to distinguish between them without the aid of electrodiagnosis. This distinction helps tailoring the ever increasing number of genetic testing needed. In many cases of HMSN, the lower extremities are involved severely leading to absent or very low amplitude CMAPs and difficult to interpret conduction velocity values. In most cases, the upper extremity nerves are less severely affected, and their velocities, particularly the median and ulnar motor conduction velocities in the forearms, have proven to be very useful in guiding the clinician to the accurate genetic diagnosis of patients with CMT (Figure C22–4).

- Motor conduction velocities are reduced markedly in CMT1. Very slow conduction velocities that are less than 70% of the lower limits of normal. Commonly reported values for the peroneal and tibial nerves are

Table C22–5. Electrophysiologic Characteristics of Demyelinating Polyneuropathy

Inherited (e.g., CMT1)	Acquired (e.g., CIDP)
Diffuse slowing	Multifocal slowing
Symmetrical slowing	Asymmetrical slowing
No conduction block	Frequent conduction blocks
Slight temporal dispersion	Prominent temporal dispersion

CIDP = chronic inflammatory demyelinating polyneuropathy; CMT1 = Charcot-Marie-Tooth disease 1.

Table C22–6. Hereditary Demyelinating Peripheral Neuropathy Associated With Prominent and Uniform Slowing of Conduction Velocities

Hereditary motor and sensory neuropathy I (CMT1)

Hereditary motor and sensory neuropathy III (CMT3)

Hereditary neuropathy with liability to pressure palsy (HNPP)*

Refsum disease (phytanic acid storage disease)

Metachromatic leukodystrophy (sulfatide lipidosis, arylsulfatase deficiency)

Adrenoleukodystrophy and adrenomyeloneuropathy

Globoid cell leukodystrophy (Krabbe disease, galactosylceramide lipidosis)

Cockayne syndrome

*Often associated with multifocal slowing and/or conduction block at common entrapment sites.

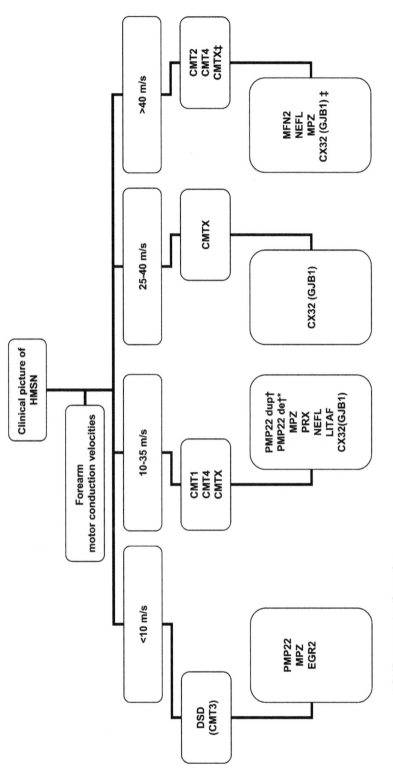

Figure C22-4. *A practical work-up for patients with hereditary motor and sensory neuropathies (HMSN) using forearm motor conduction velocities as a guide to ordering the appropriate commercially available genetic test.*

less than 25 m/s while the median and ulnar nerves are less than 35 m/s.

- Motor conduction velocities are reduced much less severely with the neuronal form (CMT2). In this condition, the velocities are either normal or slightly diminished, more so in the lower limbs. The slowing reflects the loss of large, fast-conducting axons. However, conduction slowing does not reach the values seen in CMT1. When slowing occurs in CMT2, CMAP amplitudes are reduced markedly, with velocities usually exceeding 80% of the lower limits of normal (>40 m/s in the forearms).

- In CMTX, the slowing is only moderate with values belonging to an intermediate group. Affected males have velocities that range between 25 and 38 m/s while female carriers have less slowing of velocities (>38 m/s) reaching values that resemble CMT2.

- In DSS, there is a very severe slowing of motor conduction velocities, reaching values of less than 5–10 m/s (10–20% of lower limits of normal), believed that no other peripheral nerve disorder results in such a slowing. The extreme slowing of motor conduction velocities, along with the clinical severity of the disorder and the autosomal recessive inheritance pattern, helps to distinguish this disorder from CMT1 (HMSN I).

In general, needle EMG in patients with CMT shows no specific abnormalities; results are similar in both types of the disease. Because of the slow tempo of the disease, needle EMG often reveals signs of chronic partial denervation with reinnervation. Long-duration, high-amplitude MUAPs are present bilaterally, and there is reduced recruitment of MUAPs, particularly in the distal muscles of the lower and upper limbs. Fibrillation and, less commonly, fasciculation potentials are relatively inconspicuous and are identified mainly in distal muscles. Although fibrillation potentials are more common in CMT2 (neuronal form) than CMT1 (demyelinating form), this finding does not allow differentiation of these two disorders.

FOLLOW-UP

Examination of both offspring revealed similar findings, although the patient's son had more severe manifestations, with bilateral footdrop and claw hands. DNA testing later confirmed PMP22 gene duplication on chromosome 17p11.2-12, consistent with CMT1A.

DIAGNOSIS

Charcot-Marie-Tooth disease 1A.

ANSWERS

1. D; 2. A; 3. E.

SUGGESTED READINGS

Buchthal F, Behse F. Peroneal muscular atrophy and related disorders: I. Clinical manifestations as related to biopsy findings, nerve conduction and electromyography. Brain 1977; 100:41–66.

Garcia CA et al. Clinical variability in two pairs of identical twins with the Charcot-Marie-Tooth disease type 1A duplication. Neurology 1995;45:2090–2093.

Harding AE. Inherited neuronal atrophy and degeneration predominantly of lower motor neurons. In: Dyck PJ et al., eds. Peripheral neuropathy. Philadelphia, PA: WB Saunders, 1993.

Harding AE, Thomas PK. The clinical features of hereditary motor and sensory neuropathy, types I and II. Brain 1980;103:259–280.

Lewis RA, Sumner AJ. The electrodiagnostic distinctions between chronic familial and acquired demyelinative neuropathies. Neurology 1982;32:592–596.

Scherer SS. Findings the causes of inherited neuropathies. Arch Neurol 2006;63:812–816.

Shy ME, Lupski JR, Chance PF et al. Hereditary motor and sensory neuropathies: an overview of clinical, genetic, electrophysiologic, and pathologic features. In: Dyck PJ, Thomas PK, eds. Peripheral neuropathy, 4th ed. Philadelphia, PA: WB Saunders, 2005, pp. 1623–1658.

Case 23

HISTORY AND PHYSICAL EXAMINATION

Fever, malaise, and sore throat developed in a 55-year-old woman who was otherwise in excellent health. She was treated with antibiotics and analgesics. Six days later, she first noticed that her legs had "buckled" underneath her. That afternoon, she had difficulty climbing steps and became aware of tingling in both hands. She awoke the next morning and could not stand. She was brought to the hospital and was admitted. Apart from a diuretic for mild hypertension, she was taking no other medications.

On physical examination, the patient was afebrile and in no apparent distress. She had normal vital signs, including blood pressure, pulse, and respiration. Neurologic examination revealed normal mental status and cranial nerves. Motor examination was relevant for weakness of the neck flexors (Medical Research Council [MRC] 4+/5), the proximal pelvic muscles (MRC 3/5), and the shoulder muscles (MRC 4–/5). Distally, she performed much better (5–/5). Deep tendon reflexes were absent throughout. Sensory examination was normal, except for mild impairment of touch and pin sensation in both hands. She was unable to sit or stand independently.

An electrodiagnostic (EDX) examination was performed 3 days after admission and 6 days after the onset of neurologic symptoms. This was repeated later, on the 12th day after admission, which corresponded to day 15 from the onset of neurologic symptoms. Needle electromyography was not performed due to the acute nature of the symptoms.

Please now review the Nerve Conduction Studies tables.

QUESTIONS

1. The following features make the diagnosis of Guillain-Barré syndrome (GBS) doubtful *except:*
   A. Asymmetrical weakness.
   B. Well-demarcated sensory level.
   C. Severe and persistent bowel and bladder dysfunction.
   D. Less than 10 mononuclear cells/mm^3 in the cerebrospinal fluid (CSF).
2. Common EDX patterns in GBS include:
   A. Normal nerve conduction studies.
   B. Low compound muscle action potential (CMAP) amplitudes.
   C. Conduction blocks and slowing of distal latencies.
   D. All of the above.
3. The best EDX predictor of poor neurological outcome in GBS is:
   A. The presence of fibrillation potentials.
   B. Low mean CMAP amplitude.
   C. Slowing of conduction velocities.
   D. Decreased recruitment of voluntary motor unit action potentials (MUAPs).

EDX FINDINGS AND INTERPRETATION OF DATA

The first set of nerve conduction studies (NCS), performed on day 6 from the onset of neurologic symptoms, revealed the following:

1. Low amplitude median and borderline radial sensory nerve action potentials (SNAPs), with normal sural SNAP.
2. Low-amplitude distal median, ulnar, and peroneal CMAPs with no definite evidence of proximal conduction blocks. The mean distal CMAP amplitude (all distal CMAP amplitudes obtained, divided by the number of nerves studied) is 2.29 mV, and the mean lower limit of normal (all lower limit values of CMAP amplitudes, divided by the number of nerves studied) is 5.41 mV. Thus, the mean CMAP amplitude is 42% of the lower limit of normal values (2.29/5.41 × 100).

Case 23: Nerve Conduction Studies (First Study, Day 6)

Nerve Stimulated	Stimulation Site	Recording Site	Amplitude (m = mV, s = µV)			Distal/Peak Latency (ms)			Conduction Velocity (m/s)			F Latency (ms)	
			Right	Left	Normal	Right	Left	Normal	Right	Left	Normal	Right	Left
Sural (s)	Calf	Ankle		8	≥4.0		3.1	≤4.6		45	≥40		
Peroneal (m)	Ankle	EDB	**0.25**	**0.25**	≥2.5		5.0	≤6.0			≥40		
Peroneal (m)	Knee	EDB	**0.25**	**0.25**						46			**58.4**
Tibial (m)	Ankle	AH		5.0	≥4.0		4.6	≤6.0		46	≥40	**NR**	**NR**
Tibial (m)	Knee	AH		3.0									
H reflex	Knee	Soleus		**NR**			**NR**						
M response	Knee	Soleus		0.5			6.0						
Median (s)	Wrist	Middle finger		8	≥15		3.5	≤3.6			≥50		
Median (s)	Elbow	Middle finger		3						47			
Ulnar (s)	Wrist	Little finger		18	≥10		3.1	≤3.1					
Radial (s)	Distal forearm	Thumb base		12	≥14		2.2	≤2.7					
Median (m)	Wrist	APB	**3.0**	**2.5**	≥6	**4.0**	**4.2**	≤4.0	**44**	**41**	≥50	**NR**	**NR**
Median (m)	Elbow	APB	**2.0**	**1.8**									
Ulnar (m)	Wrist	ADM	**1.2**	**1.8**	≥7	3.0	**3.4**	≤3.1	**43**	**48**	≥50	**NR**	**NR**
Ulnar (m)	Below elbow	ADM	**1.0**	**1.0**					**39**	**44**	≥50		
Ulnar (m)	Above elbow	ADM	**0.5**	**0.5**									

ADM = abductor digiti minimi; AH = abductor hallucis; APB = abductor pollicis brevis; EDB = extensor digitorum brevis; m = motor; s = sensory. Data in bold type are abnormal.

Case 23: Nerve Conduction Studies (Second Study, Day 15)

Nerve Stimulated	Stimulation Site	Recording Site	Amplitude (m = mV, s = μV)			Distal/Peak Latency (ms)			Conduction Velocity (m/s)			F Latency (ms)	
			Right	Left	Normal	Right	Left	Normal	Right	Left	Normal	Right	Left
Sural (s)	Calf	Ankle		6	≥4.0		2.9	≤4.6		45	≥40		
Peroneal (m)	Ankle	EDB		**0.2**	≥2.5		3.9	≤6.0					
Peroneal (m)	Knee	EDB		**0.2**						48	≥40		**59.6**
Tibial (m)	Ankle	AH		4.8	≥4.0		5.7	≤6.0		46	≥40		**NR**
Tibial (m)	Knee	AH		3.5									
H reflex	Knee	Soleus		**NR**			**NR**						
M response	Knee	Soleus		0.5			6.4						
Median (s)	Wrist	Middle finger		6	≥15		**5.0**	≤3.6		**NR**	≥50		
Median (s)	Elbow	Middle finger		**NR**									
Ulnar (s)	Wrist	Little finger		**NR**	≥10		**NR**	≤3.1					
Radial (s)	Distal forearm	Thumb base		4	≥14		3.6	≤2.7					
Median (m)	Wrist	APB	**2.5**	**1.8**	≥6	6.5	6.1	≤4.0					
Median (m)	Elbow	APB	**2.0**	**1.7**					**40**	43	≥50	**NR**	**NR**
Ulnar (m)	Wrist	ADM	**1.0**	**0.8**	≥7	4.9	4.5	≤3.1					
Ulnar (m)	Below elbow	ADM	**1.0**	**0.8**					**40**	**46**	≥50	**NR**	**NR**
Ulnar (m)	Above elbow	ADM	**0.8**	**0.8**					**38**	**43**	≥50		

ADM = abductor digiti minimi; AH = abductor hallucis; APB = abductor pollicis brevis; EDB = extensor digitorum brevis; m = motor; NR = no response; s = sensory. Data in bold type are abnormal.

3. Minimal slowing of distal latencies (in the hands) and moderate slowing of conduction velocities. These values are moderate and do not reach the levels of velocity slowing that is pathognomic of demyelination in the presence of low CMAPs (<70% of the lower limit of normal; see discussion). The lowest conduction velocity obtained is 39 m/s which equals 78% of the lower limit of normal.

4. Absent F waves throughout, except for the peroneal F wave, which is prolonged.

The above findings point to pathology at the spinal roots and the peripheral sensory and motor nerves, manifesting as either axonal loss or distal conduction block (as a cause of low distal CMAPs). Only one criterion of demyelination (absent F waves) is fulfilled. The absent F waves and the sural sparing pattern (i.e., abnormal upper extremity SNAPs with normal sural SNAP) are findings that are highly suggestive of GBS (see discussion).

The second study, done 9 days later (15 days from the onset of neurologic symptoms), revealed that now all hand SNAPs (median, ulnar, and radial) are abnormally low in amplitude or absent. In contrast, the sural SNAP continues to be normal. The slowing of distal latencies now is more pronounced, which fulfills one of the criteria for acquired demyelination. The F waves are still absent, fulfilling a second criterion. However, the velocities are still moderately slowed and there is no confirmed conduction block. Thus, in the second study, two criteria of acquired demyelination are fulfilled (three are required; see discussion), and the sural sparing pattern (i.e., abnormal upper extremity SNAPs with normal sural SNAP) is confirmed. These findings are strong evidence for the diagnosis of GBS.

The prognosis here is fair because of low distal CMAPs, although at no time did the mean CMAP amplitude decrease below 20% of the lower limit of normal. The first study is less helpful because the patient had not reached plateau yet and because time for the completion of wallerian degeneration has not been allowed. The second study, done a week after the patient reached plateau, reveals a mean CMAP of 39% of the lower limit of normal.

In summary, the profile of these NCSs is consistent with an acquired demyelinating polyneuropathy as seen with acute inflammatory demyelinating polyneuropathy (AIDP), the most common type of GBS. The prognosis for recovery is fair due to modest decrease in mean CMAP amplitude. A repeat EMG 3 to 5 weeks after the onset of symptoms was recommended to confirm this prognostic prediction.

DISCUSSION

Rapidly Progressive Quadriparesis: Differential Diagnosis

Quadriparesis progressing over days to weeks is a relatively common neurological presentation. Usually, the history is one of an ascending paresis beginning in the lower limbs and progressing cephalad to trunk and upper limb muscles, and often weakening the respiratory, bulbar, and ocular muscles. Descending weakness, progressing in the opposite direction, may occur but is less common. Causes of nontraumatic rapidly progressive quadriparesis are best discussed using the neuraxis as an anatomical guideline. Since many of the disorders manifesting this presentation are due to lower motor neuron dysfunction, it is useful to use the different elements of the motor unit as a tool in setting a complete differential diagnosis (Table C23–1).

Table C23–1. Causes of Rapidly Progressive Quadriparesis

Muscle Disorders
Polymyositis
Dermatomyositis
Rhabdomyolysis (drugs, toxins, exercise, trauma, metabolic myopathies, etc.)
Critical illness myopathy
Muscle Membrane Disorders
Familial periodic paralysis
Secondary hypokalemic paralysis (thyrotoxicosis, malabsorption, barium salt poisoning, or abuse of diuretics, laxatives or licorice)
Neuromuscular Junction Disorders
Myasthenia gravis (myasthenic crisis)
Botulism
Drug-induced neuromuscular blockade
Toxic
   Organophosphate
   Nerve gas
   Tick
   Black widow spider
   Snake venoms
Metabolic
   Hypermagnesemia (toxemia of pregnancy treated with parenteral magnesium, magnesium-containing antacids, or cathartics)
   Hypophosphatemia (parenteral hyperalimentation, phosphate-bindings antacids, acute alcohol intoxication, and severe respiratory alkalosis)
Peripheral Nerve and/Root Disorders
Guillain-Barré syndrome
Acute intermittent porphyria
Diphtheritic polyneuropathy

Table C23–1. —cont'd

Critical illness polyneuropathy

Vasculitic neuropathy

Heavy metal acute poisoning (thallium, arsenic)

Diffuse polyradiculopathy (infectious, neoplastic)

Anterior Horn Cell Disorders

Acute poliomyelitis (wild polio viruses, west Nile virus, enteroviruses)

Spinal Cord Disorders

Transverse myelitis

Cord compression (disc herniation, fracture/dislocation, epidural malignancy)

Cord infarction (anterior spinal artery syndrome)

Brainstem Disorders

Central pontine myelinolysis

Pontine infarct (basilar artery thrombosis)

Adapted from Katirji B, Kaminski HJ, Preston DC et al., eds. Neuromuscular disorders in clinical practice. Boston, MA: Butterworth-Heinemann, 2002.

Certain clinical features and diagnostic studies are useful in establishing the correct diagnosis:

- *Distribution and temporal progression of weakness.* The neurological examination is most useful during the early phases of these disorders, since most ultimately result in a fairly uniform appearance in the later stages of illness, including severe quadriparesis, hyporeflexia, or areflexia, with or without respiratory failure and bulbar or ocular weakness. A detailed history or observation of the progression and distribution of the weakness is extremely useful in making a correct diagnosis. For example, the first symptom of botulism is often asymmetrical ptosis or double vision, followed rapidly by dysphagia, dysarthria, and, finally, respiratory distress and limb weakness. In contrast, in a typical GBS patient, the symptoms often begin with symmetrical weakness of the legs, imbalance and numbness, followed by trunk and upper limb weakness, which may progress into respiratory failure and, sometimes, facial diplegia or diplopia.

- *Deep tendon reflexes.* The deep tendon reflexes (DTRs) are among the most important signs in patients with rapidly progressive quadriparesis. In general, disorders of peripheral nerve are often associated with early hyporeflexia, while the DTRs are usually spared in neuromuscular junction disorders and myopathies. However, the DTRs are often absent irrespective of the site of pathology within the motor unit when the weakness becomes very severe. For example, the DTRs in botulism are normal until significant limb weakness develops, while they are often depressed or absent in mildly weak limb(s) early in the course of GBS.

- *Symmetry of weakness.* Asymmetrical weakness is also an important finding early in the course of illness since many patients go on to generalized symmetrical paralysis. In general, subacute polyneuropathies and myopathies are symmetrical from the outset, while subacute neuromuscular junction disorders, polyradiculopathies, and anterior horn cell diseases are often asymmetrical early in their course. For example, the weakness is often symmetrical from the outset in GBS, polymyositis and periodic paralysis, while ocular, bulbar, and limb muscle weakness is often asymmetrical in botulism, myasthenia gravis, carcinomatous polyradiculopathy, and acute paralytic poliomyelitis. However, there are many exceptions. For example, the weakness in vasculitic neuropathy is often asymmetrical and may be restricted to peripheral nerve distributions (mononeuropathy multiplex), while tick paralysis typically causes a rapid symmetrical quadriparesis.

- *Extraocular muscle weakness.* Extraocular muscle abnormalities are common in neuromuscular junction disorders, particularly botulism and myasthenia gravis. They are rarely found in polyneuropathies and do not occur in subacute myopathies or anterior horn cell disorders. In contrast to ocular findings, bulbar manifestations, particularly dysphagia, are common to most neuromuscular disorders.

- *Sensory manifestations.* The presence of sensory symptoms excludes all subacute myopathies, and neuromuscular junction and anterior horn cell disorders, unless accompanied by a peripheral neuropathy, such as in paraneoplastic disorders. Sensory symptoms and signs are very common in polyneuropathies and polyradiculopathies.

- *Autonomic findings.* Autonomic findings are features common to polyneuropathies, polyradiculopathies, and botulism. These include orthostatic hypotension, tachy- and bradyarrhythmias, ileus, urinary retention or incontinence, and pupillary abnormalities.

- *Serum electrolytes.* Serum electrolytes are easy to measure and may suggest a specific diagnosis. Serum potassium, magnesium, and phosphorus should be obtained promptly in all patients with rapidly progressive quadriparesis (see Table C23–1). The EKG is usually abnormal with hypokalemia (prolonged QT interval, flat T wave and prominent U wave), and hyperkalemia (peaked T waves).

- *Serum creatine kinase.* Elevated serum creatine kinase (CK) often suggests a primary muscle disorder. When acute rhabdomyolysis leads to severe weakness, the CK is markedly elevated, reaching up to 1000- to 2000-fold of the normal level. In polymyositis and dermatomyositis presenting with rapid quadriparesis, the CK is often elevated, reaching usually up to 100- to 200-fold the normal value. CK is variably elevated in critical illness myopathy, and may be slightly elevated in GBS and acute paralytic poliomyelitis.

- *Cerebrospinal fluid.* Abnormalities seen in the cerebrospinal fluid (CSF) are generally supportive of a diagnosis, but not pathognomonic. In general, all myopathies and neuromuscular junction disorders are associated with normal CSF, while the CSF is often abnormal in most subacute peripheral polyneuropathies, polyradiculopathies, and anterior horn cell disorders. Elevated CSF protein is among the most common abnormality seen, followed by pleocytosis. The latter is usually dominated by lymphocytes except in infectious disorders where there is often early polymorphonuclear pleocytosis. CSF glucose is sometimes lowered in infectious, carcinomatous or lymphomatous polyradiculopathies (leptomeningeal disease).
- *Electrodiagnostic tests.* Nerve conduction studies, repetitive nerve stimulation, and needle EMG are invaluable aids in the diagnosis of patients presenting with acute or subacute quadriparesis. In general, NCSs and repetitive nerve stimulation are more useful than needle EMG in the acute phase of these disorders. Although normal NCSs suggest disorders of muscle, neuromuscular junction, spinal roots, or anterior horn cell, many patients with subacute polyneuropathies might have normal NCSs during the first week or two of illness. CMAP amplitudes may be low in botulism, drug-induced neuromuscular blockade, severe myasthenia gravis, or severe necrotizing myopathies. Sensory nerve action potentials (SNAPs) are usually abnormal in patients with subacute neuropathies, but this may be delayed also.

Clinical Features

Guillain-Barré syndrome (GBS), also known as Landry-Guillain-Barré-Strohl syndrome, is the most common cause of subacute flaccid paralysis in the world. It is a generalized disorder of the peripheral nervous system that is characterized by multiple limb and cranial muscle weakness with areflexia. It has an incidence of slightly less than 2 per 100 000 population. Guillain-Barré syndrome is frequently preceded by a viral or bacterial illness, usually an upper respiratory infection or gastroenteritis.

Typically, GBS develops over the course of a few days. Limb weakness appears simultaneously with a slight tingling and impairment of sensation in the hands and feet. The sensory symptoms are rarely painful while myalgia and back pain are common. Weakness usually ascends from the lower limbs to the upper limbs and, sometimes, to the cranial nerves. Less commonly, the weakness in GBS is descending. Facial weakness occurs in approximately one half of patients, and respiratory failure requiring

mechanical ventilation occurs in one-third. Typically, progression lasts up to 4 weeks, while progression exceeding 4 weeks suggests an alternative diagnosis, such as chronic inflammatory demyelinating polyneuropathy (CIDP). Cerebrospinal fluid protein usually rises during the second week of illness, without pleocytosis *(albuminocytologic dissociation)*. The presence of CSF pleocytosis is not incompatible with GBS, but if it is significant (>50 cells), other diagnoses, particularly infection with the human immunodeficiency virus (HIV), should be suspected. The frequency of various GBS manifestations is shown in Table C23–2.

Because of its similarity to its animal analogue, experimental allergic neuritis, GBS was considered to be a single disorder characterized by an acute immune attack on

Table C23–2. Frequency of Features and Clinical Variants of Acute Guillain-Barré Syndrome

	Frequency (%)	
Condition	**Initially**	**In Fully Developed Illness**
Features of Syndrome		
Paresthesias	70	85
Weakness		
Arms	20	90
Legs	60	95
Face	35	60
Oropharynx	25	50
Ophthalmoparesis	5	15
Sphincter dysfunction	15	5
Ataxia	10	15
Areflexia	75	90
Pain	25	30
Sensory loss	40	75
Respiratory failure	10	30
CSF protein >0.55 g/L	50	90
Abnormal electrophysiologic findings	95	99
Clinical variants*		
Fisher syndrome		5
Weakness without paresthesias or sensory loss		3
Pharyngeal-cervical-brachial weakness		3
Paraparesis		2
Facial paresis with paresthesias		1
Pure ataxia		1

*Variants are associated with diminished reflexes, demyelinating features as detected on electrophysiologic studies, and elevated cerebrospinal concentrations of fluid protein. Frequencies shown are those found in fully developed illness.
From Ropper AH. The Guillain-Barré syndrome. N Engl J Med 1992;326:1130–1136, with permission.

myelin, hence the term *acute inflammatory demyelinating polyneuropathy (AIDP)*. As the name implies, AIDP is characterized by prominent demyelination and inflammatory infiltrates in the spinal roots and nerves. Criteria for the diagnosis of GBS are based on the AIDP prototype and include both clinical and laboratory findings (Table C23–3). Until recently, AIDP had been used interchangeably with GBS. However, it is now well recognized that axonal forms of GBS exist. Several studies during the last two decades have documented that, although most cases of GBS are characterized by segmental demyelination, many patients with typical GBS have evidence of primary axonal degeneration ("axonal" GBS). GBS may be due to a pure motor axonopathy, named

Table C23–3. Diagnostic Criteria for Guillain-Barré Syndrome (Mainly Acute Inflammatory Demyelinating Polyradiculoneuropathy)

Features Required for Diagnosis
Progressive multiple limb and cranial muscle weakness of variable degree
Distal areflexia, with variable degrees of proximal areflexia
Features Strongly Supporting the Diagnosis
Clinical features supportive of diagnosis
Progression of symptoms from days to 4 weeks; nadir attained by 2 weeks in 50%, 3 weeks in 80%, and 4 weeks in 90%
Demonstration of relative limb symmetry regarding paresis
Mild to moderate sensory signs
Cranial nerve involvement: facial nerve 50% and typically bilateral; occasional involvement of cranial nerves III, IV, VI, X, XI, and XII
Recovery typically begins 2 to 4 weeks after the plateau phase
Autonomic dysfunction may include tachycardia, other arrhythmias, postural hypotension, hypertension, and other vasomotor symptoms
Absence of fever at onset of neurologic symptoms
Cerebrospinal fluid supportive of diagnosis
Elevated or serial elevation of CSF protein
CSF cell counts <10 mononuclear cells/mm^3
Electrodiagnostic Features Supportive of Diagnosis
80% of patients have evidence of NCV slowing/conduction block at some time during disease process
Patchy reduction in NCV to values lower than 60% of normal
Distal motor latency increase may reach 3 times normal values
F waves indicate proximal NCV slowing
Approximately 15–20% of patients have normal NCS findings
No abnormalities on NCS may be seen for several weeks
Features Atypical of the Diagnosis
Fever present during initial phase of neurologic symptoms
Profound disturbance of sensation with or without pain
Disease continues to progress beyond 4 weeks, rarely accompanied by a clinical relapse
Disease no longer progresses, but recovery is minimal

Table C23–3. —cont'd

Transient sphincteric dysfunction
Possible CNS involvement
Absence of CSF protein elevation
CSF cell count >11–50 mononuclear cells/mm^3
Features Making the Diagnosis Doubtful
Asymmetrical weakness
Well-demarcated sensory level
Severe and persistent bowel and bladder dysfunction
More than 50 mononuclear cells/mm^3 in CSF
CSF contains polymorphonuclear cells
Features excluding the diagnosis
History of hexacarbon abuse in recent-past sniffing of glue or lacquer vapor
Findings suggestive of abnormal porphyrin metabolism
Recent diphtheria infection
Clinical suspicion of lead or acute arsenic intoxication
Diagnosis of poliomyelitis, myasthenia, botulism, toxic neuropathy

CSF = cerebrospinal fluid; CSN = central nervous system; NCV = nerve conduction velocity; NCS = nerve conduction studies.
Modified from Asbury AK, Cornblath DR. Assessment of current diagnostic criteria for Guillain-Barré syndrome. Ann Neurol 1990;27(Suppl): S21–S24.

acute motor axonal neuropathy (AMAN), or a mixed sensorimotor axonopathies, named *acute motor sensory axonal neuropathy (AMSAN)* (Table C23–4). In addition to their electrophysiologic characteristics, the subtypes of GBS have characteristic pathological findings, with evidence of vesicular demyelination in AIDP and axonal phagocytosis in AMAN and AMSAN. Also, there is a strong association between GBS, particularly the AMAN form, with a preceding *Campylobacter jejuni* infection and the presence of serum antibodies directed toward ganglioside M1 (anti-GM1).

Table C23–4. Classification of Guillain-Barré Syndrome

Types
Acute inflammatory demyelinating polyradiculoneuropathy (AIDP)
Acute motor-sensory axonal neuropathy (AMSAN)
Acute motor axonal neuropathy (AMAN)
Variants
Miller-Fisher syndrome
Pharyngeal–cervical–brachial form
Ataxic form
Pure sensory form
Pure autonomic form (acute dysautonomia)

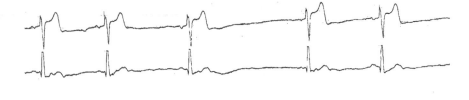

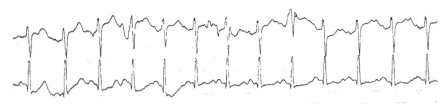

Figure C23–1. *Bardycardia alternating with tachycardia in 35-year-old man with severe quadriplegia and bifacial weakness due to GBS.*

In addition to the three major subtypes of GBS, many variants of the typical GBS presentation exist. Among them, Miller-Fisher syndrome is the most widely known. It consists of ophthalmoplegia, ataxia, and areflexia. Others include a pure sensory form, an ataxic form, a pharyngeal–cervical–brachial regional form, and a pure autonomic form. Thus, GBS is a syndrome that encompasses many disorders with similar clinical presentations but likely with different etiologies and pathophysiologies (Tables C23–2 and C23–4).

Plasma exchange (PE) is the first and only treatment that has been proven to be superior to supportive treatment alone in GBS. This is based on six randomized trials, all comparing PE versus supportive treatment alone. The number of effective PEs was compared in two randomized trials. In mild GBS, two PEs are significantly superior to none, and in moderate or severe GBS, four sessions are significantly superior to two, while additional PEs (such as six) do not provide any additional benefit. Plasma exchange is more beneficial when started within seven days after disease onset rather than later, but is still beneficial in patients treated up to 30 days after disease onset. *Intravenous immunoglobulin (IVIG)* also hastens recovery from GBS and is equivalent to plasma exchange, based on three randomized trials that compared IVIG to plasma exchange. Administering IVIG after plasma exchange is not significantly better than plasma exchange alone. Also, corticosteroids are ineffective and adding methylprednisolone to IVIG treatment provides no additional benefit.

Most patients with GBS ultimately recover, but the prognosis is extremely variable. The plateau phase usually lasts several days or weeks but may persist for months in severe cases with quadriplegia and respiratory failure. The mortality rate has declined with the advent of critical care

units and has ranged from 2 to 10%, mostly due to pulmonary embolism and cardiac arrhythmia (Figure C23–1). Approximately 20% of patients have permanent disability, and 10% of these are severely disabled. *Advanced age, history of preceding diarrheal illness, recent CMV infection, rapid evolution of weakness, prolonged plateau before recovery, and ventilator dependency predicts a poor prognosis.* Patients with AMSAN have the worst prognosis, while patients with AMAN surprisingly have a prognosis and recovery rate similar to patients with AIDP, despite electrophysiologic and pathologic evidence of axonal degeneration. This is best explained by a distal motor axonal loss (intramuscular motor nerve terminals) and rapid reinnervation. *The best prognostic indicator of poor outcome is an average CMAP amplitude at plateau of less than 20% of the lower limit of normal.* To rule out distal demyelination (i.e., distal conduction block) as a cause of low CMAP amplitudes, sequential EDX studies are often required.

Electrodiagnostic Features

Diagnostic Role of Electrodiagnostic Evaluation

The EDX study, and in particular its nerve conduction studies (NCS) component, is the most important ancillary method available to confirm the diagnosis of GBS. Yet, the electrodiagnosis of GBS continues to be a challenging task and is subject to errors that depend on the number of nerves studied and the experience of the electromyographer. The electrophysiologic evaluation of patients with GBS reveals a wide range of abnormalities caused by multifocal demyelination, axonal degeneration, or both. However, because of the patchy nature of demyelination in AIDP and its predilection to very proximal and very distal nerve segments (spinal roots and intramuscular branches, retrospectively), the EDX studies are not infrequently normal or reveal nonspecific neuropathic findings that are insufficient for a definite diagnosis, particularly when done during the first few days or weeks of disease onset. Also, the diagnosis of the axonal forms of GBS, AMAN and AMSAN, depends mostly on findings evidence of axonal loss without significant demyelination. In AMAN, which is associated with normal SNAPs, it is difficult to distinguish the disorder from a subacute axonal polyradiculopathies that also spare the SNAPs such as carcinomatous meningitis. In AMSAN, the presence of a mixed sensorimotor axonal polyneuropathy may be impossible to distinguish, based on EDX studies only, from other causes of subacute axonal polyneuropathies such as critical illness polyneuropathy or polyneuropathies associated with porphyria, or drug or environmental toxins.

The *prompt and early diagnosis* of GBS is warranted by the need to initiate early treatment. Hence, the EDX studies are most useful and often requested during the first 1–2 weeks of illness, soon after presentation or admission to the hospital. During this critical period, 5–10% of patients unfortunately have normal studies (despite severe weakness). Another 5–10% have only nonspecific nerve conduction abnormalities, such as mild slowing, absent and/or prolonged H reflexes or F waves (due to spinal root demyelination), or low-amplitude CMAPs (due to intramuscular motor nerve terminals involvement).

AIDP, the most common form of GBS, is characterized by multifocal demyelination, a required finding for definite diagnosis. Electrodiagnosis of AIDP has traditionally relied on abnormal motor NCS, such as conduction block, CMAP dispersion, delayed or absent F waves, and slowing of latencies and velocities. It is now clear that sensory NCSs are also important in providing electrodiagnostic evidence that might distinguish primary demyelinating from primary axonal polyneuropathy.

Motor Nerve Conduction Studies

Electrophysiologic evidence of definite demyelination requires the presence of demyelination in at least two motor nerves with no evidence of coexisting entrapment syndromes. During the first two weeks of illness, slowing of conduction velocity in the demyelinating range (e.g., less than 70–80% of the lower limits of normal) is present in less than 25% of patients. Conduction block in one or more motor nerves, a strong evidence for acquired demyelination, is present in less than 30% of patients (Figure C23–2).

Sensory Nerve Conduction Studies

There is relative preservation of the SNAPs compared to the CMAPs, especially in the first 2–3 weeks of illness.

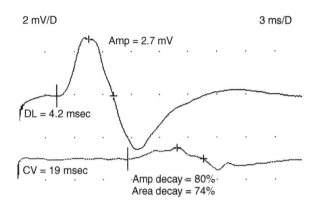

Figure C23–2. *Median motor conduction block and slowing on day 4 in a 25-year-old patient with GBS. Note the significant drop of CMAP amplitude (80%) and area (74%) between distal stimulation (upper tracing) and proximal stimulation (lower tracing) with marked slowing of proximal conduction velocity (19 m/s).*

The most common abnormalities seen in GBS are reduced SNAP amplitudes associated with variable slowing of the sensory distal latencies. The combination of normal sural SNAPs and low-amplitude or absent upper-extremity SNAPs (*"sural-sparing pattern"*) is common and distinctive of acquired demyelinating polyneuropathy, including AIDP. This finding, which is highly specific (96% specific) for the diagnosis of AIDP, is present in about half of the patients with AIDP and in about two-thirds of patients younger than 60 years. The exact cause of relative preservation of sural SNAP compared to the median and ulnar SNAPs may be due to relative resistance of the larger-diameter myelinated fibers in the sural trunk compared to the smaller tapering nerve fibers in the digital nerves of the hands. Also, this finding may reflect the lack of length-dependent axonal degeneration as seen with axonal polyneuropathy.

Limitations of the sural sparing pattern include that a pre-existing carpal tunnel syndrome may result in abnormally low amplitude or absent median and normal sural SNAPs. Hence, the *sural sparing pattern should depend on at least two abnormally low-amplitude or absent hand SNAPs and normal sural SNAPs.* Another limitation is that the sural SNAP is either low in amplitude or absent in elderly or obese patients, and in those with polyneuropathy. Technical considerations in hospitalized patients, especially those with quadriparesis or on mechanical ventilation in the intensive care units, also render studying sural SNAP difficult. In these cases, it is useful to assess the radial SNAP, since the median and ulnar SNAPs are more preferentially affected that the radial and sural SNAP. We found that *a high sensory ratio (sural + radial SNAPs/median + ulnar SNAPs >1)* is also strong evidence that support the diagnosis of AIDP. For example, we found that AIDP is 12 times more likely to have a sensory ratio of greater than 1 compared to diabetic neuropathy.

Late Responses

An absent tibial H reflex is the most common finding in patients with AIDP, being detected in about 95–100%. However, an absent H reflex is equivalent to an absent ankle jerk and is not specific (35% specificity) for AIDP as it is absent in most polyneuropathies as well as S1 radiculopathies and elderly subjects. Absent or impersistent F waves or delayed minimal F wave latencies are present in 40–80% of patients with AIDP but are, similar to the H reflex, nonspecific (33% specificity), since they accompany most peripheral polyneuropathies as well as radiculopathies and mononeuropathies. Absent or delayed minimal F wave latencies are most valuable when accompanied by normal or relatively preserved motor nerve conduction studies, a finding that is considered evidence of proximal demyelination (Figure C23–3). Another useful abnormality is the identification of A (axon) waves. Though A waves may be seen in up to 5% of asymptomatic individuals, particularly while studying the tibial nerve, recording multiple or complex A waves from several nerves is commonly associated with demyelinating polyneuropathies

such as AIDP (Figures C23–4 and C23–5). The exact pathway of the A wave is unknown but it may be generated as a result of ephaptic transmission between two axons with the action potential conducting back down the nerve fiber to the muscle.

Diagnostic Criteria

Since AIDP is the most common type of GBS, the EDX criteria of GBS depend mostly on identifying segmental demyelination of peripheral nerves. The presence of conduction block, significant temporal dispersion, marked slowing of motor distal latencies, conduction velocities or F wave latencies are necessary findings for definite segmental demyelination. When the findings are multifocal or associated with conduction blocks or both, they are strong evidence for an acquired demyelinating neuropathy such as AIDP. Several NCS patterns emerge in patients with GBS ranging from normal studies to studies that are diagnostic of AIDP (Table C23–5).

Several criteria have been proposed and none are universally accepted, some with strict definitions for demyelination and others with less rigid demands (Table C23–6). There are several limitations to the various EDX criteria for GBS. First, the exact cutoff of conduction velocities and distal latencies for establishing the diagnosis of primary

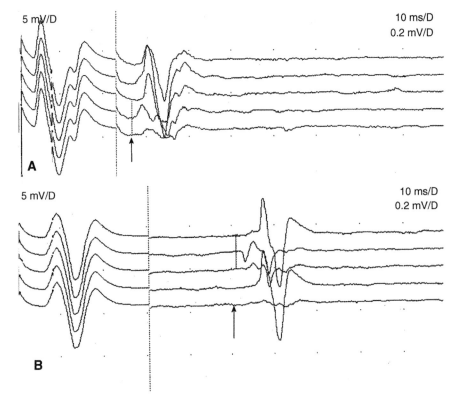

Figure C23–3. *Median minimal F wave latencies in a 30-year-old healthy subject (**A**) and a 35-year-old patient with GBS (**B**). Note the marked slowing of minimal F wave latencies (arrows) in the patient compared to control.*

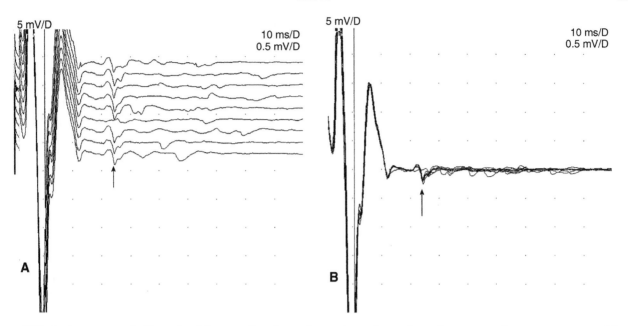

Figure C23–4. *A wave recorded from the abductor pollicis brevis (arrows) stimulating the median nerve at the wrist in a 65-year-old man with GBS. The A waves shown in a raster mode (**A**) and superimposed mode (**B**) have a constant morphology and latency, best explained by the fixed point of ephapse. Note the absence of median F waves.*

demyelination and excluding axon loss disorders continues to be controversial. This is particularly true when the distal CMAPs are diminished below the lower limit of normal (LLN). It is clear that using the LLN for velocities or upper limit of normal for distal latencies as cutoffs is incorrect since many axonal neuropathies result in some degree

of slowing. The available criteria were mostly based on consensus among groups of physicians. Earlier criteria assessed only velocities with no regards to CMAP amplitudes. More recently, Alberts and Kelly have used conduction velocity slowing of less than 90% of the LLN when CMAP amplitude is above 50% of LLN and less than 80%

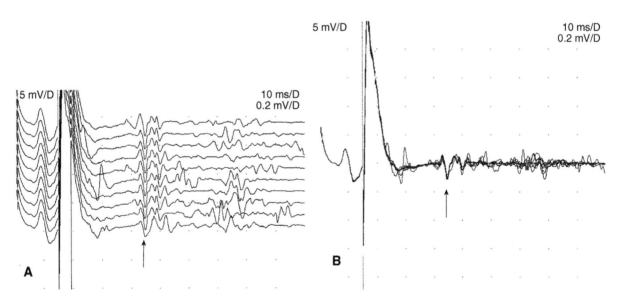

Figure C23–5. *Complex A wave recorded from the abductor hallucis (arrows), stimulating the tibial nerve at the ankle in a 65-year-old man with GBS. The A waves are shown in a raster mode (**A**) and superimposed mode (**B**).*

Table C23–5. Common Nerve Conduction Patterns in Guillain-Barré Syndrome

Normal nerve conduction studies

Absent H reflexes

Prolongation or absent F waves

Patchy, mild slowing of distal latencies and conduction velocities

Low-amplitude CMAPs and SNAPs

Distal CMAPs dispersion

Absent/low-amplitude upper extremity SNAPs, with normal sural SNAP

Sensory ratio (sural + radial SNAPs/median + ulnar SNAPs) more than 1

Single conduction block/temporal dispersion

Prominent multifocal motor and sensory slowing, with multifocal conduction blocks

CMAP = compound muscle action potential; SNAP = sensory nerve action potential.

of the LLN when CMAP amplitude is below 50% of LLN. Asbury and Cornblath suggested conduction velocity slowing of less than 80% of LLN if the CMAP amplitude is greater than 80% of LLN and less than 70% of LLN if CMAP amplitude is greater than 80% LLN. There are no available criteria for the cutoff slowing when CMAP amplitude is very low, such as less than 20% of LLN, in order to distinguish severe axonal loss from segmental demyelination.

Because of the differences of these EDX criteria, there is a considerable varaiation in the number of patients who would fulfill the criteria for AIDP (Figure C23–6). This has also resulted in disagreements between physicians and, sometimes, unfortunate misdiagnoses. The second limitation to these criteria is that the available criteria considers only the motor nerve conduction studies despite good evidence that sensory studies are important in the diagnosis of GBS and their use should be emphasized. These include the sural sparing pattern and an increased sensory ratio (sural + radial SNAPs/median + ulnar SNAPs) of more than 1.

It is clear that criteria with graded probability and various level of certainty for AIDP are needed, since the disorder has a wide range of EDX manifestations that may also change with time due to ongoing disease or due to the effect of remyelination or wallerian degeneration. Our recently published graded criteria utilized, in addition to one criteria of definite demyelination by Asbury and Cornblath, other nerve conduction abnormalities including absent/slowed F waves and sural sparing pattern. These criteria confirmed the diagnosis of AIDP in the first 2 weeks of illness with high specificity and a positive predictive value of 95–100% and with moderate sensitivity in about 65% of patients (Table C23–7).

Sequential studies, particularly in the first several weeks of illness, are valuable tools in GBS. The pathological process in GBS is dynamic during the early few weeks that

Table C23–6. Two Commonly Used Electrodiagnostic Criteria for Definite Acquired Demyelinating Polyneuropathy Including AIDP

Criteria	Albers and Kelly	Asbury and Cornblath
Required	≥3 criteria	≥3 criteria
Conduction block and/or temporal dispersion	? Number of nerve*	in ≥1 nerve*
Slowing of MCV	in ≥2 nerves <90% LLN if CMAP amplitude >50% LLN <80% LLN if CMAP amplitude <50% LLN	in ≥2 nerves <80% LLN if CMAP amplitude >80% LLN <70% LLN if CMAP amplitude <80% LLN
Slowing of MDL	in ≥2 nerves >115% ULN if CMAP amplitude is normal >125% ULN if CMAP amplitude is <LLN	in ≥2 nerves >125% ULN if CMAP amplitude >80% LLN >150% ULN if CMAP amplitude <80% LLN
F wave latency	in ≥1 nerve >125% ULN	in ≥2 nerves Absent, or latency >120% ULN if CMAP >80% LLN >150% ULN if CMAP >80% LLN

CMAP = compound muscle action potential; LLN = lower limit of normal; MCV = motor conduction velocity; MDL = motor distal latency; ULN = upper limit of normal.
*Conduction block = >30% decrease in CMAP amplitude between distal and proximal stimulations. Conduction block = >20% decrease in CMAP area or amplitude between distal and proximal stimulations, with <15% increase in CMAP duration; temporal dispersion = >20% decrease in CMAP area or amplitude between distal and proximal stimulations, with >15% increase in CMAP duration.
Adapted from Brown WF. Acute and chronic inflammatory demyelinating neuropathies. In: Brown WF, Bolton CF, eds. Clinical electromyography. Boston, MA: Butterworth-Heinemann, 1993.

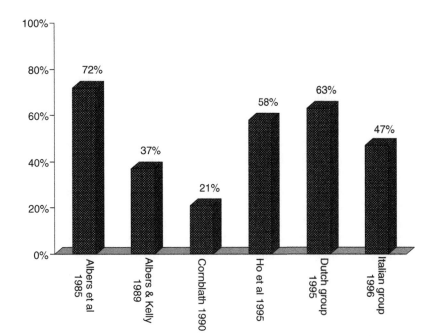

Figure C23–6. *The percentage of patients with GBS fulfilling six various EDX criteria for AIDP (see Suggested Radings list) from a total of 43 patients with GBS in the first 4 weeks of illness. (Adapted from Alam TA, Chaudhry V, Cornblath DR. Electrophysiological studies in the Guillain-Barré syndrome: distinguishing subtypes by published criteria. Muscle Nerve 1998;21:1275–1279.)*

Table C23–7. Diagnostic Power of Findings on Nerve Conduction Studies in Guillain-Barré Syndrome

	Abnormalities	**Sensitivity (%)**	**Specificity (%)**
Nondiagnostic study	Nonspecific abnormalities including a borderline or low CMAPs and/or SNAPs, minimal slowing or isolated absent H reflex, without definite demyelination	4.5	19
Suggestive study	Sural sparing pattern or absent *or* Absent or prolonged minimal F wave latencies (at least 2 motor nerves) with absent H responses	26	86
Highly suggestive study*	Sural sparing pattern *and* Absent or prolonged minimal F wave latencies (at least 2 motor nerves) with absent H responses	29	96
Definite study	Signs of multifocal demyelination (fulfilling criteria of Asbury and Cornblath; see Table C23–6) including: 1. Marked slowing of motor conduction velocity, distal latency, temporal dispersion, and conduction blocks in at least 2 motor nerves 2. Absent or prolonged minimal F wave latencies in at least 2 motor nerves with absent H responses	35	100
Highly suggestive or definite study	–	64	96–100

CMAP = compound muscle action potential; SNAP = sensory nerve action potential.
*Rapid recovery of low distal CMAPs and SNAPs on sequential studies is considered, in retrospect, highly suggestive of distal demyelination and block.
Adapted from Al-Shekhlee A, Hachwi R, Preston DC, Katirji B. New criteria for early electrodiagnosis of acute inflammatory demyelinating polyneuropathy. Muscle Nerve 2005;32:66–72.

a single EDX sampling may not be sufficient to establish the diagnosis. Unfortunately, many patients are now discharged to rehabilitative facilities before the third week of illness, and sequential studies are often not requested because clinical decisions have already been made and treatment has begun. However, there are several advantages of sequential studies:

1. During the first 2 weeks of illness, only 30 to 50% of patients with AIDP fulfill the criteria for demyelination, compared with 85% by the third week (Figure C23–7). About 10% of patients with AIDP never fulfill the criteria for demyelination.

2. Low or absent CMAPs and/or SNAPs are considered signs of axonal loss as seen with AMAN and AMSAN. However, a rapid improvement of CMAP or SNAPs amplitudes over a few weeks is occasionally observed on sequential studies. This finding is consistent with distal motor or sensory nerve demyelination and subsequent remyelination. These AIDP patients, who have good prognosis, will have early EDX studies that are misdiagnosed as axonal GBS unless sequential studies are performed.

3. In AMAN and AMSAN, the motor CMAPs are low in amplitudes with no or minimal slowing of distal latencies and conduction velocities. Occasionally, conduction block may be detected early on which suggest demyelination and a diagnosis AIDP. However, sequential studies prove in these patients that the conduction block was due to axonal loss (axonal noncontinuity, early axon loss, or axon-discontinuity conduction block) and the disorder is in fact an axonal GBS (Figure C23–8).

A small percentage of patients have *axonal GBS*, namely AMAN and AMSAN. These axonal subtypes of GBS are typified by the loss of CMAP (and SNAP in cases of AMSAN) amplitudes without significant slowing of distal latencies, F wave latencies, or conduction velocities, and by the absence of conduction blocks or temporal dispersion. This contrasts with AIDP which is characterized by slowing of both distal latencies and conduction velocities, with conduction blocks and temporal dispersion and relative preservation of CMAP and SNAP amplitudes.

Prognostic Role of Electrodiagnostic Evaluation

Another important role of EDX evaluation is its usefulness in predicting the prognosis of GBS, particularly because the clinical findings are relatively less precise predictors of outcome in GBS. The main prognostic goal is the identification of axonal degeneration, which by itself is a poor indicator for recovery that requires a long time because it is dependent on regeneration. Indicators of axonal loss that affect prognosis have included:

1. *Fibrillation potentials.* Earlier studies suggested that the "quantity" of fibrillation potentials is directly proportional to the length of hospital stay, and is inversely proportional to the rate of respiratory recovery. This has proved to be incorrect because fibrillation potentials may take up to 5 to 7 weeks from disease onset to appear. Also, fibrillation potentials are insensitive indicators of axonal loss, and only a small proportion of axonal degeneration is required to occur before fibrillations are seen.

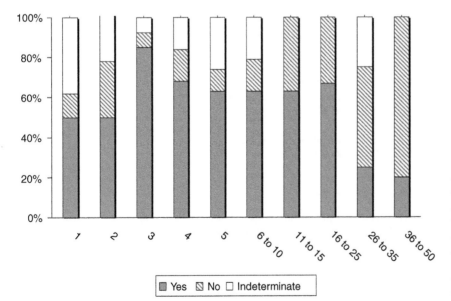

Figure C23–7. *Electrodiagnostic power of sequential nerve conduction studies in the diagnosis of AIDP during 50 weeks of illness. Note that the study is often diagnostic in the third and fourth weeks of illness and is least diagnostic after 25 weeks. (Adapted from Albers JW, Donofrio PD, McGonagle TK. Sequential diagnostic abnormalities in acute inflammatory demyelinating polyradiculopathy. Muscle Nerve 1985;8:528–539.)*

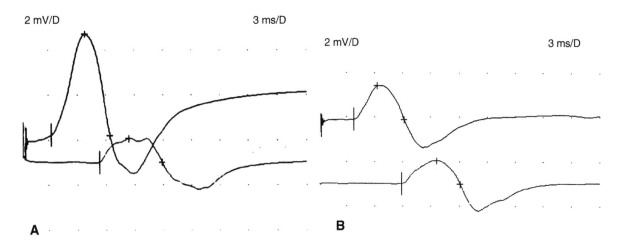

Figure C23–8. *Median motor conduction study in a 75-year-old patient with axonal GBS, compatible with AMAN, done 5 days (**A**) and 30 days (**B**) after the onset of ascending quadriparesis that reached its nadir on day 7. Note the median conduction block in the forearm on day 5 (**A**) with significant (>50%) drop in CMAP amplitude and area between distal stimulation (upper tracing) and proximal stimulation (lower tracing). Subsequent study on day 30 (**B**) showed a significant decline of the distal motor CMAP which now almost equals the proximal CMAP. The initial block is consistent with the so-called axonal noncontinuity, early axon loss, or axon-discontinuity conduction block. This type of conduction block is only confirmed after a repeat study following the completion of wallerian degeneration. Recall that in wallerian degeneration, the distal CMAP decreases in amplitude starting 1–2 days after acute nerve insult and reaches its nadir in 5–6 days.*

2. *CMAP amplitudes.* Several studies have shown that the best outcome indicator in GBS is the mean CMAP amplitude of motor nerves. A very low mean CMAP amplitude (below 20% of the LLN) at plateau is a poor prognostic indicator. However, this assessment should be done cautiously since the effect of axonal loss and wallerian degeneration on nerve conduction studies is delayed. Also, distal conduction block, caused by segmental demyelination, may result in inexitable nerves or in low distal CMAPs that mimics axonal loss. Hence, for the individual patient with low mean CMAP amplitude, the process might involve distal demyelination or axonal loss. Sequential studies, done over the first few weeks of illness, are very useful since many patients with distal conduction block may reveal some rapid improvement of CMAP amplitude consistent with segmental demyelination, while in others the CAMP amplitudes do not change or decline further due to axonal loss and wallerian degeneration. Hence, a low mean CMAP amplitude of less than 20% of the LLN, recorded more than 2 weeks after the patient reaches his/her neurological nadir, is a sensitive indicator of poor outcome.

In contrast to CMAP amplitudes, there is a very poor correlation between conduction velocities and outcome. In fact, patients with significant slowing on conduction studies tend to recover more quickly than those with normal or near-normal velocities. In the latter group, the abnormalities are likely to be low CMAPs, which reflect axonal loss rather than segmental demyelination.

FOLLOW-UP

Vital capacity on presentation was borderline at 2.6 L. Lumbar puncture was performed on the admission date, 2 days after the onset of neurologic symptoms. Cerebrospinal fluid protein was 57 mg/dL without pleocytosis. The patient was treated with a plasma exchange the next morning, 3 days after the onset of symptoms. A total of four plasma exchanges were administered over one week. Despite this, the patient's neurologic condition deteriorated to complete quadriplegia and mild bilateral facial weakness. However, respiration was maintained without the need for mechanical ventilation. Vital capacity reached a nadir of 1.8 L. Repeat CSF examination 2 weeks after the onset of neurologic symptoms revealed markedly elevated CSF protein at 753 mg/dL without pleocytosis.

The patient lingered at a plateau for approximately 1 week before showing early signs of recovery. With rehabilitation, she improved gradually, first in the distal hand and foot muscles, then in the upper limbs, and finally in the lower limbs. She was able to feed herself 6 weeks after the onset of illness, sat independently at 2 months, and ambulated with a walker at 3 months. Four months after onset, the patient was ambulating independently but demonstrated mild residual hip flexor weakness (MRC 4+/5). She still was diffusely areflexic.

DIAGNOSIS

Severe Guillain-Barré syndrome, highly suggestive of an acute inflammatory demyelinating polyneuropathy, with fair prognosis for recovery.

ANSWERS

1. D; 2. D; 3. B.

SUGGESTED READINGS

General

Asbury AK, Cornblath DR. Assessment of current diagnostic criteria for Guillain-Barré syndrome. Ann Neurol 1990;27: (Suppl):S21–S24.

Feasby TE et al. An acute axonal form of Guillain-Barré polyneuropathy, Brain 1986;109:1115–1126.

Griffin JW et al. Guillain-Barré syndrome in Northern China. The spectrum of neuropathological changes in clinically defined cases. Brain 1995;118:577–595.

Griffin JW et al. Pathology of the motor-sensory axonal Guillain-Barré syndrome. Ann Neurol 1996;39:17–28.

Ho MJ et al. Guillain-Barré syndrome in Northern China. Relationship to Campylobacter jejuni infection and anti-glycolipid antibodies. Brain 1995;118:597–605.

Ho TW et al. Guillain-Barré syndrome in Northern China. The spectrum of neuropathological changes in clinically defined cases. Brain 1995;118:577–595.

Hughes RA, Cornblath DR. Guillain-Barré syndrome. Lancet 2005;366:1653–1966.

Illa I et al. Acute axonal Guillain-Barré syndrome with IgG antibodies against motor axons following parental ganglioside. Ann Neurol 1995;38:218–222.

Katirji B, Kaminski HJ, Preston DC et al., eds. Neuromuscular disorders in clinical practice. Boston, MA: Butterworth-Heinemann, 2002.

McKhann GM et al. Plasmapheresis and Guillain-Barré syndrome: analysis of prognostic factors and the effect of plasmapheresis. Ann Neurol 1988;23:347–353.

McKhann GM et al. Acute motor axonal neuropathy: a frequent cause of acute flaccidity in China. Ann Neurol 1993;33:333–342.

Oomes PG et al. Anti GM1 IgG antibodies and Campylobacter bacteria in Guillain-Barré syndrome: evidence of molecular mimicry. Ann Neurol 1995;38:170–175.

Ropper AH. The Guillain-Barré syndrome. N Engl J Med 1992;326:1130–1136.

Electrodiagnosis

Alam TA, Chaudhry V, Cornblath DR. Electrophysiological studies in the Guillain-Barré syndrome: distinguishing subtypes by published criteria. Muscle Nerve 1998;21:1275–1279.

Albers JW, Donofrio PD, McGonagle TK. Sequential diagnostic abnormalities in acute inflammatory demyelinating polyradiculopathy. Muscle Nerve 1985;8:528–539.

Albers JW, Kelly JJ Jr. Acquired inflammatory demyelinating polyneuropathy: clinical and electrodiagnostic features. Muscle Nerve 1989;12:435–451.

Al-Shekhlee A, Hachwi R, Preston DC, Katirji B. New criteria for early electrodiagnosis of acute inflammatory demyelinating polyneuropathy. Muscle Nerve 2005;32:66–72.

Al-Shekhlee A, Robinson J, Katirji B. Sensory sparing patterns and sensory ratio in acute inflammatory demyelinating polyneuropathy. Muscle Nerve 2007;35:246–250.

Asbury AK, Cornblath DR. Assessment of current diagnostic criteria for Guillain-Barré syndrome. Ann Neurol 1990;27(Suppl):S21–S24.

Bansal R, Kalita J, Misra UK. Pattern of sensory conduction in Guillain-Barré syndrome. Electromyogr Clin Neurophysiol 2001;41:433–437.

Bromberg MB, Albers JW. Patterns of sensory nerve conduction abnormalities in demyelinating and axonal peripheral nerve disorders. Muscle Nerve 1993;16:262–266.

Cornblath DR. Electrophysiology in Guillain-Barré syndrome. Ann Neurol 1990;27(Suppl):S17–S20.

Cornblath DR et al. Motor conduction studies in Guillain-Barré syndrome: description and prognostic value. Ann Neurol 1988;23:354–359.

Cleland JC et al. Acute inflammatory demyelinating polyneuropathy: contribution of a dispersed distal compound muscle action potential to electrodiagnosis. Muscle Nerve 2006;33:771–777.

Gordon PH, Wilbourn AJ. Early electrodiagnostic findings in Guillain-Barré syndrome. Arch Neurol 2001;58:913–917.

Italian Guillain-Barré Study Group. The prognosis and main prognostic indicators of Guillain-Barré syndrome. Brain 1996;119:2053–2061.

Meulstee J, van der Meche FG. Electrodiagnostic criteria for polyneuropathy and demyelination: application in 135 patients with Guillain-Barré syndrome. Dutch Guillain-Barré Study Group. J Neurol Neurosurg Psychiatry 1995;59:482–486.

Miller RG et al. Prognostic value of electrodiagnosis in Guillain-Barré syndrome. Muscle Nerve 1988;11:769–774.

Ropper AH, Wijdicks EFM, Shahani BT. Electrodiagnostic changes in early Guillain-Barré. A prospective study in 113 patients. Arch Neurol 1990;47:881–887.

Triggs WJ et al. Motor nerve inexcitability in Guillain-Barré syndrome: the spectrum of distal conduction block and axonal degeneration. Brain 1992;115:1291–1302.

Van Der Meche FGA et al. Patterns of conduction failure in the Guillain-Barré syndrome. Brain 1988;111:405–416.

Treatment

Dutch Guillain-Barré Study Group. Treatment of Guillain-Barré syndrome with high-dose immune globulins combined with methylprednisolone: a pilot study. Ann Neurol 1994;34: 749–752.

French Cooperative Group on Plasma Exchange in Guillain-Barré syndrome. Efficiency of plasma exchange in Guillain-Barré syndrome: role of replacement fluids. Ann Neurol 1987;22:753–761.

French Cooperative Group on Plasma Exchange in Guillain-Barré syndrome. Plasma exchange in Guillain-Barré syndrome: one-year follow-up. Ann Neurol 1992;32:94–97.

French Cooperative Group on Plasma Exchange in Guillain-Barré syndrome. Appropriate number of plasma exchanges in Guillain-Barré syndrome. Ann Neurol 1997;41:298–306.

Hughes RAC et al. Controlled trial of prednisone in acute polyneuropathy. Lancet 1978;2:750–753.

Guillain-Barré Syndrome Steroidal Trial Group. Double-blind study of intravenous methylprednisolone in Guillain-Barré syndrome. Lancet 1993;341:586–590.

Guillain-Barré Syndrome Study Group. Plasmapheresis and acute Guillain-Barré syndrome. Neurology 1985;35: 1096–1104.

Plasma Exchange/Sandoglobulin Guillain-Barré Syndrome Trial Group. Randomized trial of plasma exchange, intravenous immunoglobulin, and combined treatments in Guillain-Barré syndrome. Lancet 1997;349:225–230.

Van Der Mech FGA, Schmitz PIM, the Dutch Guillain-Barré Study Group. A randomized trial comparing intravenous immune globulin and plasma exchange in Guillain-Barré syndrome. N Engl J Med 1992;326:1123–1129.

Case 24

HISTORY AND PHYSICAL EXAMINATION

A 36-year-old white man awoke with binocular diplopia; later that day, he noted blurred vision and lid ptosis. The next morning, he had nausea and vomited twice, and then he had slurred speech and difficulty swallowing. He was admitted to the hospital where magnetic resonance imaging (MRI) of the brain and cerebral angiography were normal. By the third day, he had developed complete ophthalmoplegia, severe dysarthria and dysphagia, and upper extremity weakness. Respiratory failure followed; the patient had to be intubated and required assisted ventilation. The Tensilon test was equivocal.

On examination on day 4, the patient was alert and intubated, and followed commands well. He had bilateral complete ophthalmoplegia to all gaze directions with bilateral ptosis (Figure C24–1). Pupils were dilated and unreactive to light or attempted accommodation. Corneal reflexes were depressed. The patient had bilateral peripheral facial weakness. His tongue was extremely weak, with no fasciculations. His palate did not move volitionally or to gagging. Neck flexors and extensors were weak (Medical Research Council [MRC] 3/5), as were proximal pelvic and shoulder girdle muscles (4/5). However, distal muscles were normal. Deep tendon reflexes were depressed (1/4). Sensation was normal. Cerebellar function also was normal.

An electrodiagnostic (EDX) examination was requested.

Please now review the Nerve Conduction Studies and Needle EMG tables.

QUESTIONS

1. All of the following clinical manifestations are compatible with myasthenia gravis *except:*
   A. Ophthalmoplegia.
   B. Proximal muscle weakness.
   C. Pupillary dilatation.
   D. Neck flexor weakness.
   E. Bulbar palsy.
2. The most common type of botulism in the United States is:
   A. Food-borne botulism.
   B. Wound botulism.
   C. Infantile botulism.
3. The effect of botulinum toxin on the neuromuscular system is caused by:
   A. Conduction block of terminal axons.
   B. Irreversible blockade of postsynaptic acetylcholine (ACH) receptors.
   C. Irreversible blockade of presynaptic ACH receptors.
   D. Prevention of ACH release from the presynaptic terminal by binding to proteins essential for the release of ACH.
   E. Blockade of voltage-gated calcium channels at the presynaptic terminal.

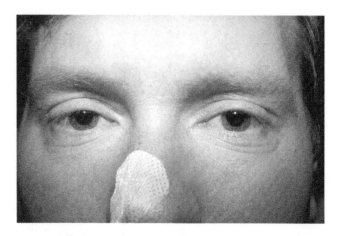

Figure C24–1. *Pupillary dilatation and ptosis in this patient at the time of diagnosis. The patient also had a complete ophthalmoplegia (not shown).*

Case 24: Nerve Conduction Studies

Nerve Stimulated	Stimulation Site	Recording Site	Amplitude (m = mV, s = µV)			Distal/Peak Latency (ms)			Conduction Velocity (m/s)			F Latency (ms)	
			Right	Left	Normal	Right	Left	Normal	Right	Left	Normal	Right	Left
Sural (s)	Calf	Ankle	15		≥5	3.7		≤4.5					
Peroneal (m)	Ankle	EDB	5		≥3	5.0		≤5.5		48	≥40	50.4	
Peroneal (m)	Ankle	EDB	4										
Median (s)	Wrist	Index finger	35		≥20	2.7		≤3.4		57	≥50		
Median (s)	Elbow	Index finger	16										
Median (m)*†	Wrist	APB	**4.2†**		≥6			≤3.9		56	≥50	29.5	
Median (m)*†	Wrist	APB	**3.8**										
Ulnar (m)	Wrist	ADM	**4.5†**		≥7	3.0		≤3.1		53	≥50	30.5	
Ulnar (m)	Elbow	ADM	**4.0**										
Spinal accessory (m)*†	Neck	Trapezius	**3.0†**		≥4	3.5		≤3.5					

ADM = abductor digiti minimi; APB = abductor pollicis brevis; EDB = extensor digitorum brevis; m = motor; s = sensory. Data in bold type are abnormal.

*Decrement on slow repetitive stimulation at rest and following exercise (see Figure C24–3).

†Increment on fast, repetitive stimulation (see Figure C24–4).

‡Compound muscle action potential (CMAP) facilitation following exercise (see Figure C24–2).

See EDX findings and interpretation of data.

Case 24: Needle EMG

| Muscle | Insertional Activity | Spontaneous Activity | | Voluntary Motor Unit Action Potentials (MUAPs) | | | | | | | |
| | | Fibs | Fascs | Recruitment | | | | Configuration | | | |
				Normal	Activation	Reduced	Early	Duration	Amplitude	% Polyphasia	Others
L. tibialis anterior	Normal	0	0	X				Normal	Normal	Normal	
Medial gastrocnemius	Normal	0	0	X				Normal	Normal	Normal	
Vastus lateralis	Normal	0	0	X				Normal	Normal	Normal	
Gluteus medius	Normal	0	0	X				Normal	Normal	Normal	
L. brachioradialis	Normal	0	0	X				Normal	Normal	Normal	
Biceps	Normal	0	0	X				Normal	Normal	Normal	
Triceps	Normal	0	0	X				Normal	Normal	Normal	
Deltoid	Normal	0	0	X				Normal	Normal	Normal	

Fascs = fasciculations; Fibs = fibrillations.

4. The EDX findings in botulism include all of the following *except:*
   A. Low-amplitude compound muscle action potentials (CMAPs).
   B. Normal sensory nerve action potential (SNAP).
   C. Slowing of motor conduction velocities.
   D. Decrement of CMAP amplitude with slow repetitive stimulation.
   E. Increment of CMAP amplitude with rapid repetitive stimulation.
   F. Increment of CMAP amplitude after a brief period of exercise.
5. The following are correct statements regarding botulism and Lambert-Eaton myasthenic syndrome (LEMS), *except:*
   A. Ocular manifestations are prominent in botulism but subtle in Lambert-Eaton Myasthenic syndrome.
   B. After 50 Hz stimulation of motor nerves, the increment of CMAP amplitude generally is more prominent in botulism than in LEMS.
   C. The CMAP increment is present in all motor nerves in LEMS but may be restricted to the affected muscles in botulism.
   D. In both disorders, there is impairment of ACH release from the presynaptic terminal.

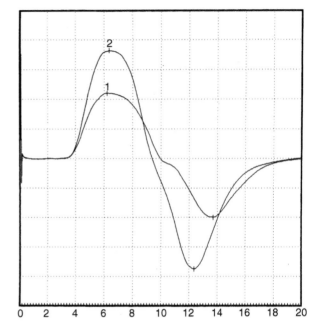

Figure C24–2. *Median compound muscle action potential (CMAP) at rest (waveform 1), and after a brief (10 seconds) period of exercise (waveform 2). Note the significant (90%) facilitation following exercise. Sensitivity = 2 mV/division.*

EDX FINDINGS AND INTERPRETATION OF DATA

The relevant EDX findings in this case are:

1. Normal sensory nerve action potentials (SNAPs).
2. Borderline or low-amplitude CMAPs.
3. Increment of the median CMAP recording abductor pollicis brevis, after a short period (10 seconds) of exercise measuring 90% (Figure C24–2).
4. Decrement of the median and spinal accessory CMAP after slow repetitive stimulation at rest (13%), with significant postexercise (post-tetanic) facilitation (Figure C24–3).
5. Increment of the CMAP amplitude after rapid, repetitive stimulation (50 Hz) measuring 100% (Figure C24–4).

The EDX findings are consistent with a neuromuscular junction disorder of the presynaptic type, as supported by the borderline or low-amplitude baseline CMAPs, and the significant increment (>50%) of the CMAP amplitude after brief exercise and rapid repetitive stimulation of motor nerves. This case is consistent with botulism based on subacute progression of a descending muscle paralysis (ocular to bulbar to limbs), the muscarinic involvement (pupillary dilatation), and the EDX findings

(presynaptic blockade). It is not consistent with Lambert-Eaton myasthenic syndrome because of the rapid evolution of symptoms, the prominent oculobulbar muscle weakness, and the relatively modest increment on rapid repetitive stimulation and after brief exercise (see electrodiagnosis).

DISCUSSION

Physiology and Pathophysiology

Botulinum toxin is produced by the anaerobic bacterium *Clostridium botulinum.* Eight immunologically distinct subtypes of the toxin have been identified (A, B, C1, C2, D, E, F, and G). Five serotypes are associated with human disease, with types A and B being the most common. Botulinum toxin type A is the most common in the United States, accounting for 60% of reported cases; it is the predominant type west of the Mississippi and is the most toxic of all subtypes. Type B serotype causes 30% of US cases and is the most common in Europe. It is the major type east of the Mississippi and tends to cause a milder illness.

Botulinum toxin is an extremely potent toxin with doses as small as 0.05 to 0.1 µg causing death in humans. The toxin has significant affinity to both muscarinic and nicotinic cholinergic nerve terminals resulting in

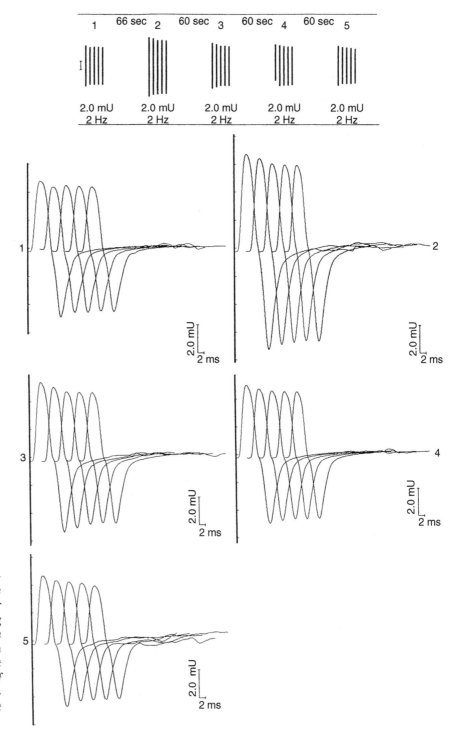

Figure C24–3. *Slow repetitive stimulation (2 Hz) of the median nerve. Train 1 is at rest, and Trains 2 through 5 are after 1 minute of exercise. The upper tracing shows all five stimulations. Although a decrement of the compound muscle action potential (CMAP) was evident at rest (13%), there is a dramatic facilitation of CMAP immediately after exercise (compare Train 1 to Train 2), with a subsequent return to baseline.*

autonomic failure and skeletal muscle paralysis. The toxin results in failure of ACH release from the presynaptic terminal and ultimately leads to destruction of the presynaptic terminal. Botulinum toxin first attaches irreversibly to the axonal terminal, and enters via endocytosis without interfering with the calcium channel (calcium entry is not blocked by botulinum toxin). The toxin then interferes with the calcium-dependent intracellular cascade that is responsible for ACH release, by cleaving proteins essential for docking and fusion of the presynaptic vesicles at the presynaptic active zones. Electron microscopy of nerve endings exposed to the toxin reveal a "log jam" of

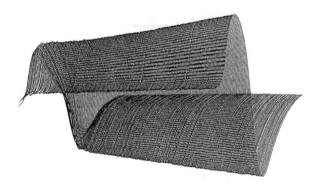

Figure C24–4. *Increment of compound muscle action potential (CMAP) (100%) after rapid (50 Hz) repetitive stimulation of the spinal accessory nerve (sensitivity = 1 mV).*

vesicles in the presynaptic terminals. It is now known that various serotypes bind to different presynaptic proteins: botulinum toxin A and E hydrolyze synaptosomal-associated protein-25 (SNAP-25), a protein of the presynaptic membrane; botulinum toxins B, D, F, and G specifically cleave synaptobrevin, a membrane protein of the neurotransmitter-containing vesicles; botulinum toxin C cleaves both SNAP-25 and syntaxin, a nerve plasmalemma protein (Figure C24–5). Because the ultimate result of this intoxication is interference with neurotransmitter release (exocytosis of synaptic vesicles) and destruction of the nerve terminals, recovery of neurologic function is protracted since it is dependent on the regrowth of sprouts from the injured nerve terminal.

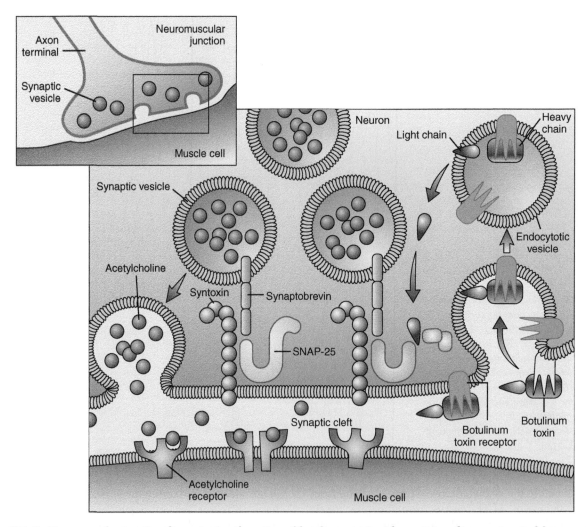

Figure C24–5. *Neuromuscular junction demonstrating the action of botulinum toxin. After entering the axon terminal by means of the botulinum toxin and endocytosis, the protease action of the toxin cleaves synaptic proteins leading to the compromise of synaptic vesicle release. Botulinum toxins A, C, and E cleave synaptosomal-associated protein (SNAP-25), shown in this illustration. Types B, D, F, and G cleave a synaptobrevin vesicle-associated membrane protein (VAMP), and type C cleaves syntaxin. (Reprinted from Hallet M. One man's poison: clinical applications of botulinum toxin. N Engl J Med 1999;341:118-120, with permission. Copyright © 1999 Massachusetts Medical Society.)*

Clinical Features

Botulism is a rare but serious and potentially fatal illness. The clinical picture and severity of botulism are variable since they are dependent on the type of toxin, the dose ingested, and the mode of entry. Although both skeletal muscle weakness and autonomic dysfunction occur in most cases, neuromuscular symptoms tend to overshadow type A intoxication, while dysautonomia dominates disease caused by types B and E. Depending on the mode of entry of the toxin into the bloodstream, botulism is classified into four clinically distinct forms.

1. *Food-borne (classic) botulism.* This is the most severe and debilitating form. It is caused by ingestion of food contaminated by the preformed toxin, which is then absorbed from the gut and distributed by the blood. Home canned foods (fish, vegetables, potatoes, garlic in oil, sautéed onions, etc.) are common vehicles for food-borne botulism. Factors that enhance spore germination and toxin production are low oxygen, low acidity, and high water content, while foods with high acid content, such as vinegar and tomato, are rarely associated with botulism. Classic botulism may manifest as an outbreak (such as restaurant-associated outbreaks), although two-thirds of reported cases have affected single individuals. Boiling food thoroughly should destroy the toxin.

   The presentation of food-borne botulism is stereotypical. The onset of symptoms is within 2 to 36 hours after ingestion and their peak is at 4 to 5 days. Muscle weakness become often generalized and evolves in a distinctive way. Symptoms begin in the ocular and bulbar musculature with blurred vision, double vision, ptosis, dysarthria, and dysphagia. Weakness then descends, usually symmetrically, to involve muscles of the trunk and limbs, and in severe cases, the respiratory muscles. Proximal muscles are weaker than distal ones, and the upper extremities usually are more involved than lower ones. Autonomic manifestations include diarrhea, nausea, and vomiting early in the illness and later dry mouth, blurred vision, constipation, ileus, and urinary retention. Dilated, fixed, or poorly reactive pupils are common but may be delayed.

2. *Infant botulism.* First described in 1976, this is the most common form of botulism in the United States. It occurs in infants, younger than 1 year of age, with a peak incidence at 2 to 4 months. Infant botulism is caused by ingestion of *Clostridium botulinum* spores that colonize the intestinal tract, leading to in vivo production of toxin and its absorption into the bloodstream. The infant gut is hospitable to the growth of the bacterium because it often lacks both the protective bacterial flora and the clostridium-inhibiting bile acids found in normal adult intestinal tract. Honey consumption as a significant risk factor for infant botulism and, hence, should not be fed to infants under the age of 1 year. Breast-feeding as a risk factor or a protective variable is a controversial issue.

   Constipation is often the first symptom in infantile botulism, followed by poor feeding, weak cry, and loss of head control. This may be followed, in 1–3 days, by a symmetrical descending paralysis that involves the cranial muscles, the proximal limb muscles, and, rarely, the diaphragm.

   Adult variations of infant botulism have been described. This form usually occurs in patients with gastrointestinal disorders, such as Crohn's disease, achlorhydria, prior gut surgery, or antibiotic treatment, who may allow the bacteria to germinate in their intestinal tract. The diagnosis is confirmed by culturing *Clostridium botulinum* in feces of these adult patients.

3. *Wound botulism.* This form is extremely rare. It is caused by anaerobic wound infection by *Clostridium botulinum*, with in vivo production of toxin and absorption into the bloodstream. Usually, the site of infection is a traumatic or surgical wound. Subcutaneous abscesses at injection sites of intravenous drug abusers or sinusitis of intranasal cocaine abusers may also be the source of *Clostridium botulinum* infection. Neurologic manifestations of wound botulism are similar to those of food-borne botulism; fever from wound infection might occur. In up to a half of patients with wound botulism, the toxin is not detected in the serum and the bacteria cannot be isolated from the wound.

4. *Iatrogenic (inadvertent) botulism.* Botulinum toxin has had an increasing role in treating several neurological disorders including dystonias, spasticity, migraine, and back pain. It has also become a popular agent in the field of cosmetics and plastic surgery. A common adverse effect of the injected toxin using therapeutic doses is its spread from an injected muscle to adjacent muscles. For example, patients with cervical dystonia may develop transient dysphagia when the sternocleidomastoid muscle is injected, and diplopia is a common adverse effect of orbicularis oculi injection in patients with blepharospasm. In addition, the toxin circulates in the blood and produces asymptomatic blockade of transmitter release at distant neuromuscular junctions and in the autonomic nervous system. This has been confirmed by finding prolonged jitter with blocking on single fiber EMG and morphologic abnormalities from muscles distant from the injection. Cases of inadvertent injection of systemically toxic doses of toxin are increasingly being reported. This has resulted in generalized weakness and a disorder that is very similar to classic food-born botulism.

The *diagnosis* of botulism may be difficult and requires a high index of suspicion. Many cases go unrecognized and are diagnosed with various neuromuscular, medical, and

Table C24–1. Diagnosis of 31 Previously Unrecognized Canadian Patients With Botulism After the Identification of Two Teenaged Sisters With Type B Botulism*

Discharge Diagnosis	Number of Patients
Myasthenia gravis	7
Psychiatric illness[†]	4
Viral syndrome	4
Botulism[‡]	3
Stroke	3
Guillain-Barré syndrome	3
Inflammatory myopathy	2
Diabetic complications	1
Hyperemesis gravidarum	1
Hypothyroidism	1
Laryngeal trauma	1
Overexertion	1

*The outbreak was subsequently identified as spoiled commercial chopped garlic in soybean oil.
[†]Includes hysteria, agitated depression, separation reaction, and factitious weakness.
[‡]All three patients were family members whose diagnosis represented the initial recognition of the outbreak.
Data from St. Louis ME et al. Botulism from chopped garlic: delayed recognition of a major outbreak. Ann Intern Med 1988;108:363–368.

even psychiatric diagnoses (Table C24–1). The diagnosis is relatively easy in epidemics, or if two or more cases are identified simultaneously. Botulism should be suspected when there is:

- Rapid, usually descending, muscular weakness (ocular to bulbar to extremities).
- Subacute bilateral ophthalmoplegia, particularly when it is associated with pupillary dilatation.
- Generalized weakness associated with autonomic symptoms (constipation, dry mouth, urinary retention).
- A history of ingestion of possibly contaminated food (canned food, restaurant food, etc.), the presence of a wound, or subacute poor feeding and constipation in infants.

The diagnosis of botulism is confirmed by:

- Electrodiagnostic testing (see following section). This is a rapid, readily available method of identification because the findings are pathognomonic.
- Identification of the toxin in serum, using mouse bioassay studies with antitoxin neutralization. This is usually performed by injecting mice with serum, with or without antitoxin, and observing for death due to paralysis. The sensitivity of serum testing declines if there is a delay in the collection of the specimens; Only one-third of serum samples collected more than 2 days after toxin ingestion are positive.

- Identification of the organism in stool cultures (especially in infantile cases) or wound culture (in wound botulism). *Clostridium botulinum* is found in the stool of 60% of patients with botulism, but this also depends on the timing of samples collection; only one-third of stool cultures are positive after 3 days of acute exposure.

Treatment of botulism should be initiated as soon as the diagnosis is suspected and confirmed by electrophysiologic findings. Specific treatment for botulism is limited, and therapy is primarily supportive.

- Supportive treatment is an essential component in survival. This includes prolonged, artificial ventilation, feeding, prophylaxis for deep vein thrombosis, and physical therapy for prevention of muscle and tendon contractures.
- Efforts to neutralize the toxin should be made. Antitoxin administration is controversial because of the lack of definite efficacy in many cases and the danger of allergic reactions (20% of patients with 2% rate of anaphylaxis). A trivalent antitoxin (A, B, and E) should be administered early, since it is most effective early in the disease while the toxin is still in the blood and before it is bound at the nerve terminals. The antitoxin is unlikely to be effective 3 days or more after toxic exposure. Cleansing the gastrointestinal tract by enema or lactulose and neomycin also is useful, particularly in infantile botulism.
- Agents that enhance the release of ACH can be used as adjuncts. Drugs that potentially help include guanidine and 3,4-diaminopyridine.

The *prognosis* for botulism has been influenced by great advances in critical care and respiratory support. Mortality from botulism in the United States has declined from about 50% before 1950 to 7.5% between 1976 and 1984. Heightened awareness, better recognition, and earlier administration of antitoxin might have played a role in this dramatic improvement in outcome. Recovery of neurologic function is usually protracted because it is dependent on regeneration of new endplates, which may continue for as long as 5 years.

Electrodiagnosis

The EDX studies provide a rapid evidence of botulism awaiting the bioassay and stool cultures. The latter two tests may also be negative. The EDX findings in botulism are compatible with a presynaptic defect of the neuromuscular junction (see electrodiagnosis in Cases 17 and 21). The findings are as follows:

1. Normal sensory nerve conduction studies.
2. Low CMAP amplitudes in 85% of cases, particularly when recording from clinically affected (weak) muscles

Table C24–2. Electrophysiological Differences Between Two Common Presynaptic Neuromuscular Disorders (Botulism and Lambert-Eaton Myasthenic Syndrome)

Electrophysiology	Botulism	Lambert-Eaton Myasthenic Syndrome
Baseline CMAPs	Low in amplitudes, particularly in proximal and weak muscles	Low in amplitudes in all muscles
CMAP increment	Present in clinically affected muscles	Present in all muscles
Degree of CMAP increment	Moderate (30–100%)	Marked (>200%)

(usually proximal), since many muscle fibers do not reach threshold after a single stimulus because of the inadequate release of quanta (vesicles). This is the most consistent EDX finding in botulism. Motor distal latencies and conduction velocities are, however, normal.

3. Decrement of CMAP after slow repetitive stimulation (2 to 3 Hz). This finding is uncommon and is usually mild, not exceeding 8 to 15% of baseline. It is explained by the progressive depletion of the immediately available ACH stores.

4. Increment of CMAP after rapid repetitive stimulation (30 to 50 Hz), or after a brief (10 seconds) of exercise CMAP. With tetanic stimulation, Ca^{2+} influx is greatly enhanced resulting in larger releases of quanta. This leads to increasing number of muscle fibers reaching the threshold required for the generation of muscle action potentials. The CMAP increment in botulism is modest, between 30 and 100%, when compared to the increment in LEMS, which usually is greater than 200% (Table C24–2). This increment may be absent, especially in severely affected muscles particularly when botulism is due to type A toxin.

5. Normal needle EMG or evidence of increased number of short-duration, low-amplitude, and polyphasic motor unit action potentials on needle EMG, with fibrillation potentials in severely weakened muscles. This is best explained by the physiologic blocking of neuromuscular transmission and denervation of many muscle fibers.

6. Increased jitter with blocking on single-fiber EMG. Jitter improves following rapid stimulation owing to enhancement of ACH release by the influx of Ca^{2+} into the presynaptic terminal.

Although the clinical presentations of LEMS and botulism are quite different, their EDX findings are similar, but with certain distinctions, since both are due to a presynaptic defect of ACH release (see Table C24–2).

FOLLOW-UP

After EDX confirmation, the patient's family recalled that the patient had lunch with a friend at a local restaurant the day before the onset of symptoms. Both had a "homemade" soup. The friend became ill that night with severe nausea and vomiting, but subsequent neurologic symptoms did not develop.

The patient was given trivalent antitoxin within 24 hours of diagnosis. However, he continued to worsen over the ensuing days to complete paralysis of all voluntary muscles on days 5 to 7 (except for flicker movements of the hands and feet). Deep tendon reflexes became unelicited. On days 8 to 10, paralytic ileus developed, and the patient lost sphincteric control. Repeated EDX examinations showed a decline in baseline CMAP amplitudes. Bioassay of serum and stool cultures at the Centers for Disease Control (CDC) confirmed the diagnosis of botulism due to *Clostridium botulinum* type A.

Recovery was protracted. The patient was completely paralyzed, except for finger flickers, until day 15. Between days 15 and 30, he showed gradual improvement: strength returned, first in the distal muscles and then proximally. Later, he regained his ability to write and started communicating this way. Paralytic ileus resolved, but ventilation dependency was unchanged, with vital capacity ranging between 500 and 700 mL. Between months 2 and 3, his strength improved such that he could sit and feed himself. Extraocular movements returned gradually to full range. Pupils were still large but started reacting to light. Swallowing and speech improved gradually. During month 4, ventilation improved to allow extubation and then discharge for physical rehabilitation.

When the patient was seen 6 months after the onset of illness, he complained of easy fatigability and poor endurance. He had no appreciable muscle atrophy and minimal weakness of proximal and neck muscles (MRC 5–/5), and he had regained all deep tendon reflexes. Pupils were normal. The patient returned to work 1 month later. Examination 1 year later revealed no abnormality. Baseline CMAPs returned to normal, with absence of increment after rapid repetitive stimulation or postexercise facilitation (Figure C24–6).

DIAGNOSIS

Food-borne botulism.

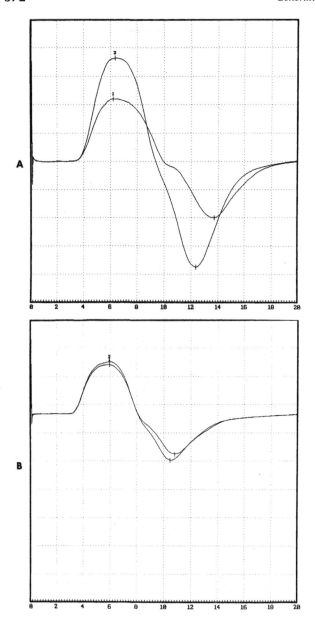

1. C; 2. C; 3. D; 4. C; 5. B

SUGGESTED READINGS

Cherrington M. Botulism. Ten-year experience. Arch Neurol 1974;30:432–437.

Cherrington M. Electrophysiologic methods as an aid in diagnosis of botulism: a review. Muscle Nerve 1982;5:528–529.

Cherington M. Botulism: update and review. Semin Neurol 2004;24:155–163.

Cornblath DR, Sladky JT, Sumner AJ. Clinical electrophysiology of infantile botulism. Muscle Nerve 1983;6:448–652.

Hallet M. One man's poison: clinical applications of botulinum toxin. N Engl J Med 1999;341:118–120.

Hunter WB. Snappy exocytoxins. Nature 1993;365:104–105.

Katirji B, Kaminski HJ. Electrodiagnostic approach to the patient with suspected neuromuscular junction disorder. Neurol Clin 2002;20:557–586.

Pickett JB. Infant botulism: the first five years. Muscle Nerve 1982;5:S26–S27.

Pickett J et al. Syndrome of botulism in infancy: clinical and electrophysiologic study. N Engl J Med 1976;295:770–772.

Robinson RF. Management of botulism. Ann Pharmacother 2003;37:127–131.

Shapiro RL, Hatheway C, Swerdlow DL. Botulism in the United States: a clinical and epidemiologic review. Ann Intern Med 1998;129:221–228.

St. Louis ME et al. Botulism from chopped garlic: delayed recognition of a major outbreak. Ann Intern Med 1988; 108:363–368.

Figure C24–6. *Median compound muscle action potential (CMAP) at rest (waveform 1) and after exercise (waveform 2), during acute illness (**A**) and after recovery (**B**). Sensitivity in (**A**) is 2 mV/division, and in (**B**) it is 5 mV/division. Note the significant increment of CMAP on the first study (90%) and the lack of increment on the second. Note also that the baseline CMAP has improved significantly from 4.2 mV to 9 mV (compare waveforms 1 in (**A**) and (**B**)).*

Case 25

HISTORY AND PHYSICAL EXAMINATION

A 70-year-old woman had a slowly progressive motor weakness, which started 20 years ago. At 50 years of age, she noted weakness of the right hand, which did not respond to surgical carpal tunnel release. Right hand weakness progressed to the point that she could not flex her thumb and index finger. She was relatively stable until age 65, when she began to trip and realized that her left foot was weak. Neurologic examination revealed weakness of left foot eversion and dorsiflexion (Medical Research Council [MRC] 4–/5), significant weakness of the right hand long finger flexors, particularly those to the thumb and index finger. There was atrophy of the right thenar muscles. Deep tendon reflexes and sensory examination were normal. Plantar responses were flexors.

During the next few years, she had further worsening that was slightly more rapid than the earlier course. At 68 years of age, the patient noted weakness of the left hand and right shoulder. She has had increasing difficulty abducting her right arm, using her left hand, and controlling her left foot. There have been no bulbar or sphincteric symptoms.

Neurologic examination at 70 years of age revealed normal cranial nerves and sensation. There was atrophy of the right thenar eminence. No fasciculations were observed. Tone was normal. Muscle strength was as follows (modified MRC scale):

	Right	Left
Shoulder abduction	2/5	5/5
Elbow flexion	3/5	5/5
Elbow extension	4–/5	5/5
Pronation	0/5	3/5
Fingers flexion	0/5	3/5
Wrist flexion	1/5	1/5
Wrist extension	2/5	5/5
Finger extension	3/5	4–/5
Finger abduction	4–/5	3/5

	Right	Left
Hip flexion	5/5	5/5
Hip extension	5/5	5/5
Knee extension	5/5	5/5
Knee flexion	5/5	5/5
Foot dorsiflexion	5/5	1/5
Toe dorsiflexion	5/5	0/5
Plantar flexion	5/5	5/5
Ankle inversion	5/5	5/5
Ankle eversion	5/5	1/5

Deep tendon reflexes revealed absent right brachioradialis and biceps reflexes, as well as both ankle jerks. All other reflexes were normal. Sensation was normal. Gait was impaired by left footdrop. Romberg test was negative. An electrodiagnostic (EDX) study was performed.

Please now review the Nerve Conduction Studies and Needle EMG tables.

QUESTIONS

1. Based on clinical grounds, the differential diagnosis should include all of the following *except:*
   A. Motor neuron disease.
   B. Chronic inflammatory demyelinating polyneuropathy.
   C. Neuropathy associated with anti-myelin-associated glycoprotein (anti-MAG) antibodies.
   D. Neuropathy associated with anti-HU antibodies.
   E. Neuropathy associated with immunoglobulin M (IgM) gammopathy.
2. Laboratory abnormalities that are potentially associated with this disorder include all of the following *except:*
   A. IgM monoclonal gammopathy.
   B. Anti-ganglioside M1 (anti-GM1) antibody.
   C. Anti-YO antibody.
   D. Anti-MAG antibody.

Case 25: Nerve Conduction Studies

Nerve Stimulated	Stimulation Site	Recording Site	Amplitude (m = mV, s = μV)			Distal/Peak Latency (ms)			Conduction Velocity (m/s)			F Latency (ms)	
			Right	Left	Normal	Right	Left	Normal	Right	Left	Normal	Right	Left
Median (s)	Wrist	Index finger	14	12	≥10	3.0	3.1	≤3.8	55		≥50		
Median (s)	Elbow	Index finger	5	4									
Median (s)	Wrist	Middle finger	15	14	≥10	3.0	3.0	≤3.8	62		≥50		
Median (s)	Elbow	Middle finger	6	6									
Ulnar (s)	Wrist	Little finger	12	14	≥5	2.7	2.9	≤3.2	59		≥50		
Ulnar (s)	Elbow	Little finger	6	4									
Radial (s)	Forearm	Dorsum of hand	24	20	≥10	2.6	2.4	≤2.8					
Median (m)	Wrist	APB	**1.6**	**4.0**	≥5.0	3.7	**4.5**	≤4.0	**NR**	**29**	≥50	**NR**	**NR**
Median (m)	Elbow	APB	**NR**	**0.4**									
Ulnar (m)*	Wrist	ADM	6.1	6.4	≥7.0	2.0	2.4	≤3.1	51	49	≥50	32.5	**NR**
Ulnar (m)*	Elbow	ADM	5.6	6.4					52	48	≥50		
Ulnar (m)*	Axilla	ADM	4.0	5.8					50	44	≥50		
Ulnar (m)*	Erb point	ADM	3.2	**1.5**									
Radial (m)*	Elbow	EDC	**3.4**	14.0	≥5.0	2.4	2.6	≤3.1	42	62	≥50		
Radial (m)*	Ab. Spiral gr.	EDC	**0.4**	13.5									
Musculo. (m)*	Axilla	Biceps	6.6		≥3.0	3.8		≤3.5	65		≥50		
Musculo. (m)*	Erb point	Biceps	**0.3**										
Super peron (s)	Leg	Ankle		8	≥3		4.5	≤4.6		46	≥40		
Peroneal (m)	Ankle	EDB		**NR**	≥2.5	4.5	**NR**	≤6.0					**NR**
Peroneal (m)	Knee	EDB		**NR**						**NR**	≥40		
Peroneal (m)	Bel. fib. head	Tibialis anterior	3.8	**2.9**	≥3.0	4.5	3.6	≤4.5					
Peroneal (m)	Knee	Tibialis anterior	3.1	**NR**					53	**NR**	≥40		
Tibial (m)	Ankle	AH		5.0	≥4.0		5.5	≤6.0					48.5
Tibial (m)	Knee	AH		3.9						49	≥40		

Ab. spiral gr. = above spiral groove; ADM = abductor digiti minimi; AH = abductor hallucis; APB = abductor pollicis brevis; Bel. fib. head = below fibular head; EDB = extensor digitorum brevis; EDC = extensor digitorum communis; m = motor; Musculo. = musculocutaneous; NR = no response; s = sensory; Super peron = superficial peroneal.
Data in bold type are abnormal.
*See Figures C25–1, C25–2, and C25–3.

Case 25: Needle EMG

| Muscle | Insertional Activity | Spontaneous Activity | | Voluntary Motor Unit Action Potentials (MUAPs) | | | | | | | |
		Fibs	Fasces	Recruitment Normal	Activation	Reduced	Early	Duration	Amplitude	% Polyphasia	Others
R. abductor pollicis brevis	↓	Rare	0			↓↓↓		↑	↑	Normal	
Flexor pollicis longus	↓	Rare	0			↓↓↓		↑	↑	Normal	1 MUAP
Pronator teres	↓	Rare	0			↓↓		↑	↑	↑	
First dorsal interosseous	Normal	0	0	X				Normal	Normal	Normal	
Abductor digiti minimi	Normal	0	0	X				Normal	Normal	Normal	
Extensor indicis proprius	↑	+/-	0			↓↓↓		↑	Normal	↑	
Extensor dig. communis	↑	+/-	0			↓↓		↑	Normal	↑	
Brachioradialis	↑	+/-	0			↓↓		↑	Normal	↑	
Biceps	↑	+/-	0			↓↓↓		↑	Normal	↑	
Triceps	Normal	0	0			↓		↑	Normal	Normal	
Deltoid	↑	+/-	0			↓↓		↑	Normal	Normal	
Midcervical paraspinal	Normal	0	0	—							

Extensor dig. communis = extensor digitorum communis; Fasces = fasciculations; Fibs = fibrillations; L. = left; R. = right; ↑ = increased; ↓ = reduced; ↓↓ = moderately reduced; ↓↓↓ = severely reduced.

3. The EDX findings observed in this patient are seen least commonly in:
   A. Classic amyotrophic lateral sclerosis.
   B. Chronic inflammatory demyelinating polyneuropathy.
   C. Acute inflammatory demyelinating polyneuropathy.
   D. Multifocal motor neuropathy.

EDX FINDINGS AND INTERPRETATION OF DATA

Relevant EDX findings in this case include:

1. Normal sensory nerve action potentials (SNAPs) amplitudes, distal latencies, and conduction velocities throughout.
2. Multifocal conduction blocks, some partial and others near complete. The motor nerves with conduction blocks are the following:
   • Both median nerves in the forearms.
   • Right radial nerve between the elbow and upper arm (Figure C25–1).
   • Left ulnar nerve between the axilla and Erb point (Figure C25–2).
   • Right musculocutaneous nerve between the axilla and Erb point (Figure C25–3).
   • Left peroneal nerve between the knee and fibular head.

3. Severe impairment of recruitment with scattered fibrillation potentials and increased motor unit action potential (MUAP) duration and polyphasia in muscles that follow multiple peripheral nerve distribution; this correlates anatomically with the sites of conduction block.

In summary, this patient has evidence of multifocal motor neuropathy, with multiple definite conduction blocks. Conduction blocks are common in the chronic acquired demyelinating neuropathies, such as chronic inflammatory demyelinating polyneuropathy (CIDP). However, the preservation of sensory nerve conductions, particularly through nerve segments with motor conduction blocks (such as of the median nerves in the forearms), is a unique feature which is diagnostic of multifocal motor neuropathy (MMN). This motor disorder is not consistent with anti-HU or anti-YO antibody-associated paraneoplastic syndromes associated usually with a sensory neuronopathy (ganglionopathy) or subacute cerebellar degeneration, respectively.

DISCUSSION

Definition and Pathogenesis

Multifocal motor neuropathy (MMN), described in the mid-1980s, is a rare disorder with a prevalence of 1 to

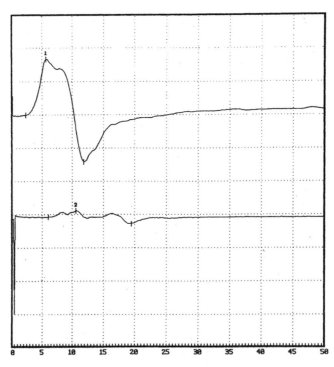

Figure C25–1. *Right radial nerve motor conduction studies, recording the extensor digitorum communis. Note the severe conduction block (>50% CMAP amplitude reduction and >50% CMAP area reduction) between the elbow (waveform 1) and spiral groove (waveform 2) stimulations. Sensitivity = 2 mV/division.*

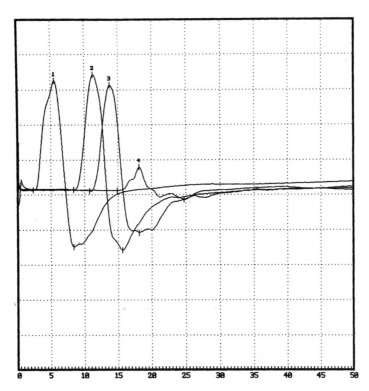

Figure C25–2. *Left ulnar nerve motor conduction studies, recording the abductor digiti minimi, shown superimposed. Waveform 1 = wrist; waveform 2 = elbow; waveform 3 = axilla; waveform 4 = Erb point. Note the conduction block (>50% CMAP amplitude reduction and >50% CMAP area reduction) between the axilla and Erb point stimulation. Sensitivity = 2 mV/division.*

2 individuals per 100 000. It is characterized by specific EDX finding, i.e., motor conduction blocks, which is the gold standard for diagnosis. The disorder is important to recognize since it is treatable and responsive to immunomodulating therapies, and may mimic amyotrophic lateral sclerosis (ALS) which has a poor prognosis for survival.

Many patients with MMN have circulating IgM antibodies to ganglioside M1 (GM1), a glycosphingolipid-incorporating sialic acid residue that is present in both the axolemma and the myelin sheath. Anti-GM1 antibodies frequently recognize the terminal disaccharide moiety of GM1, Gal(1-3)GalNAc, which possesses sialic acid. Although anti-GM1 antibodies bind to motor neurons and the spinal cord, there is ample evidence that the node of Ranvier may be the major site of the effects of anti-GM1 antibodies on peripheral nerves. These antibodies may interfere with sodium channel function localized at the node of Ranvier, as evidenced by the diffuse impairment of nodal resting Na^+ conductance.

Multifocal motor neuropathy is an immune-mediated neuropathy based on the frequent association with anti-GM1 antibodies and the improvement observed in most patients after immune therapies, particularly intravenous

immunoglobulin (IVIG). Also, human sera from patients with MMN produce conduction block when injected in vivo into the peripheral nerves of animals. Pathologic findings at the site of the conduction block include evidence of endoneurial edema, a variable degree of lymphocytic infiltration, demyelination, and onion bulb formation.

CLINICAL FEATURES

Multifocal motor neuropathy presents insidiously with asymmetrical weakness often in the distribution of individual nerves. The age of onset of first symptoms is between 20 and 50 years of age in about 80% of patients, and the disorder is more common in men than women (ratio of 2.6/1). In more than 80% of patients, the weakness starts in the upper limbs, usually hand and forearm muscles. Other than the hypoglossal nerve, cranial nerve involvement is rare. Unilateral or bilateral phrenic nerve palsy causing respiratory failure may occur and is occasionally the presenting symptom. The disorder is slowly progressive, usually for more than 6 months and often years. Sometimes, the history is one of a stepwise progression with episodes of rapid

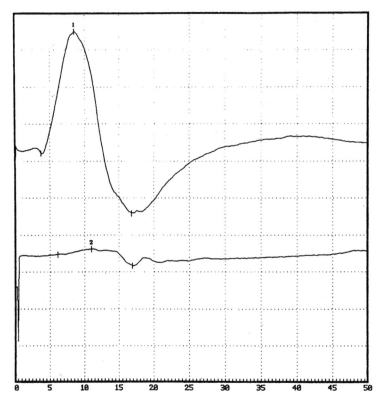

Figure C25–3. *Right musculocutaneous motor conduction studies, recording the biceps. Note the severe conduction block (>50% CMAP amplitude reduction and >50% CMAP area reduction) between the axilla (waveform 1) and Erb point (waveform 2) stimulations. Sensitivity = 2 mV/division.*

worsening followed by prolonged periods of stabilization. The deep tendon reflexes are variable; they are usually depressed or absent diffusely or in weak limbs only. They may be normal or even brisk in one-third of patients, leading to confusion with ALS. Muscle atrophy is not prominent in weak muscles, despite the degree and chronicity of weakness; it may be present over the long term in the distribution of one or more affected nerves, implicating motor axon loss and predicting poor response to therapy. Mild sensory complaints may be present, but the sensory examination is usually normal except for minor vibration sense abnormalities in the lower extremities. A high titer of anti-GM1 antibody is present in approximately 50% of patients, although this varies between 30 and 80%, probably due to the different methodology utilized for antibody measurement. The cerebrospinal fluid protein is usually normal, but may be elevated in one-third of patients without exceeding 100 mg/dL.

Multifocal motor neuropathy should be distinguished from amyotrophic lateral sclerosis, particularly in patients with predominant or exclusive lower motor neuron findings. Clues on clinical examination of patients with MMN include the distribution of weakness, which follows peripheral nerves rather than spinal segments, the insidious course over many years, and the lack of pyramidal signs. It should be cautioned that preserved or brisk reflexes may be present in one-third of patients with MMN. Also, other forms of anterior horn cell disorders, such the spinal muscular atrophies, brachial amyotrophic diplegia (the flail arm syndrome) and monomelic amyotrophy (Hirayama disease) should be excluded. The flail arm syndrome (brachial amyotrophic diplegia), a variant of the progressive muscular atrophy form of ALS, is characterized by progressive proximal and distal upper limb weakness and ultimate variable involvement of the lower limbs. Monomelic amyotrophy (Hirayama disease) affects young men between the age of 15 and 22 and presents with an asymmetrical wasting and weakness of distal upper limb muscles. The disorder is benign, initially progressive over several years and then becoming static. Finally, MMN should be distinguished from other chronic acquired demyelinating peripheral polyneuropathies that may be associated with conduction block or predominantly motor including chronic inflammatory demyelinating polyradiculoneuropathy (CIDP) and its variant the Lewis-Sumner syndrome (multifocal acquired demyelinating sensory and motor neuropathy, MADSAM), osteosclerotic myeloma (POEMS syndrome), and MGUS neuropathy.

Diagnostic criteria for MMN were proposed. The aim of these criteria is to strengthen the diagnosis of MMN and exclude other disorders that may mimic it. They mostly emphasize the mononeuropathy multiplex-like distribution of weakness, presence of multifocal motor conduction block, lack of sensory loss and lack of pyramidal signs. Table C25–1 shows recently accepted criteria for accurate diagnosis of MMN.

The *treatment* options of MMN are limited. In contrast to CIDP, MMN does not respond, or may even worsen, to corticosteroids or plasma exchange. Human intravenous immunoglobulin (IVIG) is highly effective in almost 80% of patients and is shown to be superior to placebo in four randomized, controlled, double-blind studies. Typically, improvement of strength starts 3 to 10 days after infusion; it peaks at approximately 2 weeks and lasts an average of 2 months. Most respondents become dependent on IVIG therapy because the effect of treatment dosage is short-lived and last several weeks only. Thus, periodic IVIG infusion usually is required, usually every 4 to 8 weeks. The recommended dosage is 2 g/kg infused over 2 to 5 consecutive days, although smaller doses may be sufficient to maintain remission. Improvement is more evident in the distribution of recently affected nerves and those without significant muscle atrophy. Also, improvement is variably associated with a demonstrable decrease in the conduction block in some but not all nerves. Sometimes the effectiveness of IVIG decline slightly over the years, probably due to secondary axonal degeneration. The exact mechanism of the beneficial effect of IVIG is not clear. It is possible that the immune attack is altered, allowing recovery of conduction block by unblocking of the sodium channels at the nodes of Ranvier. In patients who do not respond to IVIG, uncontrolled studies have shown that some patients have also responded to monthly high-dose intravenous pulse cyclophosphamide followed by oral cyclophosphamide as a maintenance therapy. Also, Rituximab, a CD20 monoclonal antibody, may also result in modest and delayed improvement (after a year).

Table C25–1. Criteria for the Diagnosis of Multifocal Motor Neuropathy

Core Criteria

1. Slowly progressive asymmetric limb weakness in the distribution of at least two named nerves, for more than one month but usually more than 6 months
2. Conduction blocks in motor nerves outside entrapment sites
3. No objective sensory loss
4. Normal sensory nerve conduction studies (of at least 3 nerves), particularly across the same segments with demonstrated motor conduction block

Exclusion Criteria

1. Upper motor signs (spasticity, clonus, extensor plantar responses and pseudobulbar palsy)
2. Marked bulbar involvement
3. Objective sensory loss except for minor vibration sense abnormalities in the legs
4. Diffuse symmetric weakness during the early stages of symptomatic weakness
5. Markedly elevated cerebrospinal fluid protein (>1 g/L)

Supportive Clinical Criteria

1. Predominant upper limb involvement
2. Reduced or absent deep tendon reflexes in a patchy way or diffusely, but sometimes normal or even brisk reflexes
3. Absence of cranial nerve involvement other than the XIIth cranial nerve
4. Cramps and fasciculations

Other Supportive Criteria

1. Elevated serum IgM anti-GM1 antibodies
2. Gadolinium enhancement and/or hypertrophy of the brachial plexus or peripheral nerve sites of conduction block
3. Clinical improvement to IVIG treatment

Definite multifocal motor neuropathy. Core and exclusion criteria with definite conduction block in two or more motor nerves.
Probable multifocal motor neuropathy. Core and exclusion criteria with (1) probable conduction block in two or more motor nerves, or (2) definite conduction block in one motor nerve and probable conduction block in another motor nerve, or (3) definite conduction block in one motor nerve and at least one of the "other supportive criteria."

Adopted with revisions from European Federation of Neurological Societies/Peripheral Nerve Society. Guideline on management of multifocal motor neuropathy. J Periph Nerv Syst 2006:11;1–8; Olney RK, Lewis RA, Putnam TD et al. Consensus criteria for the diagnosis of multifocal motor neuropathy. Muscle Nerve 2003;27:117–121.

Electrodiagnosis

Multifocal conduction block of motor axons is the hallmark of MMN. The conduction blocks may be seen at any segment of any motor nerve, usually asymmetrically and with predilection to upper extremity nerves. Conduction block, however, is not specific for MMN since it may accompany entrapment and compressive mononeuropathies and most acquired demyelinating polyneuropathies; Hence, finding conduction block on EDX studies should be interpreted in the context of the clinical and other electrophysiological findings. Conduction blocks across common entrapment sites are excluded during the evaluation of MMN. The conduction blocks in MMN are often chronic and persistent for several years. Sometimes, the conduction block is dynamic; it may gradually increase over time or it may occasionally decrease due to decline in distal CMAP amplitude, suggesting secondary axonal degeneration or the appearance of additional very distal conduction blocks. Other EDX signs of demyelination may accompany conduction block. However, these motor nerve abnormalities, such as slowed motor conduction velocities, prolonged distal motor latencies, and prolonged or absent F waves, are not prominent or necessary for the diagnosis of MMN.

There are no uniformly accepted criteria for the identification of conduction block. *Conduction block* is defined as a decrease in the compound muscle action potential (CMAP) amplitude and area on proximal versus distal nerve stimulation, without evidence of significant temporal dispersion (i.e., prolongation of the CMAP duration; Figure C25–4).

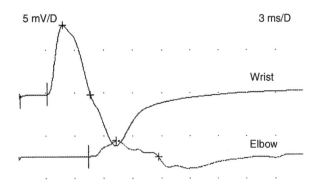

5 mV/D   3 ms/D

Wrist

Elbow

Figure C25–4. *Right median motor nerve conduction study, recording abductor pollicis brevis, in a 52-year-old man with more than 10 years of bilateral asymmetrical hand weakness due to multifocal motor neuropathy. Note the definite conduction block of the median nerve in the forearm (outside common entrapment site).*

Table C25–2 lists recommended practical criteria for the diagnosis of conduction block, particularly in patients with suspected MMN. A detailed and meticulous nerve conduction study of multiple nerves and along many segments of these nerves are essential for the diagnosis of conduction block, which is a prerequisite for establishing the diagnosis of MMN. In general, CMAP amplitude and area decay should be less stringent when evaluating short nerve segments such as with the inching technique (Figure C25–5). This technique may allow precise localization of conduction block by finding an abrupt and focal reduction of CMAP area and amplitude over a very short segment of the nerve. It also helps excluding pseudoconduction block that may be associated with axonal loss and phase cancellation.

It is also important to emphasize avoiding over diagnosing conduction block. Table C25–3 reveals some common errors that are made in the EDX laboratory when attempting to diagnose conduction block. Two situations remain the most challenging and controversial. (1) Differentiating conduction block from abnormal temporal dispersion causes the most difficulty since temporal dispersion may result in CMAP amplitude and area reduction, due to the effects of phase cancellation. Computer analysis studies had suggested that a *reduction of CMAP area of greater than 50% is always caused by a degree of conduction block.* (2) Evaluating for conduction block in the context of axonal loss, such as in peripheral nerves with very low distal CMAPs (<20% of the lower limit of normal or <1 mV) is subject to error. Most proposed criteria intentionally restrict including these nerves to avoid confusion between conduction block and phase cancellation associated with axonal loss.

A finding that is unique to MMN is that *sensory conductions across segments with motor conduction block are normal* (Figure C25–6). Also, despite severe conduction block of the motor nerves, sensory conduction studies, which typically are performed in distal nerve segments (hand or foot), are normal. This distinctive characteristic helps to differentiate MMN from CIDP (and other acquired demyelinating neuropathies), in which the disruption of impulses usually affects both sensory and motor fibers.

Unsettled Issues

Are Antiglycolipid Antibodies Essential for Diagnosis?

High titers of anti-GM1 antibodies are often associated with MMN and decrease with successful treatment. However, the role of these antibodies in the pathogenesis of MMN remains unclear for several reasons. First, only about 50% of the patients with definite MMN have elevated antibodies. Second, elevated anti-GM1 antibodies are not specific for MMN since they may be seen in a

Table C25–2. Electrodiagnostic Criteria for Partial Conduction Block in Multifocal Motor Neuropathy*

Definite Conduction Block[†‡]

>50% CMAP amplitude reduction *and* >50% CMAP area reduction with <30% prolongation of CMAP duration

>30% CMAP amplitude reduction *and* >30% CMAP area reduction with <30% prolongation of CMAP duration over a short nerve segment (such as with the inching technique)

Probable Conduction Block[†‡]

20–50% CMAP amplitude reduction *and* 20–50% CMAP area reduction, with <30% prolongation of CMAP duration

>50% CMAP amplitude reduction *and* >50% CMAP area reduction with 30 to 60% prolongation of CMAP duration

>50% CMAP amplitude reduction *and* >50% CMAP area reduction with <30% prolongation of CMAP duration on stimulations between ankle and knee for the tibial nerve

>50% CMAP amplitude reduction *and* >50% CMAP area reduction with <30% prolongation of CMAP duration on stimulations between axilla and Erb point (for the median, ulnar, radial or musculocutaneous nerves)

---

*All amplitudes, areas, and durations reflect negative-peak areas, amplitudes, and durations comparing responses of proximal to distal stimulations.
[†]Conduction blocks at common entrapment sites are excluded.
[‡]These requirements should be more stringent and sometimes cannot be included in nerves with very low distal CMAP amplitudes (<20% of the lower limit of normal or <1 mV).

variety of neuromuscular disorders, including Guillain-Barré syndrome, amyotrophic lateral sclerosis, and lower motor neuron disease. Third, sera from patients with MMN with or without anti-GM1 antibodies produce conduction block in animals. Fourth, most seronegative patients respond to IVIG and immune therapies in a fashion similar to GM1-positive patients. Hence, elevated titers of anti-GM1 antibodies are not considered a core component of the diagnostic criteria of MMN (see Table C25–1).

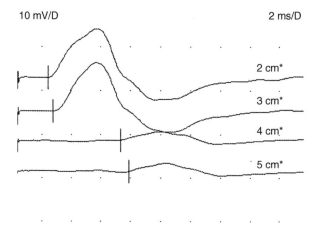

10 mV/D   2 ms/D

2 cm*

3 cm*

4 cm*

5 cm*

Figure C25–5. *Left ulnar motor nerve conduction study, recording abductor digiti minimi, in the distal forearm utilizing the inching technique in a 45-year-old woman with indolent weakness in the distribution of the left ulnar nerve and elevated anti-GM1 antibodies. The distances marked with asterisks depict the distance of the site of stimulation to the styloid process of the ulna. Note the marked sudden drop in CMAP amplitude and area (with a shift in latency) between 3 cm and 4 cm proximal to the ulnar styloid process.*

Is Conduction Block Mandatory for Diagnosis?

Although multifocal partial conduction block is considered the hallmark of the disease, there are increasing reports of patients with MMN who do not have identifiable motor conduction blocks on EDX studies and who respond similarly to IVIG when compared to those with conduction block. These patients are sometimes referred to as "axonal MMN" or "multifocal acquired motor axonopathy." Although these cases may represent patients with primary axonopathies, several other alternative explanations for the absence of conduction block may exist. First, some of these cases may be caused by failure to study several different nerves at several levels such as proximal stimulation at Erb point. Second, underdiagnosis of MMN with conduction block may be due to a stringent criterion of conduction block, such as requiring greater than 50% reduction in CMAP amplitude and area regardless of segment length. Third, some patients with long standing illness were shown to have typical conduction blocks in nerves that decrease or disappear after several years due to progressive decrease in distal CMAP, due to secondary axonal degeneration or the appearance of additional very distal conduction blocks. Since MMN patients without conduction block respond to IVIG, a trial of IVIG is recommended for all patients with MMN with or without conduction block.

CIDP and Its Variants

Though MMN is a purely motor disorder, sensory symptoms are sometimes reported by patients and objective sensory loss may be seen in about 20% of patients. Also, subtle abnormalities in sensory NCSs and sural nerve biopsies may be noted in a few patients. These sensory abnormalities may suggest alternative diagnosis particularly

Table C25–3. Common False-Positive Results in the Diagnosis of Conduction Block

Failure to reach supramaximal percutaneous stimulation (proximal sites, obesity, edema)
Evaluation of long peripheral nerves (tibial nerve, tall subjects)
Abnormal temporal dispersion with phase cancellation
Evaluation of peripheral nerves with very low distal CMAPs (<20% of the lower limit of normal or <1 mV) suggestive of axonal loss

the Lewis-Sumner syndrome (MADSAM), a variant of CIDP. In general, if the sensory nerve action potentials are unelicitable or are grossly abnormal, other demyelinating neuropathies, particularly the Lewis-Sumner syndrome and CIDP, must be interpreted (Table C25–4). The distinction between MMN and CIDP and the Lewis-Sumner syndrome is important since plasma exchange and corticosteroids are usually effective in CIDP and the

Lewis-Sumner syndrome, while ineffective and sometimes harmful in MMN.

FOLLOW-UP

Antibody to GM1 was elevated moderately in the serum, with a titer of 1/1600 (normal = <1/800). Serum protein

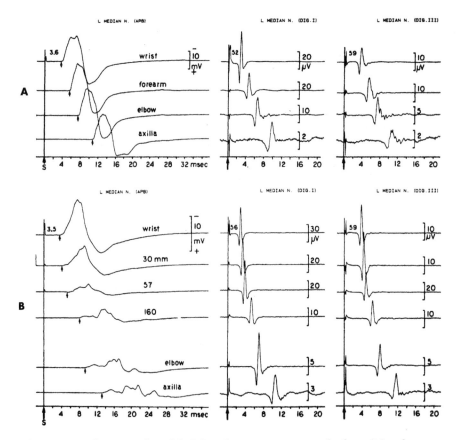

Figure C25–6. *Motor and sensory conduction studies of the left median nerve in a control subject (**A**) and a patient with multifocal motor neuropathy with conduction block (**B**). The site of stimulation is indicated above the traces in the left column. The median nerve was stimulated in the patient at the wrist; 30 mm, 57 mm, and 160 mm proximal to the wrist; at the elbow; and at the axilla. The sensory nerve action potentials (SNAPs) evoked at digit I (middle column) and digit III (right column) were recorded at the same recording sites. The distal motor latencies and sensory conduction velocities are indicated above the uppermost trace in each column. Despite severe conduction block and dispersion of motor responses in the patient, the decrease in amplitude of the SNAP was not different from that in the control. (From Krarup C et al. A syndrome of asymmetric limb weakness with motor conduction block. Neurology 1990;40:118–127, with permission.)*

Table C25–4. Comparison of Three Different Acquired Demyelinating Polyneuropathies: CIDP, Lewis-Sumner Syndrome, and Multifocal Motor Neuropathy

Feature	Chronic Inflammatory Demyelinating Polyneuropathy	Lewis-Sumner Syndrome	Multifocal Motor Neuropathy
Age at onset	Adults of all ages, children rarely	Adults of all ages	Adults of all ages
Sex	Slight male predominance	Males much more common	Males much more common
Duration of illness at presentation	Varies widely – days to years. Usually months	Usually years	Usually years
Weakness	Symmetric	Asymmetric, in the distribution of peripheral nerves. Upper > lower extremities; distal > proximal	Asymmetric, in the distribution of peripheral nerves. Upper > lower extremities; distal > proximal
Sensory impairment	Symmetric	Asymmetric, in the distribution of sensory nerves	Minimal or none
Reflexes	Generally absent	Focally decreased or absent	Focally decreased or absent
Sensory nerve studies	Usually abnormal	Usually abnormal	Normal
Motor nerve studies	Acquired demyelination. Conduction block, abnormal temporal dispersion, slowed conduction velocities, prolonged distal latencies, prolonged F wave latencies	Acquired demyelination. Conduction block, abnormal temporal dispersion, slowed conduction velocities, prolonged distal latencies, prolonged F wave latencies	Acquired demyelination. Conduction block, abnormal temporal dispersion, slowed conduction velocities, prolonged distal latencies, prolonged F wave latencies
Anti-GM1 antibodies	May be present, usually not at high titers	Usually absent	High titers in about half
CSF protein	Usually elevated	Usually elevated	Usually normal. May be elevated to <100 mg/dL
Sensory nerve biopsy	Demyelination, axonal degeneration, mononuclear inflammation, endoneurial edema	Demyelination	Normal or minor abnormalities
Usual treatments	Prednisone, IVIG, plasma exchange	Prednisone, IVIG	IVIG, cyclophosphamide, rituximab
Course	Relapsing, monophasic, or progressive	Progressive until treated	Progressive until treated

Adapted with revisions from Simmons Z, Albers JW. In: Katirji B, Kaminski HJ, Preston DC, Ruff RL, Shapiro EB, eds. Neuromuscular disorders in clinical practice. Boston, MA: Butterworth-Heinemann, 2002, pp. 567–588.

electrophoresis and immunofixation were normal. Cerebrospinal fluid examination revealed normal protein. The patient was infused with IVIG (total 2 g/kg), which resulted in dramatic improvement of the right shoulder and wrist and the left hand. This effect was maximal in 10 days and stabilized for 2 weeks, but the patient's strength worsened again. She was given periodic IVIG every 4 weeks, with good results. Neurologic examination 6 months after the institution of therapy revealed significant improvement of the right upper extremity, particularly the biceps and wrist extensors, and of the left median innervated muscles. Repeat motor conduction showed significant improvement in conduction blocks (Figure C25–7). The patient has been maintained for the last 10 years on periodic IVIG every 6 to 8 weeks with no loss of effectiveness.

DIAGNOSIS
Multifocal motor neuropathy with conduction block.

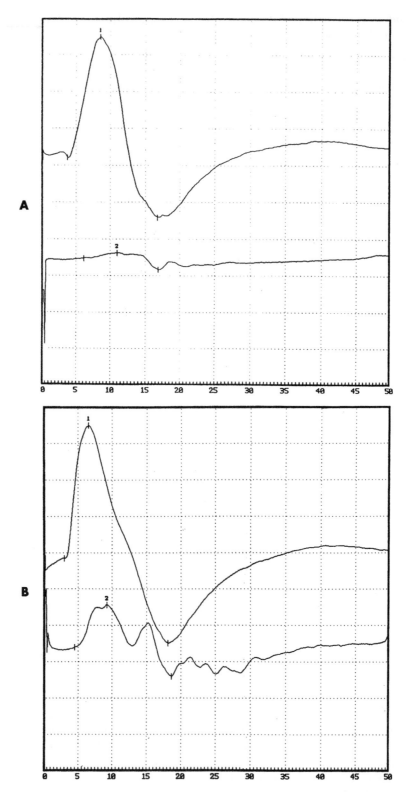

Figure C25–7. *Right musculocutaneous motor conduction studies, recording the biceps, while stimulating at the axilla (1) and Erb point (2), before (**A**) and 6 months after treatment with intravenous immunoglobulin (**B**). Note that the severe conduction block noted with Erb point (2) stimulations initially improved significantly, though not completely, after therapy. Sensitivity = 2 mV/division.*

ANSWERS

1. D; 2. C; 3. A.

SUGGESTED READINGS

American Association of Electrodiagnostic Medicine. Consensus criteria for the diagnosis of partial conduction block. Muscle Nerve 1999;22:S225–S229.

Boonyapisit K, Katirji B. Multifocal motor neuropathy with conduction block presenting with respiratory failure. Muscle Nerve 2000;23:1887–1890.

Chaudhry V et al. Multifocal motor neuropathy: response to human immune globulin. Ann Neurol 1993;33:237–242.

Chaudhry V, Corse AM, Cornblath DR et al. Multifocal motor neuropathy: electrodiagnostic features. Muscle Nerve 1994; 17:198–205.

Delmont E, Azulay JP, Girogi et al. Multifocal motor neuropathy with or without conduction block: a single entity? Neurology 2006;67:592–596.

European Federation of Neurological Societies/Peripheral Nerve Society. Guideline on management of multifocal motor neuropathy. J Periph Nerv Syst 2006;11:1–8.

Kaji R et al. Pathological findings at the site of conduction block in multifocal motor neuropathy. Ann Neurol 1993;33: 152–158.

Katirji B. Chronic relapsing axonal neuropathy responsive to intravenous immunoglobulins. Neurology 1997;48:1690–1694.

Katz JS, Wolfe GI, Bryan WW et al. Electrophysiologic findings in multifocal motor neuropathy. Neurology 1997;48:700–707.

Kornberg AJ, Pestronk A. Chronic motor neuropathies: diagnosis, therapy, and pathogenesis. Ann Neurol 1995;37(S1): S43–S50.

Krarup C et al. A syndrome of asymmetric limb weakness with motor conduction block. Neurology 1990;40:118–127.

Lewis RA. Multifocal motor neuropathy and Lewis-Sumner syndrome. Two distinct entities. Muscle Nerve 199;22: 1738–1739.

Lewis RA et al. Multifocal demyelinating neuropathy with persistent conduction block. Neurology 1982;32:958–964.

Nobile-Orazio E, Cappellari A, Priori A. Multifocal motor neuropathy: current concept and controversies. Muscle Nerve 2005;31:663–680.

Oh SJ et al. Multifocal demyelinating motor neuropathy: pathologic evidence of inflammatory demyelinating polyradiculoneuropathy. Neurology 1995;45:1828–1832.

Olney RK, Lewis RA, Putnam TD et al. Consensus criteria for the diagnosis of multifocal motor neuropathy. Muscle Nerve 2003;27:117–121.

Parry GJ. Antiganglioside antibodies do not necessarily play a role in multifocal motor neuropathy. Muscle Nerve 1994; 17:97–99.

Parry GJ, Clarke S. Multifocal acquired demyelinating neuropathy masquerading as motor neuron disease. Muscle Nerve 1988;11:103–107.

Pestronk A. Motor neuropathies, motor neuron disorders and antiglycolipid antibodies. Muscle Nerve 1991;14:927–936.

Robers M et al. Multifocal motor neuropathy human sera block distal motor nerve conduction in mice. Ann Neurol 1995;38:111–118.

Terenghi F, Cappellari A, Bersano A et al. How long is IVIG effective in multifocal motor neuropathy? Neurology 2004;62:666–668.

Van Schaik IN, Bossuyt PM, Brand A et al. Diagnostic value of GM1 antibodies in motor neuron disorders and neuropathies: a meta-analysis. Neurology 1995;45:1570–1577.

Van Schaik IN, Van den Berg LH, de Haan R et al. Intravenous immunoglobulin for multifocal motor neuropathy. Cochrane Database of Systematic Reviews 2005;2.

Case 26

HISTORY AND PHYSICAL EXAMINATION

A 45-year-old man noted numbness in both toes for almost two years prior. The numbness had ascended to the ankles and lower legs. More recently, he noted numbness in the tips of his fingers. Burning pain followed in the same distribution. He also had mild imbalance. Upon review of systems, he admits to a 30 pounds weight loss over 3–4 years. He had mild hypertension and was on metoprolol. He smoked half a pack of cigarette a day and drank 1–2 pints of whiskey a day. There was no history of other toxic exposures or megavitamin consumption. There was no family history of neurological disease.

On examination, he was 6 ft 1 in tall and weighed 140 pounds. His lying and standing blood pressures were 140/85 and 138/80, respectively. His general physical examination was normal except for slight discoloration of skin in both feet with brittle toenails. Peripheral pulses were normal. On neurological examination, the mental status and cranial nerves were normal. The motor examination reveals atrophy of intrinsic muscles of foot bilaterally with mild weakness of ankle dorsiflexors and plantar flexors as well as toe extensors and flexors. There was no weakness or atrophy of hand muscles or proximal muscles. Sensory examination revealed a symmetrical decrease in pain, touch, and temperature sensations in both legs and fingers in a distal to proximal gradient. Position and vibration sense were diminished at the toes but normal elsewhere. Deep tendon reflexes were +2 and symmetrical in the upper extremities and at the knees while the ankle jerks were absent. Plantar responses were normal. Gait was normal but tandem gait was slightly impaired. Romberg test was negative. Electrodiagnostic (EDX) study was requested.

Please now review the Nerve Conduction Studies and Needle EMG tables.

QUESTIONS

1. All the following represent axonal polyneuropathies *except*:
   A. Diabetic polyneuropathy.
   B. Charcot-Marie-Tooth disease type 1.
   C. Alcoholic polyneuropathy.
   D. Critical illness polyneuropathy.
   E. Charcot-Marie-Tooth disease type 2.

2. Electrodiagnostic features of axonal polyneuropathies include all the following *except*:
   A. Conduction velocities greater than 80% of lower limits of normal.
   B. Low compound muscle action potential (CMAP) amplitudes.
   C. Low or absent sensory nerve action (SNAP) potentials.
   D. Distal latencies greater than 120% of upper limits of normal.

3. Characteristics of alcoholic polyneuropathy include all the following *except*:
   A. It is a chronic symmetric sensorimotor peripheral polyneuropathy.
   B. It is easily distinguished from diabetic and uremic polyneuropathy.
   C. It is often nutritional in origin.
   D. It may respond to abstinence and vitamin supplementation.

EDX FINDINGS AND INTERPRETATION OF DATA

The abnormal EDX findings in this case include:

1. Absent sensory nerve action potentials (SNAP) in both lower extremities and low SNAP amplitudes in the

Case 26: Nerve Conduction Studies

Nerve Stimulated	Stimulation Site	Recording Site	Amplitude (m = mV, s = µV)			Distal/Peak Latency (ms)			Conduction Velocity (m/s)			F Latency (ms)	
			Right	Left	Normal	Right	Left	Normal	Right	Left	Normal	Right	Left
Sural (s)	Calf	Ankle	NR	NR	>5	NR	NR	<4.5					
Superficial peroneal (s)	Leg	Ankle	**NR**	**NR**	>5	**NR**	**NR**	<4.5					
Peroneal (m)	Ankle	EDB	**1.0**	**0.9**	>2.5	5.6	5.7	<5.6				**49**	**47.5**
Peroneal (m)	Bel. Fib. head	EDB	**0.8**	**0.7**					39	38	>40		
Peroneal (m)	Knee	EDB	**0.7**	**0.6**					37	38	>40		
Tibial (m)	Ankle	AH	**3.5**	**3.8**	>8	**6.1**	**6.0**	<6.0				**52**	**51.4**
Tibial (m)	Knee	AH	**2.5**	**2.6**					37	38	>40		
Peroneal (m)	Bel. Fib. head	Tibialis anterior	**3.8**		>4	3.8		<4.0					
Peroneal (m)	Knee	Tibialis anterior	**3.6**						42		>40		
Median (s)	Wrist	Index	10	**8**	>20	3.3	**3.4**	<3.4					
Ulnar (s)	Wrist	Little Finger	**5**	**5**	>12	3.1	3.2	<3.1					
Radial (s)	Forearm	Snuffbox	16		>18	2.8		<2.7					
Median (m)	Wrist	APB	**4.0**		>6	3.8		<3.9					30
Median (m)	Elbow	APB	**3.8**						49		>50		
Ulnar (m)	Wrist	ADM	**4.4**		>7	3.0		<3.1					31
Ulnar (m)	Below elbow	ADM	**4.0**						51		>50		
Ulnar (m)	Above elbow	ADM	**3.8**						50		>50		

ADM = abductor digiti minimi; AH = abductor hallucis; APB = abductor pollicis brevis; EDB = extensor digitorum brevis; L. = left; NR = no response; R. = right. Data in bold type are abnormal.

Case 26: Needle EMG

Muscle	Insertional Activity	Spontaneous Activity		Voluntary Motor Unit Action Potentials (MUAPs)							
		Fibs	Fascs	Recruitment				Configuration			
				Normal	Activation	Reduced	Early	Duration	Amplitude	% Polyphasia	Others
Right Abductor hallucis	↑	1+	0			↓↓↓		↑↑↑	↑	Normal	
Extensor digitorum brevis	↑	1+	0			↓↓↓		↑↑↑	↑	Normal	
Extensor hallucis longus	↑	1+	0			↓↓		↑↑	↑	Normal	
Tibialis posterior	↑	1+	0			↓↓		↑↑	↑	Normal	
Tibialis anterior	↑	+/−	0			↓		↑↑	Normal	Normal	
Medial gastrocnemius	↑	+/−	0			↓		↑	↑	↑	
Vastus lateralis	Normal	0	0	X						Normal	
Left Tibialis anterior	↑	+/−	0			↓		↑	↑	Normal	
Medial gastrocnemius	↑	+/−	0			↓↓		↑	↑	Normal	
Vastus lateralis	Normal	0	0	X				Normal	Normal	Normal	
Right first dorsal interosseous	↑	+/−	0			↓		↑	↑	Normal	
Abductor pollicis brevis	↑	+/−	0			↓		↑	↑	Normal	
Flexor pollicis longus	Normal	0	0	X				↑	Normal	Normal	
Pronator teres	Normal	0	0	X				Normal	Normal	Normal	
Biceps	Normal	0	0	X				Normal	Normal	Normal	
Triceps	Normal	0	0	X				Normal	Normal	Normal	
Deltoid	Normal	0	0	X				Normal	Normal	Normal	
Left first dorsal interosseous	↑	+/−	0			↓		↑	↑	Normal	
Biceps	Normal	0	0	X				Normal	Normal	Normal	

Fascs = Fasciculations; Fibs = Fibrillations; ↑, ↑↑, ↑↑↑ = mildly, moderately, markedly increased, respectively; ↓, ↓↓, ↓↓↓ = mildly, moderately, markedly decreased, respectively.

upper extremities. This is symmetrical and worse in the lower than the upper extremities.

2. Low compound muscle action potential (CMAP) amplitudes with either normal or borderline distal latencies, conduction velocities and F wave minimal latencies. This is symmetrical in the lower extremities and worse in the lower than the upper extremities. Also, it is worse distally in the lower extremities by comparing the peroneal motor conduction study recording extensor digitorum brevis to the study recording tibialis anterior.

3. Fibrillation potentials and decrease in motor unit action potential (MUAP) recruitment in the lower and upper extremities, worse in the lower and distally. The recruited MUAPs in the affected muscles are long in duration and, sometimes, high in amplitude and polyphasic.

The above findings are consistent with a generalized disorder affecting the sensory and motor fibers, worse distally. The recorded SNAPs and CMAPs are characterized by being low in amplitudes, but with either no or minimal slowing of distal latencies, conduction velocities, and F wave minimal latencies. These findings are diagnostic of a generalized, axonal, dying-back, sensorimotor, peripheral polyneuropathy, chronic with active (ongoing) denervation and reinnervation. This polyneuropathy is compatible with a wide range of disorders including alcoholic polyneuropathy, diabetic polyneuropathy, uremic polyneuropathy, nutritional polyneuropathy, or toxic polyneuropathy.

DISCUSSION

Definition and Pathogenesis

Peripheral Polyneuropathy

Peripheral neuropathy is a relatively common disorder with a prevalence that may reach up to 10% of the general population. Peripheral neuropathy is often a manifestation of a systemic disease such as diabetes, alcohol abuse, or leprosy. However, about 20% of neuropathies remain idiopathic; a significant number of these cases are likely inherited in nature.

The myriad of etiologies of peripheral neuropathy pose a daunting task for the clinician. Investigating peripheral neuropathy has included several approaches. First, is the *pattern recognition approach* where a diagnosis of a polyneuropathy is based on highly specific associated findings such as the Mee line in arsenic or thallium poisoning, red tongue in vitamin B12 deficiency, or predilection of the sensory loss to cool areas of the body (such as earlobes, nipples, and buttock) in leprosy. Unfortunately, this

approach applies to a minority of patients usually with advanced disease, requires a vast clinical experience and is mostly accomplished by senior neurologists. The second approach frequently used by many physicians (including some neurologists) is a *"shotgun" approach* by ordering a battery of tests on every patient with a neuropathy. This irrational approach is costly and may result in incorrect diagnosis secondary to incidental abnormalities, such as elevated blood glucose in a patient with CIDP. The third recommended approach is a *systematic approach* that utilizes mainly the clinical findings and EDX studies to generate a more limited differential diagnosis and help guide the laboratory investigations necessary for establishing a final diagnosis (Table C26–1). Additional studies that are useful in the accurate diagnosis of peripheral neuropathy include autonomic testing, quantitative sensory testing, antibody testing, and skin or cutaneous nerve biopsy.

It is important to try defining the predominant pathophysiologic mechanism of the polyneuropathy, though the clinical examination is often unable to discriminate between a primarily axonal and demyelinating polyneuropathy. Demyelinating polyneuropathies have a limited number of etiologies, while the causes of axonal polyneuropathies, particularly those that are chronic and affect the sensory and motor axons, are numerous (Table C26–2).

Alcoholic Polyneuropathy

Chronic alcoholism is a relatively common cause of generalized sensorimotor polyneuropathy. The incidence of alcoholic polyneuropathy is unknown, but is likely underestimated since many asymptomatic alcoholic patients have physical or EDX signs of polyneuropathy. The incidence ranges from 9 to 30% among hospitalized alcoholics, and up to 90% of ambulatory alcoholics may have EDX evidence of neuropathy. Alcoholic polyneuropathy almost always occurs on a background of nutritional deficiency, particularly thiamine (vitamin B1) deficiency, and its clinical features are almost identical to beriberi. A history of poor nutrition is often present, and the diet of alcoholics is usually high in carbohydrates and low in vitamins. Moreover, alcoholics have a reduced capacity to absorb thiamine. Since the total lifetime dose of alcohol is an important factor in neuropathy, a direct neurotoxic effect of alcohol on peripheral nerves remain a possibility and cannot be totally excluded.

The clinical manifestations of alcoholic polyneuropathy are typical of a length-dependent generalized, sensorimotor polyneuropathy. The neuropathy is often asymptomatic and only detected by clinical or EDX examination. The symptoms begin usually symmetrically with numbness, paresthesias, and burning feet, followed by cramps, weakness, and sensory ataxia. The symptoms are chronic and

Table C26–1. Essential Steps in the Classification and Etiologic Diagnosis of Peripheral Polyneuropathy

The Temporal Profile of the Polyneuropathy
Is the polyneuropathy subacute or chronic?

If chronic, is the disorder progressive, relapsing and remitting, or stepwise?

Subacute – consider Guillain-Barré syndrome, porphyria, diphtheria, critical illness, and drugs/toxins

Chronic relapsing and remitting – consider CIDP and drugs/toxins

Chromic progressive – consider CIDP, metabolic disorder*, nutritional deficiency, and toxins

The Anatomic Pattern of the Polyneuropathy
Is the polyneuropathy distal, proximal, or both?

Are there any foot or spine deformities (pes cavus or kyphoscoliosis)?

Is the polyneuropathy symmetric or asymmetric?

If asymmetric, do the findings follow specific peripheral nerve distribution?

Distal – consider metabolic disturbance*, vitamin deficiency, toxins, drugs, critical illness, hereditary

Distal and proximal – consider Guillain-Barré syndrome, CIDP, porphyria

Asymmetric – consider vasculitis, CIDP, HNPP

Mononeuropathy multiplex – consider multifocal motor neuropathy, Lewis-Sumner syndrome, HNPP, vasculitis, leprosy

Pes cavus or kyphoscoliosis – consider CMT, HNPP

The Type(s) of Nerve Fiber Involvement
Is the polyneuropathy sensory, motor, or mixed?

If sensory, is it small fiber, large fiber, or both?

Are the autonomic fibers involved?

Large fiber sensory – consider Sjögren syndrome, anti-HU paraneoplastic disease, vitamin E deficiency, and vitamin B6 intoxication

Small fiber sensory – consider diabetes, amyloidosis, HIV, metabolic disturbance*, toxins, drugs, or amyloidosis

Autonomic – consider Guillian-Barré syndrome, metabolic disturbance*, amyloidosis, HIV infection

Family History of Polyneuropathy
Is there a family history of polyneuropathy?

Is there a family history of foot deformities (pes cavus) or the spine (kyphoscoliosis)?

Autosomal dominant – consider CMT 1, CMT2, CMT3, HNPP

X-linked – consider CMTX

Autosomal recessive – consider CMT4, CMT3

Medical Illness and Exposure to Drugs or Toxins
Is the exposure time locked to the onset of symptoms?

Did eliminating the exposure stop progression of polyneuropathy?

Medical illness – consider diabetes mellitus, chronic renal insufficiency, hypothyroidism, HIV infection, connective tissue disease, myeloproliferative disorders (+/– paraproteinemia), celiac disease, and paraneoplastic disease

Drugs – consider vincristine, paclitaxil, cisplatin, amiodarone, hydralazine, isoniazid, metronidazole, nitrofurantoin, disulfiram, thalidomide, gold, and pyridoxine (toxicity)

Toxins – consider ethyl alcohol, arsenic, thallium, acrylamide, nitric oxide, ethylene oxide, n-hexane, perhexiline, and methyl n-butyl ketone

Primary Pathology (Axonal or Demyelinating)
Is the polyneuropathy primarily axonal or demyelinating?

If demyelinating, is it segmental (multifocal) or uniform?

Axonal – consider metabolic disturbance,* toxins, drugs, critical illness, CMT2, CMT4

Demyelinating and segmental (multifocal) – consider Guillain-Barré syndrome, CIDP, CIDP with paraproteinemia, HNPP

Demyelinating and uniform – consider CMT1, CMT3, CMTX

CIDP = chronic inflammatory demyelinating polyradiculoneuropathy; CMT = Charcot-Marie-Tooth disease; HIV = human immunodeficiency virus; HNPP = hereditary neuropathy with liability to pressure palsy.

*Include diabetes mellitus, uremia, thyroid disorders.

Table C26–2. Common Causes of Chronic Symmetrical Axonal Peripheral Polyneuropathies

Metabolic disorders	HTLV1	Gold
Diabetes	Lyme disease	Hydralazine
Hypothyroidism	Hereditary disorders	Metronidazole
Acromegaly	CMT2	Nitrofurantoin
Deficiency states	CMTX	Phenytoin
Vitamin B12	Toxins	Thalidomide
Vitamin B1	Alcohol	Vincristine
Gastric bypass surgery	Arsenic	Malignancies (paraneoplastic)
Paraproteinemia	Thallium	Others
MGUS associated (IgA/IgG)	n-Hexane	Celiac disease/sprue
Multiple myeloma	Acrylamide	Whipple disease
Amyloidosis	Carbon disulfide (CS2)	Vasculitis
Connective tissue disorders	Organophosphate	Sarcoidosis
SLE	Ethylene oxide	Cryptogenic
Sjögren syndrome	Drugs	
Rheumatoid arthritis	Amiodarone	
Mixed connective tissue disorder	Chloroquine	
Infections	Colchicine	
HIV	Disulfuram	

CMT = Charcot-Marie-Tooth disease; HIV = human immunodeficiency virus; HTLV1 = human T lymphotropic virus type 1; MGUS = monoclonal gammopathy of unknown significance; SLE = systemic lupus erythematosus.

usually evolve slowly over months or years. Overt manifestations of autonomic dysfunction, such as orthostatic hypotension, are relatively uncommon. Weight loss, often in the range of 30–40 pounds or about 10% of body weight, is common but not always present. The neurological examination discloses a sensory loss to most modalities and muscle weakness in the lower extremities in a distal to proximal gradient. Allodynia and calf tenderness may also be present. Areflexia or hyporeflexia is also worse distally. Findings of other neurological alcoholic-nutritional deficiency states may coexist, such as cerebellar degeneration or Wernicke-Korsakoff syndrome. The laboratory tests are most useful in excluding other causes of polyneuropathy. Macrocytic anemia, abnormal liver function tests, and MRI evidence of cerebellar atrophy are common supportive findings for alcoholism.

Alcoholic polyneuropathy is managed by abstinence from alcohol intake and enhancing diet with vitamin supplements including thiamine. Pain control with anticonvulsant or antidepressants may be necessary is some patients. The prognosis depends on the severity and duration of symptoms; patients with mild and recent symptoms are more likely to improve or recover.

Electrodiagnosis

The EDX testing is an essential diagnostic tool in peripheral neuropathies, being most useful when utilized as a direct extension of the neurological examination. In a patient with suspected peripheral polyneuropathy, the EDX study often:

1. Provides an unequivocal diagnosis of peripheral polyneuropathy.
2. Excludes mimickers of polyneuropathies such as L5 and S1/S2 radiculopathies, tarsal tunnel syndromes, carpal tunnel syndromes, and distal myopathies.
3. Defines the anatomic distribution of a neuropathy, as a single mononeuropathy, multiple mononeuropathies, or a generalized peripheral polyneuropathy.
4. Establish the type of fiber(s) affected (sensory, motor, or both).
5. Estimate the duration and activity of the neuropathy (acute, active (ongoing) or chronic).
6. Identify the primary pathophysiologic process (axonal loss, uniform demyelination, multifocal demyelination, or conduction block).

At the completion of the EDX study, the clinician should be able to better characterize the polyneuropathy and classify its pathophysiology. This helps establish a relatively short differential diagnosis and work-up aimed at identifying the cause of the neuropathy and planning its management (Figure C26–1).

Analyzing conduction times (velocities and latencies), as well as CMAP amplitude, area, and duration, is an essential exercise in the EMG laboratory for establishing the

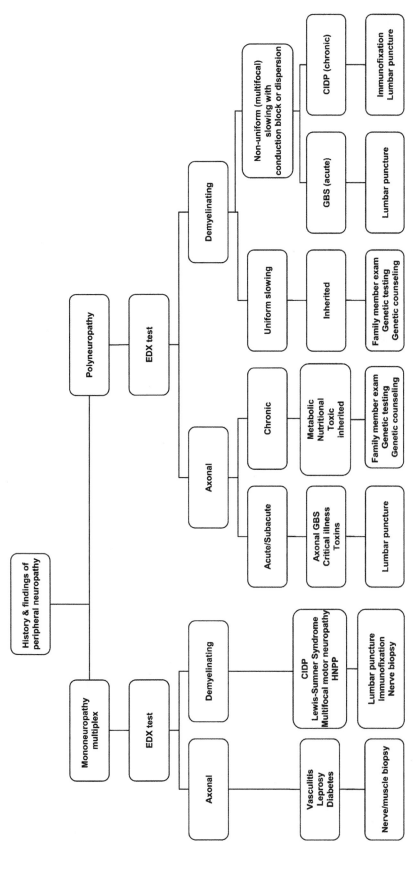

Figure C26-1. *A practical approach to peripheral neuropathy. CIDP = chronic inflammatory demyelinating polyneuropathy; HNPP = hereditary neuropathy with lia-bility to pressure palsy; GBS = Guillain-Barré syndrome. (Adapted with revisions from Asbury AK, Gilliatt RW. The clinical approach to neuropathy. In: Asbury AK, Gilliatt RW, eds. Peripheral nerve disorders. London: Butterworths, 1994).*

primary pathologic process of a polyneuropathy. In most situations, the polyneuropathy falls in one of the two categories based on which of the two primary nerve fiber components is dysfunctional: the axon or its supporting myelin. Occasionally, such as in very mild polyneuropathies or in severe situations associated with absent sensory and motor responses, it may be difficult to establish the primary pathology based on EDX studies.

- *Primary axonal polyneuropathies (axonopathies)* affect the axon primarily and produce a length-dependent dying-back degeneration of axons. These findings are first observed in the lower extremities but in more severe cases, similar alterations occur in the upper extremities. The major change on nerve conduction studies is a decrease, or absence in more advanced disease, of the CMAP and SNAP amplitudes, more marked in the lower extremities (see Figure C18–4B, Case 18). In contrast, conduction times (velocities, distal latencies, and F wave minimal latencies) are normal. Sometimes, there is a slight slowing of distal latencies, conduction velocities and F wave minimal latencies when the polyneuropathy is advanced (Figure C26–2). This is explained by the fact that the loss of axons is distributed in a random fashion, which results in survival of some thickly myelinated, fast-conducting fibers. Figure C26–3 reveals the theoretical distribution of conduction

velocity in motor nerves of healthy patients and patients with axonal polyneuropathy. The random axonal loss results in survival of some, fast-conducting fibers leading to normal velocities. It is only when axonal loss is severe, surpassing 80% of the total population of axons, that slight slowing of velocities occurs. In these situations, conduction velocities should be no less than 80% of the lower limit of normal and the distal latencies should be no more than 120% of the upper limits of normal.

- *Primary demyelinating polyneuropathies (myelinopathies)* are, in contrast, characterized by significant slowing of conduction times (velocities, distal latencies, and F wave latencies) because the pathologic process results in myelin disruption (segmental and paranodal demyelination) which impedes saltatory conduction (see Figure C18–4C, Case 18). Commonly, the CMAP amplitudes are relatively preserved distally, although conduction blocks and dispersion are common in the acquired forms (such as chronic inflammatory demyelinating polyneuropathy). With distal stimulation, the CMAP is mildly reduced in amplitude because of temporal dispersion and phase cancellation. The distal latency is slowed (>120% of upper limit of normal) because of demyelination. With more proximal stimulation, the CMAP is much lower in amplitude, which results from temporal dispersion and conduction block along some fibers. The proximal conduction

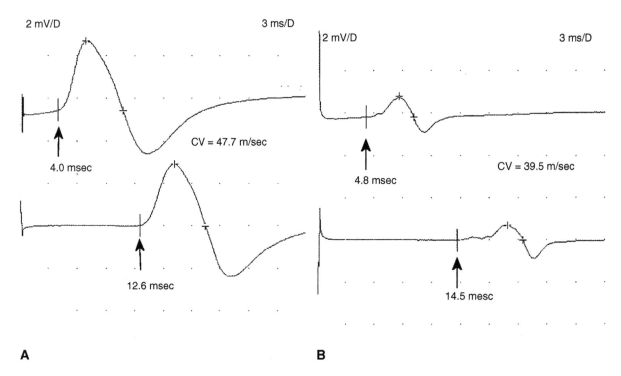

Figure C26–2. *Peroneal motor conduction nerve conduction studies recording extensor digitorum brevis in a control (**A**) and in an age-matched patient with axonal polyneuropathy due to chronic alcoholism (**B**). Note the significant decrease in CMAP amplitudes in (**B**) compared to (**A**), while there is only slight slowing of distal latencies and conduction velocities.*

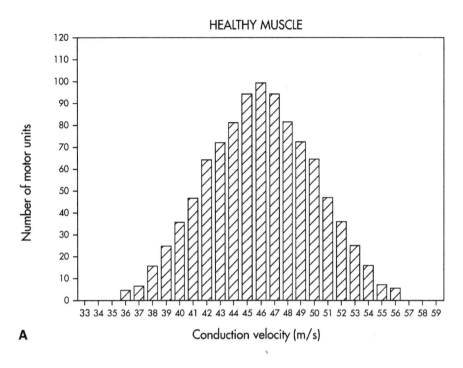

A

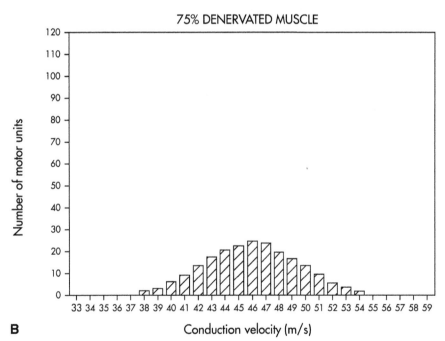

Figure C26–3. *Computer simulation of the effect on the distribution of conduction velocities of a loss of 75% of the motor units. (A) Normal. (B) Abnormal. (From Osselton JW et al., eds. Clinical neurophysiology, EMG, nerve conduction and evoked potentials. Oxford: Butterworth-Heinemann, 1995.)* **B**

velocities are markedly slow (<80% of lower limit of normal) because of increased probability for the action potentials to pass through demyelinated nerve segments (see Case 18). Caution should be taken when evaluating for conduction block and slowing in the demyelinating range in peripheral nerves with very low distal CMAPs (<20% of the lower limit of normal or <1 mV).

Needle electromyography in axonal polyneuropathy often discloses changes consistent with symmetrical motor axon loss, in a distal to proximal gradient, manifested by fibrillation potentials and reinnervation MUAPs of increased duration, amplitude, and polyphasia.

FOLLOW-UP

Complete blood count reveals large mean corpuscular volume (MCV) of 102, but was otherwise normal. The following laboratory tests were normal or negative: glucose tolerance test, hemoglobin A1C, liver function tests, BUN, creatinine, thyroid function tests, vitamin B12 level, methylmalonic acid level, serum and urine immunofixation, and hepatitis serology. Cerebrospinal fluid examination was normal except slight elevation of protein (65 mg/dL). The patient was started on multivitamins and nutritional supplement, and advised to abstain from alcohol.

DIAGNOSIS
Chronic alcoholic peripheral polyneuropathy.

ANSWERS

1. B; 2. D; 3. B.

SUGGESTED READINGS

Asbury AK, Gilliatt RW. The clinical approach to neuropathy. In: Asbury AK, Gilliatt RW, eds. Peripheral nerve disorders. London: Butterworths, 1994, pp. 1–20.

Behse F, Buchthal F. Alcoholic neuropathy: clinical, electrophysiological and biopsy findings. Ann Neurol 1977;2:95–110.

Claus D, Eggers R, Engelhardt A et al. Ethanol and polyneuropathy. Acta Neurol Scand 1985;72:312–316.

England JD, Asbury AK. Peripheral neuropathy. Lancet 2004;363:2151–2161.

Herrmmann DN, Logigian EL. Approach to peripheral nerve disorders. In: Katirji B, Kaminski HJ, Preston DC, Ruff RL, Shapiro EB, eds. Neuromuscular disorders in clinical practice. Boston, MA: Butterworth-Heinemann, 2002, pp. 501–512.

Hughes RAC. Peripheral neuropathy. BMJ 2002;324:466–469.

McLeod JG. Alcohol, nutrition, and the nervous system. Alcoholic neuropathy. Med J Aust 1982;2:274–275.

Shields RW. Alcoholic polyneuropathy. Muscle Nerve 1985; 8:183–187.

Shields RW. Nutritional AMD alcoholic neuropathies. In: Katirji B, Kaminski HJ, Preston DC, Ruff RL, Shapiro EB, eds. Neuromuscular disorders in clinical practice. Boston, MA: Butterworth-Heinemann, 2002, pp. 622–636.

Vrankcken AFJE et al. Feasibility and cost efficiency of a diagnostic guideline for chronic polyneuropathy: A prospective implementation. J Neurol Neurosurg Psychiatry 2006;77: 397–401.

Wein TH, Albers JW. Electrodiagnostic approach to the patient with suspected peripheral polyneuropathy. Neurol Clin N Am 2002;20:503–526.

Case 27

HISTORY AND PHYSICAL EXAMINATION

A 45-year-old woman developed increasing abdominal pain, nausea, and occasional vomiting. She underwent a cholecystectomy at a community hospital with no help. Pain persisted and she had increasing weight loss. Upper endoscopy was normal and laparoscopy showed minor adhesions. She then developed abdominal distention and an ileus. An exploratory laparotomy revealed a small bowel perforation and a 15 cm of small bowel was resected with primary anastomosis. Her postoperative course was complicated by fever, prolonged ileus, and abdominal infection. She required mechanical ventilation for about 3 days for sepsis and respiratory failure. She was hospitalized for a total of 10 weeks and was started on intravenous total protein nutrition due to malnutrition and severe loss of weight.

During this prolonged hospitalization, she reported rapidly progressive weakness of the right hand which became complete over one to two weeks. She was ill and obtunded and could not give better details about her leg symptoms. Severe distal weakness of both lower extremities, worse on the right was noted by treating physicians during her hospitalization, requiring bilateral ankle braces. She was diagnosed with a secondary critical illness polyneuropathy and was discharged to rehabilitation. However, she was readmitted two weeks later to our teaching hospital because of nausea and persistent abdominal pain. Upon arrival, she reported that she had developed, while in rehabilitation, abrupt weakness of the left hand, particularly the left thumb and index and middle fingers.

Her past medical history was relevant for diffuse joint pain and swelling, six months prior to the initial presentation, diagnosed as "arthritis" and treated successfully with oral prednisone for 3 months. She has not had any skin rash. The patient was receiving intravenous total protein nutrition.

On examination, she was cachectic and ill appearing woman with modest abdominal pain. She was afebrile with a blood pressure of 160/70. General physical examination was relevant for distended and moderately tender abdomen with no guarding or rebound tenderness. Bowel sounds were hypoactive. The neurological examination revealed normal mental status and cranial nerves. The motor examination revealed significant atrophy in both lower extremities below the knees, as well as the right hand and forearm and the left thenar muscles. There were no fasciculations. Muscle strength testing revealed asymmetrical weakness most notable in the upper extremities. Detailed manual muscle testing was as follows (Modified Medical Research Council [MRC] scale):

	Right	Left
Shoulder abduction	5/5	5/5
Elbow flexion	5/5	5/5
Elbow extension	2/5	5/5
Pronation	0/5	2/5
Finger flexion (digits 1, 2, and 3)	0/5	0/5
Finger flexion (digits 4 and 5)	0/5	4+/5
Wrist flexion	0/5	2/5
Wrist extension	0/5	5/5
Finger extension	0/5	4+/5
Finger abduction	0/5	4+/5

	Right	Left
Hip flexion	5/5	5/5
Hip extension	5/5	5/5
Knee extension	4+/5	4+/5
Knee flexion	4+/5	4+/5
Foot dorsiflexion	0/5	4–/5
Toe dorsiflexion	0/5	0/5
Plantar flexion	0/5	4/5
Ankle inversion	0/5	0/5
Ankle eversion	0/5	0/5

Sensation revealed a stocking glove distribution bilaterally with no clear asymmetry. There was no clear sensory loss in the left median distribution compared to the ulnar distribution on formal testing. The deep tendon reflexes were +2 at the biceps bilaterally, +2 at the left triceps, and absent at the right triceps, and absent at the brachioradialis bilaterally. The knee jerks were +1 bilaterally, while the ankle jerks were absent. Plantar responses are both flexors. Gait was not examined.

The laboratory studies revealed a white cell count of 11 000 cm^3 with no bands. Westegren sedimentation rate and C-reactive protein were elevated at 75 mm/h and 12.50, respectively. Liver function tests revealed elevated AST, ALT, and alkaline phosphatase at 84 U/L, 61 U/L, and 429 U/L, respectively. Prothrombin time and INR were slightly elevated at 12.8 and 1.3, respectively. Antinuclear antibody (ANA) and antineruonal cytoplasmic antibodies (ANCA) were negative. Hepatitis B and B core antigens were reactive. Hepatitis B and core antibodies were nonreactive. Viral DNA count was more than 8.3 millions copies. Hepatitis A and C antibodies were nonreactive. Cryoglobulins were negative. Endomysial antibody was negative. Vitamin B12 and E were normal at 662 pg/mL and 15 mg/L, respectively. Abdominal x-rays revealed dilated small bowel loops with air-fluid level. An electrodiagnostic (EDX) study was requested.

Please now review the Nerve Conduction Studies and Needle EMG tables.

QUESTIONS

1. Common neurological manifestations of this disorder include all the following except:
   A. Multiple mononeuropathies.
   B. Symmetrical polyneuropathy.
   C. Dorsal ganglionopathy.
   D. Asymmetrical polyneuropathy.
2. Peripheral nerve vasculitis is most commonly a manifestation of:
   A. Systemic lupus erythematosus.
   B. Nonsystemic vasculitic neuropathy.
   C. Rheumatoid arthritis.
   D. Sjögren syndrome.
3. The least useful test in the diagnosis of vasculitic neuropathy is:
   A. Antinuclear antibody.
   B. Muscle biopsy.
   C. Cutaneous nerve biopsy.
   D. Antineutrophil cytoplasmic antibody.
   E. Cerebrospinal fluid examination.
   F. Hepatitis B and C serology.

EDX FINDINGS AND INTERPRETATION OF DATA

The relevant EDX findings in this case include:

1. Absent routine sensory nerve action potentials (SNAPs) and routine compound muscle action potentials (CMAPs) in both lower extremities. This finding is consistent with a generalized axon-loss disorder affecting the sensory and motor fibers, such as a sensorimotor peripheral polyneuropathy.
2. Asymmetrical peroneal motor nerve conduction studies (NCSs), recording tibialis anterior, in the lower extremities. The responses were absent on the right while they were evoked with low CMAP amplitudes on the left with no conduction block or slowing of distal latency and minimal slowing of conduction velocity. This finding suggests that the disorder is asymmetrical.
3. Absent routine sensory and motor conduction studies in the right upper extremity while the left upper extremity showed absent median sensory and motor conduction studies and only borderline or slightly reduced ulnar and radial SNAP amplitudes and ulnar motor CMAP amplitude with normal distal latency, conduction velocity and F wave minimal latency. This is a very useful finding; it points to a severe left median mononeuropathy as well as an asymmetrical polyneuropathy in the upper extremities. The left median mononeuropathy could not be localized since the median motor and sensory responses were absent. Hence, a remote left carpal tunnel cannot be excluded at this point.
4. The needle examination confirms several important findings. First, the severe left median mononeuropathy is at or above the elbow as evidenced by the severe active denervation and loss of motor unit action potentials (MUAPs) of all sampled median innervated muscles in the left hand and forearm, including the pronator teres. Second, the active denervation and loss of MUAPs is asymmetrical, as noted mostly in the distal upper extremities (much worse on the right, excluding the left median nerve), but also slightly in the lower extremities (much severe denervation of the right tibialis anterior and medial gastrocnemius than the left). Third, the active denervation and loss of MUAPs in the right upper extremity suggests either overlapping and combined right median, ulnar, and radial mononeuropathies or a right middle and lower trunk brachial plexopathy. Fourth, the prominent fibrillation potentials are supportive evidence for ongoing (active) denervation.

In summary, this EDX study reveals an asymmetrical sensorimotor polyneuropathy superimposed on multiple and asymmetrical mononeuropathies. This is most consistent

Case 27: Nerve Conduction Studies

Nerve Stimulated	Stimulation Site	Recording Site	Amplitude (m = mV, s = μV)			Distal/Peak Latency (ms)			Conduction Velocity (m/s)			F Latency (ms)	
			Right	Left	Normal	Right	Left	Normal	Right	Left	Normal	Right	Left
Sural (s)	Calf	Ankle	NR	NR	>5	NR	NR	<4.5					
Superficial peroneal (s)	Leg	Ankle	NR	NR	>5	NR	NR	<4.5					
Peroneal (m)	Ankle	EDB	NR	NR	>2.5	NR	NR	<5.6					
Tibial (m)	Ankle	AH	NR	NR	>8	NR	NR	<6.0					
Peroneal (m)	Bel. Fib head	Tibialis anterior	NR	**1.2**	>4	NR	3.5	<4.0					
Peroneal (m)	Knee	Tibialis anterior	NR	**1.0**		NR	4.5			**39**	>40		
Median (s)	Wrist	Index	NR	NR	>20	NR	NR	<3.4					
Ulnar (s)	Wrist	Little finger	NR	**12**	>12	NR	2.8	<3.1					
Radial (s)	Forearm	Snuffbox	NR	**10**	>18	NR	2.5	<2.7					
Median (m)	Wrist	APB	NR	NR	>6	NR	NR	<3.9					
Median (m)	Elbow	APB	NR	NR		NR	NR						
Ulnar (m)	Wrist	ADM	NR	**3.5**	>7	NR	2.8	<3.1	NR			31	
Ulnar (m)	Below elbow	ADM	NR	**3.1**		NR			NR	53	>50		
Ulnar (m)	Above elbow	ADM	NR	**3.0**		NR			NR	54	>50		

ADM = abductor digiti minimi; AH = abductor hallucis; APB = abductor pollicis brevis; EDB = extensor digitorum brevis; L. = left; NR = no response; R. = right. Data in bold type are abnormal.

Case 27: Needle EMG

| Muscle | Insertional Activity | Spontaneous Activity | | Voluntary Motor Unit Action Potentials (MUAPs) | | | | | | | |
| | | | | Recruitment | | | | Configuration | | | |
		Fibs	Fascs	Normal	Activation	Reduced	Early	Duration	Amplitude	% Polyphasia	Others
Right tibialis anterior	↑	2+	0	No voluntary MUAPs							
Medial gastrocnemius	↑	2+	0	No voluntary MUAPs							
Extensor hallucis longus	↑	2+	0	No voluntary MUAPs							
Tibialis posterior	↑	2+	0	No voluntary MUAPs							
Vastus lateralis	Normal	0	0			↓		↑	Normal	Normal	
Left tibialis anterior	↑	1+	0			↓↓		↑↑	↑	↑	
Medial gastrocnemius	↑	1+	0			↓↓		↑↑	↑	↑	
Extensor hallucis longus	↑	2+	0	No voluntary MUAPs							
Tibialis posterior	↑	2+	0	No voluntary MUAPs							
Vastus lateralis	Normal	0	0			↓		↑	Normal	Normal	
Right first dorsal interosseous	↑	1+	0	No voluntary MUAPs							
Abductor pollicis brevis	↑	1+	0	No voluntary MUAPs							
Flexor pollicis longus	↑	1+	0	No voluntary MUAPs							
Pronator teres	↑	1+	0	No voluntary MUAPs							
Extensor indicis	↑	1+	0	No voluntary MUAPs							

Muscle							
Biceps	Normal	0	0		Normal	Normal	Normal
Triceps	↑	1+	0	↓↓↓	↑↑	↑	↑
Deltoid	Normal	0	X				
Left first dorsal interosseous	↑	+/−	0	↓			
Abductor pollicis brevis	↑	3+	0	No voluntary MUAPs			
Flexor pollicis longus	↑	3+	0	No voluntary MUAPs			
Pronator quadratus	↑	3+	0	No voluntary MUAPs			
Pronator teres	↑	2+	0	↓↓↓	↑	↑	↑↑↑
Extensor indicis	Normal	0	0	↓	↑	Normal	Normal
Biceps	Normal	0	X		Normal	Normal	Normal
Triceps	Normal	0	X		Normal	Normal	Normal
Deltoid	Normal	0	X		Normal	Normal	Normal

Fascs = Fasciculations; Fibs = Fibrillations; ↑, ↑↑, ↑↑↑ = mildly, moderately, markedly increased, respectively; ↓, ↓↓, ↓↓↓ = mildly, moderately, markedly decreased, respectively.

with an axon-loss mononeuritis multiplex becoming incompletely confluent. This case is most suggestive of a vasculitic neuropathy resulting in multiple nerve ischemia, which forms the basis for this disorder.

DISCUSSION

Definition and Classification

The vasculitides are group of disorders that are defined by the presence of inflammatory cells in the vessel wall with reactive damage to mural structures that compromises the lumen and leads to tissue ischemia or, occasionally, hemorrhage. They are classified based on the predominant size of the most commonly affected blood vessels (Table C27–1). The vasculitides may occur as a primary process where vasculitis is the defining feature of the illness (such as

polyarteritis nodosa) or may be secondary to another underlying disease such as any connective tissue disease, infection, or drug exposure. Affected organs may become symptomatic either in isolation or in combination.

The clinical manifestations of vasculitis are extremely variable due to the wide range of organs involved. The diagnosis is often delayed since the disorders mimic a large number of other illnesses such as atherosclerotic vascular disorders, systemic embolization, infection, and malignancy. A high index of suspicion is necessary and appropriate testing rendered as soon as possible. However, there is no single uniform method of evaluating patients suspected with vasculitis, since the work-up depends on the type of vasculitis suspected and the organs involved. Tests that are very useful in the diagnosis of vasculitis are listed in Table C27–2. Biopsy of nerve and muscle is often informative, but may occasionally not be necessary if there is histopathologic or angiographic evidence of vasculitis in other organs.

Vasculitis that affects the peripheral nerves may be a feature of a systemic disorder or represent an isolated peripheral nervous system vasculitis that possesses no clinical or laboratory evidence of other organ system involvement. This isolated vasculitis is usually referred to as *nonsystemic vasculitic neuropathy*. Nonsystemic vasculitic neuropathy constitutes about 30 to 40% of all cases of

Table C27–1. Major Classification of the Vasculitides

Large Vessel Vasculitis
Giant cell arteritis
Takayasu arteritis
Medium Sized Vessel Vasculitis
Polyarteritis nodosa
Kawasaki disease
Isolated central nervous system vasculitis
Small Vessel Vasculitis
ANCA-associated small vessel vasculitis
   Churg-Strauss syndrome
   Microscopic polyarteritis
   Wegener's granulomatosis
Essential cryoglobulinemic vasculitis
Hypersensitivity vasculitis
   Henoch-Schönlein purpura
   Cutaneous leukocytoclastic vasculitis
   Drug-induced vasculitis
Vasculitis secondary to connective tissue disorders
   Lupus vasculitis
   Rheumatoid vasculitis
   Sjögren syndrome vasculitis
   Behçet disease
Vasculitis secondary to viral infection
   Hepatitis B or C
   HIV
   Cytomegalovirus
   Epstein-Barr
   Parvo B19
Nonsystemic vasculitic neuropathy

ANCA = antineutrophil cytoplasmic autoantibodies; HIV = human immunodeficiency virus.

Table C27–2. Diagnostic Laboratory Tests in the Evaluation of Patients With Suspected Vasculitis in General and Vasculitic Neuropathy in Particular

Complete blood count and differential
Westegren sedimentation rate
Serum creatinine and creatinine clearance
Liver function tests
Urinalysis with microscopic examination of urinary sediment
ANA (antinuclear antibodies)
RF (rheumatoid factor)
ANCA (antineutrophil cytoplasmic antibody)
Complement components (C3 and C4)
Antibodies to double stranded DNA
Antibodies to extractable nuclear antigens
   Anti-Smith
   Anti-Ro/SS-A
   Anti-La/SS-B
   Anti RNP
Serum immunofixation
Cryoglobulins
Hepatitis B and hepatitis C serology
Chest x-rays and CT scan of chest
CT scan of sinuses
Mesenteric angiography
Cutaneous nerve and muscle biopsy

vasculitic neuropathies, while the majority of the remaining cases are peripheral nerve manifestations of a systemic disorder, mostly polyarteritis nodosa, ANCA-associated small vessel vasculitis, or rheumatoid arthritis (Table C27–3).

Clinical Features

Mononeuropathy multiplex is defined as nerve lesions in two or more named nerves in separate parts of the body. It is usually a manifestation of vasculitis, granulomatous diseases, infiltrative neoplastic conditions, infections,

Table C27–3. Clinical and Laboratory Features of the Vasculitides Associated With Vasculitic Neuropathy

Disorder	Other Organs Involved (%)	Laboratory Studies (%)	PNS/CNS Involvement (%)	Tissues to Biopsy
Polyarteritis nodosa	Kidneys ~70	↑ ESR ~90	PNS ~60	Nerve
	Skin ~50	Rheumatoid factor 40–60	CNS 10–20	Muscle
	Muscles ~40	↓ Complements ~25		Skin
	GI ~30	Hepatitis B ~30		Kidney
	Testes 5-30	Hepatitis C 5-20		Rectum
	Heart ~15	ANCA ~10		Testis
		Angiography +ve 70%		
Churg-Strauss syndrome	Lungs ~100	ANCA ~60–75 (p > c)	PNS ~70	Nerve
	Skin ~60	Eosiophilia ~100	CNS ~10–20	Skin
	GI ~50	↑ IgE ~75		Lungs
	Heart ~50	Rheumatoid factor ~50		Kidney
	Kidneys ~40			ENT
	ENT ~25			
Microscopic polyangiitis	Kidneys ~100	ANCA ~75–90 (p > c)	PNS ~60	Kidney
	Lungs 40-50	Rheumatoid Factor ~40–50	CNS ~10	Lungs
	Gut ~50	↓ Complements – rare		Skin
	Skin ~50	Hepatitis B −ve		Nerve
	Eye ~30	Angiography +ve rare		
	Spleen ~30			
	Muscles ~20			
Wegener granulomatosis	ENT > 90	ANCA ~50–90	PNS ~15	ENT
	Lungs ~85	Rheumatoid factor ~60	CNS ~4–8	Lungs
	Kidneys ~80			Kidney
	Eyes ~50			Orbit
	Skin 40–50			Skin
				Nerve
Rheumatoid vasculitis	Skin ~70	Rheumatoid factor ~ 90–95	PNS 45–50	Nerve
	Muscle ~55	↑ ESR ~85	CNS ~10–15	Muscle
	Heart 35–40	↓ Complements ~45		Skin
	Lung ~25	ANCA ~40		Rectum
	Kidney ~25	ANA ~50		Salivary gland
	Serositis ~20–25	Eosinophilia ~20		
	GI ~10			
Lupus vasculitis	Skin vasculitis ~90	ANA 90–100	PNS ~10	Skin
	Arthritis ~85	Double stranded DNA 60–70	CNS ~5–10	Nerve
	Skin rash ~75	Anti-Smith 30–40		Kidney
	Kidneys ~50	Anti-Ro/SS-A 25–40		
	Pleurisy ~35	Anti La/SS-B 10–45]		
	CNS lupus ~30	Rheumatoid factor ~30		

Continued

Table C27–3. —cont'd

Disorder	Other organs Involved (%)	Laboratory Studies (%)	PNS/CNS Involvement (%)	Tissues to Biopsy
	Raynaud ~30 Adenopathy ~25 Pericarditis ~20	ANCA ~15		
Sjögren syndrome vasculitis	Skin ~75 GI ~50 Kidneys ~50 Muscle ~50	ANA ~90 Anti-Ro/SS-A 60–70 Anti- La/SS-B 40–60 Rheumatoid factor ~60–90 ↓ Complements >50 Cryoglobulins ~15 ANCA ~10	PNS ~35 CNS – varies	Nerve Kidney
Cryoglobulinemic vasculitis	Skin ~75 Kidneys ~20 Raynaud ~20–45 GI ~10	Rheumatoid factor ~ 70–80 ↓ Complements ~90 Hepatitis C ~80–90 Hepatitis B ~5 ANA ~20 Anti-Smith ~5 ANCA <5	PNS ~50 CNS – rare	Skin Nerve Kidney
Nonsystemic vasculitic neuropathy	Muscle ~15	↑ ESR ~60	PNS 100 CNS 0	Nerve Muscle

ANCA = antineutrophil cytoplasmic autoantibodies; angiography = abdominal angiographically demonstrated microaneurysms; CNS = central nervous system; ENT = upper respiratory tract involvement; GN = glomerulonephritis; LCV = leukocytoclastic vasculitis; PNS = peripheral nervous system. Adapted with revisions from Kissel JT, Collins MP. Vasculitic neuropathies and neuropathies of connective tissue disorder. In: Katirji B, Kaminski HJ, Preston DC, Ruff RL, Shapiro EB, eds. Neuromuscular disorders in clinical practice. Boston, MA: Butterworth-Heinemann, 2002, pp. 669–702.

diabetes, and multiple entrapment neuropathy as seen in hereditary neuropathy with liability to pressure palsy (Table C27–4). Mononeuropathy multiplex is the most specific manifestation of vasculitic neuropathy, and is often referred to as mononeuritis multiplex. The typical presentation is acute or subacute onset of multifocal mononeuropathies with weakness, sensory loss, and pain. Among peripheral nerves involved, the peroneal nerve is affected in more than three-quarters of patients presenting as mononeuritis multiplex. Other nerves affected in order of frequencies are the tibial, ulnar, radial, and median nerves. In contrast to common belief, only about half of the patients with vasculitic neuropathy present with mononeuropathy multiplex. The other half of the patients manifest with either an asymmetrical or symmetrical polyneuropathy that may be difficult to distinguish from other polyneuropathies such as metabolic or toxic polyneuropathies. It is likely that the polyneuropathy presentation of vasculitis is the result of disease progression where additional nerves are involved and become overlapped, leading to an increasingly symmetric or confluent polyneuropathy.

The pathophysiology of vasculitic neuropathy is nerve infarction due to occlusion of vasa nervorum, usually of the epineurial arterioles. Pathologically, there is usually fibrinoid necrosis with inflammatory infiltrate (neutrophils and lymphocytes) within the vessel wall of small to medium-sized epineurial arterioles. Perivascular collection of inflammatory cells is a useful but less specific finding. The nerve ischemia results in axonal degeneration which may be either complete or "fascicular" depending on individual nerve blood supply.

The diagnosis of vasculitic neuropathy often requires a high index of suspicion by relying on manifestations that are common to the vasculitides (Table C27–5). Cutaneous nerve biopsy is often necessary for final diagnosis. The yield of nerve biopsy in identifying vasculitic findings improves when nerve sampling is guided by the clinical and EDX findings and when a muscle biopsy is also obtained. Commonly biopsied nerve and muscle combinations include the sural nerve and gastrocnemius muscle or the superficial peroneal nerve and peroneus brevis muscle.

Table C27–4. Causes of Mononeuropathy Multiplex

Vascular Insufficiency
Vasculitic neuropathy
Diabetic proximal neuropathy (amyotrophy)
Immune-Mediated
Multifocal motor neuropathy*
Lewis-Sumner syndrome*
Chronic inflammatory demyelinating polyneuropathy (CIDP)*
Neuralgic amyotrophy (idiopathic brachial plexitis)
Idiopathic lumbosacral plexitis
Neoplastic
Leukemia/lymphoma
Neurolymphomatosis
Infectious/Inflammatory
Leprosy
Lyme disease
Herpes zoster
Sarcoidosis
Inherited
Hereditary neuropathy with liability to pressure palsy (HNPP)*
Hereditary neuralgic amyotrophy
Hereditary high-density lipoprotein deficiency (Tangier disease)
Neurofibromatosus
Compressive/Traumatic
Multiple nerve entrapments
Multiple peripheral nerve injury

*Demyelinating neuropathies.

Electrodiagnosis

The aim of the EDX studies in patients with suspected vasculitis is to confirm the multifocal nature of the disorder, establish what nerves are involved, and guide the treating physician to the most appropriate nerve to biopsy. Confirming the presence of axon-loss multiple

Table C27–5. Manifestations That May Suggest the Presence of a Vasculitis in Patients With Peripheral Neuropathy

Mononeuropathy multiplex
Asymmetrical polyneuropathy
Palpable purpura
Ulcerating skin rash
Glomerulonephritis
Hemoptysis
Destructive upper airway lesions
Asthma
Allergic rhinitis
Nasal polyps
Abdominal pain
Small intestinal perforation

mononeuropathies (mononeuritis multiplex) is the most specific finding that is highly suggestive of vasculitic neuropathy; however, other disorders such as granulomatous diseases, infiltrative neoplastic conditions, infections, or diabetes may present in a similar fashion. The EDX study also confirms the axonal loss nature of the disorder, thus eliminating other causes of predominantly demyelinating mononeuropathy multiplex such as seen with entrapment neuropathies, hereditary neuropathy with liability to pressure palsy, Lewis-Sumner syndrome, or multifocal motor neuropathy (see Table C27–4).

The EDX study of patients with suspected vascultic neuropathy should be extensive and guided by the neurological examination. Testing multiple nerves in several limbs as well as more proximal conduction studies, such peroneal motor NCS recording tibialis anterior and radial motor study recording extensor digitorum communis, is often necessary for accurate diagnosis. The findings on NCSs are typical of an axonal neuropathy; they reveal low-amplitude or absent sensory nerve action potentials (SNAPs) and compound muscle action potentials (CMAPs). Conduction velocities are normal or mildly reduced and distal latencies normal or mildly prolonged. F-waves may be normal or mildly prolonged latencies. Occasionally, pseudoconduction blocks may be seen in acute ischemic nerve lesions, studied within 7–10 days of injury prior to the completion of wallerian degeneration. These blocks are transient and become low-amplitude CMAP responses typical of axonal degeneration. Needle electromyography (EMG) reveals fibrillation potentials in affected muscles, with decreased recruitment of motor unit action potentials (MUAPs). Long-duration and polyphasic MUAPs are observed if the disorder becomes chronic. The classic EDX studies in vasculitic neuropathy are characterized by axonal damage involving multiple individual nerves in an asymmetric fashion (typical mononeuropathy multiplex). The abnormalities may also show a less specific asymmetrical or symmetrical polyneuropathy, which may be difficult to distinguish from the more common subacute axon loss polyneuropathies such as toxic neuropathies or critical illness polyneuropathy.

FOLLOW-UP

The patient underwent a sural nerve biopsy which showed prominent necrotizing vasculitis of epineurial arterioles with fibrinoid necrosis and inflammatory infiltrates in all arteriole vessel wall layers (Figure C27–1). Immunosuppressive drugs were held because of concerns about excessive hepatitis B viral replication which may cause fulminant liver failure. The patient was given three doses of

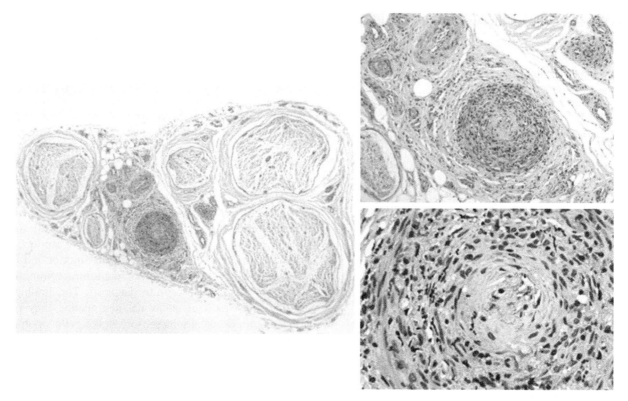

Figure C27–1. *Transverse section of the sural nerve biopsy showing a necrotizing vasculitis affecting several epineurial arterioles with fibrinoid necrosis and inflammatory infiltrates in all arteriole vessel wall layers (right, panels with higher magnifications).*

intravenous methylprednisolone and was then started on a combination of lamivudine, oral corticosteroids, and plasma exchange for three months or until hepatitis B antibody seroconversion occurs.

DIAGNOSIS
Vasculitic neuropathy due to polyarteritis nodosa associated with hepatitis B infection.

ANSWERS

1. D; 2. B; 3. E.

SUGGESTED READINGS

Collins MP, Mendell JR, Periquet MI et al. Superficial peroneal nerve/peroneus brevis muscle biopsy in vasculitic neuropathy. Neurology 2000;55:636.

Collins MP, Periquet MI. Non-systemic vasculitic neuropathy. Curr Opin Neurol 2004;17:587.

Davies L, Spies JM, Pollard JD et al. Vasculitis confined to peripheral nerves. Brain 1996;119(Pt 5):1441.

Dyck PJ, Benstead TJ, Conn DL et al. Nonsystemic vasculitic neuropathy. Brain 1987;110(Pt 4):843.

Guillevin L, Lhote F, Cohen P et al. Polyarteritis nodosa related to hepatitis B virus: a prospective study with long-term observation of 41 patients. Medicine 1995;74:238–253.

Guilleven L et al. Short-term corticosteroids then lamivudine and plasma exchanges to treat hepatitis b virus-related polyarteritis nodosa. Arthr Care Res 2004;51:482–487.

Jamieson PW, Guiliani MJ, Martinez AJ. Necrotizing angiopathy presenting with multifocal conduction blocks. Neurology 1991;41:442–444.

Jennette JC, Falk RJ. Small-vessel vasculitis. N Engl J Med 1997;337:1512.

Kissel JT, Slivka AP, Warmolts JR et al. The clinical spectrum of necrotizing angiopathy of the peripheral nervous system. Ann Neurol 1985;18:251–257.

Mathew L et al. Treatment of vasculitic peripheral neuropathy: A retrospective analysis of outcome. Q J Med 2007;100:41–51.

Olney RK. Neuropathies in connective tissue disease. Muscle Nerve 1992;15:531.

Pagnoux C, Guillevin L. Peripheral neuropathy in systemic vasculitides. Curr Opin Rheumatol 2005;17:41.

Index

Index of Cases

Index of Diagnoses

Printed and bound by CPI Group (UK) Ltd, Croydon, CR0 4YY

03/10/2024

01040301-0020